Interdisciplinary Biotechnological Advances

Series Editors

Jayanta Kumar Patra, Research Institute of Integrative Life Sciences
Dongguk University
Ilsandong, Goyang, Korea (Republic of)

Gitishree Das, Research Institute of Integrative Life Sciences
Dongguk University
Goyang, Korea (Republic of)

This series is an authoritative resource that explains recent advances and emerging directions in biotechnology, reflecting the forefront of research clearly and reliably, without excessive hype. Each volume is written by authors with excellent reputations and acknowledged expertise in the topic under discussion. The volumes span the entire field from an interdisciplinary perspective, covering everything from biotechnology principles and methods to applications in areas including genetic engineering, transgenic plants and animals, environmental problems, genomics, proteomics, diagnosis of disease, gene therapy, and biomedicine. The significance of these applications for the achievement of UN Sustainable Development Goals is highlighted. The series will be highly relevant for Master's and PhD students in Biotechnology, Nanochemistry, Biochemical Engineering, and Microbiology, medical students, academic and industrial researchers, agricultural scientists, farmers, clinicians, industry personnel, and entrepreneurs.

Sharad Kumar Tripathi
Sankhadip Bose
Abhishek Kumar Bhardwaj
Pharkphoom Panichayupakaranant
Editors

Phytoceuticals for Sustainable Medication

Springer

Editors
Sharad Kumar Tripathi
Department of Life Sciences
Arni University
Himachal Pradesh, Himachal Pradesh, India

Abhishek Kumar Bhardwaj
Department of Environmental Science
Amity University
Gwalior, Madhya Pradesh, India

Sankhadip Bose
School of Pharmacy
The Neotia University
Sarisa, West Bengal, India

Pharkphoom Panichayupakaranant
Department of Pharmacognosy and Pharmaceutical Botany, Faculty of Pharmaceutical Sciences
Prince of Songkla University
Songkhla, Thailand

ISSN 2730-7069 ISSN 2730-7077 (electronic)
Interdisciplinary Biotechnological Advances
ISBN 978-981-95-7587-9 ISBN 978-981-95-7588-6 (eBook)
https://doi.org/10.1007/978-981-95-7588-6

This Springer imprint is published by the registered company Springer Nature Singapore Pte Ltd.
The registered company address is: 152 Beach Road, #21-01/04 Gateway East, Singapore 189721, Singapore

Preface

In an era marked by the remarkable achievements of synthetic pharmaceuticals, yet shadowed by unintended side effects, environmental degradation, antimicrobial resistance, and rising healthcare burdens, the search for more sustainable and holistic therapeutic solutions has become imperative. *Phytoceuticals: An Emerging Sustainable Medication* emerges at this critical juncture, offering a compelling exploration of plant-derived bioactive compounds as a bridge between ancient medicinal wisdom and modern scientific rigor.

Phytoceuticals, sourced from the vast diversity of the world's flora, represent a convergence of tradition, innovation, and environmental responsibility. Long before the advent of industrial medicine, plants formed the foundation of human healthcare, from the neem tree celebrated in Ayurveda for its antimicrobial properties to willow bark, the precursor of aspirin. Today, advances in chemistry, pharmacology, and biotechnology allow us to rediscover and scientifically validate these natural resources, positioning them not merely as alternatives but as integral components of a sustainable paradigm shift in modern therapeutics.

This textbook systematically examines the chemical diversity, pharmacological mechanisms, and clinical potential of key classes of phytoceuticals, including polyphenols, alkaloids, terpenoids, and flavonoids. Beyond efficacy, it addresses critical challenges that define their future integration into mainstream medicine: standardized extraction methods, enhancement of bioavailability, regulatory considerations, ethical sourcing, and sustainable production from biodiverse ecosystems. By integrating ethnopharmacological knowledge with contemporary biotechnological innovations, the book outlines viable pathways toward scalable, regenerative, and eco-conscious pharmacotherapy.

What distinguishes this volume is its holistic perspective. It underscores a fundamental truth that effective healthcare need not come at the expense of planetary well-being. When studied with scientific rigor and cultivated with care, nature offers resilient, renewable solutions to pressing health challenges, including cancer, metabolic disorders, infectious diseases, and neurodegenerative conditions.

This work is the result of collaborative insights across botany, pharmacology, environmental science, and related disciplines. It is intended to serve as a valuable resource for researchers, clinicians, students, and policymakers who are committed to advancing sustainable healthcare. We hope that *Phytoceuticals* will inspire critical inquiry, responsible innovation, and a renewed appreciation of nature's role in shaping the future of medicine, one that heals both humanity and the environment.

Tanda, Himachal Pradesh, India Sharad Kumar Tripathi
Sarisa, West Bengal, India Sankhadip Bose
Gwalior, Madhya Pradesh, India Abhishek Kumar Bhardwaj
Songkhla, Thailand Pharkphoom Panichayupakaranant
November, 2025

Contents

Therapeutic Applications by Disease Category

Specific Compound Classes and Mechanisms

Editors and Contributors

About the Editors

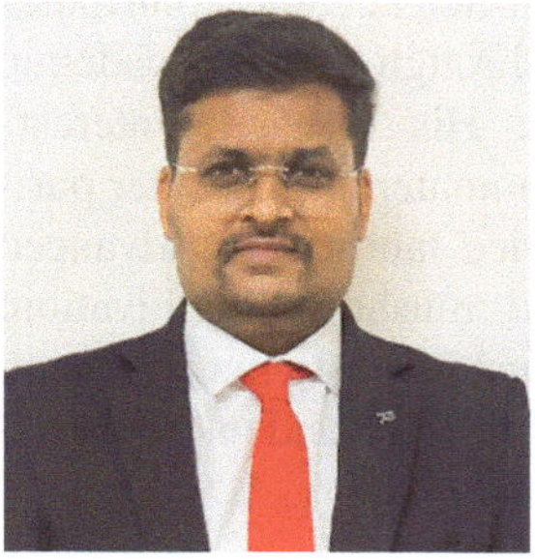

Sharad Kumar Tripathi is an Assistant Professor in the Department of Life Sciences at the Arni School of Basic Sciences & Biotechnology, Arni University, Kangra, Himachal Pradesh, India. He earned his Ph.D. from the Central University of Allahabad (Prayagraj) and completed postdoctoral research at the ICAR–Directorate of Medicinal and Aromatic Plants Research, Anand, Gujarat, focusing on the quantification, isolation, and molecular identification of phytochemicals from *Garcinia* species of North-East India. His research interests include phytochemical characterization and bioprospection of medicinal and aromatic plants. He teaches plant sciences, ethnobotany, and ethnopharmacology at undergraduate and postgraduate levels, and has supervised over 20 postgraduate projects and one Ph.D. scholar. He received the Young Scientist Award in 2019 from the Botanical Society of India and GESA India.

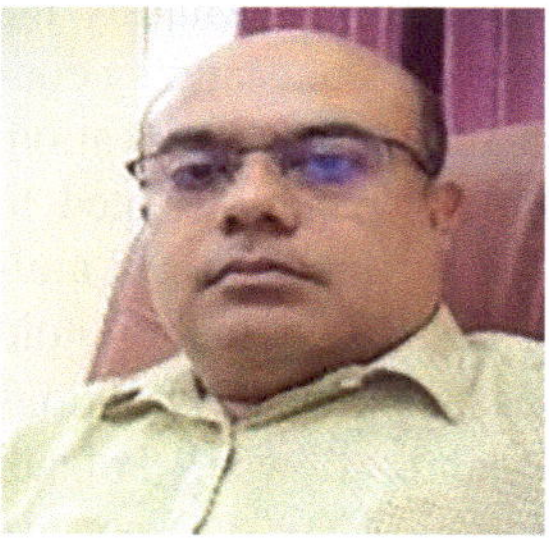

Sankhadip Bose is Professor and Head of the School of Pharmacy at The Neotia University, West Bengal, India. He has over 19 years of academic experience, including long-term service at Maulana Abul Kalam Azad University of Technology, where he guided more than 20 M.Pharm research projects. He has successfully completed a Central Government–funded research project supported by the Department of Science and Technology (DST), Government of India. One Ph.D. has been awarded under his supervision, and seven doctoral projects are currently ongoing across The Neotia University and Maulana Abul Kalam Azad University of Technology. He is a life member of SPER and serves as a CEC member of the Association of Pharmaceutical Teachers of India (APTI).

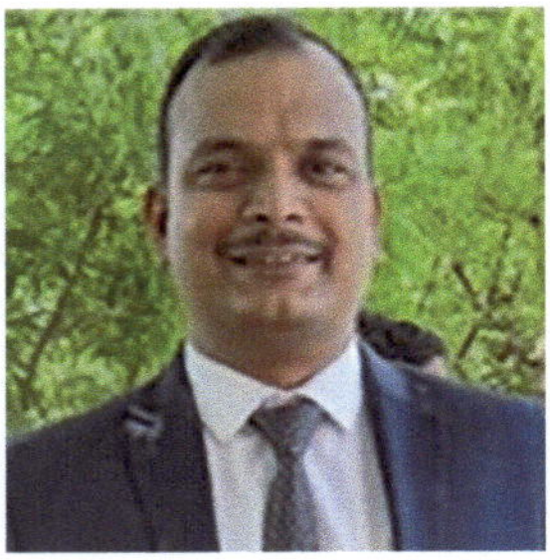

Abhishek Kumar Bhardwaj is an Assistant Professor in the Department of Environmental Science, Amity School of Life Sciences, Amity University, Gwalior, Madhya Pradesh, India. He earned his Ph.D. from the Central University of Allahabad (Prayagraj) on drinking water disinfection using green-synthesized metal nanoparticles and completed postdoctoral research in the Department of Environmental Science at VBS Purvanchal University, Jaunpur. He teaches postgraduate students of Environmental Science and contributes to university administration through various academic and organizing committees. His research interests include green synthesis of nanomaterials for water purification, biosensing, nanodevice fabrication, advanced water treatment, diatom and mushroom cultivation, phytoremediation, and sustainable waste management. He is a life member of several national and international scientific societies.

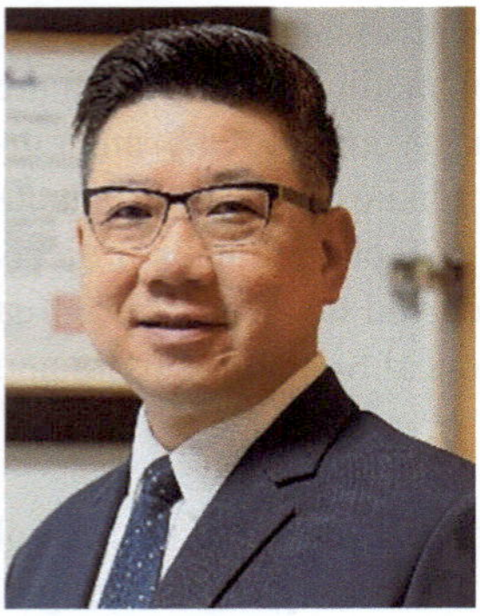

Pharkphoom Panichayupakaranant is a Professor in the Department of Pharmacognosy and Pharmaceutical Botany, Faculty of Pharmaceutical Sciences, Prince of Songkla University, Thailand. His research focuses on the development of herbal products using green extraction technologies, standardization strategies, active-constituent-enriched extracts, and medicinal plant tissue culture systems. In 2021, he received the Dushdi Mala Medal of Arts and Sciences (Pin of Scientific Arts), conferred by His Majesty the King of Thailand, in recognition of his outstanding contributions to scientific research and national innovation. He holds 17 patents and 21 petty patents related to herbal product development. His work has earned multiple international invention awards, including gold medals and special recognitions from major exhibitions in Germany, Korea, Switzerland, Taiwan, Poland, Malaysia, and Belgium.

Contributors

Ajaya Acharya Department of Pharmacy, Herbal Research Laboratory, School of Science, Kathmandu University, Dhulikhel, Nepal

Sankhadip Bose School of Pharmacy, The Neotia University, Sarisha, West Bengal, India

Subhadas Chatterjee School of Pharmacy, The Neotia University, Sarisha, West Bengal, India

Bengal School of Technology, Sugandha, Chuchura, Hooghly, West Bengal, India

Durgesh Nandini Chauhan Columbia Institute of Pharmacy, Raipur, Chhattisgarh, India

Nagendra Singh Chauhan Drugs Testing Laboratory Avam Anusandhan, Raipur, Chhattisgarh, India

Haixia Chen Tianjin Key Laboratory for Modern Drug Delivery & High-Efficiency, School of Pharmaceutical Science and Technology, Faculty of Medicine, Tianjin University, Tianjin, People's Republic of China

Sivaprakasam Chinnarasu Division of Endocrinology, Diabetes and Metabolism, Ohio State University Wexner Medical Center, Columbus, OH, USA

Younes Rezaee Danesh Department of Plant Protection, Faculty of Agriculture, Van Yuzuncu Yil University, Van, Türkiye

Rajeswar Das School of Pharmacy, The Neotia University, Sarisha, West Bengal, India

Sandipan Dash University Institute of Pharma Sciences, Chandigarh University, Mohali, Punjab, India

Arghya Kusum Dhar School of Pharmacy, The Neotia University, Sarisha, West Bengal, India

Subas Chandra Dinda School of Pharmacy, The Neotia University, Sarisha, West Bengal, India

Melford Egbujor Department of Chemistry, Federal University Otuoke, Otuoke, Bayelsa State, Nigeria

Gaurav Department of Research and Development, Hamdard Laboratories (India), Ghaziabad, Uttar Pradesh, India

Vijayalakshmi Ghosh GD Rungta College of Science & Technology, Bhilai, Chhattisgarh, India

Department of Biotechnology, Rungta International Skills University, Bhilai, Chhattisgarh, India

Anshita Gupta Department of Pharmacy, Guru Ghasidas Vishwavidyalaya, Bilaspur, Chhattisgarh, India

Rajendra Gyawali Department of Pharmacy, Herbal Research Laboratory, School of Science, Kathmandu University, Dhulikhel, Nepal

Priti Jana School of Pharmacy, The Neotia University, Sarisha, West Bengal, India

Suvechchha Jana School of Pharmacy, The Neotia University, Sarisha, West Bengal, India

Lim Eng Keat Tianjin Key Laboratory for Modern Drug Delivery & High-Efficiency, School of Pharmaceutical Science and Technology, Faculty of Medicine, Tianjin University, Tianjin, People's Republic of China

Mayank Krishna Kulshrestha Shri Narayan Prasad Awasthi Govt. Ayurved College, Raipur, Chhattisgarh, India

Vijay Kumar Department of Pharmaceutics, SPER, Jamia Hamdard, New Delhi, India

Deepshikha Kushwaha Centre for Microbiology, Ewing Christians College Prayagraj, Allahabad, Uttar Pradesh, India

Yiping Li Tianjin Key Laboratory for Modern Drug Delivery & High-Efficiency, School of Pharmaceutical Science and Technology, Faculty of Medicine, Tianjin University, Tianjin, People's Republic of China

Aachal Lonhare GD Rungta College of Science & Technology, Bhilai, Chhattisgarh, India

Department of Biotechnology, Rungta International Skills University, Bhilai, Chhattisgarh, India

Ramkumar Muthu Department of Biotechnology, Sri Kaliswari College (Autonomous), Sivakasi, Tamil Nadu, India

Partha Palit Drug Discovery Research Laboratory, Assam University, Silchar, Department of Pharmaceutical Sciences, Silchar, Assam, India

Pharkphoom Panichayupakaranant Department of Pharmacognosy and Pharmaceutical Botany, Faculty of Pharmaceutical Sciences, Prince of Songkla University, Songkhla, Thailand

Phytomedicine and Pharmaceutical Biotechnology Excellence Center, Faculty of Pharmaceutical Sciences, Prince of Songkla University, Songkhla, Thailand

Shraddha Patel Centre of Experimental Medicine and Surgery, Institute of Medical Sciences, Banaras Hindu University, Varanasi, Uttar Pradesh, India

Prem Narayan Paudel Department of Chemical Science and Engineering, School of Engineering, Kathmandu University, Dhulikhel, Nepal

Eldho Paul One Clinical Research, Mentor Education, Perth, WA, Australia

Marika Pellegrini Department of Life, Health and Environmental Sciences, University of L'Aquila, L'Aquila, Italy

Rajkumar Prabhakaran Department of Biochemistry, Karpagam Academy of Higher Education, Deemed to be University, Coimbatore, Tamil Nadu, India

Chandrabhan Prajapati Centre of Experimental Medicine and Surgery, Institute of Medical Sciences, Banaras Hindu University, Varanasi, Uttar Pradesh, India

Anu Shri Rai Department of Life Sciences, I.E.S University, Bhopal, Madhya Pradesh, India

Manasi Rai Department of Microbiology, Central University of Rajasthan, Dist-Ajmer, Rajasthan, India

Sachchida Nand Rai Centre of Experimental Medicine and Surgery, Institute of Medical Sciences, Banaras Hindu University, Varanasi, Uttar Pradesh, India

Shalini Rai Department of Microbiology, DSMNRU University, Lucknow, Uttar Pradesh, India

Samiran Sadhukhan School of Pharmacy, The Neotia University, Sarisha, West Bengal, India

Netaji Subhash Chandra Bose Institute of Pharmacy, Chakdaha, West Bengal, India

Sheetal S. Samant Department of Pharmacognosy, Yashwantrao Bhonsale College of Pharmacy, University of Mumbai, Mumbai, Maharashtra, India

Prabodh Satyal Aromatic Plant Research Center, Lehi, UT, USA

Santosh Kumar Singh Centre of Experimental Medicine and Surgery, Institute of Medical Sciences, Banaras Hindu University, Varanasi, Uttar Pradesh, India

Manoj Kumar Solanki Department of Life Sciences, I.E.S University, Bhopal, Madhya Pradesh, India

Deependra Soni School of Pharmacy, MATS University, Aarang, Chhattisgarh, India

R. S. Suresh Kumar College of Natural and Computational Sciences, Arba Minch University, Southern Ethiopia, Ethiopia

Wiwit Suttithumsatid Prince of Songkla University, Faculty of Pharmaceutical Sciences, Department of Pharmacognosy and Pharmaceutical Botany, Hat-Yai, Thailand

Prince of Songkla University, Phytomedicine and Pharmaceutical Biotechnology Excellence Center, Hat-Yai, Thailand

Maruthanayagam Veerabadhran Bioprospecting Research Unit, Department of General Surgery, Saveetha Medical College and Hospital, Saveetha Institute of Medical and Technical Sciences (SIMATS), Thandalam, Chennai, Tamil Nadu, India

Siyu Wang Tianjin Key Laboratory for Modern Drug Delivery & High-Efficiency, School of Pharmaceutical Science and Technology, Faculty of Medicine, Tianjin University, Tianjin, People's Republic of China

Wen Zhang Tianjin Key Laboratory for Modern Drug Delivery & High-Efficiency, School of Pharmaceutical Science and Technology, Faculty of Medicine, Tianjin University, Tianjin, People's Republic of China

Foundations and Production Technologies

Green Technology for Phytochemicals

Pharkphoom Panichayupakaranant

Abstract The integration of green technologies into phytochemical research marks an important step toward environmentally sustainable methods for obtaining natural products. Phytochemicals, plant-derived compounds with biological activity, have gained growing attention for their medicinal value and wide-ranging applications in drug development, health supplements, and cosmetic formulations. Nevertheless, conventional extraction methodologies are frequently characterized by the utilization of hazardous organic solvents and substantial energy requirements, which in turn exacerbate environmental burdens, compromise phytochemical integrity, and introduce safety concerns. Techniques categorized as green extraction, encompassing microwave-assisted extraction (MAE), ultrasound-assisted extraction (UAE), supercritical fluid extraction (SFE), pressurized liquid extraction (PLE), and pulsed electric field (PEF), provide sustainable alternatives that lower energy requirements, reduce reliance on solvents, and curtail waste generation, all while enhancing process efficiency and safeguarding bioactive compounds. Recent progress highlights the application of environmentally benign solvent systems, including bio-derived solvents, pharmaceutically acceptable excipients, ionic liquids (ILs), and deep eutectic solvents (DESs), all of which exhibit biodegradability, renewability, and low toxicity. Despite these promising developments, challenges persist in the standardization, selectivity, and scalability of green extraction methods. Addressing these issues requires interdisciplinary collaboration, regulatory support, and continuous technological innovation. Novel computational approaches, including artificial intelligence (AI) and machine learning (ML), provide promising avenues for optimizing extraction conditions, improving reproducibility, and expediting process development. The present chapter delivers a detailed exploration of eco-friendly

P. Panichayupakaranant (✉)
Department of Pharmacognosy and Pharmaceutical Botany, Faculty of Pharmaceutical Sciences, Prince of Songkla University, Hat-Yai, Songkhla, Thailand

Phytomedicine and Pharmaceutical Biotechnology Excellence Center, Faculty of Pharmaceutical Sciences, Prince of Songkla University, Hat-Yai, Songkhla, Thailand
e-mail: pharkphoom.p@psu.ac.th

S. Kumar Tripathi et al. (eds.), *Phytoceuticals for Sustainable Medication*, Interdisciplinary Biotechnological Advances,
https://doi.org/10.1007/978-981-95-7588-6_1

technological innovations within phytochemical production, underscoring their relevance to research, industry, and sustainability. Framed within the Bio-Circular-Green (BCG) economic model, green extraction technologies are positioned as key drivers of sustainable growth, resource conservation, and global competitiveness in the herbal and natural product industries.

Keywords Green extraction · Natural products · Phytochemicals · Sustainability · Therapeutic applications

1 Introduction

Naturally occurring plant metabolites with biological activity, known as phytochemicals, hold significant importance in traditional therapeutic practices and modern phytopharmaceutical studies. These compounds, including polyphenols, naphthoquinones, anthraquinones, flavonoids, coumarins, alkaloids, terpenes, steroids, and their glycosides, serve essential physiological and defensive functions in plants. Importantly, they also demonstrate a broad spectrum of therapeutic activities that are beneficial to human health. Scientific evidence has increasingly emphasized their role in combating chronic and degenerative pathologies, which is linked to their wide spectrum of biological functions encompassing anti-diabetic, anti-hyperlipidemic, antioxidant, anti-inflammatory, anticancer, and antimicrobial potentials (Forni et al. 2019; Choudhari et al. 2020; Khameneh et al. 2021; Majrashi et al. 2023; Nisar et al. 2023; Alum 2025).

The growing global demand for herbal and plant-based products reflects a paradigm shift toward natural alternatives to synthetic pharmaceuticals. This trend is fueled by increased health awareness and consumer concern over the long-term safety of chemical drugs. Consequently, the phytopharmaceutical, nutraceutical, and botanical supplement industries are experiencing unprecedented growth. To meet this demand, there is a pressing requirement for extraction and production methodologies that combine high efficiency, scalability, and ecological sustainability (Balkrishna et al. 2024; Chaachouay and Zidane 2024).

Phytochemicals have traditionally been obtained through established extraction techniques such as Soxhlet extraction, reflux, maceration, percolation, and hydrodistillation. While effective, these methods typically require large quantities of organic solvents, high energy inputs, and extended processing times. Such conditions can lead to the degradation of heat-sensitive compounds and contribute to excessive waste generation, posing environmental and regulatory concerns.

To address these limitations, environmentally friendly extraction technologies have been developed as novel and sustainable solutions. Aligned with the principles of green chemistry, these methods, such as ultrasound-assisted extraction (UAE), supercritical fluid extraction (SFE), pressurized liquid extraction (PLE), microwave-assisted extraction (MAE), enzyme-assisted extraction (EAE), and biotransformation through fermentation, offer numerous advantages. These include reduced solvent consumption, lower energy requirements, shortened processing times, enhanced selectivity, and minimized environmental impact (Osorio-Tobón 2020; Santos and Santana 2022; Martins et al. 2023; Mungwari et al. 2025).

Globally, there is increasing governmental and institutional support for the adoption of green technologies in the herbal and phytochemical industries. For example, the BCG Economy Model in Thailand synergizes biotechnological advances, circular economy principles, and eco-innovative approaches to support environmentally sustainable and socially inclusive development (Panichayupakaranant 2024). Within this framework, the application of green technologies in phytochemical production is not merely a technical enhancement but rather a strategic imperative. These technologies enable industrial scalability, compliance with international standards, and environmental stewardship. Such approaches contribute to cost reduction, ensure the integrity and safety of products, and bolster the competitiveness of herbal-based industries on a global scale. Furthermore, by fostering sustainable resource management, they contribute to both local economic development and biodiversity preservation.

This chapter provides a comprehensive overview of the role of green technologies in advancing phytochemical research and production. It examines the driving forces behind their adoption, current global trends, key technological approaches, relevant case studies, and future directions. Through this analysis, the chapter highlights how green extraction technologies not only represent scientific and industrial progress but also act as catalysts for sustainable economic transformation, particularly within models such as the BCG economy.

2 The Necessity of Green Technology in Phytochemical Extraction

Plants serve as rich reservoirs of bioactive constituents, including phenolics, alkaloids, terpenoids, steroids, and their glycosides, which constitute vital raw materials for nutraceutical, pharmaceutical, and cosmeceutical applications. The efficient isolation of these phytochemicals is crucial for maintaining the efficacy, safety, and consistency of herbal-derived products (Bommakanti et al. 2023; Kumar et al. 2023; Wang et al. 2023; Valisakkagari et al. 2024). Employing appropriate extraction techniques ensures the preservation of molecular integrity and biological functionality, thereby optimizing therapeutic potential while minimizing unwanted or potentially toxic compounds.

Nevertheless, traditional extraction techniques, including heat reflux, Soxhlet extraction, and maceration, exhibit several inherent limitations. These traditional techniques typically rely on large volumes of hazardous organic solvents, including methanol, chloroform, dichloromethane, and hexane. These solvents are classified as Class II by the International Council for Harmonisation (ICH) due to their potential toxicity, and their use is strictly regulated in pharmaceutical products (ICH 2021). Even more concerning are Class I solvents, such as benzene and carbon tetrachloride, which are prohibited due to their high toxicity and environmental persistence. Residual traces of these solvents can be difficult to eliminate completely, raising concerns over carcinogenicity, neurotoxicity, and other adverse health effects in consumers.

Beyond chemical safety, conventional methods are also inefficient and environmentally burdensome. Techniques such as Soxhlet and reflux extraction require prolonged heating, often for several hours, which leads to high energy consumption and operational costs. Prolonged exposure to high temperatures may induce thermal decomposition of heat-sensitive phytochemicals, including alkaloids and polyphenols, leading to decreased extract yield and loss of bioactivity (Zhang et al. 2018; Chemat et al. 2020; Kumar et al. 2023).

Amidst these concerns and the heightened global focus on ecological and health impacts, there is a pressing requirement for extraction technologies that combine efficiency with environmental and safety considerations. Today's consumers increasingly favor herbal products manufactured using eco-friendly methods and free from harmful chemical residues. At the same time, global governance frameworks such as the SDGs, the EGD, and Thailand's BCG economy model highlight the promotion of sustainable industrial development, conscientious resource management, and ethical manufacturing processes (United Nations 2015; APEC 2022; Edyvean et al. 2023; Panichayupakaranant 2024; Palmisano et al. 2025).

Green extraction technologies have thus emerged as scientifically sound and forward-thinking solutions to these challenges. Techniques such as MAE, UAE, and SFE, coupled with bio-based or natural deep eutectic solvents (NADES), provide significant advantages, including minimized use of toxic solvents, shorter processing times, reduced energy consumption, increased selectivity, and better protection of thermolabile phytochemicals. The integration of biocompatible and renewable solvents, such as ethanol, glycerol, and plant oils, further reinforces the safety and environmental sustainability of these extraction processes (Gil-Martín et al. 2022; Bitwell et al. 2023; Didion et al. 2023; Cannavacciuolo et al. 2024).

In conclusion, the adoption of green extraction technologies represents more than a response to regulatory or ethical imperatives; it reflects a strategic shift toward innovation, sustainability, and long-term competitiveness in the herbal product industry. These technologies enable efficient utilization of natural resources, minimize environmental impact, and align with global sustainability objectives, while meeting the expectations of increasingly informed and health-conscious consumers.

3 Gains from Green Technology in Phytochemical Extraction

The adoption of green technologies in phytochemical extraction has garnered substantial attention in recent years, driven by the global demand for safer, more sustainable, and efficient processing methods. Such innovative approaches serve to both minimize ecological impact and optimize the quality, safety, and market potential of herbal-derived products. Accordingly, green extraction techniques are gaining recognition as key enablers of industrial competitiveness in harmony with international sustainability goals. Their principal benefits are outlined in the following section.

3.1 Improved Efficiency and Selectivity

Green extraction strategies such as MAE, SFE, and PLE provide superior efficiency compared to conventional extraction techniques. By promoting cell wall rupture and accelerating mass transfer, these methods enable the targeted recovery of phytochemicals in higher yields while preserving their chemical integrity. Their shorter processing times are especially beneficial for preserving thermolabile compounds such as phenolics and flavonoids (Awad et al. 2021; Martins et al. 2023; Usman et al. 2023; Bhadange et al. 2024; Cannavacciuolo et al. 2024; Valisakkagari et al. 2024). MAE has been reported to efficiently extract phenolic compounds, often providing superior yields in a fraction of the time required by traditional methods (Osorio-Tobón 2020; Tsevdou et al. 2024).

3.2 Lower Energy Consumption and Minimized Waste Production

One of the most significant advantages of green technologies is their contribution to energy conservation and waste minimization. These approaches commonly operate under milder thermal conditions and make use of eco-friendly solvents, thereby lowering energy requirements and decreased emissions of greenhouse gases. Furthermore, they minimize the degradation of sensitive phytochemicals, thereby improving product quality and process sustainability (Chemat et al. 2012, 2019b; Martins et al. 2023). For instance, supercritical carbon dioxide (SC-CO_2) extraction eliminates the need for organic solvents and operates under moderate conditions, offering an environmentally benign alternative (Yıldırım et al. 2024). Similarly, MAE reduces energy input and extraction time while maintaining the structural integrity of bioactive compounds (López-Salazar et al. 2023). UAE also enhances extraction rates and lowers solvent consumption, effectively decreasing chemical waste and improving operational efficiency (Shen et al. 2023).

3.3 Reduced Use of Toxic Solvents

One of the key advantages of green extraction is the minimization or total elimination of hazardous solvents, which enhances the safety of the final formulations. Eco-friendly solvents, including ethanol, glycerol, and water, classified as Generally Recognized as Safe (GRAS), are progressively adopted for their favorable toxicological and environmental properties (Burdock and Carabin 2004; Chemat et al. 2012). This practice supports compliance with international regulations on residual solvents (e.g., ICH Q3C), minimizes environmental pollution, and reduces occupational health risks. Consequently, extracts obtained via non-toxic solvents are more acceptable to consumers and suitable for use in food, pharmaceutical, and cosmetic products.

3.4 Enhanced Marketability and Consumer Acceptance

In an era of increased environmental and health awareness, consumers are more inclined toward products that are natural, sustainably sourced, and transparently processed. Green extraction technologies enhance the market appeal of herbal products by aligning with these consumer expectations. Products manufactured using eco-friendly processes can be marketed as premium, ethical, and sustainable, attributes that improve brand value and consumer trust (Majeed et al. 2022; Huang et al. 2024; Lopes et al. 2024). Furthermore, certifications related to sustainability and green processing can offer competitive advantages in global markets where regulatory, environmental, and ethical standards are stringent.

3.5 Promotion of a Sustainable and Circular Bioeconomy

Green extraction technologies support the development of a circular bioeconomy by maximizing the value derived from natural resources and minimizing waste generation. These approaches enable the utilization of agricultural by-products, plant residues, and underexploited biomass to create high-value phytochemical products. Such valorization strategies align with zero-waste principles and contribute to economic sustainability while reducing pressure on natural ecosystems (Sharma et al. 2022). Incorporating green extraction techniques aligns with major international sustainability agendas, including the United Nations SDGs, the European Green Deal, and Thailand's BCG economy strategy (Roobab et al. 2025; Panichayupakaranant 2024). By integrating environmental stewardship with economic innovation, these methods advance both ecological sustainability and industrial competitiveness.

In summary, green extraction technologies offer multifaceted advantages that go beyond environmental sustainability. These technologies improve extraction efficiency, lower energy demands, reduce reliance on hazardous solvents, and facilitate adherence to international safety regulations. Such advantages enhance both the quality and safety of phytochemical products while bolstering their market competitiveness and consumer acceptance. Furthermore, by aligning with global sustainability objectives, these approaches serve as pivotal tools in advancing a circular and bio-based economy.

4 Advantages and Challenges of Green Extractions

The utilization of environmentally friendly extraction technologies in the preparation of phytochemical products has garnered attention, owing to their sustainability, cost-effectiveness, and market-related advantages. These methods present a promising alternative to conventional techniques, aligning with the global shift toward sustainability. However, the implementation of green extractions is not without its limitations and technical challenges (Martins et al. 2023; Usman et al. 2023; Bhadange et al. 2024; Irianto et al. 2025). This section provides a critical overview of the key advantages and potential obstacles associated with green extraction technologies.

4.1 Advantages of Green Technologies

(a) *Environmental sustainability:* One of the most notable advantages of green extraction technologies is their reduced environmental impact. Unlike traditional methods, which often rely on hazardous solvents and energy-intensive processes, green extractions utilize environmentally friendly solvents, renewable energy sources, and cleaner techniques. These practices significantly decrease emissions and waste generation. Techniques such as UAE and MAE demonstrate reduced solvent usage and lower energy demands, positioning them as environmentally sustainable alternatives (Chemat et al. 2017; Sadeghi et al. 2017; Bagade and Patil 2021).

(b) *Long-term cost efficiency:* Although green extraction systems typically require substantial initial investment in advanced equipment, they offer considerable long-term economic benefits. These include higher extraction yields, reduced processing times, lower energy demands, and minimized solvent usage, all contributing to lower overall production costs. Additionally, the use of renewable solvents and the reduction of waste lessen disposal costs and regulatory burdens (Sridhar et al. 2021; Gil-Martín et al. 2022; Imamoglu 2024). Over time, these savings can offset the upfront expenses, making green technologies financially viable for many industries.

(c) *Alignment with clean-label product demands:* There is a growing global interest in products that are natural, sustainable, and transparent, commonly referred to as "clean-label" products. Green extraction technologies are especially suitable for manufacturers seeking organic certifications or eco-friendly branding, as they avoid synthetic chemicals and emphasize environmentally responsible practices. The use of non-toxic, biodegradable solvents enhances compliance with organic standards and builds consumer trust, thereby improving product marketability in health-conscious and regulated markets (Rocca et al. 2022; Cam 2023; Couceiro et al. 2025).

4.2 Challenges of Green Technologies

(a) *High capital requirements:* The substantial initial expenditure necessary for advanced extraction technologies, including SFE, MAE, and PLE, represents a major barrier to their large-scale adoption. These systems involve high-end, precision-engineered equipment that may be financially inaccessible for small and medium-sized enterprises (SMEs), particularly in developing regions with limited access to capital (Picot-Allain et al. 2021; Fahad et al. 2022; Putra et al. 2023).
(b) *The complexity of the technology and the necessity for skilled staff:* Green extraction processes often require careful control of operational parameters and specialized knowledge to achieve optimal efficiency. For instance, SFE with supercritical CO_2 demands precise manipulation of temperature and pressure, while PLE requires the accurate calibration of solvent composition and thermal settings. These complexities necessitate trained personnel and advanced operational expertise, posing a barrier in contexts where technical skills or infrastructure are lacking (Picot-Allain et al. 2021; Cannavacciuolo et al. 2024). Moreover, limited access to technical support and maintenance services can hinder reliable operation, especially in low-resource settings.
(c) *Lack of standardization and comparative data:* Despite the increasing interest in green technologies, the industry currently lacks comprehensive and standardized protocols for evaluating and comparing these methods across different plant matrices and target compounds. The absence of harmonized methodologies complicates reproducibility and limits data comparability between studies. Additionally, many green extraction techniques remain confined to laboratory or pilot-scale investigations, with few established guidelines for their industrial implementation. As a result, these factors hinder regulatory compliance and limit the implementation of green extraction methods within tightly controlled sectors, including the food, cosmetic, and pharmaceutical industries (Usman et al. 2023; Irianto et al. 2024; Irianto et al. 2025).
(d) *Scalability and industrial integration:* Green extraction methods exhibit promising outcomes at the bench scale; however, achieving efficient scale-up for industrial manufacturing remains a major obstacle. Issues such as solvent

recovery, process optimization, equipment cost, and energy requirements become increasingly complex at larger scales. Maintaining product quality and extraction efficiency while adhering to green principles during upscaling is a demanding task that often requires substantial investment in both equipment and process engineering (Usman et al. 2023; Bouizgma et al. 2025; Irianto et al. 2025; Panda and Gorantla 2025).

Overall, green extraction technologies present a promising and impactful framework for advancing the sustainable development of products derived from phytochemicals. They offer substantial benefits in terms of environmental impact, economic efficiency, and consumer appeal. Nevertheless, the successful transition from traditional to green extraction methods is contingent on overcoming several practical barriers, including high initial costs, operational complexity, and the lack of standardization. Strategic investments in technology, infrastructure, training, and regulatory harmonization are essential to fully harness the potential of green extraction. Addressing these obstacles enables the herbal industry to progress toward enhanced sustainability and strengthened international competitiveness.

5 Global Trends in Green Technology for Herbal Extracts and Phytochemicals

Global industries related to herbal extracts and phytochemicals are currently transitioning toward new paradigms in response to increasing demand for eco-friendly and health-conscious products. This evolution is further reinforced by supportive regulatory frameworks, public and private investments, and innovations in green technology. These developments indicate a broader recognition of the environmental and health challenges posed by classical extraction techniques and affirm the capacity of green extraction technologies to support sustainable production pathways. This section explores major global trends influencing the adoption and proliferation of green technologies within the sector.

5.1 The Rise of Clean-Label and Sustainable Product Movements

Recent years have witnessed a significant change in consumer behavior, characterized by a pronounced preference for clean-label and sustainably produced goods. Consumers are increasingly discerning about product origins, processing methods, and ecological impact. This trend is especially pronounced in industries such as pharmaceuticals, food, and cosmetics, where clean-label products, characterized by transparency, avoidance of synthetic additives, and reliance on natural components, are steadily increasing their market share.

The clean-label movement aligns closely with the principles of green extraction. These technologies employ non-toxic solvents, renewable feedstocks, and energy-efficient processes that preserve phytochemical integrity while reducing environmental harm. As a result, products derived via green extraction methods not only meet consumer expectations for safety and sustainability but also offer companies competitive advantages in terms of branding, market access, and regulatory compliance (Martins and Marto 2023; Ajayi et al. 2024; Couceiro et al. 2025).

A compelling illustration of this trend is provided by a recent study on turmeric-based products in the United States. Contrary to initial assumptions that curcumin content was the primary purchasing factor, the study found that product origin and organic certification were more influential in shaping consumer decisions. Respondents showed strong preferences for domestically sourced and organically certified turmeric, underscoring the growing importance of local and sustainable sourcing strategies (Nguyen et al. 2024). These findings signal a need for manufacturers to align extraction practices and sourcing protocols with consumer values related to transparency, environmental stewardship, and health consciousness.

5.2 Policy Initiatives Promoting Sustainable Production

The global shift toward green technologies is further supported by national and international policies designed to promote sustainable industrial practices. Many of these initiatives are embedded within larger policy agendas, including the United Nations SDGs, which highlight the importance of responsible manufacturing, biodiversity preservation, and fair access to healthcare resources. The World Health Organization (WHO) has acknowledged the role of herbal medicines in supporting these goals by integrating them into health systems, preserving traditional knowledge, and enhancing rural economic development (Pathak et al. 2024).

Regionally, the European Union (EU) has been particularly proactive through its European Green Deal (EGD), which aims to make Europe the first climate-neutral continent by 2050. Key components of this initiative include investments in green innovation, regulatory incentives for clean manufacturing, and sustainability-focused industrial reforms. The accompanying Circular Economy Action Plan further supports these efforts by promoting waste reduction, resource efficiency, and the adoption of renewable and biodegradable materials in manufacturing, including phytochemical extraction processes (Hereu-Morales et al. 2024; Palmisano et al. 2025).

Beyond Europe, countries such as the United States and Canada have implemented complementary measures, including tax credits for green research and development (R&D), public funding for sustainable technology startups, and stringent environmental standards that pressure industries to reduce emissions and adopt cleaner processes. These evolving policy environments are not only fostering innovation but also creating economic incentives and regulatory imperatives that catalyze the transition toward green technologies in the phytochemical sector.

5.3 *Growth in Investment for Green Extraction Technologies*

The increasing market and policy momentum toward sustainability has spurred a surge in global investment in green extraction technologies. Venture capitalists, private equity firms, and governmental funding bodies are increasingly channeling resources into companies developing and commercializing sustainable extraction solutions, such as SFE, MAE, and EAE (Takacs 2023; Gucciardi 2024; Cannavacciuolo et al. 2024).

Increased investment flows are fostering the rapid development of SMEs focused on environmentally friendly technologies and are likewise prompting major firms in pharmaceuticals, nutraceuticals, and cosmetics to incorporate sustainable extraction practices into their broader corporate social responsibility (CSR) and environmental commitments. Such investments not only facilitate the scale-up of green technologies but also accelerate their adoption across global markets, creating a positive feedback loop of innovation, competitiveness, and environmental performance (Appiah-Kubi et al. 2024).

5.4 *Expansion of R&D and Intellectual Property in Green Extraction*

A parallel trend to the rise in investment is the significant increase in R&D activity focused on improving the efficiency, selectivity, and sustainability of green extraction methods. This trend is evidenced by the increasing number of patents granted for innovations in solvent-free extraction, the utilization of deep eutectic solvents, energy-efficient equipment configurations, and hybrid extraction strategies that integrate multiple green methodologies (Nameroff et al. 2004; Santos et al. 2011; Llompart et al. 2019; de María et al. 2022; Drannikov et al. 2024).

Academic and industrial research is increasingly exploring novel applications and cross-disciplinary techniques. For example, integrating MAE with EAE is emerging as a promising strategy for improving both yield and selectivity of bioactive compounds. These innovations not only enhance extraction performance but also reduce environmental impact, making them attractive for commercial application. The expansion of patent activity and research initiatives is promoting stronger collaboration among academic institutions, industry stakeholders, and government agencies, thereby cultivating an ecosystem that supports innovation and facilitates the broad implementation of green technologies.

6 Common Green Extraction Used for Phytochemicals

The rise of green technologies has revolutionized the way phytochemicals and herbal extracts are produced. Compared with traditional methods, these advanced techniques deliver enhanced operational efficiency, greater selectivity, and significant ecological benefits. This section discusses the most widely used green technologies that are making significant contributions to the herbal extract and phytochemical innovation landscape. Each of these technologies demonstrates how the sector is adopting more sustainable, safer, and energy-efficient processes to meet consumer and regulatory demands for eco-friendly production.

6.1 Supercritical Fluid Extraction

Supercritical fluid extraction (SFE) represents an environmentally friendly and highly effective method for isolating bioactive compounds from plant matrices. By leveraging the distinctive physicochemical properties of supercritical fluids, particularly carbon dioxide (CO_2), this technique enables selective extraction of both polar and non-polar phytochemicals while minimizing thermal degradation (Uwineza and Waśkiewicz 2020; Arumugham et al. 2021; Herzyk et al. 2024; Mungwari et al. 2025).

A supercritical fluid is defined as a substance maintained above its critical temperature and pressure, wherein it exhibits characteristics of both gaseous and liquid phases. Supercritical carbon dioxide (SC-CO_2), the most commonly employed fluid for extraction, attains its critical point at 31.1 °C and 73.8 bar. In its supercritical form, CO_2 exhibits gas-like penetration into plant matrices while simultaneously dissolving target compounds in a liquid-like manner. This unique combination of properties renders SC-CO_2 highly effective for the selective extraction of bioactive constituents from complex botanical materials. Typically, the SFE technique involves directing SC-CO_2 through botanical materials while maintaining controlled operational parameters. The supercritical fluid solubilizes the target phytochemicals, which are then separated from CO_2 in a dedicated separator by lowering the pressure or temperature. This phase change returns CO_2 to its gaseous state, enabling its recovery and reuse in subsequent extraction cycles (Uwineza and Waśkiewicz 2020; Kamjam et al. 2024).

The effectiveness of SFE is largely determined by the solubility of the target phytochemicals within the supercritical medium. Given that SC-CO_2 is naturally non-polar, it is particularly efficient for extracting non-polar compounds such as essential oils, terpenoids, and fatty acids. To enhance the extraction of polar constituents, including flavonoids, alkaloids, and glycosides, co-solvents (modifiers) such as ethanol or methanol are commonly introduced. These co-solvents increase the polarity of the supercritical phase, thereby expanding the spectrum of extractable compounds. However, careful optimization of the type and proportion of the co-solvent is essential to maximize selectivity and minimize the extraction of undesired components (Aili et al. 2024; Herzyk et al. 2024; Kamjam et al. 2024).

Precise control of operational parameters, particularly temperature and pressure, is crucial in maintaining the supercritical state and targeting specific compounds of interest. While this need for high-pressure equipment and rigorous control systems adds technical complexity and financial cost, these challenges are increasingly mitigated by advances in process automation and predictive modeling. Additionally, various matrix-related factors, including particle size, moisture content, and packing density, can significantly influence extraction performance. Nevertheless, modern SFE systems have evolved to become more robust and scalable, supporting their application in the development of high-value herbal products (Uwineza and Waśkiewicz 2020).

SFE provides multiple advantages compared to traditional extraction methods, rendering it particularly suitable for isolating bioactive compounds from herbal matrices. One of its most notable strengths is its environmental sustainability. By utilizing non-toxic CO_2 as the primary solvent, SFE reduces the need for hazardous organic solvents commonly used in traditional methods. Additionally, the process is highly selective and tunable: critical extraction parameters, such as pressure, temperature, and co-solvent composition, can be precisely adjusted to target specific phytochemicals.

A further notable benefit of SFE is its compatibility with thermolabile compounds. By operating at relatively low temperatures, the technique reduces the risk of thermal degradation and helps maintain the chemical integrity of heat-sensitive phytochemicals. Furthermore, SFE is known for its process efficiency, offering shorter extraction times and often higher yields compared to conventional techniques. The resulting extracts are typically free from residual solvents, a critical quality attribute for pharmaceutical and nutraceutical applications (Uwineza and Waśkiewicz 2020; Arumugham et al. 2021; Herzyk et al. 2024; Mungwari et al. 2025).

Despite its benefits, SFE also presents certain limitations. The high capital cost associated with specialized high-pressure equipment remains a significant barrier, particularly for small- and medium-scale operations. The non-polar character of SC-CO_2 inherently limits its efficacy in extracting highly polar phytochemicals, necessitating the use of co-solvents like ethanol or methanol. The selection and proportion of these modifiers, along with their compatibility with the supercritical fluid, must be meticulously adjusted, adding operational complexity. Extraction efficiency is also influenced by a variety of matrix-related factors, including plant material characteristics, particle size, moisture content, and solvent flow rate. These parameters require meticulous optimization for each specific application, necessitating both technical expertise and thorough process development (Kamjam et al. 2024).

The adaptability and efficiency of SFE for extracting a wide array of herbal bioactive compounds have been well-documented. Notably, SC-CO_2 has been successfully employed to recover ginsenosides, pharmacologically active saponins, from both *Panax ginseng* and *P. quinquefolius*. The inclusion of methanol or ethanol as co-solvents significantly improved the extraction of these polar constituents while maintaining their structural stability (Samimi et al. 2014; Razgonova et al. 2020).

Another successful application is the production of γ-oryzanol-enriched extracts from rice bran, which exhibit antioxidant and antiproliferative properties. Under conditions optimized at 500 bar and 62 °C, the process produced a 17.3% mass yield, containing 78.45% fatty acids and 3.66% γ-oryzanol, successfully reconciling extraction efficiency with the retention of bioactive compounds (Baixinho et al. 2025).

In the case of ginger (*Zingiber officinale*), SC-CO_2 extraction performed at 15 MPa, 35 °C, and a CO_2 flow rate of 15 g/min successfully yielded ginger oil containing 20.7% [6]-gingerol, with an overall oil yield of 3.1%. A subsequent scale-up using a commercial-scale system (2 × 50 L extraction vessels) resulted in a 50-fold increase in batch size, with an oil yield of 3.8% and a slightly lower [6]-gingerol content of 18.0% (Salea et al. 2017).

These examples underscore the wide applicability of SFE in the extraction of high-value herbal compounds and its potential to produce clean, potent extracts suitable for use in pharmaceuticals, functional foods, and cosmetics.

In conclusion, the use of SFE offers both efficiency and sustainability, positioning it as a superior alternative to conventional extraction methods for herbal and phytochemical applications. While technical complexity and investment costs remain challenges, the advantages in terms of extract purity, process efficiency, and environmental safety are substantial. With ongoing innovations in process parameters, co-solvent application, and apparatus design, SFE is poised to assume a key role in the future development of industries focused on natural products.

6.2 Microwave-Assisted Extraction

Microwave-assisted extraction (MAE) has become a highly effective and efficient approach for isolating bioactive compounds from herbal matrices, providing multiple advantages compared to traditional extraction techniques. The underlying mechanism of MAE involves the rapid and intense generation of thermal energy through ionic conduction and dipole rotation within phytochemical molecules and surrounding solvents. This localized heating plays a critical role in accelerating cell wall rupture and enhancing the mass transfer of phytochemicals into the extraction solvent. MAE promotes concurrent heat and mass transfer, generating a synergistic effect that increases extraction efficiency, shortens extraction time, and lowers solvent requirements. It is especially effective for extracting thermolabile compounds that are prone to degradation with traditional heating approaches (Zhang et al. 2018; López-Salazar et al. 2023).

While MAE can employ a wide range of solvents, the choice of solvent is critical given the chemical heterogeneity of phytochemicals, spanning from highly polar compounds (e.g., phenolic compounds, glycosides, and quaternary alkaloids) to non-polar compounds such as chamuangone, α-mangostin, and rhinacanthins. Polar solvents, including ethanol, methanol, and water, are frequently employed in MAE for the extraction of polar phytochemicals due to their high dielectric constants and strong microwave absorption properties. Conversely, non-polar phytochemicals often require solvent mixtures or pretreatment steps to facilitate extraction, as non-polar solvents like hexane have low microwave absorption efficiency. To address this, co-solvent systems (e.g., ethanol/water or methanol/hexane) are frequently optimized to balance polarity, dielectric properties, and extraction efficiency. A major limitation of MAE lies in the need for accurate regulation of extraction parameters, including temperature, microwave power, extraction duration, and solvent-to-solid ratio, as these variables critically determine both extraction efficiency and the stability of bioactive compounds (Puttarak and Panichayupakaranant 2013; Lateh et al. 2019; Sae-Lim et al. 2019; Meah and Panichayupakaranant 2020; Sampaopan and Suksaeree 2022; Suttithumsatid et al. 2025).

One of the well-documented applications of MAE is its effectiveness in isolating curcuminoids from turmeric (*Curcuma longa*). Under optimized MAE conditions with ethanol, significantly enhanced yields of curcumin, demethoxycurcumin, and bisdemethoxycurcumin have been achieved in a reduced time (Lateh et al. 2019, 2022; Pengjam et al. 2021). An additional noteworthy application is the extraction of chamuangone from *Garcinia cowa* leaves, demonstrating the method's broad applicability, where MAE not only preserved the compound's anticancer activity more effectively due to shorter heat exposure but also reduced production costs (Sae-Lim et al. 2019, 2020; Rahman et al. 2025). MAE has also been successfully applied for extracting a broad range of phytochemicals with varying polarities, including:

- [6]-Gingerol from *Zingiber officinale* rhizomes (Promdam and Panichayupakaranant 2022; Promdam et al. 2022),
- Artocarpin from *Artocarpus heterophyllus* heartwoods (Bazmi and Panichayupakaranant 2022; Bazmi et al. 2022),
- Cannabinoids such as Δ^9-tetrahydrocannabinol (THC) and cannabidiol (CBD), which are primarily derived from *Cannabis sativa* (Suttithumsatid et al. 2022, 2023).
- Pentacyclic triterpenoids from *Centella asiatica* such as asiaticoside, madecassoside, asiatic acid, and madecassic acid (Puttarak and Panichayupakaranant 2013; Puttarak et al. 2016),
- Phenylbutenoids from *Zingiber cassumunar* rhizomes, including (*E*)-1-(3,4-dimethoxyphenyl)but-3-en-1-ol (compound D) and its acetate derivative and (*E*)-(3,4-dimethoxyphenyl)butadiene (DMPBD) (Gundom et al. 2024, 2025),
- Rhinacanthins, namely rhinacanthin-C, -D, and -N from *Rhinacanthus nasutus* leaves (Suksawat and Panichayupakaranant 2023, 2024), and
- α-Mangostin from *Garcinia mangostana* peels (Bundeesomchok et al. 2016; Meah and Panichayupakaranant 2020; Suttithumsatid et al. 2024).

Collectively, these cases demonstrate the ability of MAE to maintain the chemical integrity of bioactive compounds while enhancing extraction efficiency.

In conclusion, MAE represents a significant advancement in phytochemical extraction technologies. With proper optimization of solvent systems and operational parameters, MAE offers a rapid, efficient, and scalable approach suitable for both polar and non-polar phytochemicals. Despite challenges in parameter control and scale-up, its advantages in compound preservation, reduced environmental impact, and process efficiency make MAE a valuable tool in modern herbal research and natural product industries.

6.3 Ultrasound-Assisted Extraction

Ultrasound-assisted extraction (UAE) represents an advanced technique that offers high efficiency in recovering bioactive constituents from plants. When ultrasonic waves at frequencies of 20–100 kHz are applied, they induce structural damage to plant cells, leading to improved solvent infiltration and enhanced mass transfer of phytochemicals into the extraction medium (Gouda et al. 2021; Kumar et al. 2021; Shen et al. 2023). This mechanism is driven by acoustic cavitation, characterized by the generation, expansion, and eventual implosion of microscopic bubbles within a liquid medium. Upon their collapse, these bubbles produce transient hotspots characterized by elevated temperature and pressure, thereby promoting the degradation of cellular matrices and enhance the release of intracellular constituents. Consequently, UAE constitutes an attractive alternative to conventional extraction techniques, offering superior efficiency, shorter processing times, and reduced solvent requirements.

The overall performance of UAE is strongly influenced by the meticulous adjustment of both physical and operational conditions (Xue et al. 2022; Hao et al. 2023; Shen et al. 2023; Chumanee et al. 2024; Andriana et al. 2025; Li et al. 2025). Several critical factors influence the extraction outcome:

- Ultrasound frequency and intensity: These parameters determine the nature and extent of cavitation. Lower frequencies (20–40 kHz) typically produce more intense cavitation and are thus more effective in disrupting plant tissues. Conversely, higher frequencies may be more suitable for the extraction of thermolabile compounds due to their milder effects.
- Extraction temperature: Moderate temperature elevation can increase the solubility and diffusion rate of phytochemicals. However, excessive heat may degrade heat-sensitive bioactive compounds, underscoring the need for temperature control.
- Solvent type and polarity: The selection of solvent plays a pivotal role in determining both the selectivity and yield of the desired compounds. Commonly employed solvents, such as aqueous ethanol and methanol, are favored for their intermediate polarity and strong interactions with plant cellular constituents.
- Solvent-to-solid ratio: A higher solvent volume relative to plant material generally enhances the concentration gradient, promoting mass transfer. However, beyond a certain threshold, increases in solvent volume may yield diminishing returns.
- Extraction time and ultrasonic power: An appropriate balance of these factors is essential to achieve optimal extraction efficiency without inducing the degradation of target compounds. Prolonged sonication or excessive power input can damage sensitive phytochemicals or alter their structure.
- Particle size of plant material: Smaller particle sizes increase surface area, promoting higher extraction efficiency. Nevertheless, overly fine powders may impede solvent flow and reduce extraction efficiency.

A well-informed adjustment of these parameters is essential to ensure high extraction efficiency, compound integrity, and sustainability. Owing to its adaptability and potential for scale-up, UAE represents a valuable approach for herbal product development, especially when aligned with environmentally sustainable extraction practices.

Different classes of phytochemicals, such as polyphenols, alkaloids, flavonoids, and terpenoids, exhibit diverse sensitivities to heat, oxidation, and solvent polarity. For instance, phenolic acids and anthocyanins are highly susceptible to thermal degradation and generally require extraction at mild temperatures below 50 °C to preserve their stability. Flavonoids, on the other hand, may necessitate the use of moderately polar solvents to achieve efficient solubilization and recovery.

In order to precisely tailor the extraction conditions for individual classes of phytochemicals, statistical modeling techniques such as Response Surface Methodology (RSM) are frequently employed. Common RSM approaches include the Box–Behnken Design (BBD) and the three-level full factorial design (TFFD), which facilitate the systematic evaluation of multiple variables and their interactions. These methods help identify the optimal combination of parameters, such as temperature, time, solvent type, and ultrasonic power, that maximize yield, purity, and preservation of bioactivity (Wang et al. 2020; Hefied et al. 2023; Sanou et al. 2023; Andrade et al. 2024; Hiranpradith et al. 2025; Kim et al. 2025).

Despite its many advantages, the practical implementation of UAE poses technical challenges. This process responds strongly to variations in operating conditions, where small shifts in ultrasonic intensity, extraction time, or temperature may significantly impact yield and reproducibility. Transitioning from lab-scale to industrial-scale production introduces additional challenges, particularly in ensuring uniform energy distribution throughout larger volumes (Shen et al. 2023). Additionally, the initial cost of ultrasonic equipment and its associated energy consumption must be carefully evaluated against the benefits in extraction performance.

In contrast to conventional extraction methods, UAE offers faster processing, less solvent consumption, and improved yields of thermally sensitive compounds, protecting volatile and labile phytochemicals from degradation. UAE is often recognized for its cost-effectiveness, operational simplicity, and broad compatibility with various solvents. These characteristics make UAE an attractive option for both academic research and industrial applications, especially when resources are limited. Advanced techniques, such as SFE and MAE, offer advantages that may be more suitable for particular extraction purposes. SFE stands out for its selectivity and environmental compatibility, thanks to the use of supercritical CO_2, making it ideal for producing extracts of high purity without solvent contamination. As a result, SFE is especially effective for obtaining high-purity extracts while avoiding the presence of harmful solvent residues. On the other hand, MAE has demonstrated superior efficiency in extracting phenolic compounds from *Camellia japonica*, especially under conditions of high temperature and short extraction times. These comparisons highlight the importance of selecting an extraction technique based on a clear understanding of the specific objectives, available resources, and the phytochemical characteristics of the plant material in question. By carefully aligning method selection with the intended application, whether for maximizing yield, ensuring eco-friendliness, or simplifying operation, researchers can optimize the extraction process in the development of herbal-based products (Pereira et al. 2023).

Several successful applications of UAE in herbal extraction underscore its efficiency, selectivity, and practical relevance across various plant species. For instance, UAE has been effectively employed to isolate silymarin flavonolignans from *Silybum marianum* (milk thistle), achieving significantly higher yields than traditional maceration methods. Using optimized conditions, 54.5% aqueous ethanol, 36.6 kHz ultrasound frequency, and a 60-minute extraction at 45 °C, this method produced extracts that complied with AOAC standards for precision and accuracy (Drouet et al. 2019). The extracted compounds maintained significant antioxidant activity and exhibited notable inhibition of collagenase and elastase, enzymes associated with skin aging, indicating promising applications in cosmetics. This case exemplifies how UAE can serve as a sustainable and efficient platform for producing high-quality herbal extracts tailored for functional and therapeutic purposes.

In a similar vein, optimized UAE protocols have been developed for extracting bioactive triterpenoids from *Centella asiatica*, such as asiaticoside and madecassoside. Using response surface methodology, the study found that extraction yields were strongly affected by ethanol concentration and solvent volume, whereas ultrasonic power and extraction duration had more limited or specific impacts (Hiranpradith et al. 2025). The optimized conditions yielded extract concentrations that closely matched predicted values from the statistical model, further validating the robustness of UAE for use in the production of functional food ingredients or nutraceuticals derived from *C. asiatica*.

The use of UAE enabled efficient extraction of alkaloids such as mitragynine and 7-hydroxymitragynine from *Mitragyna speciosa* (Kratom) leaves. Optimal conditions, 0.5:10 g/mL sample-to-solvent ratio, 70% methanol, 175 W ultrasonic power, and a 10-minute extraction, resulted in maximum alkaloid yield, highlighting its practical utility for developing standardized kratom products.

Taken together, these examples underscore the exceptional ability of UAE to improve the extraction of various phytochemical groups while maintaining their structural integrity and biological activity. Whether targeting flavonolignans, triterpenoids, or alkaloids, UAE offers a reliable, scalable, and eco-friendly alternative to conventional extraction techniques.

In conclusion, UAE represents a powerful and versatile technique for the extraction of phytochemicals from botanical matrices. While challenges such as process optimization, reproducibility, and industrial scale-up remain, the advantages of this method, in terms of speed, efficiency, and preservation of thermolabile compounds, make it highly attractive for both academic research and commercial production. Future advancements in UAE, including hybrid technologies (e.g., ultrasound combined with enzymatic treatment or microwave heating) and intelligent process control systems, may further expand its utility and reliability across diverse applications in the pharmaceutical, cosmetic, and functional food industries.

6.4 Pressurized Liquid Extraction

Pressurized liquid extraction (PLE), also referred to as accelerated solvent extraction (ASE) or subcritical solvent extraction (SSE), has become a highly effective and eco-friendly approach for isolating bioactive compounds, particularly phytochemicals, from medicinal and aromatic plants. This technique uses conventional solvents at elevated temperatures (typically 50–200 °C) and high pressures (usually 10–15 MPa), allowing the solvent to remain in a liquid state above its normal boiling point. Under these subcritical conditions, the solvent's physical properties, including viscosity and surface tension, are significantly decreased, enhancing the solubility of target compounds and improving mass transfer. Consequently, the solvent can penetrate the plant matrix more efficiently, facilitating faster and deeper extraction of phytochemicals. Compared with traditional extraction methods, PLE offers notable benefits, such as lower solvent consumption, shorter extraction durations, and higher extraction efficiency.

The efficiency of PLE depends on several critical operational factors, including temperature, pressure, solvent selection, extraction time, and the number of extraction cycles. These parameters should be carefully optimized according to the physicochemical properties and thermal stability of the target phytochemicals. For example, thermolabile compounds such as polyphenols and flavonoids are vulnerable to prolonged high-temperature exposure. In such cases, milder extraction conditions using solvents such as aqueous ethanol, methanol, or environmentally friendly alternatives such as deep eutectic solvents are recommended to maintain their bioactivity. Conversely, more thermally stable compounds, such as alkaloids, phytosterols, and triterpenoids, may require more intense extraction conditions to maximize yield. In such cases, higher temperatures and pressures can be employed without significant risk of compound degradation (Okiyama et al. 2018; Allcca-Alca et al. 2021; Supasatyankul et al. 2022; Dobroslavić et al. 2022; Cegledi et al. 2023; da Cunha Rodrigues et al. 2023; Huamán-Castilla et al. 2023; Višnjevec et al. 2024).

PLE represents a notable advancement in phytochemical extraction technologies, offering a well-balanced combination of extraction efficiency, environmental sustainability, and product integrity. This technique is particularly relevant for developing herbal and plant-based products, where maintaining bioactivity is essential. PLE also holds strong potential for innovation in natural product research and the production of functional ingredients.

In comparison with traditional methods like Soxhlet extraction, PLE provides notable advantages, including shorter extraction times, reduced solvent usage, higher yields, and improved selectivity. Additionally, when combined with environmentally friendly solvents such as ethanol or water, PLE adheres to green chemistry principles, making it particularly suitable for sustainable product development (Hirondart et al. 2020).

Among advanced extraction techniques including SFE, MAE, and UAE, PLE demonstrates moderate performance. SFE operates at lower temperatures (around

40 °C), whereas MAE and UAE provide shorter extraction times than both PLE and SFE. For phenolic compound extraction, the typical order of total phenolic content is MAE > PLE > UAE > SFE (Osorio-Tobón 2020).

Despite these advantages, several limitations may affect the broader application of PLE. One major constraint is the relatively high cost of instrumentation. The equipment must endure high pressure and temperature conditions, necessitating the use of specialized, corrosion-resistant materials, both in research laboratories and industrial-scale operations (Perez-Vazquez et al. 2023; Palos-Hernández et al. 2025).

Another issue is selectivity, since unwanted substances are often co-extracted from intricate plant matrices, which can make downstream purification more difficult and compromise product quality. Furthermore, reproducibility remains a concern, especially when working with heterogeneous plant materials. Factors such as matrix variability, particle size, and moisture content can significantly influence extraction behavior, requiring meticulous sample preparation and strict protocol standardization.

Nonetheless, recent technological advancements have improved the usability and precision of PLE systems. Modern instruments now incorporate programmable pressure and temperature settings, automated solvent delivery, and enhanced safety features. These developments allow for greater control and repeatability in extraction processes, even when applied to diverse and complex botanical samples.

One notable use of PLE involves the valorization of wine production by-products. In this case, phenolic compounds were recovered from Cannonau grape pomace, a waste material rich in bioactive compounds. The effects of key extraction factors, such as temperature, ethanol concentration, and extraction time, were evaluated using a Central Composite Design with Response Surface Methodology. The optimal extraction conditions were identified as 130 °C, 55% ethanol, and 22 minutes. Under these settings, PLE achieved higher yields and superior phenolic recovery compared to conventional extraction techniques, demonstrating its effectiveness in the sustainable revalorization of agro-industrial residues (Perra et al. 2023).

Similarly, PLE has been shown to efficiently produce high-quality extracts from *Moringa oleifera* leaves, which are well known for their therapeutic properties. By optimizing parameters such as the liquid-to-solid ratio (70 mL/g), temperature (150 °C), pressure (around 1700 psi), and extraction time (15 minutes) using deionized water as a green and cost-effective solvent, the resulting extracts contained substantial amounts of total flavonoids (19.8 mg RtE/g dw), total polyphenols (24.6 mg GAE/g dw), and ascorbic acid (4.6 mg/g dw). These findings demonstrate PLE's capability to recover diverse bioactive compounds efficiently while maintaining environmentally sustainable practices (Chatzimitakos et al. 2024).

Such examples emphasize the effectiveness of PLE in enhancing the quality and standardization of herbal extracts, essential for use in pharmaceuticals, nutraceuticals, and functional foods. The technique's precise control over extraction parameters allows consistent recovery of compounds with desired bioactivity and stability.

In conclusion, PLE stands as a pivotal development in phytochemical extraction technologies. Its capacity to efficiently recover a wide spectrum of bioactive compounds under tunable and relatively mild subcritical conditions positions it as a valuable tool in contemporary natural product research and product development. However, successful implementation necessitates a comprehensive understanding of the chemical nature of target compounds as well as the influence of extraction parameters on yield, selectivity, and compound stability. As advancements in equipment design and green solvent systems continue to evolve, PLE is poised to play an increasingly important role in the sustainable and standardized production of high-value botanical extracts.

6.5 Pulsed Electric Field Extraction

Emerging as a non-thermal extraction method, pulsed electric field (PEF) has shown strong potential for isolating bioactive compounds from plants. By applying brief high-voltage pulses (0.5–45 kV/cm) to plant tissues, electroporation occurs, disrupting cell membranes and improving mass transfer. This allows intracellular compounds to be efficiently released into the solvent with minimal heat-induced degradation (Ranjha et al. 2021; Naliyadhara et al. 2022; Athanasiadis et al. 2023; Chatzimitakos et al. 2023).

The effectiveness of PEF-assisted extraction depends on several factors, including electric field strength, pulse duration, number and shape of pulses, treatment time, and temperature. Careful optimization of these parameters is crucial, particularly when dealing with thermolabile or oxidation-sensitive plant pigments, including carotenoids, betalains, anthocyanins, and chlorophylls, which can easily degrade if conditions are not properly controlled. To maximize the recovery of natural pigments and other phytochemicals, structured optimization strategies must be employed. Key parameters such as electric field intensity, energy input per unit mass, pulse count, exposure time, and processing temperature directly govern electroporation efficiency. Enhancing these parameters can improve the permeability of plant cell membranes, facilitating more effective release and diffusion of bioactive compounds into the solvent. PEF extraction efficiency is highly dependent on the properties of the plant material. Variations such as differences between peel and pulp structure, the chemical and physical stability of target pigments, their localization within cells, and their interaction with the surrounding matrix all affect the overall yield. In some instances, overly aggressive PEF conditions may actually decrease efficiency or cause degradation of the desired compounds (Arshad et al. 2020; Arruda et al. 2021; Bocker and Silva 2022).

PEF extraction presents several compelling advantages over traditional methods such as maceration and Soxhlet extraction. Notably, PEF enables rapid processing, reduces solvent usage, and minimizes thermal degradation, thereby preserving thermolabile bioactive compounds. In comparison with contemporary technologies like MAE and UAE, PEF distinguishes itself through superior energy efficiency and suitability for continuous, large-scale processing. Despite these strengths, PEF has inherent limitations. It is generally not sufficient for exhaustive extraction on its own, often necessitating a subsequent solvent-based step to achieve complete recovery of phytochemicals (Jintawiwat et al. 2023). Furthermore, the high capital investment required for PEF equipment poses a significant barrier to widespread adoption, particularly when compared to more accessible alternatives (Arshad et al. 2020; Bocker and Silva 2022). These considerations underscore the importance of evaluating both the technical and economic feasibility of PEF in the context of specific extraction objectives and resource availability.

As a non-thermal method, PEF technology shows great potential for improving the recovery of bioactive compounds from plant matrices. For instance, the extraction of polyphenols from *Elaeagnus pungens* leaves was optimized by adjusting key process variables, including the ethanol–water solvent ratio and PEF settings such as pulse duration, interval, and field strength. When applied at 10 µs pulses, 1000 µs intervals, 0.85 kV/cm electric field, and 50% ethanol, the polyphenol content was enhanced by 58% relative to conventional methods without PEF (Pappas et al. 2022). This underscores the critical role of fine-tuning extraction parameters to maximize yield and efficiency.

Yang et al. (2024) studied the impact of PEF on the performance and quality of extra virgin olive oil extracted from the Koroneiki variety. The application of PEF led to a 5.6% increase in oil yield while maintaining essential quality indicators such as saponification value and UV absorbance. Moreover, PEF-treated oil exhibited elevated levels of health-promoting compounds, including total phenolics, flavonoids, oleuropein, and tocopherols, resulting in improved antioxidant capacity. These findings highlight PEF's potential to enhance both yield and nutritional value in edible oil processing.

Further evidence of PEF's efficacy comes from its application in the extraction of phenolic compounds from mangosteen (*Garcinia mangostana*) pericarp. Applying different electric field strengths and pulse counts markedly enhanced both the total phenolic content (TPC) and antioxidant activity, as assessed by the FRAP assay, relative to conventional water maceration. Notably, the treatment with 6 kV/cm and 5000 pulses resulted in a 4-times increase in TPC, along with the strongest antioxidant response (Alide et al. 2020).

Collectively, these studies demonstrate the versatility and effectiveness of PEF as a green extraction technology, particularly in the valorization of plant-derived polyphenols for use in functional foods, nutraceuticals, and herbal product development. Parameter optimization remains a critical factor in achieving maximum recovery and bioactivity of target compounds, and future research should focus on scaling up PEF processes for industrial applications while maintaining bioactive integrity.

In conclusion, PEF offers a green and efficient method for improving the extraction yield and quality of plant-derived phytochemicals. Its non-thermal operation safeguards heat-sensitive compounds, and its flexibility for scaling and combining with other extraction approaches makes it a valuable technology for the formulation of functional ingredients in nutraceutical, cosmetic, and pharmaceutical sectors. However, to fully realize the potential of PEF technology, further investigations are necessary, particularly in the areas of process standardization, long-term stability of extracted compounds, and industrial-scale implementation. Continued research in these directions will be crucial for optimizing performance and facilitating the broader adoption of PEF in herbal product innovation.

6.6 Enzyme-Assisted Extraction

EAE, or enzyme-assisted extraction, is increasingly recognized as a valuable method that exploits enzymes to degrade plant cell wall components. This disruption facilitates the penetration of extraction solvents and enhances the release of intracellular phytochemicals. EAE utilizes a range of enzymes, such as cellulases, hemicellulases, pectinases, and proteases, to break down the proteins and polysaccharides that constitute plant cell structures. By breaking down these components, EAE not only increases extraction yields but also improves the bioavailability and preserves the functional integrity of the target phytochemicals. Serving as a more eco-conscious and affordable option compared with conventional extraction techniques, EAE is increasingly acknowledged within both academic research and industrial applications (Gil-Martín et al. 2022; Lubek-Nguyen et al. 2022; Streimikyte et al. 2022). Its sustainable character resonates with contemporary priorities in natural product innovation, notably the value addition to medicinal plants and agricultural by-products.

Key variables affecting the success of EAE include enzyme type and concentration, physicochemical conditions (pH and temperature), incubation period, solvent environment, and the intrinsic features of the substrate. These factors must be carefully optimized according to the specific properties of the target phytochemicals. Importantly, while enzymatic hydrolysis enhances extraction efficiency, excessively harsh enzymatic conditions may lead to degradation of sensitive bioactive compounds. Accordingly, precise adjustment of operational variables plays a vital role in maximizing recovery while safeguarding the stability of phytochemicals.

For instance, Zuorro et al. (2019) demonstrated that pretreatment of corn husks with cellulase, followed by aqueous ethanol extraction, significantly improved the recovery of flavonoids. The optimization of enzyme concentration (0.3–0.5% w/w), incubation period (1.5–2.5 h), liquid-to-solid ratio (30–40 mL/g), and ethanol concentration (60–80% v/v) was conducted using a four-factor, three-level Box–Behnken design with RSM, resulting in a flavonoid recovery of about 1.3% w/w.

In another example, Polo-Castellano et al. (2023) applied a combination of Plackett–Burman and Box–Behnken experimental designs to optimize EAE conditions for flavonoid and phenolic compound extraction from *Moringa oleifera* leaves. Key parameters included temperature (58.9 °C), agitation speed (50 rpm), pH (4.0), ethanol concentration (32.5%), sample-to-solvent ratio (0.2 g in 15 mL), and a pectinase dose of 106 U/g derived from *Aspergillus niger*. Remarkably, this optimized protocol allowed for efficient extraction within just two minutes, yielding extracts with high antioxidant activity and phenolic content. The method also demonstrated good precision and repeatability, underscoring its potential for reliable phytochemical extraction.

Controlling the enzymatic extraction process is generally feasible under laboratory and pilot-scale conditions, primarily due to the well-characterized activity profiles of commercially available enzymes (Tarafdar et al. 2021). However, scaling up EAE for industrial applications poses several challenges. These include the relatively high cost of enzymes, the gradual loss of enzymatic activity during extended processing times, and the inherent variability in raw plant materials. Moreover, the efficiency of enzyme-mediated hydrolysis is often constrained by the limited accessibility of target substrates, necessitating mechanical pre-treatments, such as milling, grinding, or homogenization, to increase the available surface area and enhance enzyme–substrate interactions.

In comparison with established approaches like maceration, decoction, and Soxhlet extraction, EAE offers several superior features. It typically operates under milder processing conditions, uses less organic solvent, and is more environmentally friendly. Importantly, EAE is highly suitable for extracting thermolabile or oxidation-sensitive phytochemicals, which might degrade under the harsher conditions of traditional methods.

When evaluated alongside other modern extraction technologies, such as SFE, MAE, and UAE, EAE is generally more cost-effective and energy-efficient. It does not require high pressures, temperatures, or specialized instrumentation, making it attractive for applications in resource-limited settings. Nonetheless, EAE is not without limitations. The extraction process can be time-consuming, and the specificity of enzymes may restrict their effectiveness when dealing with the complex and heterogeneous structures of certain plant matrices (Cannavacciuolo et al. 2024; Cao et al. 2025; Shawky et al. 2025).

An illustrative case of EAE application is its role in improving the extraction of bioactive compounds from eggplant (Solanum melongena) peel, encompassing overall yield, anthocyanins, phenolics, and antioxidant activity. Optimization through response surface methodology identified enzyme concentration, temperature, and extraction duration as critical parameters. Under the optimal conditions, 37.3 °C, 5% enzyme loading, and 1 h incubation, substantially greater amounts of all targeted phytochemicals were obtained relative to conventional techniques, highlighting the superior potential of EAE in the valorization of agro-waste (Amulya and Ul Islam 2023).

EAE was also applied to mulberry fruits, where optimized extraction (0.15 g fruit, 70% ethanol, pH 4.0, 40 °C, 38.5 enzyme units/g, 5 min at 200 rpm) yielded reproducible results with less than 5% variation. *Morus nigra* showed the highest anthocyanin concentration, whereas *Morus rubra* contained the most phenolics. The extracts exhibited notable antioxidant and antimicrobial effects, supporting their application in nutraceuticals and pharmaceuticals (Tizón Alba et al. 2023).

Recent innovations have expanded the scope of EAE through integration with modern extraction techniques to enhance selectivity and efficiency. One such approach is enzyme-assisted ultrasonic extraction (EUAE), which was successfully applied to *Abelmoschus manihot*, a traditional Chinese medicinal plant. Under optimized conditions, 3% enzyme concentration using a 1:1 cellulase to pectinase ratio in a 70% ethanol–buffer solution at 50 °C for 40 minutes, the method achieved a flavonoid yield of 3.5%. EUAE markedly improved both flavonoid and polysaccharide yields compared to conventional UAE, confirming its synergistic efficiency (Chu et al. 2024).

Another hybrid approach, enzyme-assisted supercritical fluid extraction (EA-SFE), has proven highly effective for isolating bioactive compounds from complex matrices. Mikšovsky et al. (2024) developed an EA-SFE method to recover flavonoids from apple pomace using snailase, a multi-enzyme preparation. The enzymes facilitated the hydrolysis of flavonoid glycosides into aglycone forms such as quercetin and phloretin, which were subsequently extracted using supercritical CO_2 with a minimal amount of methanol as co-solvent. The process achieved a 96% enzymatic conversion rate and a 90% extraction yield, and was equally effective on both fresh and dried pomace. These results highlight the scalability, efficiency, and environmental compatibility of EA-SFE as a next-generation green extraction technique.

As a novel and sustainable extraction approach, EAE provides a mild yet effective means of isolating phytochemicals from plants and herbs. Its capacity to boost yields, safeguard sensitive bioactive compounds, and reduce dependence on toxic solvents supports the vision of green chemistry and circular bioeconomy. Furthermore, the technique's flexibility allows broad application across plant systems and seamless integration with advanced methods such as ultrasound and supercritical fluid extraction, enabling synergistic gains in both efficiency and selectivity.

However, to fully exploit the potential of EAE, ongoing research is necessary. Areas requiring further development include enzyme engineering for broader substrate specificity, strategies to reduce enzyme cost, and process integration to enable continuous, scalable operations. Innovations in these domains will be critical for translating the laboratory success of EAE into robust industrial applications that support sustainable natural product development.

7 Alternative Green Solvents for Phytochemical Extraction

The isolation of bioactive constituents from plant sources represents a fundamental step in the production of herbal medicines, nutraceuticals, functional foods, and cosmetic formulations. Historically, organic solvents, including hexane, dichloromethane, chloroform, acetone, and methanol, have been widely used due to their capacity to dissolve a broad spectrum of phytochemicals. However, these solvents are associated with significant drawbacks, including environmental persistence, human toxicity, and high flammability. These concerns have prompted a shift toward more sustainable extraction practices, resulting in the development and application of green solvents as environmentally friendly alternatives (Chemat et al. 2019a).

This section explores the foundational principles of green solvent use, highlights various types of alternative green solvents, and discusses their respective advantages, limitations, and successful applications in the field of phytochemical extraction.

7.1 Principles of Green Solvent Use

The notion of green solvents originates from the overarching principles of green chemistry, which seek to reduce or eliminate the use and production of hazardous chemicals. Green solvents are designed to fulfill multiple criteria that make them more sustainable than conventional organic solvents. Ideally, they should be:

- Derived from renewable or bio-based sources
- Biodegradable, minimizing environmental persistence
- Non-toxic to humans and ecosystems
- Efficient in extracting target bioactive compounds
- Compatible with downstream purification or formulation processes
- Economically feasible for applications ranging from lab-scale experiments to large-scale industrial processes.

Using green solvents is consistent with several of the Twelve Principles of Green Chemistry proposed by Anastas and Warner (1998), particularly those related to solvent choice:

- Principle 2: Atom Economy—Maximizing the utilization of all process inputs in the end product.
- Principle 3: Less Hazardous Chemical Syntheses—Avoiding or reducing the use of toxic substances.
- Principle 4: Designing Safer Chemicals—Reducing toxicity in the chemicals used.
- Principle 6: Design for Energy Efficiency—Enabling lower-temperature and lower-pressure processes.
- Principle 7: Use of Renewable Feedstocks—Favoring solvents derived from plant-based or waste-derived sources.
- Principle 10: Design for Degradation—Ensuring chemicals break down into non-harmful components after use.
- Principle 12: Inherently Safer Chemistry for Accident Prevention—Reducing risks by avoiding flammable and volatile substances.

Adhering to these principles, the adoption of green solvents not only mitigates environmental impact and enhances process safety but also supports the development of more sustainable and circular chemical manufacturing practices.

7.2 Types of Alternative Green Solvents

Various green solvents, such as agro-based solvents, pharmaceutical excipients, ionic liquids, and deep eutectic solvents, have been studied for herbal extraction. Their effectiveness and suitability depend on the target phytochemicals and the purpose of the extract.

7.2.1 Agro-based Solvents

Agro-based solvents are obtained from renewable agricultural sources, including plant biomass, by-products from the food industry, and residues from essential oil production. These solvents are generally biodegradable, non-toxic, renewable, and considered environmentally sustainable. Common examples include ethanol, glycerol, propylene glycol, vegetable oils, and D-limonene (Usman et al. 2023; Darwin et al. 2025; dos Santos et al. 2025).

Ethanol, commonly obtained from the fermentation of sugarcane, corn, or other carbohydrate-rich crops, is one of the most widely used plant-derived solvents.

Advantages:

- Effective in recovering diverse polar and moderately non-polar plant compounds
- Food-grade, safe for oral and topical formulations
- Biodegradable and environmentally friendly

Limitations:

- May co-extract unwanted compounds such as chlorophyll, waxes, or pigments
- Highly flammable, requiring stringent safety measures during handling and processing
- Often requires evaporation or dilution in final product formulations

Glycerol is a secondary product obtained from biodiesel manufacturing and is commonly used in the pharmaceutical and cosmetic industries as a solvent and humectant.

Advantages:

- Excellent solvent for highly polar and water-soluble compounds
- Non-toxic and suitable for oral, dermal, and cosmetic applications
- Acts as a humectant, enhancing the moisture retention of end-products

Limitations:

- High viscosity can hinder mass transfer and reduce extraction efficiency
- Ineffective for extracting non-polar compounds such as essential oils
- Slower extraction kinetics compared to lower-viscosity solvents like ethanol

Propylene glycol, while often synthetically produced, is also available from bio-based feedstocks. It is commonly used as a co-solvent in pharmaceutical and cosmetic products.

Advantages:

- Capable of solubilizing both polar and some non-polar constituents
- Low volatility and chemical stability under a range of conditions
- Broadly accepted in regulatory frameworks for food and cosmetic use

Limitations:

- Bio-based production remains limited and more costly than synthetic counterparts
- Sometimes perceived as less natural compared to other agro-based solvents
- Not ideal for products aiming for "100% natural" certification

Edible oils from various plant sources, e.g., coconut oil, palm oil, and rice bran oil, are used for the extraction of lipophilic compounds.

Advantages:

- Excellent solvents for lipophilic phytochemicals such as essential oils, terpenes, and carotenoids
- Safe for human consumption and topical applications
- Inexpensive, widely available, and biodegradable

Limitations:

- Poor extraction efficiency for hydrophilic or polar compounds
- Susceptible to oxidation and rancidity; requires proper storage conditions
- Oily texture may limit applicability in certain formulation types

D-limonene is a terpene solvent obtained from citrus peel waste, particularly from orange or lemon processing industries.

Advantages:

- Highly effective at solubilizing non-polar, lipophilic compounds, including essential oils, resins, and waxes
- Naturally derived from citrus waste; supports circular bioeconomy principles
- Possesses intrinsic antimicrobial and aromatic properties that may enhance product quality

Limitations:

- Potential allergenic or irritant effects in sensitive individuals.
- Volatile and flammable; requires appropriate handling precautions.
- Narrow polarity range; not effective for polar or hydrophilic compound extraction.

7.2.2 Pharmaceutical Excipients

Selecting an effective extraction method is essential for the commercialization of herbal products. Traditional approaches such as Soxhlet extraction, maceration, and heat reflux require considerable labor and time, as well as substantial amounts of organic solvents that are environmentally hazardous and potentially toxic, thereby limiting their practicality for industrial applications.

To address these challenges, recent studies have increasingly focused on green extraction technologies that emphasize environmental protection, human safety, and economic viability. Microwave-assisted extraction (MAE) has emerged as a particularly promising approach. By applying microwave energy to rapidly heat both the plant matrix and solvents, MAE improves extraction efficiency while markedly reducing solvent usage, energy consumption, and processing time.

A particularly innovative advancement in this field involves the use of pharmaceutical excipients, non-active ingredients commonly found in creams, lotions, dermal patches, and pastilles, as alternative green solvents in MAE (Panichayupakaranant 2023). These excipients are generally recognized as safe (GRAS) and are used in pharmaceutical formulations to improve stability, bioavailability, and delivery of active compounds. Their known safety profiles and compatibility with human use make them ideal candidates for green extraction of herbal bioactive compounds.

Crucially, these excipients serve a dual function: they act as eco-friendly extraction media and can be directly incorporated into final formulations. This eliminates the need for solvent evaporation, reduces production costs, and streamlines manufacturing processes for herbal-based therapeutics and cosmeceuticals.

Several case studies illustrate the effectiveness of this approach:

Cetyl alcohol and isopropyl myristate, frequently employed in cream formulations, were used as alternative solvents for the extraction of α-mangostin from mangosteen (*Garcinia mangostana*, Clusiaceae) pericarp powder. This method produced an extract containing 2.0% w/w α-mangostin, which was directly applied in the formulation of anti-acne creams and oral-ulcer gels, with no requirement for solvent removal (Panichayupakaranant and Bundeesomchok 2015).

In another study, a deep eutectic mixture of sucrose and citric acid and glycerin, excipients commonly employed in pastilles, was utilized to extract [6]-gingerol from powdered ginger (*Zingiber officinale*, Zingiberaceae). The resulting extract, containing 1.7% w/w [6]-gingerol, was deemed suitable for direct incorporation into anti-emetic pastille formulations (Promdam et al. 2022).

Polyethylene glycol 400 (PEG 400), a co-solvent widely used in ultrasound gels, was applied as a green solvent for extracting phenylbutenoids from *Cassumunar ginger* (*Zingiber cassumunar*, Zingiberaceae). The extraction produced a total phenylbutenoid content of 1.4% w/w, consisting of DMPBD (0.9% w/w), compound D (0.3% w/w), and compound D acetate (0.2% w/w). This extract was directly formulated into an anti-inflammatory ultrasound gel for phonophoresis in the treatment of musculoskeletal disorders (Gundom et al. 2024, 2025).

These examples underscore the potential of MAE combined with pharmaceutical-grade excipients to transform the landscape of herbal product development. By eliminating toxic solvents and simplifying post-extraction processing, this approach supports the creation of scalable, safe, and sustainable herbal formulations in alignment with green chemistry principles.

7.2.3 Ionic Liquids

Ionic liquids (ILs) have emerged as an advanced category of solvents for extracting phytochemicals from herbal matrices. These salts, which remain liquid at or near ambient temperature, comprise organic cations paired with a variety of anions. Their distinctive physicochemical characteristics, such as high thermal and chemical stability, negligible vapor pressure, and adjustable solvation properties, render them promising alternatives to traditional organic solvents in natural product extraction.

One major benefit of ILs is their effectiveness in breaking down plant cell walls and solubilizing diverse phytochemicals. Their strong hydrogen-bonding capability, polarity, and interaction with both polar and non-polar molecules make them particularly suited for extracting alkaloids, flavonoids, terpenoids, and phenolics (Ventura et al. 2017; Xiao et al. 2018; Flieger and Flieger 2020).

The efficiency of phytochemical extraction using ionic liquids depends critically on the careful optimization of several parameters. These include the choice of ILs (cation and anion type), its concentration, extraction temperature, pH, duration, and the solid-to-liquid ratio. For instance, the use of 1-butyl-3-methylimidazolium bromide ([C_4mim]Br) in the extraction of resveratrol from *Polygonum cuspidatum* resulted in significantly higher yields compared to conventional solvent systems (Zhao et al. 2024). Such optimization improves extraction yield while maintaining the structural integrity and biological activity of the target phytochemicals.

Ionic liquids offer several compelling advantages over traditional solvents:

- Enhanced extraction efficiency: ILs can dissolve a wide variety of phytochemicals, often leading to improved yields.
- Environmental compatibility: Their negligible volatility minimizes the release of volatile organic compounds, aligning well with green chemistry principles.
- Reusability: The recoverable and reusable nature of many ILs reduces solvent waste and contributes to more sustainable processes.

Despite their potential, certain limitations must be addressed before ionic liquids can be widely adopted in industrial applications:

- Toxicity: Some ILs exhibit ecotoxicity, particularly toward aquatic organisms, raising environmental safety concerns.
- Cost and availability: The synthesis and large-scale production of ILs can be costly, limiting their accessibility.
- High viscosity: The relatively high viscosity of some ILs may hinder mass transfer, especially in large-scale extraction processes.

Recent studies have highlighted the successful integration of ILs with modern extraction technologies such as UAE and MAE, both of which significantly improve process efficiency and reduce solvent consumption.

A notable example is the MAE-based extraction of ten flavonoid glycosides from *Chrysanthemum morifolium* using a series of imidazolium-based ILs ([$C_n$mim]Br, where n = 2–16). It was found that [C_{12}mim]Br offered the highest extraction efficiency. The research also investigated how microwave power, IL concentration, the ratio of matrix to solvent, and extraction duration affect the extraction process, highlighting the importance of each factor in achieving optimal results (Zhou et al. 2015).

Similarly, lycopene was efficiently extracted from *Psidium guajava* fruits using an IL-UAE approach. Among 13 ILs tested, 1-butyl-3-methylimidazolium chloride ([C_4mim]Cl) achieved the highest yield. By applying optimal conditions, including 33 min extraction, 3.0 mol/L IL, 22 mL/g solvent-to-solid ratio, 225 W ultrasonic power, and three extraction cycles, lycopene yield reached 9.4 mg/g, which was higher than that obtained through conventional techniques (Wang et al. 2024).

Ionic liquids represent a versatile and powerful medium for the selective extraction of phytochemicals from herbal materials. Their customizable molecular structures allow researchers to tailor solvent properties for specific target compounds, potentially achieving superior yields and environmental performance compared to traditional organic solvents. Nevertheless, challenges such as environmental toxicity, economic feasibility, and process scalability must be addressed to fully realize the industrial potential of ILs. Advancing the field will require the development of biodegradable, low-toxicity ionic liquids, affordable synthesis techniques, and intensified process strategies. Addressing these areas is vital for integrating ILs into eco-friendly, large-scale herbal extraction practices.

7.2.4 Deep Eutectic Solvents

Deep eutectic solvents (DESs) constitute a novel class of green solvents, recognized for their environmental friendliness, versatility, and customizable physicochemical features. These solvents are generally prepared by combining two or more substances, most often a hydrogen bond donor (HBD) and a hydrogen bond acceptor (HBA), which form hydrogen-bonded eutectic mixtures with melting points considerably lower than those of the individual components. DESs can exist as binary or ternary systems and commonly include quaternary ammonium salts, metal salts, or organic compounds (Hikmawanti et al. 2021; Kaoui et al. 2023; Li et al. 2023; Ferreira and Sarraguça 2024; Stanisz et al. 2024; Yeow et al. 2024).

Unlike conventional solvents, DESs are not single, well-defined chemical entities but rather mixtures whose properties are governed by intermolecular interactions among their constituents. This unique nature allows researchers to tailor DESs by varying the types and ratios of HBDs and HBAs, thus adjusting parameters such as polarity, viscosity, pH stability, and solvation capacity to suit specific applications.

Among DESs, natural deep eutectic solvents (NADESs) stand out due to their composition of biocompatible, naturally occurring compounds such as sugars, organic acids, amino acids, and polyols. NADESs are increasingly recognized as sustainable and high-performing alternatives to traditional organic solvents for plant-based phytochemical extraction.

DESs possess several properties that make them especially attractive for applications in natural product extraction, catalysis, pharmaceuticals, and materials science:

- Low Volatility: Most DESs have negligible vapor pressure, reducing hazards associated with inhalation and flammability, as compared to volatile organic solvents like methanol or acetone.
- Environmental Compatibility: Many DESs, especially NADESs, are derived from biodegradable and non-toxic compounds, offering a greener alternative for sustainable processing.
- Thermal and Chemical Stability: DESs exhibit high stability over a broad range of temperatures and pH levels, making them suitable for processing heat- or acid-sensitive phytochemicals.
- Customizability: The physicochemical properties of DESs can be tuned by selecting specific HBDs and HBAs in different molar ratios, enabling the development of task-specific solvents.

However, a common limitation of DESs is their relatively high viscosity at room temperature, which can hinder mass transfer during extraction. This limitation can be addressed through moderate heating or by adding small quantities of water, which lowers viscosity without compromising the solvent's extraction performance.

The efficacy of DESs in extracting bioactive plant compounds is largely attributed to their extensive hydrogen-bonding networks and strong solvation capabilities. Such properties allow for the solubilization of a broad spectrum of secondary metabolites, including flavonoids, phenolic acids, alkaloids, and terpenoids.

The careful selection of DES components and their molar ratios is crucial for optimizing extraction efficiency. For example, choline chloride-based NADESs paired with polyalcohols such as glycerol have shown excellent performance in the extraction of flavonoids and other polar phytochemicals. These systems not only enhance extraction yields but also offer an environmentally friendly alternative to conventional solvent systems.

To achieve high extraction efficiency and preserve phytochemical structures, it is important to fine-tune parameters such as DES composition, water proportion, extraction temperature and duration, as well as the solid-to-liquid ratio. Research has indicated that changes in water content within DESs can strongly affect both solubility and compound stability.

For example, Gómez-Urios et al. (2023) assessed eight NADESs for their effectiveness in extracting bioactive compounds from orange peel, evaluating antioxidant capacity, ascorbic acid, total phenolic content, and total flavonoid content. Among the NADESs tested, choline chloride:malic acid (ChCl:MA) and choline chloride:glycerol (ChCl:Gly) exhibited the highest extraction efficiencies. ChCl:MA was especially effective in preserving ascorbic acid and phenolic compounds, whereas ChCl:Gly led to the highest flavonoid yields. Both NADESs demonstrated enhanced antioxidant stability and maintained antioxidant capacity over a 12-day storage period, highlighting their potential as non-toxic, food-grade extraction solvents that obviate the need for solvent removal.

Another study by Hikmawanti et al. (2024) focused on optimizing NADES-based ultrasound-assisted extraction (UAE) of antioxidant polyphenols from

Pluchea indica leaves using ChCl:urea in a 1:3 molar ratio. Under conditions of 26% water, 52 °C, and 15 min, the extraction considerably improved phenolic and flavonoid contents. Antioxidant activity was enhanced by approximately 1.2- and 3.1-fold over extractions with 50% ethanol and methanol, respectively, indicating the enhanced efficiency of this method.

Oomen et al. (2020) investigated flavonoid extraction from *Scutellaria baicalensis* bark using NADESs as environmentally friendly alternatives to organic solvents. Four formulations, all citric acid-based with β-alanine, glucose, xylitol, or proline, were studied at water contents between 20% and 60%. Results indicated that flavonoid aglycones were extracted 2–6 times more effectively with NADESs than with aqueous methanol, while glycosides exhibited a more modest improvement (1.5–1.8-fold). Notably, aglycones, despite being less hydrophilic than their glycosylated counterparts, were more efficiently extracted, underscoring the selective extraction capabilities of NADESs.

In comparison with conventional organic solvents like ethanol and methanol, DESs offer several notable advantages, including lower toxicity, greater biodegradability, and tunable physicochemical properties. In contrast to certain ionic liquids, DESs are frequently composed of naturally derived, non-toxic components, making them more environmentally acceptable. Nonetheless, their high viscosity remains a key limitation, often impeding mass transfer during extraction processes. This issue can be alleviated by incorporating controlled amounts of water or by applying assisted techniques such as ultrasound, which enhances mass transfer and extraction kinetics.

Over the last 20 years, DESs have become a central topic in green chemistry owing to their exceptional versatility, sustainability, and the nearly limitless possibilities for combining hydrogen bond donors (HBDs) and acceptors (HBAs) in their synthesis. These tunable and modular systems offer several advantages over conventional ionic liquids, including lower toxicity, enhanced biodegradability, ease of preparation, and lower cost.

DESs have shown outstanding performance in a variety of industrial and scientific applications. In ionothermal synthesis, DESs function not only as solvents but also as structure-directing agents, facilitating the formation of novel porous and crystalline materials. In environmental applications, they help reduce reliance on volatile organic compounds, thereby mitigating environmental and health-related risks.

In the pharmaceutical field, DESs have shown substantial promise both as drug delivery systems and, in some cases, as active pharmaceutical ingredients themselves. The ability of these systems to increase solubility, stability, and bioavailability in poorly soluble drugs has established them as effective carriers for better pharmacokinetic performance. Furthermore, their role as dual-function solvents and co-catalysts, combined with recyclability, supports the development of more sustainable and efficient industrial processes.

Looking ahead, continued innovation in DESs is anticipated to impact a range of emerging areas, including biomass conversion, medicinal chemistry, and optoelectronics. Notably, the extension of the eutectic concept to include electronic and photonic properties, such as modulation of band gaps, opens new opportunities for the design of DESs with application-specific functionalities. To fully realize this potential, further molecular-level studies are needed to deepen the understanding of intermolecular interactions and enable precise, task-specific DES design (Mannu et al. 2021).

8 Conclusions

The adoption of green technologies in phytochemical research represents a pivotal move toward sustainable and environmentally conscious practices in the extraction and utilization of natural products. Phytochemicals, plant-derived bioactive compounds, have attracted considerable attention due to their therapeutic properties and diverse applications in pharmaceuticals, nutraceuticals, and cosmetics. Conventional extraction techniques frequently rely on toxic solvents and energy-intensive processes, raising environmental and safety concerns. Green extraction methods seek to overcome these challenges by using eco-friendly solvents, lowering energy consumption, and reducing waste production.

Recent developments in green extraction methods, including MAE, PEF, SFE, PLE, and UAE, have shown improved efficiency and selectivity in isolating phytochemicals. These approaches not only enhance extraction yields but also maintain the structural integrity and bioactivity of the compounds. In addition, the use of green solvents, such as bio-based solvents, pharmaceutical excipients, ILs, and DESs, has further promoted the sustainability of extraction processes. These solvents are characterized by low toxicity, biodegradability, and renewability, in line with green chemistry principles.

Despite these advancements, several challenges persist in the widespread implementation of green technologies for phytochemical extraction. Standardization and reproducibility remain critical issues, as variations in extraction protocols can lead to inconsistent results. Enhancing the selectivity of green extraction methods to target specific phytochemicals without co-extracting unwanted compounds is another area requiring attention. Additionally, scaling up these techniques from laboratory to industrial levels poses technical and economic hurdles that need to be addressed through interdisciplinary collaboration and innovation.

Future applications of advanced tools like AI and ML are expected to optimize extraction conditions and forecast outcomes, improving both the efficiency and consistency of processes. The development of modular and versatile extraction systems can facilitate scalability and adaptability across different applications. Moreover, encouraging dialogue between scientists, industry representatives, and policymakers is essential to create regulatory guidelines and standards that support the adoption of sustainable extraction methods. Such collaborative efforts will ensure that the benefits of phytochemicals are harnessed in a manner that is both effective and environmentally sustainable.

In summary, green technology in phytochemical research is expected to experience substantial growth in the coming years, driven by the imperative for sustainable practices and the potential health benefits of plant-derived compounds. Continued research and innovation are vital to overcome existing challenges and to fully realize the advantages of green extraction methods. By embracing environmentally friendly technologies and fostering interdisciplinary collaboration, the field can advance towards more sustainable and responsible utilization of phytochemicals.

References

Aili Q, Cui D, Li Y, Zhige W, Yongping W, Minfen Y, Dongbin L, Xiao R, Qiang W (2024) Composing functional food from agro-forest wastes: selectively extracting bioactive compounds using supercritical fluid extraction. Food Chem 455:139848. https://doi.org/10.1016/j.foodchem.2024.139848

Ajayi SA, Oluwaseun OO, Tunbosun OO, Nneka DA, Folashade GO (2024) Sustainable sourcing of organic skincare ingredients: a critical analysis of ethical concerns and environmental implications. Asian J Adv Res Reports 18(1):65–91. https://doi.org/10.9734/ajarr/2024/v18i1598

Alide T, Wangila P, Kiprop A (2020) Effect of cooking temperature and time on total phenolic content, total flavonoid content and total in vitro antioxidant activity of garlic. BMC Res Notes 13:564. https://doi.org/10.1186/s13104-020-05404-8

Allcca-Alca EE, León-Calvo NC, Luque-Vilca OM, Martínez-Cifuentes M, Pérez-Correa JR, Mariotti-Celis MS, Huamán-Castilla NL (2021) Hot pressurized liquid extraction of polyphenols from the skin and seeds of *Vitis vinifera* L. cv. Negra Criolla Pomace a Peruvian native pisco industry waste. Agronomy 11(5):866. https://doi.org/10.3390/agronomy11050866

Alum EU (2025) Role of phytochemicals in cardiovascular disease management: insights into mechanisms, efficacy, and clinical application. Phytomed Plus 5(1):100695. https://doi.org/10.1016/j.phyplu.2024.100695

Amulya PR, Ul Islam R (2023) Optimization of enzyme-assisted extraction of anthocyanins from eggplant (*Solanum melongena L.*) peel. Food Chem X 18:100643. https://doi.org/10.1016/j.fochx.2023.100643

Anastas PT, Warner JC (1998) Green chemistry: theory and practice. Oxford University Press, New York, p 30. https://www.acs.org/green-chemistry-sustainability/principles/12-principles-of-green-chemistry.html

Andrade AC, Borsoi FT, Saliba ASMC, de Alencar SM, Pastore GM, Arruda HS (2024) Optimization of ultrasonic-assisted extraction of phenolic compounds and antioxidant activity from Araticum peel using response surface methodology. Plants 13(18):2560. https://doi.org/10.3390/plants13182560

Andriana Y, Abdurrahman MF, Haryanti P, Pangestuti R, Kurnianto D, Sefrienda AR, Apriyati E, Wungkana J, Indriati A, Litaay C (2025) Optimization of ultrasonic-assisted extraction (UAE) for phenolics and antioxidant activity from cocoa (*Theobroma cacao*) leaves and phytochemical profiling using GC-MS and LC-HRMS. Biocatal Agric Biotechnol 65:103557. https://doi.org/10.1016/j.bcab.2025.103557

APEC (2022) Understanding the Bio-Circular-Green (BCG) Economy Model. Asia-Pacific Economic Cooperation, SOM Steering Committee on Economic and Technical Cooperation: Singapore. https://www.apec.org/publications/2022/08/understanding-the-bio-circular-green-(bcg)-economy-model. Accessed 2 May 2025

Appiah-Kubi E, Koranteng FO, Dura CC, Mihăilă AA, Drigă I, Preda A (2024) Green financing and sustainability reporting among SMEs: the role of pro-environmental behavior and digitization. J Clean Prod 478:143939. https://doi.org/10.1016/j.jclepro.2024.143939

Arruda HS, Silva EK, Peixoto Araujo NM, Pereira GA, Pastore GM, Marostica Junior MR (2021) Anthocyanins recovered from agri-food by-products using innovative processes: trends, challenges, and perspectives for their application in food systems. Molecules 26(9):2632. https://doi.org/10.3390/molecules26092632

Arshad RN, Abdul-Malek Z, Munir A, Buntat Z, Ahmad MH, Jusoh YMM, Bekhit AE, Roobab U, Manzoor MF, Aadil RM (2020) Electrical systems for pulsed electric field applications in the food industry: an engineering perspective. Trends Food Sci Technol 104:1–13. https://doi.org/10.1016/j.tifs.2020.07.008

Arumugham T, Rambabu K, Hasan SW, Show PL, Rinklebe J, Banat F (2021) Supercritical carbon dioxide extraction of plant phytochemicals for biological and environmental applications - a review. Chemosphere 271:129525. https://doi.org/10.1016/j.chemosphere.2020.129525

Athanasiadis V, Chatzimitakos T, Kotsou K, Kalompatsios D, Bozinou E, Lalas SI (2023) Polyphenol extraction from food (by) products by pulsed electric field: a review. Int J Mol Sci 24(21):15914. https://doi.org/10.3390/ijms242115914

Awad AM, Kumar P, Ismail-Fitry MR, Jusoh S, Ab Aziz MF, Sazili AQ (2021) Green extraction of bioactive compounds from plant biomass and their application in meat as natural antioxidant. Antioxidants (Basel) 10(9):1465. https://doi.org/10.3390/antiox10091465

Bagade SB, Patil M (2021) Recent advances in microwave assisted extraction of bioactive compounds from complex herbal samples: a review. Crit Rev Anal Chem 51(2):138–149. https://doi.org/10.1080/10408347.2019.1686966

Baixinho JP, Cardeira M, Bento-Silva A, Partidário AMC, Serra AT, Bronze MDR, Fernández N (2025) Optimization of supercritical fluid extraction for the recovery of γ-oryzanol-rich extracts with improved bioactivity from rice bran. Antioxidants (Basel) 14(2):206. https://doi.org/10.3390/antiox14020206

Balkrishna A, Sharma N, Srivastava D, Kukreti A, Srivastava S, Arya V (2024) Exploring the safety, efficacy, and bioactivity of herbal medicines: bridging traditional wisdom and modern science in healthcare. Future Integr Med 3(1):35–49. https://doi.org/10.14218/FIM.2023.00086

Bazmi RR, Panichayupakaranant P (2022) Synergistic interactions between artocarpin-rich extract, lawsone methyl ether and ampicillin on anti-MRSA and their antibiofilm formation. Lett Appl Microbiol 74:777–786

Bazmi RR, Asif M, Yaseen HS, Panichayupakaranant P (2022) Comparison of anti-inflammatory and analgesic effects of artocarpin-rich *Artocarpus heterophyllus* extract and artocarpin. J Angiother 6:V601–V611

Bhadange YA, Carpenter J, Saharan VK (2024) A comprehensive review on advanced extraction techniques for retrieving bioactive components from natural sources. ACS Omega 9(29):31274–31297. https://doi.org/10.1021/acsomega.4c02718

Bitwell C, Sen IS, Luke C, Kakoma M (2023) A review of modern and conventional extraction techniques and their applications for extracting phytochemicals from plants. Sci Afr 19:e01585. https://doi.org/10.1016/j.sciaf.2023.e01585

Bocker R, Silva EK (2022) Pulsed electric field assisted extraction of natural food pigments and colorings from plant matrices. Food Chem 15:100398. https://doi.org/10.1016/j.fochx.2022.100398

Bommakanti V, Puthenparambil Ajikumar A, Sivi CM, Prakash G, Mundanat AS, Ahmad F, Haque S, Prieto MA, Rana SS (2023) An overview of herbal nutraceuticals, their extraction, formulation, therapeutic effects and potential toxicity. Separations 10(3):177. https://doi.org/10.3390/separations10030177

Bouizgma K, Rabbah N, Abbas Z, Abourriche A (2025) Unlocking sustainable extraction of natural antioxidants: green solvents, smart technologies, scalability and future directions. Sep Sci Technol 60(6):657–683. https://doi.org/10.1080/01496395.2025.2452411

Bundeesomchok K, Filly A, Rakotomanomana N, Panichayupakaranant P, Chemat F (2016) Extraction of α-mangostin from *Garcinia mangostana* L. using alternative solvents: computational predictive and experimental studies. LWT 65:297–303. https://doi.org/10.1016/j.lwt.2015.08.036
Burdock GA, Carabin IG (2004) Generally recognized as safe (GRAS): history and description. Toxicol Lett 150(1):3–18. https://doi.org/10.1016/j.toxlet.2003.07.004
Cam LNT (2023) A rising trend in eco-friendly products: A health-conscious approach to green buying. Heliyon 9(9):e19845. https://doi.org/10.1016/j.heliyon.2023.e19845
Cannavacciuolo C, Pagliari S, Celano R, Campone L, Rastrelli L (2024) Critical analysis of green extraction techniques used for botanicals: trends, priorities, and optimization strategies-A review. TrAC Trends Anal Chem 173:117627. https://doi.org/10.1016/j.trac.2024.117627
Cao S, Liang J, Chen M, Xu C, Wang X, Qiu L, Zhao X, Hu W (2025) Comparative analysis of extraction technologies for plant extracts and absolutes. Front Chem 13:1536590. https://doi.org/10.3389/fchem.2025.1536590
Cegledi E, Repajić M, Balbino S, Peričić M, Dragović-Uzelac V (2023) Sterols and pentacyclic triterpenoids from nettle root: content and composition as affected by pressurized liquid extraction. J Sci Food Agric 103(8):4058–4067. https://doi.org/10.1002/jsfa.12373
Chaachouay N, Zidane L (2024) Plant-derived natural products: A source for drug discovery and development. Drugs Drug Cand 3(1):184–207. https://doi.org/10.3390/ddc3010011
Chatzimitakos T, Athanasiadis V, Kalompatsios D, Mantiniotou M, Bozinou E, Lalas SI (2023) Pulsed electric field applications for the extraction of bioactive compounds from food waste and by-products: a critical review. Biomass 3(4):367–401. https://doi.org/10.3390/biomass3040022
Chatzimitakos T, Athanasiadis V, Kotsou K, Mantiniotou M, Kalompatsios D, Makrygiannis I, Bozinou E, Lalas SI (2024) Optimization of pressurized liquid extraction (PLE) parameters for extraction of bioactive compounds from *Moringa oleifera* leaves and bioactivity assessment. Int J Mol Sci 25(9):4628. https://doi.org/10.3390/ijms25094628
Chemat F, Vian MA, Cravotto G (2012) Green extraction of natural products: concept and principles. Int J Mol Sci 13(7):8615–8627. https://doi.org/10.3390/ijms13078615
Chemat F, Rombaut N, Sicaire AG, Meullemiestre A, Fabiano-Tixier AS, Abert-Vian M (2017) Ultrasound assisted extraction of food and natural products. Mechanisms, techniques, combinations, protocols and applications. A review. Ultrason Sonochem 34:540–560. https://doi.org/10.1016/j.ultsonch.2016.06.035
Chemat F, Abert Vian M, Ravi HK, Khadhraoui B, Hilali S, Perino S, Tixier AF (2019a) Review of alternative solvents for green extraction of food and natural products: panorama, principles, applications and prospects. Molecules 24(16):3007. https://doi.org/10.3390/molecules24163007
Chemat F, Abert-Vian M, Fabiano-Tixier AS, Strube J, Uhlenbrock L, Gunjevic V, Cravotto G (2019b) Green extraction of natural products. Origins, current status, and future challenges. TrAC Trends Anal Chem 118:248–263. https://doi.org/10.1016/j.trac.2019.05.037
Chemat F, Vian MA, Fabiano-Tixier A-S, Nutrizio M, Jambrak AR, Munekata P, Lorenzo J, Barba F, Binello A, Cravotto G (2020) A review of sustainable and intensified techniques for extraction of food and natural products. Green Chem 22(8):2325–2353
Choudhari AS, Mandave PC, Deshpande M, Ranjekar P, Prakash O (2020) Phytochemicals in cancer treatment: from preclinical studies to clinical practice. Front Pharmacol 11:175. https://doi.org/10.3389/fphar.2020.00175
Chu Q, Xie S, Wei H, Tian X, Tang Z, Li D, Liu Y (2024) Enzyme-assisted ultrasonic extraction of total flavonoids and extraction polysaccharides in residue from *Abelmoschus manihot* (L). Ultrason Sonochem 104:106815. https://doi.org/10.1016/j.ultsonch.2024.106815
Chumanee S, Thunta J, Khoomsab R, Winyakul C (2024) Optimizing ultrasound-assisted extraction for enhanced quantification of 7-hydroxymitragynine and mitragynine in kratom. Creat Sci 17(1):258707. https://doi.org/10.55674/cs.v17i1.258707
Couceiro B, Hameed H, Vieira ACF, Singh SK, Dua K, Veiga F, Pires PC, Ferreira L, Paiva-Santos AC (2025) Promoting health and sustainability: exploring safer alternatives in cosmet-

ics and regulatory perspectives. Sustain Chem Pharm 43:101901. https://doi.org/10.1016/j.scp.2024.101901

da Cunha Rodrigues L, Bodini RB, Caneppele FL, Dacanal GC, Crevelin EJ, de Moraes LAB, de Oliveira AL (2023) Pressurized liquid extraction (PLE) in an intermittent process as an alternative for obtaining passion fruit (*Passiflora edulis*) leaf hydroalcoholic extract (Tincture). Processes 11(8):2308. https://doi.org/10.3390/pr11082308

Darwin R, Valmon S, Chithanna SH, Galla SH, Syed SH, Billah AAM, Reddy KTK, Arjun UVNV (2025) Sustainable extraction and purification of phytochemicals: A review of green solvents and techniques. Chem Method 9(5):356–385. https://doi.org/10.48309/CHEMM.2025.504050.1892

de María PD, Guajardo N, González-Sabín J (2022) Recent granted patents related to deep eutectic solvents. Curr Opin Green Sustain Chem 38:100712. https://doi.org/10.1016/j.cogsc.2022.100712

Didion YP, Tjalsma TG, Su Z, Malankowska M, Pinelo M (2023) What is next? The greener future of solid liquid extraction of biobased compounds: novel techniques and solvents overpower traditional ones. Sep Purif Technol 320:124147. https://doi.org/10.1016/j.seppur.2023.124147

Dobroslavić E, Elez Garofulić I, Šeparović J, Zorić Z, Pedisić S, Dragović-Uzelac V (2022) Pressurized liquid extraction as a novel technique for the isolation of *Laurus nobilis* L. Leaf Polyphenols. Molecules 27(16):5099. https://doi.org/10.3390/molecules27165099

dos Santos LC, Grisales-Mejía JF, Strieder MM, Mendiola JA, Ibáñez E (2025) Innovative sample preparation techniques in Food Analysis: the rise of Compressed Fluids and Novel Solvents. Adv Sample Prepar:100191. https://doi.org/10.1016/j.sampre.2025.100191

Drannikov AA, Trusova ME, Martino AD (2024) Reviewing twenty years of patents on ultrasonic-assisted pectin extraction from food and food waste. Chimica Techno Acta 11(2):202411213

Drouet S, Leclerc EA, Garros L, Tungmunnithum D, Kabra A, Abbasi BH, Lainé É, Hano C (2019) A green ultrasound-assisted extraction optimization of the natural antioxidant and anti-aging flavonolignans from milk thistle *Silybum marianum* (L.) Gaertn. fruits for cosmetic applications. Antioxidants (Basel) 8(8):304. https://doi.org/10.3390/antiox8080304

Edyvean RGJ, Apiwatanapiwat W, Vaithanomsat P, Boondaeng A, Janchai P, Sophonthammaphat S (2023) The bio-circular green economy model in Thailand - a comparative review. Agric Nat Resour 57(1):51–64

Fahad S, Alnori F, Su F, Deng J (2022) Adoption of green innovation practices in SMEs sector: evidence from an emerging economy. Econ Res 35(1):5486–5501. https://doi.org/10.1080/1331677X.2022.2029713

Ferreira C, Sarraguça M (2024) A comprehensive review on deep eutectic solvents and its use to extract bioactive compounds of pharmaceutical interest. Pharmaceuticals 17(1):124. https://doi.org/10.3390/ph17010124

Flieger J, Flieger M (2020) Ionic liquids toxicity-benefits and threats. Int J Mol Sci 21(17):6267. https://doi.org/10.3390/ijms21176267

Forni C, Facchiano F, Bartoli M, Pieretti S, Facchiano A, D'Arcangelo D, Norelli S, Valle G, Nisini R, Beninati S, Tabolacci C, Jadeja RN (2019) Beneficial role of phytochemicals on oxidative stress and age-related diseases. Biomed Res Int 2019:8748253. https://doi.org/10.1155/2019/8748253

Gil-Martín E, Forbes-Hernández T, Romero A, Cianciosi D, Giampieri F, Battino M (2022) Influence of the extraction method on the recovery of bioactive phenolic compounds from food industry by-products. Food Chem 378:131918. https://doi.org/10.1016/j.foodchem.2021.131918

Gómez-Urios C, Viñas-Ospino A, Puchades-Colera P, Blesa J, López-Malo D, Frígola A, Esteve MJ (2023) Choline chloride-based natural deep eutectic solvents for the extraction and stability of phenolic compounds, ascorbic acid, and antioxidant capacity from Citrus sinensis peel. LWT 177:114595. https://doi.org/10.1016/j.lwt.2023.114595

Gouda M, El-Din Bekhit A, Tang Y, Huang Y, Huang L, He Y, Li X (2021) Recent innovations of ultrasound green technology in herbal phytochemistry: a review. Ultrason Sonochem 73:105538. https://doi.org/10.1016/j.ultsonch.2021.105538

Gucciardi G (2024) Do venture capital investments contribute to the achievement of the sustainable development goals? Bus Strateg Environ 33(8):8716–8746. https://doi.org/10.1002/bse.3942

Gundom T, Amnuaikit T, Panichayupakaranant P (2024) Formulation of gel containing phenylbutenoid extract for pain relief. J Health Sci Med Res 42(1):e2023986. https://doi.org/10.31584/jhsmr.2023986

Gundom T, Sukketsiri W, Panichayupakaranant P (2025) Phytochemical analysis and biological effects of *Zingiber cassumunar* extract and three phenylbutenoids: targeting NF-κB, Akt/MAPK, and caspase-3 pathways. BMC Complement Med Ther 25:180. https://doi.org/10.1186/s12906-025-04907-w

Hao J, Wang Z, Jia Y, Sun L, Fu Z, Zhao M, Li Y, Yuan N, Cong B, Zhao L, Ge G (2023) Optimization of ultrasonic-assisted extraction of flavonoids from *Lactuca indica* L. cv. Mengzao and their antioxidant properties. Frontiers. Nutrition 10:1065662. https://doi.org/10.3389/fnut.2023.1065662

Hefied F, Ahmed ZB, Yousfi M (2023) Optimization of ultrasonic-assisted extraction of phenolic compounds and antioxidant activities from *Pistacia atlantica* Desf. galls using response surface methodology. J Appl Res Med Arom Plants 32:100449. https://doi.org/10.1016/j.jarmap.2022.100449

Hereu-Morales J, Segarra A, Valderrama C (2024) The European (Green?) Deal: a systematic analysis of environmental sustainability. Sustain Dev 32(1):647–661. https://doi.org/10.1002/sd.2671

Herzyk F, Piłakowska-Pietras D, Korzeniowska M (2024) Supercritical extraction techniques for obtaining biologically active substances from a variety of plant byproducts. Foods. 13(11):1713. https://doi.org/10.3390/foods13111713

Hikmawanti NPE, Ramadon D, Jantan I, Mun'im A (2021) Natural deep eutectic solvents (nades): phytochemical extraction performance enhancer for pharmaceutical and nutraceutical product development. Plants (Basel) 10(10):2091. https://doi.org/10.3390/plants10102091

Hikmawanti NPE, Saputri FC, Yanuar A, Jantan I, Ningrum RA, Juanssilfero AB, Mun'im A (2024) Choline chloride-urea-based natural deep eutectic solvent for highly efficient extraction of polyphenolic antioxidants from *Pluchea indica* (L.) less leaves. Arab J Chem 17(2):105537. https://doi.org/10.1016/j.arabjc.2023.105537

Hiranpradith V, Therdthai N, Soontrunnarudrungsri A, Rungsuriyawiboon O (2025) Optimisation of ultrasound-assisted extraction of total phenolics and flavonoids content from *Centella asiatica*. Foods 14(2):291. https://doi.org/10.3390/foods14020291

Hirondart M, Rombaut N, Fabiano-Tixier AS, Bily A, Chemat F (2020) Comparison between pressurized liquid extraction and conventional Soxhlet extraction for rosemary antioxidants, yield, composition, and environmental footprint. Foods 9(5):584. https://doi.org/10.3390/foods9050584

Huamán-Castilla NL, Gajardo-Parra N, Pérez-Correa JR, Canales RI, Martínez-Cifuentes M, Contreras-Contreras G, Mariotti-Celis MS (2023) Enhanced polyphenols recovery from grape pomace: a comparison of pressurized and atmospheric extractions with deep eutectic solvent aqueous mixtures. Antioxidants 12(7):1446. https://doi.org/10.3390/antiox12071446

Huang L, Solangi YA, Magazzino C, Solangi SA (2024) Evaluating the efficiency of green innovation and marketing strategies for long-term sustainability in the context of environmental labeling. J Clean Prod 450:141870. https://doi.org/10.1016/j.jclepro.2024.141870

ICH (2021) Impurities: Guideline for residual solvents Q3C(R8). International council for harmonisation of technical requirements for pharmaceuticals for human use; April 22

Imamoglu E (2024) Green extraction processes from renewable biomass to sustainable bioproducts. Bioresour Technol Rep 27:101952. https://doi.org/10.1016/j.biteb.2024.101952

Irianto I, Naryaningsih A, Trisnawati NW, Astuti A, Komariyah K, Qomariyah L, Chaidir C, Saputri A, Wulandari R, Rizkiyah DN, Putra NR (2024) From sea to solution: A review of green extraction approaches for unlocking the potential of brown algae. South Afr J Chem Eng 48:1–21. https://doi.org/10.1016/j.sajce.2024.01.001

Irianto I, Putra NR, Yustisia Y, Abdullah S, Syafruddin S, Paesal P, Irmadamayanti A, Herawati H, Raharjo B, Agustini S, Asmaliyah A, Krismawati A, Airlangga B (2025) Green technologies in food colorant extraction: a comprehensive review. South Afr J Chem Eng 51:22–34. https://doi.org/10.1016/j.sajce.2024.10.013

Jintawiwat R, Punamorntarakul N, Hirunyasiri R, Jarupoom P, Pankasemsuk T, Supasin S, Kawee-ai A (2023) Testing the efficacy of a prototype that combines ultrasound and pulsed electric field for extracting valuable compounds from *Mitragyna speciosa* leaves. AgriEngineering 5(4):1879–1892. https://doi.org/10.3390/agriengineering5040115

Kamjam M, Ngamprasertsith S, Sawangkeaw R, Charoenchaitrakool M, Privat R, Jaubert J-N, Molière M (2024) The great versatility of supercritical fluids in industrial processes: A focus on chemical, agri-food and energy applications. Processes 12(11):2402. https://doi.org/10.3390/pr12112402

Kaoui S, Chebli B, Zaidouni S, Basaid K, Mir Y (2023) Deep eutectic solvents as sustainable extraction media for plants and food samples: a review. Sustain Chem Pharm 31:100937. https://doi.org/10.1016/j.scp.2022.100937

Khameneh B, Eskin NAM, Iranshahy M, Fazly Bazzaz BS (2021) Phytochemicals: A promising weapon in the arsenal against antibiotic-resistant bacteria. Antibiotics (Basel) 10(9):1044. https://doi.org/10.3390/antibiotics10091044

Kim KC, Kim JH, Kim JS, Lee DS (2025) Optimization of ultrasonic-assisted extraction of anthocyanins from *Prunus yedoensis* fruit and evaluation of antioxidant and anti-inflammatory activity. Food Sci Biotechnol 34:2039–2049. https://doi.org/10.1007/s10068-025-01843-w

Kumar K, Srivastav S, Sharanagat VS (2021) Ultrasound assisted extraction (UAE) of bioactive compounds from fruit and vegetable processing by-products: a review. Ultrason Sonochem 70:105325. https://doi.org/10.1016/j.ultsonch.2020.105325

Kumar A, Kumar M, Jose A, Tomer V, Oz E, Proestos C, Zeng M, Elobeid T, Oz F (2023) Major phytochemicals: recent advances in health benefits and extraction method. Molecules 28(2):887. https://doi.org/10.3390/molecules28020887

Lateh L, Yuenyongsawad S, Chen H, Panichayupakaranant P (2019) A green method for preparation of curcuminoid-rich *Curcuma longa* extract and evaluation of its anticancer activity. Pharmacogn Mag 15:730–735. https://doi.org/10.4103/pm.pm_162_19

Lateh L, Kaewnopparat N, Yuenyongsawad S, Panichayupakaranant P (2022) Enhancing the water-solubility of curcuminoids-rich extract using a ternary inclusion complex system: preparation, characterization, and anti-cancer activity. Food Chem 368:130827. https://doi.org/10.1016/j.foodchem.2021.130827

Li M, Rao C, Ye X, Wang M, Yang B, Wang C, Guo L, Xiong Y, Cui X (2023) Applications for natural deep eutectic solvents in Chinese herbal medicines. Front Pharmacol 13:1104096. https://doi.org/10.3389/fphar.2022.1104096

Li W, Zhang Y, Wei Y, Sun J, Zhao X, Xie J (2025) Ultrasound-assisted extraction and antioxidant activity of triterpenoid saponins from *Platycodon grandiflorum* roots: optimization, purification, and molecular insights. Ind Crop Prod 223:119877. https://doi.org/10.1016/j.indcrop.2024.119877

Llompart M, Celeiro M, Dagnac T (2019) Microwave-assisted extraction of pharmaceuticals, personal care products and industrial contaminants in the environment. TrAC Trends Anal Chem 116:136–150. https://doi.org/10.1016/j.trac.2019.04.029

Lopes JM, Gomes S, Trancoso T (2024) Navigating the green maze: insights for businesses on consumer decision-making and the mediating role of their environmental concerns. Sustain Account Manage Policy J 15(4):861–883

López-Salazar H, Camacho-Díaz BH, Arenas Ocampo ML, Jiménez-Aparicio AR (2023) Microwave-assisted extraction of functional compounds from plants: a review. Bioresources 18(3):6614–6638. https://ojs.bioresources.com/index.php/BRJ/article/view/22613

Lubek-Nguyen A, Ziemichód W, Olech M (2022) Application of enzyme-assisted extraction for the recovery of natural bioactive compounds for nutraceutical and pharmaceutical applications. Appl Sci 12(7):3232. https://doi.org/10.3390/app12073232

Majeed MU, Aslam S, Murtaza SA, Attila S, Molnár E (2022) Green marketing approaches and their impact on green purchase intentions: mediating role of green brand image and consumer beliefs towards the environment. Sustainability 14(18):11703. https://doi.org/10.3390/su141811703

Majrashi TA, Alshehri SA, Alsayari A, Muhsinah AB, Alrouji M, Alshahrani AM, Shamsi A, Atiya A (2023) Insight into the biological roles and mechanisms of phytochemicals in different types of cancer: targeting cancer therapeutics. Nutrients 15(7):1704. https://doi.org/10.3390/nu15071704

Mannu A, Blangetti M, Baldino S, Prandi C (2021) Promising technological and industrial applications of deep eutectic systems. Materials 14(10):2494. https://doi.org/10.3390/ma14102494

Martins AM, Marto JM (2023) A sustainable life cycle for cosmetics: from design and development to post-use phase. Sustain Chem Pharm 35:101178. https://doi.org/10.1016/j.scp.2023.101178

Martins R, Barbosa A, Advinha B, Sales H, Pontes R, Nunes J (2023) Green extraction techniques of bioactive compounds: a state-of-the-art review. PRO 11(8):2255. https://doi.org/10.3390/pr11082255

Meah MS, Panichayupakaranant P (2020) A-Mangostin-rich extract: A potential oral antibacterial agent prepared by green extraction. Int J Pharmacogn Chin Med 4:000201. https://doi.org/10.23880/ipcm-16000201

Mikšovsky P, Kornpointner C, Parandeh Z, Goessinger M, Bica-Schröder K, Halbwirth H (2024) Enzyme-assisted supercritical fluid extraction of flavonoids from apple pomace (Malus×domestica). ChemSusChem 17(7):e202301094. https://doi.org/10.1002/cssc.202301094

Mungwari CP, King'ondu CK, Sigauke P, Obadele BA (2025) Conventional and modern techniques for bioactive compounds recovery from plants: review. Sci Afr 27:e02509. https://doi.org/10.1016/j.sciaf.2024.e02509

Naliyadhara N, Kumar A, Girisa S, Daimary UD, Hegde M, Kunnumakkara AB (2022) Pulsed electric field (PEF): Avant-Garde extraction escalation technology in food industry. Trends Food Sci Technol 122:238–255. https://doi.org/10.1016/j.tifs.2022.02.019

Nameroff TJ, Garant RJ, Albert MB (2004) Adoption of green chemistry: an analysis based on US patents. Res Policy 33(6–7):959–974. https://doi.org/10.1016/j.respol.2004.03.001

Nguyen L, Govindasamy R, Mentreddy SR (2024) Turmeric trends: analyzing consumer preferences and willingness to pay. Front Sustain Food Syst 8:1359040. https://doi.org/10.3389/fsufs.2024.1359040

Nisar A, Jagtap S, Vyavahare S, Deshpande M, Harsulkar A, Ranjekar P, Prakash O (2023) Phytochemicals in the treatment of inflammation-associated diseases: the journey from preclinical trials to clinical practice. Front Pharmacol 14:1177050. https://doi.org/10.3389/fphar.2023.1177050

Okiyama DCG, Soares ID, Cuevas MS, Crevelin EJ, Moraes LAB, Melo MP, Oliveira AL, Rodrigues CEC (2018) Pressurized liquid extraction of flavanols and alkaloids from cocoa bean shell using ethanol as solvent. Food Res Int 114:20–29. https://doi.org/10.1016/j.foodres.2018.07.055

Oomen WW, Begines P, Mustafa NR, Wilson EG, Verpoorte R, Choi YH (2020) Natural deep eutectic solvent extraction of flavonoids of *Scutellaria baicalensis* as a replacement for conventional organic solvents. Molecules 25(3):617. https://doi.org/10.3390/molecules25030617

Osorio-Tobón JF (2020) Recent advances and comparisons of conventional and alternative extraction techniques of phenolic compounds. J Food Sci Technol 57(12):4299–4315. https://doi.org/10.1007/s13197-020-04433-2

Palmisano GO, Rocchi L, Negri L, Piscitelli L (2025) Evaluating the progress of the EU countries towards implementation of the European Green Deal: a multiple criteria approach. Land 14(1):141. https://doi.org/10.3390/land14010141

Palos-Hernández A, González-Paramás AM, Santos-Buelga C (2025) Latest advances in green extraction of polyphenols from plants, foods and food by-products. Molecules 30(1):55. https://doi.org/10.3390/molecules30010055

Panda S, Gorantla S (2025) Green analytical approaches and eco-friendly solvents: advancing industrial applications and environmental sustainability: a comprehensive review. 41(2):616–627. https://doi.org/10.13005/ojc/410231

Panichayupakaranant P (2023) Pharmaceutical excipients as alternative solvents for green microwave extraction of herbs. J CAM Res Progr 2(1):111. https://doi.org/10.33790/jcrp1100111

Panichayupakaranant P (2024) Development of natural product innovation based on the bio-circular- green (BCG) economy model. J Nutraceut Health 2(1):3–5

Panichayupakaranant P, Bundeesomchok K (2015) Preparation of a mangosteen fruit pericarp extract containing α-mangostin made into a formulation of a gel and cream for treating oral mucositis. Brussels Expo 2015, November 19–21, Brussels

Pappas VM, Palaiogiannis D, Athanasiadis V, Chatzimitakos T, Bozinou E, Makris DP, Lalas SI (2022) Optimization of pulsed electric-field-based total polyphenols' extraction from *Elaeagnus pungens* 'Limelight' leaves using hydroethanolic mixtures. Oxygen 2(4):537–546. https://doi.org/10.3390/oxygen2040035

Pathak A, Gupta AP, Pandey P (2024) Herbal medicine and sustainable development challenges and opportunities. In: Izah SC et al (eds) Herbal medicine phytochemistry, reference series in phytochemistry. Springer Nature, Cham. https://doi.org/10.1007/978-3-031-21973-3_48-11

Pengjam Y, Syazwani N, Inchai J, Numit A, Yodthong T, Pitakpornpreecha T, Panichayupakaranant P (2021) High water-soluble curcuminoids-rich extract regulates osteogenic differentiation of MC3T3-E1 cells: involvement of Wnt/β-catenin and BMP signaling pathway. Chin Herb Med 13:534540

Pereira AG, Cruz L, Cassani L, Chamorro F, Lourenço-Lopes C, Freitas V, Otero P, Fraga-Corral M, Prieto MA, Simal-Gandara J, Perez-Gregorio R (2023) Comparative study of microwave-assisted extraction and ultrasound-assisted extraction techniques (MAE vs. UAE) for the optimized production of enriched extracts in phenolic compounds of *Camellia japonica* var Eugenia de Montijo. Eng Proc 37(1):124. https://doi.org/10.3390/ECP2023-14615

Perez-Vazquez A, Carpena M, Barciela P, Cassani L, Simal-Gandara J, Prieto MA (2023) Pressurized liquid extraction for the recovery of bioactive compounds from seaweeds for food industry application: a review. Antioxidants (Basel) 12(3):612. https://doi.org/10.3390/antiox12030612

Perra M, Leyva-Jiménez FJ, Manca ML, Manconi M, Rajha HN, Borrás-Linares I, Segura-Carretero A, Lozano-Sánchez J (2023) Application of pressurized liquid extraction to grape by-products as a circular economy model to provide phenolic compounds enriched ingredient. J Clean Prod 402:136712. https://doi.org/10.1016/j.jclepro.2023.136712

Picot-Allain C, Mahomoodally MF, Ak G, Zengin G (2021) Conventional versus green extraction techniques - a comparative perspective. Curr Opin Food Sci 40:144–156. https://doi.org/10.1016/j.cofs.2021.02.009

Polo-Castellano C, Mateos RM, Visiedo F, Palma M, Barbero GF, Ferreiro-González M (2023) Optimizing an enzymatic extraction method for the flavonoids in moringa (*Moringa oleifera* Lam.) leaves based on experimental designs methodologies. Antioxidants (Basel) 12(2):369. https://doi.org/10.3390/antiox12020369

Promdam N, Panichayupakaranant P (2022) Quantitative HPLC method and alternative green solvents for extraction of [6]-gingerol from ginger. Pak J Pharm Sci 35(3):851–857

Promdam N, Khuituan P, Panichayupakaranant P (2022) Effects of standardized [6]-gingerol extracts and [6]-gingerol on isolated ileum and lower esophageal sphincter contractions in mice. Food Chem 378:132077. https://doi.org/10.1016/j.foodchem.2022.132077

Putra NR, Yustisia Y, Heryanto RB, Asmaliyah A, Miswarti M, Rizkiyah DN, Yunus MAC, Irianto I, Qomariyah L, Rohman GAN (2023) Advancements and challenges in green extraction techniques for Indonesian natural products: a review. South Afr J Chem Eng 46:88–98. https://doi.org/10.1016/j.sajce.2023.08.002

Puttarak P, Panichayupakaranant P (2013) A new method for preparing pentacyclic triterpene rich *Centella asiatica* extracts. Nat Prod Res 27(7):684–686. https://doi.org/10.1080/14786419.2012.686912

Puttarak P, Brantner A, Panichayupakaranant P (2016) Biological activities and stability of a standardized pentacyclic triterpene enriched *Centella asiatica* extract. Nat Prod Sci 22(1):20–24. https://doi.org/10.20307/nps.2016.22.1.20

Rahman AU, Khan NU, Panichayupakaranant P, Ni J (2025) A standardized chamuangone enriched extract shows anticancer efficacy in allograft models of metastatic breast cancer. J Funct Foods 127:106730

Ranjha MMAN, Kanwal R, Shafique B, Arshad RN, Irfan S, Kieliszek M, Kowalczewski PŁ, Irfan M, Khalid MZ, Roobab U, Aadil RM (2021) A critical review on pulsed electric field: a novel technology for the extraction of phytoconstituents. Molecules 26(16):4893. https://doi.org/10.3390/molecules26164893

Razgonova M, Zakharenko A, Shin T-S, Chung G, Golokhvast K (2020) Supercritical CO_2 extraction and identification of ginsenosides in Russian and North Korean ginseng by HPLC with tandem mass spectrometry. Molecules 25(6):1407. https://doi.org/10.3390/molecules25061407

Rocca R, Acerbi F, Fumagalli L, Taisch M (2022) Sustainability paradigm in the cosmetics industry: state of the art. Clean Waste Syst 3:100057. https://doi.org/10.1016/j.clwas.2022.100057

Roobab U, Aadil RM, Kurup SS, Maqsood S (2025) Comparative evaluation of ultrasound-assisted extraction with other green extraction methods for sustainable recycling and processing of date palm bioresources and by-products: a review of recent research. Ultrason Sonochem 114:107252. https://doi.org/10.1016/j.ultsonch.2025.107252

Sadeghi A, Hakimzadeh V, Karimifar B (2017) Microwave assisted extraction of bioactive compounds from food: a review. Int J Food Sci Nutr Eng 7(1):19–27. https://doi.org/10.5923/j.food.20170701.03

Sae-Lim P, Yuenyongsawad S, Panichayupakaranant P (2019) Chamuangone-enriched *Garcinia cowa* leaf extract with rice bran oil: extraction and cytotoxic activity against cancer cells. Pharmacogn Mag 15:183–188. https://doi.org/10.4103/pm.pm_472_18

Sae-Lim P, Seetaha S, Tabtimmai L, Suphakun P, Kiriwan D, Panichayupakaranant P, Choowongkomon K (2020) Chamuangone from *garcinia cowa* leaves inhibits cell proliferation and migration and induces cell apoptosis in human cervical cancer in vitro. J Pharm Pharmacol 72:470–480. https://doi.org/10.1111/jphp.13216

Salea R, Veriansyah B, Tjandrawinata RR (2017) Optimization and scale-up process for supercritical fluids extraction of ginger oil from *Zingiber officinale* var. Amarum. J Supercrit Fluids 120:285–294. https://doi.org/10.1016/j.supflu.2016.05.035

Samimi R, Xu WZ, Alsharari Q, Charpentier PA (2014) Supercritical fluid chromatography of North American ginseng extract. J Supercrit Fluids 86:115–123. https://doi.org/10.1016/j.supflu.2013.12.004

Sampaopan Y, Suksaeree J (2022) Microwave-assisted extraction and content determination of astilbin in *Lysiphyllum strychnifolium* stems. Brazil J Pharm Sci 58. https://doi.org/10.1590/s2175-97902022e20577

Sanou A, Konaté K, Kabakdé K, Dakuyo R, Bazié D, Hemayoro S, Dicko MH (2023) Modelling and optimisation of ultrasound-assisted extraction of roselle phenolic compounds using the surface response method. Sci Reports 13(1):358. https://doi.org/10.1038/s41598-023-27434-5

Santos TRJ, Santana LCLA (2022) Conventional and emerging techniques for extraction of bioactive compounds from fruit waste. Brazil J Food Technol 25:e2021130. https://doi.org/10.1590/1981-6723.13021

Santos DT, Angela A, Meireles M (2011) Extraction of volatile oils by supercritical fluid extraction: Patent survey. Rec Pat Eng 59(1):17–22. https://doi.org/10.2174/187221211105010017

Sharma M, Sridhar K, Gupta VK, Dikkala PK (2022) Greener technologies in agri-food wastes valorization for plant pigments: step towards circular economy. Curr Res Green Sustainable Chem 5:100340. https://doi.org/10.1016/j.crgsc.2022.100340

Shawky E, Zhu W, Tian J (2025) A review of innovative extraction technologies for protein recovery from plant-based by-products: a step toward zero-waste processing. Int J Biol Macromol 315:144301. https://doi.org/10.1016/j.ijbiomac.2025.144301

Shen L, Pang S, Zhong M, Sun Y, Qayum A, Liu Y, Rashid A, Xu B, Liang Q, Ma H, Ren X (2023) A comprehensive review of ultrasonic assisted extraction (UAE) for bioactive components: principles, advantages, equipment, and combined technologies. Ultrason Sonochem 101:106646. https://doi.org/10.1016/j.ultsonch.2023.106646

Sridhar A, Ponnuchamy M, Kumar PS, Kapoor A, Vo DN, Prabhakar S (2021) Techniques and modeling of polyphenol extraction from food: a review. Environ Chem Lett 19(4):3409–3443. https://doi.org/10.1007/s10311-021-01217-8

Stanisz M, Stanisz BJ, Cielecka-Piontek J (2024) A comprehensive review on deep eutectic solvents: their current status and potential for extracting active compounds from adaptogenic plants. Molecules 29(19):4767. https://doi.org/10.3390/molecules29194767

Streimikyte P, Viskelis P, Viskelis J (2022) Enzymes-assisted extraction of plants for sustainable and functional applications. Int J Mol Sci 23(4):2359. https://doi.org/10.3390/ijms23042359

Suksawat T, Panichayupakaranant P (2023) Variation of rhinacanthin content in *Rhinacanthus nasutus* and its health products. J Pharm Biomed Anal 224:115177. https://doi.org/10.1016/j.jpba.2022.115177

Suksawat T, Panichayupakaranant P (2024) Enhanced rhinacanthin production in *Rhinacanthus nasutus* roots using a hydroponics and elicitation system. J Young Pharm 16(2):216–222. https://doi.org/10.5530/jyp.2024.16.28

Supasatyankul B, Saisriyoot M, Klinkesorn U, Rattanaporn K, Sae-Tan S (2022) Extraction of phenolic and flavonoid compounds from mung bean (*Vigna radiata* L.) seed coat by pressurized liquid extraction. Molecules 27(7):2085. https://doi.org/10.3390/molecules27072085

Suttithumsatid W, Shah MA, Bibi S, Panichayupakaranant P (2022) α-Glucosidase inhibitory activity of cannabidiol, tetrahydrocannabinol and standardized cannabinoid extracts from *Cannabis sativa*. Curr Res Food Sci 5:1091–1097

Suttithumsatid W, Sukketsiri W, Panichayupakaranant P (2023) Cannabinoids and standardized cannabis extracts inhibit migration, invasion, and induce apoptosis in MCF-7 cells through FAK/MAPK/Akt/NF-κB signaling. Toxicol In Vitro 93:105667. https://doi.org/10.1016/j.tiv.2023.105667

Suttithumsatid W, Toriumi T, Sukketsiri W, Nagasaki Y, Panichayupakaranant P (2024) Enhanced stability of α-mangostin-rich extract and selective cytotoxicity against cancer cells via encapsulation in antioxidant nanoparticles (AME@NanoAOX). ACS Biomater Sci Eng J 10(8):5027–5038. https://doi.org/10.1021/acsbiomaterials.4c00997

Suttithumsatid W, Sukketsiri W, Panichayupakaranant P (2025) A green microwave-assisted extraction of *Cannabis sativa* L. extract and its cytotoxic activity against cancer cells. Turk J Pharm Sci 22(1):64–70. https://doi.org/10.4274/tjps.galenos.2025.33490

Takacs A (2023) The positive effects of green technology investments on growth expectations. Technol Soc 75:102407. https://doi.org/10.1016/j.techsoc.2023.102407

Tarafdar A, Sirohi R, Gaur VK, Kumar S, Sharma P, Varjani S, Pandey HO, Sindhu R, Madhavan A, Rajasekharan R, Sim SJ (2021) Engineering interventions in enzyme production: lab to industrial scale. Bioresour Technol 326:124771. https://doi.org/10.1016/j.biortech.2021.124771

Tizón Alba A, Aliaño-González MJ, Palma M, Fernández Barbero G, Carrera C (2023) Enhancing efficiency of enzymatic-assisted extraction method for evaluating bioactive compound analysis in mulberry: an optimization approach. Agronomy 13(10):2548. https://doi.org/10.3390/agronomy13102548

Tsevdou M, Ntzimani A, Katsouli M, Dimopoulos G, Tsimogiannis D, Taoukis P (2024) Comparative study of microwave, pulsed electric fields, and high pressure processing on the extraction of antioxidants from olive pomace. Molecules 29(10):2303. https://doi.org/10.3390/molecules29102303

United Nations (2015) Department of Economic and Social Affairs -Sustainable Development. https://sdgsunorg/goals. Accessed 2 May 2025

Usman M, Nakagawa M, Cheng S (2023) Emerging trends in green extraction techniques for bioactive natural products. Processes 11(12):3444. https://doi.org/10.3390/pr11123444

Uwineza PA, Waśkiewicz A (2020) Recent advances in supercritical fluid extraction of natural bioactive compounds from natural plant materials. Molecules 25(17):3847. https://doi.org/10.3390/molecules25173847

Valisakkagari H, Chaturvedi C, Rupasinghe HPV (2024) Green extraction of phytochemicals from fresh vegetable waste and their potential application as cosmeceuticals for skin health. Processes 12(4):742. https://doi.org/10.3390/pr12040742

Ventura SPM, E. Silva FA, Quental MV, Mondal D, Freire MG, Coutinho JAP (2017) Ionic-liquid-mediated extraction and separation processes for bioactive compounds: past, present, and future trends. Chem Rev 117(10):6984–7052. https://doi.org/10.1021/acs.chemrev.6b00550

Višnjevec AM, Barp L, Lucci P, Moret S (2024) Pressurized liquid extraction for the determination of bioactive compounds in plants with emphasis on phenolics. TrAC Trends Anal Chem 173:117620. https://doi.org/10.1016/j.trac.2024.117620

Wang Y, Zhao L, Zhang R, Yang X, Sun Y, Shi L, Xue P (2020) Optimization of ultrasound-assisted extraction by response surface methodology, antioxidant capacity, and tyrosinase inhibitory activity of anthocyanins from red rice bran. Food Sci Nutr 8(2):921–932. https://doi.org/10.1002/fsn3.1371

Wang H, Chen Y, Wang L, Liu Q, Yang S, Wang C (2023) Advancing herbal medicine: enhancing product quality and safety through robust quality control practices. Front Pharmacol 14:1265178. https://doi.org/10.3389/fphar.2023.1265178

Wang J, Zhao H, Xue X, Han Y, Wang X, Sheng Z (2024) Application of ionic liquid ultrasound-assisted extraction (IL-UAE) of lycopene from guava (*Psidium guajava* L.) by response surface methodology and artificial neural network-genetic algorithm. Ultrason Sonochem 106:106877. https://doi.org/10.1016/j.ultsonch.2024.106877

Xiao J, Chen G, Li N (2018) Ionic liquid solutions as a green tool for the extraction and isolation of natural products. Molecules 23(7):1765. https://doi.org/10.3390/molecules23071765

Xue Y, Wang F, Zhou C (2022) Optimization of ultrasonic extraction of triterpenes from loquat peel and pulp and determination of antioxidant activity and triterpenoid components. Foods 11(17):2563. https://doi.org/10.3390/foods11172563

Yang S, Li S, Li G, Li C, Li W, Bi Y, Wei J (2024) Pulsed electric field treatment improves the oil yield, quality, and antioxidant activity of virgin olive oil. Food Chem 22:101372. https://doi.org/10.1016/j.fochx.2024.101372

Yeow ATH, Hayyan A, Hayyan M, Junaidi MUM, Saleh J, Basirun WJ, Nor MRM, Abdulmonem WA, Salleh MZM, Zuki FM, Hamid MD (2024) A comprehensive review on the physicochemical properties of deep eutectic solvents. Results Chem 7:101378. https://doi.org/10.1016/j.rechem.2024.101378

Yıldırım M, Erşatır M, Poyraz S, Amangeldinova M, Kudrina NO, Terletskaya NV (2024) Green extraction of plant materials using supercritical CO_2: insights into methods, analysis, and bioactivity. Plants 13(16):2295. https://doi.org/10.3390/plants13162295

Zhang QW, Lin LG, Ye WC (2018) Techniques for extraction and isolation of natural products: a comprehensive review. Chin Med 13:20. https://doi.org/10.1186/s13020-018-0177-x

Zhao H, Wang J, Han Y, Wang X, Sheng Z (2024) Optimization of process conditions for ionic liquid-based ultrasound-enzyme-assisted extraction of resveratrol from *Polygonum Cuspidatum*. Ultrason Sonochem 108:106973. https://doi.org/10.1016/j.ultsonch.2024.106973

Zhou Y, Wu D, Cai P, Cheng G, Huang C, Pan Y (2015) Special effect of ionic liquids on the extraction of flavonoid glycosides from *Chrysanthemum morifolium* Ramat by microwave assistance. Molecules 20(5):7683–7699. https://doi.org/10.3390/molecules20057683

Zuorro A, Lavecchia R, González-Delgado ÁD, García-Martinez JB, L'Abbate P (2019) Optimization of enzyme-assisted extraction of flavonoids from corn husks. PRO 7(11):804. https://doi.org/10.3390/pr7110804

Approaches of Biotechnology in Phytochemicals

Anu Shri Rai, Manoj Kumar Solanki, Shalini Rai, Deepshikha Kushwaha, and Manasi Rai

Abstract Biologically active substances with specific therapeutic qualities are known as phytochemicals, and prior research has shown that these substances are frequently employed in traditional medicine to treat certain illnesses. These compounds have been shown to play an indispensable role in medical science, particularly in physiological regulation, healthcare, and disease prevention through their actions in lipid profile regulation, cardiovascular protection, immunity regulation, neuroprotection, antioxidation, anti-inflammation, anti-aging, antivirus, anticancer, and antithrombosis. They also improve metabolic functions. These chemicals are often categorized as compounds that contain sulfur, nitrogen, terpenes, polyphenols, and other components and are utilized as industrial chemicals, medicines, health-promoting agents, and biopesticides. With the development of contemporary science and technology, the researcher is more interested in the possible applications of these physiologically active substances. This study's main goal is to identify the various characteristics of phytochemicals used in biotechnology, food, and medicine. The emergence of phytochemicals, their use in different fields, and biotechnological methods for producing them are the main topics of the current study. Biotechnology, which encompasses metabolic engineering, genetic engineering, and plant tissue culture techniques to boost phytochemical yields, stabilize them, and develop novel functions, is essential to improving the production and use of phytochemicals. Additionally, biotechnology makes it possible to create more effec-

A. S. Rai · M. K. Solanki
Department of Life Sciences, I.E.S University, Bhopal, Madhya Pradesh, India

S. Rai (✉)
Department of Microbiology, DSMNRU University, Lucknow, Uttar Pradesh, India

D. Kushwaha
Centre for Microbiology, Ewing Christians College Prayagraj, Allahabad, Uttar Pradesh, India

M. Rai
Department of Microbiology, Central University of Rajasthan, Dist-Ajmer, Rajasthan, India

S. Kumar Tripathi et al. (eds.), *Phytoceuticals for Sustainable Medication*, Interdisciplinary Biotechnological Advances,
https://doi.org/10.1007/978-981-95-7588-6_2

tive extraction and purification techniques for the commercial production of beneficial phytochemicals.

Keywords Phytochemicals · Biotechnological approaches · Plant tissue culture · Pharmaceuticals · Genetic engineering · Disease treatment

1 Introduction

A wide range of compounds known as phytochemicals is created by plants throughout their growth and metabolism. They may be found in several foods, including fruits, vegetables, cereals, nuts, cocoa, chocolate, juice, tea, coffee, and wine. In 1891, these substances were dubbed "secondary metabolites" since most of them do not directly contribute to the growth, development, and reproduction of plants (Ahmed et al. 2017). In contrast, primary metabolites, which include carbohydrates, acyl lipids, phytosterols, and organic acids, are found in all plant tissues and carry out the metabolic processes required for plant growth and development. Remarkably, the glycolysis system produces several secondary metabolites that change into aromatic amino acids, including tryptophan, phenylalanine, and tyrosine. The distinction between primary and secondary metabolites is therefore still unclear and cannot be clearly classified according to chemical structure, precursor molecules, or biosynthetic origin (Kumar et al. 2023). Crucially, research conducted in the last several decades has demonstrated the effectiveness of these secondary metabolites in reducing the risk of conditions including diabetes, obesity, cancer, and inflammation, in addition to scavenging free radicals (Huang et al. 2019).

Recent studies on the possible health advantages of phytochemicals in mammalian systems have drawn a lot of attention to them. Carotenoids, isoprenoids, polyphenols, dietary fibers, phytosterols, saponins, and certain polysaccharides are a few of the important phytochemicals. These phytochemicals contain substantial antioxidant properties and display antibacterial, antidiarrheal, anthelmintic, antiallergic, antispasmodic, and antiviral effects (Sharma et al. 2018). Additionally, they support immunity, increase gap junction communication, control gene transcription, and offer defense against prostate and lung malignancies (Rowles and Erdman 2020; Shikov et al. 2022). Maceration, percolation, decoction, reflux, and Soxhlet extraction are a few of the commonly used conventional methods. The newer techniques include pressurized liquid extraction (PLE), high hydrostatic pressure extraction (HHP), microwave-assisted extraction (MAE), ultrasound-assisted extraction (UAE), pulsed electric field extraction (PEF), vibro-cavitation extraction, extraction under vacuum-oscillating boiling conditions, mill extractions, rotary-pulsation apparatus (RPE), liquid gas extraction (LGS), enzyme-assisted extraction (EAE), supercritical fluid extraction (SFE), and natural deep eutectic solvent extraction (NADES) (Quitério et al. 2022). Furthermore, the species that have important phytochemicals may be endangered if plants from their native habitats are overharvested for their compounds (Canter et al. 2005). Therefore, biotechnological methods have been used as a source of secondary metabolites in an effort to find new ways to generate these chemicals. Several technological techniques are used to improve the phytochemical substances, including fermentation, plant tissue culture, adventitious root culture, metabolic engineering, genetic alteration, in vitro synthesis, and gene editing. One of the most promising approaches to creating biotechnological processes for the industrial production of high-value phytochemicals is likely the use of metabolic engineering techniques that include altering endogenous pathways. We suggest research avenues to further the field's investigation of phytochemicals, the role of biotechnology in the production of phytochemicals, and the potential for innovative treatments for a range of illnesses.

2 Overview of Important Phytochemicals, Biotechnological Approaches, and Associated Health Advantages

Crop type, variety, soil, and cultivation environment (region, altitude, and season) are examples of extrinsic and intrinsic variables that affect the type and concentration of phytochemicals in the source crop. This section covers the main phytochemicals, their properties, the biotechnological methods used to produce them, and the related health advantages. Additionally, Table 1 lists the main phytochemicals, their sources, and their health advantages.

3 Approaches of Biotechnology in Phytochemicals

The synthesis, extraction, and modification of phytochemicals or bioactive substances made by plants, many of which have practical uses in medicine, nutrition, or industry, are greatly aided by biotechnology. Here are some important biotechnological research and manufacturing strategies for phytochemicals:

3.1 Plant Tissue Culture and Micropropagation

Customers' growing awareness of lifestyle choices has increased the demand for natural and organic products. Due to their cost-effectiveness and safety advantages over synthetic pharmaceuticals, medicinal plants have gained popularity over the past 20 years (Anand et al. 2019). The herbal medicine sector is currently one of the fastest-growing in the world. In 2000, the global commerce in medical plants and their metabolites was valued at US$60 billion. It is expected to expand at an average annual rate of 7% to reach US$5 trillion by 2050 (ISMH 2000). A number of medicinal plants are in danger of losing their natural environment due to population growth, rising demand for plant products, and illegal trading.

Table 1 Major phytochemicals, their sources, active parts of plants, biotechnological approaches, and the related health benefits

Phytochemicals	Active part of plants	Sources	Biological benefits	Biotechnological approaches for production	References
Carotenoids					
Lycopene	Skin and pulp of tomato, grapefruit, watermelon, apricot, guava	Tomato, sweet potato, pink grapefruit, pink guava, watermelon, apricot, papaya, rosehip	Improves eyesight, reduces pain, and strengthens bones	Fermentation technology, Plant tissue culture	Saubenova et al. (2024), Paul et al. (2023), and Murthy et al. (2025)
Fucoxanthin	Chloroplasts of brown seaweeds	Brown seaweeds, Bacillariophyta, Chromophyta, Macroalgae, Microalgae	Antioxidant, anti-inflammatory, antihypertensive, anticancerous, antidiabetic, antiobesity and radioprotective properties	Fermentation technology, Metabolic engineering	Leong et al. (2022) and Budiarso et al. (2025)
Xanthophylls	Young leaves of papaya, pumpkin; essential oil of pepper	Pumpkin, papaya, pepper, mushroom	Antioxidant properties, boosts eye health and blood flow	Fermentation technology, Metabolic engineering, Plant tissue culture	Ozyigit et al. (2023), Siziya et al. (2022), and Wang et al. (2023)
α-carotene	Pulp of mango, tangerine, avocado, butternut squash, and pumpkin; the green part of okra, chard, collard greens	Mango, pear, peach, pumpkin, butternut squash, green bean, okra, avocado, chard, collard greens, tangerine, banana	Regulates gene transcription, protects against lung and prostate cancer, good for eye health	Fermentation technology, Metabolic engineering, Plant tissue culture	Wang et al. (2023)
β-carotene	Green parts of plants, flowers, roots, and stems of plants; pulp of mango, grapefruit, papaya, etc.	Red pepper, carrot, spinach, peaches, brussel sprout, grapefruit, sour cherries, papaya, mango, romaine lettuce	Enhancement of gap junction communication, enhances immunity	Fermentation technology, Metabolic engineering	Almagro et al. (2022) and Paul et al. (2023)

Isoprenoids					
Myrcene	Essential oil extract of lemongrass, juniper, cardamom	Mango, guava, thyme, parsley, bay leaves, lemongrass, cardamom, sweet basil, juniper	Anxiolytic, antioxidant, anti-aging, anti-inflammatory, and analgesic properties	Genetic engineering	Li and Wang (2016)
Limonene	Oil of orange	Lemon, lime, orange	Anti-inflammatory, antioxidant, and anti-stress properties, as well as a neuroprotective role in Alzheimer's disease	Synthetic biology, Fermentation technology	Immethun et al. (2013)
Polyphenols					
Flavanols	Green and black tea leaves	Chocolate, tea, grapes	Action against free radicals, prevention of inflammation and allergies	Genetic engineering, Fermentation technology	Lasinskas et al. (2023) and Siller-Sánchez et al. (2024)
Flavones	Essential oils of spices, pulp of watermelon and pumpkin	Parsley, oregano, rosemary, green olive, pumpkin, watermelon, bell pepper, honey, fava beans, chickpea, field pea	Action against free radicals, protective effects against cardiovascular diseases, cancers, and other age-related diseases	Fermentation technology, Metabolic engineering	Yiakoumetti et al. (2023)
Anthocyanidins and anthocyanins	Flesh of berries, skin of grapes, corn fiber	Blueberry, cranberry, pomegranate, red grapes, black soybean, purple corn, red cabbage, raspberry	Protective effects against cardiovascular diseases, prevention of inflammation and allergies	Plant tissue culture, Fermentation technology, Metabolic engineering	Murthy et al. (2024) and Xu et al. (2022)

(continued)

Table 1 (continued)

Phytochemicals	Active part of plants	Sources	Biological benefits	Biotechnological approaches for production	References
Phytosterols					
Sitosterol	Oil of hazelnut, walnut, olive, canola, soybean	Avocado, hazelnut, walnut, soybean, olive, canola	Used in the treatment of an enlarged bladder; reduces the risk of cardiovascular disease, promotes anti-cancer properties	Plant tissue culture, Fermentation technology, Metabolic engineering	Pereira et al. (2023) and Gu et al. (2021)
Campestanol	Oil of soybean, olive, hazelnut, flax, and cashew	Soybean, olive, hazelnut, flax, cashew	Prostate health, hair growth, reduce LDL cholesterol	Plant tissue culture, Fermentation technology	Xu et al. (2023)
Stigmasterol	Oil of soybean, Calabar bean, and rapeseed	Soybean, Calabar bean, and rapeseed	Has a protective effect against gastric and duodenal ulcers, neurological disorders	Plant tissue culture, Fermentation technology, Metabolic engineering	Bapat et al. (2023) and Li et al. (2025)
Stigmastanol	Oil of hazelnut and olive, as well as corn fiber	Hazelnut, olive, corn	Reduces chance of heart attack and stroke, antioxidant activity	Plant tissue culture, Fermentation technology, Metabolic engineering	Jiang et al. (2023)
Saponins					
Dammarane	Middle lamella of peas and legumes	Black gram, garden pea, pigeon pea	Exhibits hypoglycemic, virucidal, and antifungal activity	Fermentation technology, Metabolic engineering	Chen et al. (2024)
Oleanane	Middle lamella of legumes and oil of almond	Common bean, black gram, almond	Antimicrobial and hypolipidemic activities; aids in the treatment of chronic diseases	Fermentation technology, Metabolic engineering	Cheng et al. (2024)
Tirucallane	Oil of almond, sunflower, and walnut	Sunflower, almond, walnut	Has an effect on the transverse tubular system and sarcoplasmic reticulum at lower concentration (10 μg/mL), affects skin inflammation and diarrhea	Fermentation technology, Metabolic engineering	Lee et al. (2018)

Plant metabolites may be extracted from naturally occurring plants; however, geographical and environmental limitations limit their economic production (Yue et al. 2016). It takes years for plants to mature to the point where they can produce the appropriate amount of metabolite; therefore, conventional approaches are time-consuming. The technology of plant tissue culture (PTC) and micropropagation has shown promise as a substitute for the extraction of valuable bioactive components from plants in order to conserve endangered species and generate the necessary quantities of plant material (Chandran et al. 2020). The production of plant compounds in a variety of medicinal plants has been improved and enhanced via considerable research on various plant tissue culture systems (Yue et al. 2016). This chapter thus emphasizes on the benefits of employing PTC approaches for the synthesis of secondary metabolites, as well as the distribution of several types of plant secondary metabolites throughout plant families, significant medical applications, and methods to enhance their production in order to boost output. Table 2 provides a summary of a few significant medicinal plants and their commercially significant secondary metabolites.

Table 2 Production of therapeutic phytochemicals from medicinal plants by using plant tissue culture and micropropagation and their applications

S. No.	Plant name	Active phytochemical(s)	Application(s)
1	Ginkgo biloba	Kaempferol, isorhamnetin, quercetin, bilobalide, ginkgolide A, B, C, ginsenoside	Antidiabetes, anti-inflammatory, cancer therapy, cardiovascular diseases,
2	Catharanthus roseus	Catharanthine, indole alkaloids	Cancer therapy
3	Ruta species	Alkaloids, acridone, quinolone, flavonoids furanocoumarins	Contraceptive preparations, antioxidant, natural fungicides and pesticides, antiplasmodial, analgesic, anti-inflammatory, antipyretic, antiviral,
4	Rauwolfia species	Ajmaline, solasodine, alstonine, α-solanine, ajmalicine, serpentine and reserpine, rescinnamine, β-carboline, reserpiline	Natural tranquilizer, hypertension, insomnia, epilepsy, schizophrenia, antidote against snake bite
5	Datura stramonium	Tropane alkaloids (atropine, hyoscyamine, and scopolamine)	Relive pain of rheumatism and gout, hallucinogenic drug, treat epilepsy and depression, powerful mind-altering drug, anti-inflammatory, antimicrobial
6	Taxus species	Essential oils, paclitaxel, flavonoids, baccatin III, taxol, lignans	Treatment of epilepsy, rheumatism, analgesic, aphrodisiac, antiepileptic, anti-inflammatory, anticancer, antidote for snake bite, antipyretic, immunomodulatory, antimicrobial activities.

(continued)

Table 2 (continued)

S. No.	Plant name	Active phytochemical(s)	Application(s)
7	Thymus species	Borneol, geraniol, α-terpineol, carotenoids, carvacrol, thymol, rosmarinic acid	Anti-inflammatory, gastroprotective, antiulcer, hepatoprotective, antimicrobial, antihyperlipidemic activity, anti-HIV-1 activity, hypoglycemic, antioxidative capacity, flavoring agent
8	Dioscorea doryphora	Diosgenin	Cancer therapy, hypercholesterolemia, inflammation
9	Scopolia parviflora	Scopalamine, hyoscyamine	Anticholinergic drug, antispasmodic drug hallucinogenic agent, treat motion sickness
10	Stevia rebaudiana	Stevioside, essential oils steviol rebaudioside	Anti-diabetes, obesity, cancer, renal disease, cardiovascular disease, dental caries, treating inflammatory bowel disease,
11	Panax ginseng	Ginsenosides (dammarane and oleanane)	Tonic for gastro enteric disorders, diabetes, anti-stress agents, cardioprotective, antioxidant, anxiolytic, anticancer, aphrodisiac
12	Beta vulgaris	Betalains, apigenin flavonoids like vitexin, vitexin-2-O-rhamnoside, vitexin-2-O-xyloside	Antihypertensive, hypoglycemic, antioxidant, anticancer agent, natural dye in food industry
13	Atropa belladona	Tropane alkaloids (atropine, hyoscyamine, and scopolamine)	Treatment of Parkinson's disease, hallucinogenic agent, treatment of ulcers, motion sickness, inflammation, antidote for snake bites
14	Punica granatum	Pelletierine, ellagic acid, phenol, flavonoid	Anti-cancer, anti-diabetes, cardiovascular disease, immune modulatory activity, treat dental problems
15	Coleus blumei	Rosmarinic acid, cavacrol, β-sitosterol, apigenin, forskolin, chavicol, eugenol, quercetin	Antigalucomic, antimetastatic, antidepressant, cardiotonic, anticancer, nervous system depressant, vasodialator, immunosuppressant, antioxidant

3.2 *In Vitro Systems for Metabolite(s) Production—PTC*

The process of producing secondary metabolites in vitro involves two steps: (i) biomass aggregation and (ii) secondary metabolite synthesis (Murthy et al. 2014). Secondary metabolite synthesis has allegedly been facilitated by organized structures such as calli, cell suspension, shoots, and roots. (Hussain et al. 2012).

In vitro, stimulated plant cells create a disorganized mass of cells called a callus. High doses of auxin or a combination of auxin and cytokinin are frequently employed to induce callus. Commercial potential for the production of therapeutically significant secondary metabolites has increased with callus cultures (Ogita 2015). According to reports, callus cultivation is a more dependable method of harvesting medicinal compounds than gathering plant materials from the wild. They may be utilized to create single-cell suspension cultures utilizing batch or continuous fermentation to generate the desired secondary metabolites, as well as to create numerous plant clones using micropropagation (Wu et al. 2016). Callus and suspension cultures can then produce secondary metabolites and manipulate the pathways involved in the creation of secondary metabolites. Reserpine, tropane alkaloids, ajmaline, α-tocopherol, stilbene, serpentine, paclitaxel, flavonoids, scopolamine, anthocyanins, and resveratrol have all been reported to be produced from callus cultures (Efferth 2019).

According to Tošić et al. (2025), metabolite synthesis from differentiated organ cultures, such as shoots or roots, has been documented and can resemble the metabolite profile of natural plants. According to Karuppusamy (2009), plant hairy root cultures are the most promising alternative technique for creating chemicals that are generated in plant roots. By causing hairy roots in plants, Agrobacterium rhizogenes-mediated transformation has made it possible to create secondary metabolites in vitro that are produced in plant roots (Chen et al. 2018). They have developed a useful biological framework to investigate the production of a number of bioactive substances, including ginsenosides (Ha et al. 2016), anthraquinones (Perassolo et al. 2017), nicotine and tropane alkaloids (Yu et al. 2005), and artemisinin (Patra and Srivastava 2016). Hairy roots are advantageous for compound formation because of their high production, consistency, and competence (Thakore et al. 2017; Cardoso et al. 2019).

3.3 Metabolic Engineering

The process of altering an organism's metabolic pathways utilizing contemporary scientific methods such as proteomics, metabolomics, and genomics in order to generate metabolites of economic significance is known as metabolic engineering (Della Penna 2001). Therefore, it permits the control of natural biochemical processes. Using recombinant DNA technology, it includes rerouting common precursors, enzymes, and regulatory proteins to either overexpress or downregulate metabolic pathways. Many metabolic pathways found in plants are responsible for the manufacture of intricate metabolites. In order to isolate and overproduce commercially significant plant metabolites, these pathways can be reproduced in heterologous hosts.

The shikimate, polyketide, and terpenoid pathways are the biosynthetic pathways that plants use to produce secondary metabolites. According to reports, the primary source of phenylpropanoids and aromatic chemicals is the highly conserved shikimate pathway. Given that about 30% of fixed carbon is anticipated to be fixed by this system, it is regarded as a crucial metabolic pathway in plants for carbon flow (Maeda and Dudareva 2012). Through the process of shikimate biosynthesis, phenylalanine is converted into phenolic secondary metabolites in plants. Flavonoids, betalains, gallic acid, vanillin, coumarins, lignans, stilbenoids, catechins, and other metabolites are formed from the intermediate pcoumaroyl-CoA. The isoprenoid route is another name for the terpenoid pathway. Mevalonic acid (MVA) and methyl-D-erythritol (MEP) are two independent routes used in plants for terpenoid biosynthesis. Triterpenoids, brassinosteroids, polyprenols, phytosterols, and sesquiterpenoids are all synthesized by the MVA route. Gibberellins, tocopherols, plastoquinones, monoterpenoids, diterpenoids, hemiterpenoids, and plant growth regulators like cytokinins are all produced via the MEP route. The polyketide pathway plays a crucial part in the production of fatty acids. Either acetyl CoA or malonyl CoA is the source of them. Jasmonates 6-methylsalicylic acid, acetogenins, plumbagin, anthraquinones, and coniine are examples of secondary metabolites that have been identified from the polyketide route (Verpoorte et al. 2002).

3.3.1 Up-Regulating Pathways

Transcription factors are proteins that attach to particular DNA regions, such as promoters or enhancers, to regulate the transcription or expression of target genes. They alter the rate of transcription and decode information in the genome (Albert et al. 2014). An activator domain and a DNA-binding domain are their two functional areas. While activator domains have binding sites known as activation functions and trans-activation domains for other proteins (transcription coregulators), DNA binding domains have amino acids that recognize certain DNA bases on the regulatory element.

The generation of secondary metabolites has been linked to a number of transcription factors. In a number of plant species, MYB transcription factors have been identified as the regulators of many metabolic pathways. It has been reported that anthocyanin accumulation and flavonoid levels in plant species such as *Solanum lycopersicum, Arabidopsis, Zea mays, Petunia hybrida, Ipomoea batatas*, and others are controlled by transcription factors such as R2R3-MYB, WD repeat (beta-transducin repeat), adenine nucleotide translocator (also known as adenine nucleotide translocase or Ant) type 1, APETALA2/ethylene response factor (AP2/ERF), WRKY, NAC, and SQUAMOSA Promoter Binding Protein-Like (SPL) (Xu et al. 2015).

3.3.2 Redirecting Common Precursors

In a biosynthesis route, enzymes compete with one another for precursors. By changing the precursor towards the biosynthesis of the target metabolites, either by blocking the competitive route or by causing overexpression of genes in the precursor pathway, metabolite production can be boosted (Verpoorte et al. 2002). Increasing the expression of the gene that codes for taxadiene synthase, a precursor in the carotenoid pathway, can increase the synthesis of taxadiene in tomato mutants. According to Jadaun et al. (2017), increased terpenoidal secondary metabolite accumulation in *Withania somnifera* (withanolides) and *Pelargonium* spp. (essential oil) was caused by the overexpression of 1-deoxy-d-xylulose-5-phosphate synthase (GrDXS).

3.3.3 Targeting Metabolites to Specific Cell Compartments

The cytoplasm and organelles, such as peroxisomes, vesicles, and vacuoles, contain the enzymes and metabolites of secondary metabolic pathways. According to Jorgensen et al. (2005), the enzymes involved in secondary metabolic pathways are arranged into multifunctional enzyme complexes that have substrate channeling effects, in which the metabolic products of one enzyme serve as a substrate for the enzyme that follows.

Proteins have been reported to be targeted and retained by certain amino acid sequences in specific organelles. Enzymes involved in the manufacture of monoterpenoid indole alkaloids are found in the roots, leaves, flowers, buds, and other parts of *C. roseus*, while the metabolite builds up in unique cells known as idioblasts and laticifers. It is necessary to move the generated enzymes and metabolites across cells of various tissue types rather than to a single cell (St-Pierre et al. 1999). The processes that produce toxic metabolites are compartmentalized by cells to prevent self-toxicity. Nicotine in tobacco and the alkaloid berberine produced by *Coptis japonica* are both contained in vacuoles (Otani et al. 2005). Chalcone synthase, dihydroflavonol 4-reductase, and chalcone isomerase are among the several enzymes that work together in *Arabidopsis thaliana* to produce flavonoids (Burbulis and Winkel-Shirley 1999).

3.3.4 Down-Regulating Pathways (Silencing)

By reducing the amount of enzyme, catabolism, and carbon flow into competing pathways can be increased, reducing the synthesis of certain metabolites. By hiding genes that enhance the metabolic process or promote their catabolism, undesirable compounds can be prevented from being created (Gómez-Galera et al. 2007). Co-suppression, RNA interference (RNAi), and antisense RNA are examples of contemporary r-DNA technologies that can be utilized to phase out unwanted metabolites. Plant secondary metabolites such as terpenoids, alkaloids, and phenylpropanoids have purportedly been manipulated by RNA interference. RNA interference (RNAi) has been used to manipulate the phenylpropanoid pathway, resulting in poor pigmentation in the seed coat, abundant floral colors, etc. According to reports, it has been used to boost the opium poppy's synthesis of codeine and morphine, reduce the cyanogenic glucoside components of cassava, raise tomato flavonoids and carotenoids, control petunia flower smell, and more (Wagner and Kroumova 2008).

4 Conclusion and Perspectives

The usage of plants for medicinal reasons dates back thousands of years. Using biotechnological methods such as plant tissue culture, micropropagation, microbial fermentation, metabolic engineering, and synthetic biology, it is necessary to mass clone plants to meet the growing demand for sustainable and affordable natural phytochemicals. Comparing in vitro methods to traditional methods, a large number of therapeutic plants and their metabolites have been created quickly. Artificial selection, the generation of variant clones, gene transfer technologies, and environmental regulation have all been shown to increase the biosynthetic activity of cultivated cells. These developments have led to an unprecedented growth in the study of biotechnological methods for producing plant compounds. The commercial development of metabolites and food ingredients derived from plant cell and tissue culture is anticipated to increase in the upcoming years as more is learned about the biochemical and genetic regulation of plant secondary metabolism, as well as progress is made in the design of large-scale bioreactors and the development of yield improvement strategies. Consequently, the use of these technologies will enable more thorough research into the physiology of medicinal plants as well as better phytopharmaceutical manufacturing.

References

Ahmed E, Arshad M, Khan MZ, Amjad MS, Ahmad SJAP (2017) Secondary metabolites and their multidimensional prospective in plant life. J Pharmacogn Phytochem 6(2):205–214

Albert NW, Davies KM, Lewis DH, Zhang H, Montefiori M, Brendolise C, Boase MR, Ngo H, Jameson PE, Schwinn KE (2014) A conserved network of transcriptional activators and repressors regulates anthocyanin pigmentation in eudicots. Plant Cell 26(3):962–980

Almagro L, Correa-Sabater JM, Sabater-Jara AB et al (2022) Biotechnological production of β-carotene using plant in vitro cultures. Planta 256:41

Anand U, Jacobo-Herrera N, Altemimi A, Lakhssassi N (2019) A comprehensive review on medicinal plants as antimicrobial therapeutics: potential avenues of biocompatible drug discovery. Meta 9:258

Bapat VA, Kavi Kishor PB, Jalaja N, Jain SM, Penna S (2023) Plant cell cultures: biofactories for the production of bioactive compounds. Agronomy 13(3):858

Budiarso FS, Leong YK, Chang J-J, Chen C-Y, Chen J-H, Yen H-W, Chang J-S (2025) Current advances in microalgae-based fucoxanthin production and downstream processes. Bioresour Technol 428:132455

Burbulis IE, Winkel-Shirley B (1999) Interactions among enzymes of the *Arabidopsis* flavonoid biosynthetic pathway. Proc Natl Acad Sci USA 96:12929–12934

Canter PH, Thomas H, Ernst E (2005) Bringing medicinal plants into cultivation: opportunities and challenges for biotechnology. Trends Biotechnol 23:180–185

Cardoso JC, de Oliveira BEBS, de CI Cardoso, F (2019) Advances and challenges on the in vitro production of secondary metabolites from medicinal plants. Hortic Bras 37(2):124–132

Chandran H, Meena M, Barupal T, Sharma K (2020) Plant tissue culture as a perpetual source for production of industrially important bioactive compounds. Biotechnol Rep (Amst) 26:e00450

Chen L, Cai Y, Liu X (2018) Soybean hairy roots produced in vitro by agrobacterium rhizogenes-mediated transformation. Crop J 6:162–171

Chen Q, Wang J, Gao Y, Wang Z, Wang D, Gao X, Yan P (2024) Fermentation, identification, and antioxidant activity of Saponins produced by a wild ginseng endophytic fungus *Umbelopsis dimorpha* strain NSJG. Fermentation 10(1):9

Cheng X, Pang Y, Ban Y, Cui S, Shu T, Lv B, Li C (2024) Application of multiple strategies to enhance oleanolic acid biosynthesis by engineered *Saccharomyces cerevisiae*. Bioresour Technol 401:130716

Della Penna D (2001) Plant metabolic engineering. Plant Physiol 125(1):160–163
Efferth T (2019) Biotechnology applications of plant callus cultures. Engineering 5(1):50–59
Gómez-Galera S, Pelacho A, Gené A, Capell T, Christou P (2007) The genetic manipulation of medicinal and aromatic plants. Plant Cell Rep 26:1689–1715
Government of India, Medicinal Plants Introduction, Indian System of Medicine and Homoeopathy (ISMH), Department of ISMH, Ministry of Health and Family Welfare, Govt. of India, (2000). http://indianmedicine.nic.in/html/plants/mimain.htm
Gu Y, Jiao X, Ye L et al (2021) Metabolic engineering strategies for de novo biosynthesis of sterols and steroids in yeast. Bioresour Bioprocess 8:110
Ha LT, Pawlicki-Jullian N, Pillon-Lequart M, Boitel-Conti M, Duong HX, Gontier E (2016) Hairy root cultures of Panax vietnamensis, a promising approach for the production of ocotillol-type ginsenosides. Plant Cell Tissue Organ Cult 126:93–103
Huang W, Feng Z, Aila R, Hou Y, Carne A, Bekhit AEA (2019) Effect of pulsed electric fields (PEF) on physico-chemical properties, β-carotene and antioxidant activity of air-dried apricots. Food Chem 291:253–262
Hussain MS, Fareed S, Saba Ansari M, Rahman A, Ahmad IZ, Saeed M (2012) Current approaches toward production of secondary plant metabolites. J Pharm Bioallied Sci 4(1):10–20
Immethun CM, Hoynes O'Connor AG, Balassy A, Moon TS (2013) Microbial production of isoprenoids enabled by synthetic biology. Front Microbiol 4:75
Jadaun JS, Sangwan NS, Narnoliya LK, Singh N, Bansal S, Mishra B, Sangwan RS (2017) Over-expression of DXS gene enhances terpenoidal secondary metabolite accumulation in rose-scented geranium and *Withania somnifera*: active involvement of plastid isoprenogenic pathway in their biosynthesis. Physiol Plantarum 159:381–400
Jiang Y, Sun Z, Lu K et al (2023) Manipulation of sterol homeostasis for the production of 24-epi-ergosterol in industrial yeast. Nat Commun 14:437
Jorgensen K, Rasmussen AV, Morant M, Nielsen AH, Bjarnholt N, Zagrobelny M, Bak S, Moller BL (2005) Metabolon formation and metabolic channeling in the biosynthesis of plant natural products. Curr Opin Plant Biol 8:280–291
Karuppusamy S (2009) A review on trends in production of secondary metabolites from higher plants by in vitro tissue, organ and cell cultures. J Med Plant Res 3:1222–1239
Kumar AN, Kumar M, Jose A, Tomer V, Oz E, Proestos C, Zeng M, Elobeid T et al (2023) Major phytochemicals: recent advances in health benefits and extraction method. Molecules 28:887
Lasinskas M, Jariene E, Vaitkeviciene N, Kulaitiene J, Adamaviciene A, Hallmann E (2023) The impact of solid-phase fermentation on flavonoids, phenolic acids, tannins and antioxidant activity in *Chamerion angustifolium* (L.) Holub (fireweed) leaves. Plants 12(2):277
Lee SR, Choi E, Jeon SH, Zhi XY, Yu JS, Kim SH, Lee J, Park KM, Kim KH (2018) Tirucallane triterpenoids from the stems and stem bark of Cornus walteri that control adipocyte and osteoblast differentiations. Molecules 23:2732
Leong YK, Chen C-Y, Varjani S, Chang J-S (2022) Producing fucoxanthin from algae – recent advances in cultivation strategies and downstream processing. Bioresour Technol 344(A):126170
Li Y, Wang G (2016) Strategies of isoprenoids production in engineered bacteria. J Appl Microbiol 121(4):932–940
Li J, Zheng X, Qi J (2025) Research progress on the therapeutic mechanisms of stigmasterol for multiple diseases. Molecules 30(9):1874
Maeda H, Dudareva N (2012) The shikimate pathway and aromatic amino acid biosynthesis in plants. Annu Rev Plant Biol 63:73–105
Murthy HN, Lee EJ, Paek KY (2014) Production of secondary metabolites from cell and organ cultures: strategies and approaches for biomass improvement and metabolite accumulation. Plant Cell Tissue Organ Cult 118:1–16
Murthy HN, Joseph KS, Paek KY, Park SY (2024) Anthocyanin production from plant cell and organ cultures in vitro. Plants 13(1):117

Murthy HN, Yadav GG, Paek KY, Park SY (2025) Production of carotenoids from plant cell and organ cultures: a comprehensive review. In: Ramawat KG, Mérillon JM (eds) Natural products. Springer, Berlin/Heidelberg

Ogita S (2015) Plant cell, tissue and organ culture: the most flexible foundations for plant metabolic engineering applications. Nat Prod Commun 10(5):815–820

Otani M, Shitan N, Sakai K, Martinoia E, Sato F, Yazaki K (2005) Characterization of vacuolar transport of the endogenous alkaloid berberine in *Coptis japonica*. Plant Physiol 138:1939–1946

Ozyigit II, Dogan I, Hocaoglu-Ozyigit A, Yalcin B, Erdogan A, Yalcin IE, Cabi E, Kaya Y (2023) Production of secondary metabolites using tissue culture-based biotechnological applications. Front Plant Sci 14:1132555

Patra N, Srivastava AK (2016) Artemisinin production by plant hairy root cultures in gas-and liquid-phase bioreactors. Plant Cell Rep 35:143–153

Paul D, Kumari PK, Siddiqui N (2023) Yeast carotenoids: cost-effective fermentation strategies for health care applications. Fermentation 9:147

Perassolo M, Cardillo AB, Laura Mugas M, Núñez Montoya SC, Giulietti AM, Taloua AR (2017) Enhancement of anthraquinone production and release by combination of culture medium selection and methyl jasmonate elicitation in hairy root cultures of Rubia tinctorum. Ind Crop Prod 105:124–132

Pereira ADS, Fraga JL, Souza CPL, Torres AG, Amaral PFF (2023) β-Sitosterol Oleate synthesis by *Candida rugosa* lipase in a solvent-free mini reactor system: free and immobilized on chitosan-alginate beads. Catalysts 13(4):780

Quitério E, Grosso C, Ferraz R, Delerue-Matos C, Soares C (2022) A critical comparison of the advanced extraction techniques applied to obtain health-promoting compounds from seaweeds. Marine Drug 20:677

Rowles JL 3rd, Erdman JW Jr (2020) Carotenoids and their role in cancer prevention. Biochim Biophys Acta Mol Cell Biol Lipids 2020(1865):158613

Saubenova M, Rapoport A, Venkatachalam M, Dufossé L, Yermekbay Z, Oleinikova Y (2024) Production of carotenoids by microorganisms. Fermentation 10:502

Sharma BR, Kumar V, Gat Y, Kumar N, Parashar A, Pinakin DJ (2018) Microbial maceration: a sustainable approach for phytochemical extraction. 3 Biotech 8:401

Shikov AN, Mikhailovskaya IY, Narkevich IA, Flisyuk EV, Pozharitskaya ON (2022) Methods of extraction of medicinal plants. In: Evidence-based validation of herbal medicine. Elsevier, Amsterdam, pp 771–796

Siller-Sánchez A, Aguilar CN, Chávez-González ML, Ascacio-Valdés JA, Kumar Verma D, Aguilar-González M (2024) Solid-state fermentation-assisted extraction of flavonoids from grape pomace using co-cultures. Processes 12(9):2027

Siziya IN, Hwang CY, Seo MJ (2022) Antioxidant potential and capacity of microorganism-sourced C30 carotenoids–a review. Antioxidants 11(10):1963. https://doi.org/10.3390/antiox11101963

St-Pierre B, Vazquez-Flota FA, De Luca V (1999) Multicellular compartmentation of *Catharanthus roseus* alkaloid biosynthesis predicts intercellular translocation of a pathway intermediate. Plant Cell 11:887–900

Thakore D, Srivastava AK, Sinha AK (2017) Mass production of Ajmalicine by bioreactor cultivation of hairy roots of Catharanthus roseus. Biochem Eng J 119:84–91

Tošić SM, Ilić M, Svilar L, Nikolić J, Mitić M, Mitić V, Stankov Jovanović VP (2025) Conserved and divergent phytochemical profiles in native and micropropagated Micromeria croatica (Pers.) Schott: an LC-HRMS study across solvent extracts. Plants 14(19):2971

Verpoorte R, Contin A, Memelink J (2002) Biotechnology for the production of plant secondary metabolites. Phytochem Rev 1:13–25

Wagner GJ, Kroumova AB (2008) The use of RNAi to elucidate and manipulate secondary metabolite synthesis in plants. In: Ying SY (ed) Current perspectives in MicroRNAs (miRNA). Springer, Dordrecht

Wang N, Peng H, Yang C, Guo W, Wang M, Li G, Liu D (2023) Metabolic engineering of model microorganisms for the production of xanthophyll. Microorganisms 11:1252

Wu CF, Karioti A, Rohr D, Bilia AR, Efferth T (2016) Production of rosmarinic acid and salvianolic acid B from callus culture of salvia miltiorrhiza with cytotoxicity towards acute lymphoblastic leukemia cells. Food Chem 201:292–297

Xu W, Dubos C, Lepiniec L (2015) Transcriptional control of flavonoid biosynthesis by MYB-bHLH-WDR complexes. Trends Plant Sci 20:176–185

Xu S, Li G, Zhou J, Chen G, Shao J (2022) Efficient production of anthocyanins in Saccharomyces cerevisiae by introducing anthocyanin transporter and knocking out endogenous degrading enzymes. Front Bioeng Biotechnol 10:899182

Xu S, Teng X, Li Y (2023) Optimization of Campesterol-producing yeast strains as a feasible platform for the functional reconstitution of plant membrane-bound enzymes. ACS Synth Biol 21;12(4):1109–1118

Yiakoumetti A, Hanko EKR, Zou Y, Chua J, Chromy J, Stoney RA, Valdehuesa KNG, Connolly JA, Yan C, Hollywood KA, Takano E, Breitling R (2023) Expanding flavone and flavonol production capabilities in Escherichia coli. Front Bioeng Biotechnol 11:1275651

Yu KW, Hosakatte NM, Hahn EJ, Paek KY (2005) Ginsenoside production by hairy root cultures of Panax ginseng: influence of temperature and light quality. Biochem Eng J 23:53–56

Yue W, Ming QL, Lin B, Rahman K, Zheng CJ, Han T, Qin LP (2016) Medicinal plant cell suspension cultures: pharmaceutical applications and highyielding strategies for the desired secondary metabolites. Crit Rev Biotechnol 36:215–232

Novel Pharmaceutical Technologies in Development of Phytopharmaceuticals

Subhadas Chatterjee, Samiran Sadhukhan, Rajeswar Das, Sankhadip Bose, and Subas Chandra Dinda

Abstract Phytoceuticals are the plant-based pharmaceutical products drawing attention as integrative solutions bridging traditional medicine and modern healthcare. However, their clinical translation is often limited because of poor bioavailability, chemical instability, and lack of standardization. This chapter explores how novel drug delivery systems, including liposomes, phytosomes, nanoemulsions, solid lipid nanoparticles, nanostructured lipid carriers, dendrimers, and nanoemulgels, enhance the solubility, stability, and are utilized to develop targeted delivery of phytoconstituents. In parallel, green extraction technologies have also been found to improve the efficiency and selectivity of phytochemical isolation. A significant focus is also placed on the integration of in silico tools, such as molecular docking, ADMET profiling, network pharmacology, and molecular dynamics simulations, which accelerate the discovery, optimization, and mechanistic understanding of bioactive compounds. Together, these advances support the development of phytopharmaceuticals that are not only more effective and scalable but also aligned with the growing demands for personalized medicines and evidence-based therapeutics.

Keywords Phytoceuticals · Nano-pharmaceuticals · Liposomes · Phytosomes · Nanoemulsions · Solid lipid nanoparticles · Nanostructured lipid carriers · Polymeric nanoparticles · Dendrimers · Nanoemulgel · Green extraction

S. Chatterjee (✉)
School of Pharmacy, The Neotia University, Sarisha, West Bengal, India

Bengal School of Technology, Sugandha, Chuchura, Hooghly, West Bengal, India
e-mail: subhadaschatterjee@gmail.com

S. Sadhukhan
School of Pharmacy, The Neotia University, Sarisha, West Bengal, India

Netaji Subhash Chandra Bose Institute of Pharmacy, Chakdaha, West Bengal, India
e-mail: samiranrana05@gmail.com

R. Das · S. Bose · S. C. Dinda
School of Pharmacy, The Neotia University, Sarisha, West Bengal, India
e-mail: rajeswar.das@tnu.in; sankha.bose@gmail.com; subaschandra.dinda@tnu.in

S. Kumar Tripathi et al. (eds.), *Phytoceuticals for Sustainable Medication*, Interdisciplinary Biotechnological Advances,
https://doi.org/10.1007/978-981-95-7588-6_3

1 Introduction

Phytopharmaceuticals, a term derived from 'phyto' (plant) and 'pharmaceuticals', refer to bioactive plant-derived compounds formulated with pharmaceutical precision to deliver therapeutic effects. While often confused with phytochemicals, phytoceuticals differ in their application and processing. Phytochemicals are compounds that naturally exist in plants that may or may not have pharmacological activity, whereas phytoceuticals are standardized, often clinically validated, formulations developed for specific health outcomes (Yuan et al. 2016; Lee et al. 2008). Traditional medical systems, such as Ayurveda, Traditional Chinese Medicine (TCM), Siddha, and Unani, have long utilized plant-based formulations to manage a variety of health conditions. These systems employ pharmacologically active botanical extracts for treating ailments like diabetes, inflammation, cardiovascular disorders, and microbial infections (Yuan et al. 2016). Modern phytoceuticals have evolved from these ancient remedies, incorporating advanced technologies to enhance efficacy and safety.

The global market for herbal medicine was estimated to be worth around USD 70.57 billion in 2023. It is expected to expand at a compound annual growth rate (CAGR) of 20.91% between 2024 and 2030, potentially reaching USD 328.72 billion by 2030 (Grand View Research 2024). The World Health Organization (WHO) reports that over 80% of the global population, spanning more than 170 of its 194 Member States, currently rely on various forms of traditional medicine, including herbal remedies, yoga, Ayurveda, acupuncture, and indigenous healing practices (World Health Organization 2023). The global nutraceutical market is expected to grow from USD 418.2 billion in 2024 to USD 571.3 billion by 2029, reflecting a compound annual growth rate (CAGR) of 6.4% during the forecast period from 2024 to 2029 (BCC Research 2024). This growing reliance underscores the significance of integrating modern pharmaceutical technologies to develop effective and standardized phytoceuticals.

Despite their therapeutic promise, phytoceuticals face several development challenges, including low oral bioavailability, chemical instability, batch-to-batch variability, and lack of standardization. Many phytochemicals exhibit poor solubility and are rapidly metabolized, limiting their systemic availability and clinical efficacy (Singh et al. 2019). These challenges necessitate the application of advanced delivery and formulation technologies. To tackle these challenges, new pharmaceutical technologies have been introduced. Techniques such as nanocarriers, liposomes, phytosomes, solid lipid nanoparticles (SLNs), nanoemulsions, 3D printing, microfluidics, and AI-based drug discovery are revolutionizing phytoceutical development. These approaches improve solubility, protect active ingredients from degradation, and enable site-specific, controlled delivery (Chakraborty et al. 2016; Li et al. 2021). Additionally, recent advances in extraction techniques such as ultrasound-assisted extraction (UAE), microwave-assisted extraction (MAE), and supercritical fluid extraction (SFE) have enabled more efficient and targeted extraction of bioactive compounds from plant materials, making them highly relevant for standardized phytoceutical development (Colombo et al. 2023).

The evolving landscape of personalized medicine has significantly broadened the scope of phytoceuticals. The integration of in silico tools—including molecular docking, ADMET prediction, network pharmacology, and molecular dynamics simulations—alongside artificial intelligence, machine learning, and omics platforms, enables a thorough understanding of the interactions between plant-derived compounds, bioactivity, and safety profiles. These computational approaches accelerate the identification of promising phytochemicals and enable their tailored application in disease-specific therapeutic strategies (Kalita et al. 2025; Alotaibi et al. 2023; Abdullah et al. 2023a, b).

These developments highlight the growing need for innovation in formulation science to complement the advances in computational and personalized approaches. As consumer expectations shift towards scientifically validated, high-performance natural products, the role of novel pharmaceutical technologies becomes increasingly pivotal, not only in addressing the inherent limitations of traditional phytoformulations but also in ensuring consistent efficacy, scalability, and alignment with evolving global regulatory standards.

This chapter offers an in-depth overview of the cutting-edge pharmaceutical technologies that are advancing the formulation, delivery, and therapeutic performance of phytoceuticals. It explores a range of platforms, including nanotechnology-based systems, liposomes, phytosomes, mucosal and transdermal delivery strategies, as well as in silico tools for predictive screening and optimization. Special emphasis is placed on green extraction methods and metabolomics profiling, highlighting the future direction of this rapidly evolving field.

2 The Phytoceutical Landscape: Origins, Advances, and Limitations

Phytoceuticals have evolved from traditional plant-based remedies into scientifically backed therapeutic formulations. This shift reflects the growing integration of traditional knowledge with modern pharmaceutical science (Yuan et al. 2016).

2.1 Historical Perspective

The medicinal use of plants spans thousands of years, with early practices rooted in various ancient civilizations, including Egypt, India, and China. These cultures laid the foundation for the modern use of phytoceuticals, with many plant remedies based on empirical knowledge passed down through generations. Some of these plants have since been validated by contemporary science for their therapeutic properties (Hart 2005).

For example, ancient Egyptians used remedies like garlic and aloe vera for their antimicrobial and anti-inflammatory effects. Similarly, traditional Chinese medicine (TCM) incorporated herbs such as ginseng and ginger not only as foods but also as treatments for various ailments. Ayurveda, the traditional Indian system of medicine, includes a vast array of plant-based remedies, many of which have been rigorously studied in recent years and shown promising therapeutic potential (Ernst 2005; Khan and Balick 2001). Textual sources such as the *Charaka Samhita* and classical Materia Medica record detailed formulations, dosing guidelines, and therapeutic strategies rooted in traditional systems like Ayurveda and TCM (Paul and Ray 2023). The pharmacological principles embedded in these systems emphasized the synergy between multiple plant constituents, a concept now being explored through modern pharmacognosy and network pharmacology approaches (Li and Zhang 2013; Williamson 2001).

2.2 Present Scenario

In recent years, the field of phytoceuticals has witnessed significant growth, supported by modern pharmaceutical techniques, biotechnology, and molecular biology. Phytoceuticals have become integral to preventive health, dietary supplements, and alternative medicine.

Advancements such as high-performance liquid chromatography (HPLC), metabolomics, and artificial intelligence (AI)-assisted drug discovery are now being applied to accelerate the identification of therapeutic phytochemicals (Subramoniam 2014; Lin et al. 2022). Moreover, innovative delivery systems like nanocarriers and 3D printing have improved the bioavailability of phytoceuticals, enabling more efficient targeting of diseases (Dima et al. 2021). Personalized medicine has also influenced the development of phytoceuticals, allowing for treatments tailored to an individual's genetic profile. Plant-based compounds like turmeric and cannabidiol (CBD) have gained widespread attention for their potential benefits in managing conditions such as chronic inflammation, anxiety, and pain, with ongoing research exploring their efficacy (Singh et al. 2023).

2.3 Challenges

Despite the promising developments, the integration of phytoceuticals into mainstream medicine faces several challenges:

2.3.1 Bioavailability and Efficacy

Many plant-derived compounds have poor bioavailability, making it difficult for the body to absorb or utilize them effectively. While advances in nanotechnology and delivery systems have improved absorption, bioavailability remains a major challenge (Rombolà et al. 2020).

2.3.2 Lack of Standardization

Variability in plant cultivation, harvesting, and extraction methods makes it difficult to ensure consistent quality and potency. This inconsistency can undermine consumer trust and hinder the regulatory acceptance of phytoceuticals as therapeutic agents (Abdullah et al. 2023a, b).

2.3.3 Regulatory Challenges

Unlike pharmaceutical drugs, which are subject to rigorous clinical trials and regulatory scrutiny, phytoceuticals are often marketed as dietary supplements with less stringent regulations. This regulatory gap raises concerns about product safety, especially when phytoceuticals interact with prescription medications, leading to adverse effects or diminished efficacy (Prajapati et al. 2023).

2.3.4 Limited Clinical Evidence

Despite their deep roots in traditional medicine, many phytoceuticals still lack strong clinical validation through large-scale, randomized trials. While several plant-derived compounds demonstrate promise in early-phase studies, very few advance to comprehensive phase III trials. This is often due to constraints such as high research costs, limited intellectual property protection, and complex regulatory pathways. As a result, the absence of high-quality clinical data continues to restrict the integration of phytoceuticals into mainstream, evidence-based healthcare (Petrini 2002).

2.3.5 Herbal-Drug Interactions

Herbal medicines have been used for treating a wide range of ailments for centuries, and their use alongside prescription medications has become increasingly common. However, this combination can lead to herb–drug interactions (HDIs), which may significantly alter the effectiveness of the prescribed drugs. These interactions often occur through pharmacokinetic mechanisms, affecting how the body absorbs, distributes, metabolizes, and eliminates drugs. Many HDIs arise due to herbal medicines' influence on enzymes such as cytochrome P450 (CYP3A4, CYP2C9, CYP1A2) and transporters like P-glycoprotein. For instance, St. John's Wort, widely used for depression, increases the activity of CYP3A4 and P-glycoprotein, thereby speeding up the metabolism of certain medications. It can also cause serotonin syndrome when used in combination with serotonin reuptake inhibitors (Ghosh et al. 2018).

2.3.6 Consumer Awareness and Education

As the phytoceutical market grows, consumer education is critical. Many individuals may not be aware of the potential risks, side effects, or interactions associated with phytoceuticals. This lack of understanding can lead to misuse, such as improper dosages or combining phytoceuticals with other treatments (Asokkumar and Ramachandran 2020).

3 Novel Drug Delivery Systems

Phytoceuticals are recently gaining a lot of popularity due to their promising pharmacological action with minimal adverse effects. But the problem regarding the use of phytoceuticals is alarming due to their poor bioavailability. Several novel approaches have been proposed to improve the bioavailability and therapeutic activity of these phytoceuticals. Advancements in the nanodelivery systems have led to improved bioavailability and activity of several drugs, as the active pharmaceutical ingredient gets released and distributed more prominently. Improved action of phytoceuticals using nano drug delivery systems is now widely used. A graphical illustration of various novel drug delivery systems and their common routes of administration is depicted in Fig. 1.

3.1 Liposomes

Liposomes are the most common nano-formulations used to improve the bioavailability of various phytoceuticals. Numerous examples of preclinical studies have been reported in which various phytoceuticals have been encapsulated in liposomes to increase therapeutic activity. In an in vitro study by Ng et al. (2018), curcumin was loaded in liposomes and applied directly on bronchial epithelial cells, where reduction of pro-inflammatory cytokines was reported, supporting the better activity of a phytoceutical in alleviating disease (Ng et al. 2018). A recent study was involved the combined use of berberine and magnolol against A549 lung carcinoma cell lines. Modulation of the apoptotic pathways was observed, and liposomes enhanced the stability and release of the combined phytoceuticals, suggesting a better activity

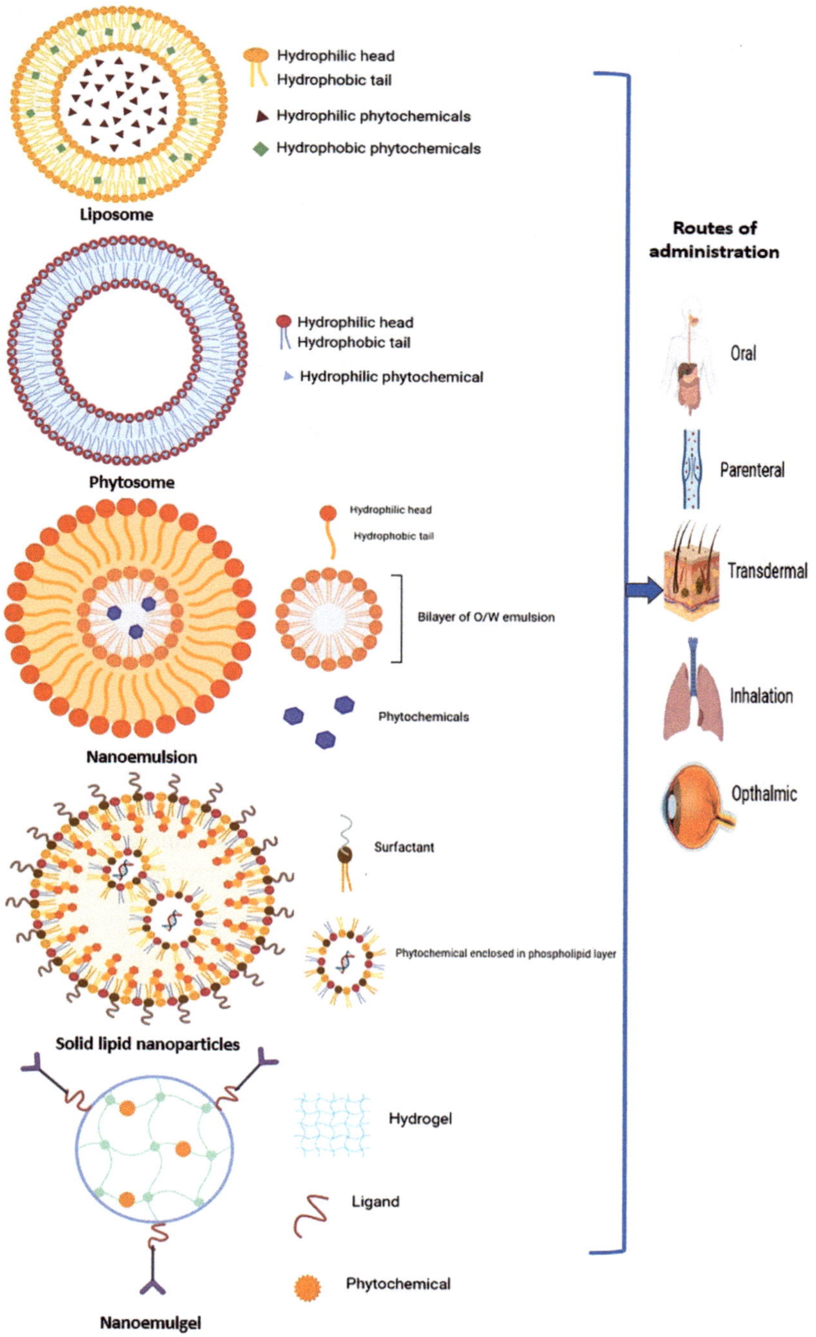

Fig. 1 Some common novel drug delivery systems of phytoceuticals

of phytoceuticals when moulded in liposomes (Ma et al. 2023). Further advancements to the previous research were also made, in which curcumin loaded in specialized liposomal bilayers efficiently induced metastasis in A549 cell lines by inhibiting cell growth and downregulating pro-oncogenic proteins expression (Singh et al. 2024).

3.2 Phytosomes

A newer and novel approach to targeted drug delivery systems is phytosomes. The basic concept of phytosomes is similar to that of liposomes. The phytoconstituents which are poorly absorbed and have less bioavailability are targeted to be delivered by phytosomes. Some major phytoconstituents like polyphenols have very low bioavailability, so to improve that condition, they are complexed with phospholipids and transformed into molecular complexes, which are lipid compatible (Vrushabh et al. 2025). Divakar and Lakshmidevi (2012) inferred that *Wrightia arborea* extract encapsulated in phytosomes have potent wound healing effect, which is better than the effect caused by *Wrightia arborea* extract itself (Divakar and Lakshmidevi 2012). Several reports of silymarin phytosomes have been reported to have better hepatoprotective effect in comparison to silymarin alone (Tedesco et al. 2004). Green tea extract encapsulated in phytosomes has shown better free radical scavenging activity rather than direct application of phytosomes (Manach et al. 2004). Other research has also been performed where several pharmacological effects were advanced after phytochemicals were administered post-entrapment in phytosomes (Kareparamban et al. 2012). Several recent studies regarding the use of phytoceuticals encapsulated in phytosomes against obesity have also emerged (Adiki et al. 2023). Topical drug delivery systems with phytoceuticals have also been improved after the use of phytosomes (Vrushabh et al. 2025).

3.3 Nanoemulsions

Another novel formulation is the nanoemulsion, where submicron colloidal particles of 20–200 nm size are made, and the active pharmaceutical ingredient is given along with the micro particles. De Rubis et al. (2023) conducted an in vitro experiment, where Agarwood oil nanoemulsion was successfully able to abate the inflammation and downregulate markers of oxidative stress in BCi-NS1.1 airway basal epithelial cells (De Rubis et al. 2023). A similar kind of recent research by Malik et al. (2023) also postulated the concept of anti-inflammatory effect exerted by Agarwood oil nanoemulsion against LPS-induced oxidative stress and inflammation in RAW264.7 mouse macrophages (Malik et al. 2023). Some other discoveries include the application of quercetin-loaded nanoemulsion against the A549 human lung carcinoma cell line, where significant reduction of growth and viability of the cells was found (Yeung et al. 2024).

3.4 Solid Lipid Nanoparticles (SLNs)

A much more precise method of drug delivery with low bioavailability is with the help of Solid Lipid Nanoparticles (SLN). This type of delivery system is appropriate for drugs which are easily biodegradable and those drugs, which have a lower retention time in the body. A study by Wang et al. (2012) implied the use of curcumin encapsulated in solid lipid nanoparticles against rat OVA cell lines. Significant improvement in asthmatic conditions by reduction of T-helper-2 type cytokines formation was noted (Wang et al. 2012). Increased bioavailability and pharmacological effect of berberine encapsulated in chitosan-coated solid lipid nanoparticle was observed against COPD in Cigarette Smoke Exposed Rats (Liu et al. 2022).

3.5 Nanostructured Lipid Carriers (NLCs)

Modern pharmaceutical formulations aim to provide a pharmacological effect directly to the target for maximum effect. Nanostructured Lipid Carriers or NLCs aim to encapsulate phytoceuticals with low bioavailability and minimal retention time in the body. Awasthi et al. (2022) used NLC technology to encapsulate curcumin and mesalamine and observe the activity in nitric oxide generation. Prominent reduction of keratinocyte proliferation with reduced inflammation was inferred when tested on keratinocytes and RAW264.7 cells in vitro (Awasthi et al. 2022). In a recent study against idiopathic pulmonary fibrosis, when ciprofloxacin and montelukast were used entrapped in NLCs much improved pharmacological effect was observed in pulmonary conditions (Suriya Prakaash and Narayansamy 2025).

3.6 Polymeric Nanoparticles

Similar approaches of targeted drug therapy using novel formulations have been implied by the use of polymeric nanoparticles. Targeting carcinogenic cells with anticancer medications has been difficult due to their low activity on the selective target. Enhancement of the anticancer drug using polymeric nanoparticles has been quite a development in the last century (Rizi et al. 2022).

3.7 Dendrimers

A much newer targeted therapy includes the application of dendrimers. They have a hooklike structure in which the phytoceuticals are attached and applied, which causes to have a direct effect on the target. Anticancer targeted therapy using phytoceuticals with dendrimers has been an area of research interest. Anticancer effect of quercetin attached with polyamidoamine dendrimers resulted in a much more potent action than quercetin alone (Madaan et al. 2016). Similarly, camptothecin, an alkaloid, has significant anticancer potential, along with severe adverse effects. Another experiment by Zolotarskaya et al. (2015) highlighted the reduced toxicity of camptothecin, with increased sustainability and targeted therapy when applied with polyamidoamine dendrimers (Zolotarskaya et al. 2015).

3.8 Nanoemulgel

Nanoemulgel comprises a nanogel, emulsified into a hydrogel for better stability of drugs and a targeted drug delivery system. Several advancements have been made in this form of novel drug delivery system for maximizing the therapeutic effect. Algahtani et al. (2021) studied the improved wound healing effect of thymoquinone nanoemulgel formulation compared to the conventional hydrogel system (Algahtani et al. 2021). Enhanced anti-nociceptive and anti-inflammatory effect of brucine-loaded nanoemulgel was observed compared to traditional hydrogel form (Saab et al. 2021). Sultan et al. (2022) investigated the improved antimicrobial effect of *Nigella sativa* oil when formulated as nanoemulgel, observed against *Staphylococcus aureus* strain (ATCC 29213) (Sultan et al. 2022).

4 Green Extraction Technologies

Common extraction methodologies have been applied for several centuries in order to isolate the active phytochemical from the respective plants. But one major drawback of conventional extraction processes includes higher consumption of energy without obtaining maximum yield. This has led to the discovery of Green Extraction technologies. Green extraction is defined as a modified process of extraction where phytochemicals are effectively extracted using the least energy, along with the application of renewable natural products and various solvents, which can be reused for producing maximum yield.

4.1 Ultrasound-Assisted Extraction (UAE)

Ultrasound-Assisted Extraction (UAE) is a novel technique for the isolation of the phytoconstituent mass from the plant extract into the respective solvent. Application of high temperatures causes an increase in the size and number of bubbles formed, which enhances the cavitation phenomena and performs the extraction process much more effectively and efficiently. *Erica australis* is a plant which has several proven pharmacological effects, and to improve the extraction process for better targeted therapy, UAE technology was applied (Carrera et al. 2021). Similarly, Dai et al. (2021) used the UAE method to isolate five potent anthraquinones from *Rheum palmatum* aqueous extract, which have been inferred to have some prominent antimicrobial effect (Dai et al. 2021).

4.2 Microwave-Assisted Extraction (MAE)

Similar to the UAE, Microwave-Assisted Extraction (MAE) is also quite common for the extraction of phytoceuticals from the respective plant extracts. Microwave is used to properly extract the phytoceutical mass as the energy consumption is much lower in comparison to other extraction techniques. Vázquez-Espinosa et al. (2019) used MAE to isolate capsinoids from peppers, which have a potent antioxidant property (Vázquez-Espinosa et al. 2019). Similarly, Patra et al. (2021) inferred that the MAE of *Anacardium occidentale* L. led to significant improvement in phytoceutical yield as compared to conventional extraction techniques (Patra et al. 2021).

4.3 Supercritical Fluid Extraction (SFE)

Compared to previous conventional extraction techniques, using a solvent with or without agitation, Supercritical Fluid Extraction (SFE) is a huge step up in the extraction domain. Supercritical CO_2 is used for the isolation of solute from the extracted solution, and the solvent can be recovered and reused more effectively. A successful SFE of caffeic acid derivatives from *Echinacea purpurea* was performed by Konar et al. (2014) that have proven to have increased phytochemical yield compared to normal solvent extraction methods (Konar et al. 2014).

4.4 Pressurized Liquid Extraction (PLE)

Pressurized Liquid Extraction (PLE) involves the extraction of phytoceuticals from their respective plant extract under high temperature (around 200 °C) and high pressure (3.5–20 MPa). Several phytochemicals, including anthocyanin's, are promisingly extracted from plants via PLE as compared to other extraction techniques, which have been proven to have potential health benefits and an adjuvant to pharmacological therapies (de Barros et al. 2024). Various polyphenolics having antimicrobial effects have also been extracted with maximum percentage of yield from the fruit pomace via PLE (dos Santos et al. 2023).

4.5 Enzyme-Assisted Extraction (EAE)

During the extraction process of several plants, it has been observed that appropriate isolation of the phytoceuticals from the respective parts of the plants cannot be performed. The reason behind such an anomaly could be the strong entrapment of the phytochemicals within the plant parts that prevents their easy release. In such cases, Enzyme-Assisted Extraction (EAE) has been proven highly advantageous. Enzymes used during this process effectively hydrolyze various plant cell wall materials, including cellulose, pectin and glycosidic esters, which potentially recover entrapped phenolics in the solvent used during the extraction procedure. Qadir et al. (2019) used EAE to isolate different phenolics from *Momordica balsamina* that have different potential therapeutic effects (Qadir et al. 2019). Phenolics present in the peel of *Punica granatum* have a promising antioxidant effect, which could be used against various diseases of high oxidative stress and free radical formation. Kumar et al. (2020) applied the same principle of EAE to efficiently extract the phenolics, which is inferred to have a more antioxidant effect as compared to the normal extraction procedure (Kumar et al. 2020).

5 Computational Drug Discovery and Optimization of Phytoceuticals

The use of computational tools has transformed the initial stages of screening, optimization, and development of phytoceuticals. These methods help minimize time, expenses, and experimental labour, while also providing molecular-level mechanistic insights (Singh and Bharadvaja 2021). This section highlights the essential computational techniques, such as target prediction, molecular docking, ADMET profiling, and dynamic simulations, that are now commonly employed to drive the discovery and enhancement of bioactive compounds derived from plants. Table 1 depicts various in silico tools and databases that can be used for the identification of phytoceuticals.

Table 1 Key in silico tools and databases for phytoceutical discovery and optimization

Tool/database	Category	Application in phytoceuticals	Website/URL
TCMSP	Phytochemical Database	Screening traditional compounds, ADME filtering	tcmsp-e.com
IMPPAT	Phytochemical Database	Indian medicinal plant data and phytochemical profiling	cb.imsc.res.in/imppat
NPASS	Natural Product Database	Bioactive natural product data	bidd.group/NPASS
SwissTargetPrediction	Target Prediction Tool	Predicts protein targets of phytocompounds	swisstargetprediction.ch
SuperPred	Target Prediction Tool	Structure-based drug–target interaction prediction	prediction.charite.de
Cytoscape	Network Pharmacology Tool	Network visualization and compound–target mapping	cytoscape.org
STRING	Interaction Database	Protein–protein interaction mapping	string-db.org
AutoDock Vina	Molecular Docking Tool	Ligand–protein docking and binding affinity prediction	vina.scripps.edu
PyRx	Virtual Screening Tool	High-throughput docking using AutoDock Vina	pyrx.sourceforge.io
SwissADME	ADMET Prediction Tool	Bioavailability and drug-likeness prediction	www.swissadme.ch
pkCSM	ADMET Prediction Tool	Predicts pharmacokinetic properties and toxicity	biosig.lab.uq.edu.au/pkcsm
GROMACS	MD Simulation Tool	Protein–ligand complex dynamics and stability analysis	gromacs.org
Desmond	MD Simulation Tool	High-speed molecular dynamics simulations	schrodinger.com/desmond
Gaussian	DFT Tool	Quantum chemical analysis and reactivity prediction	gaussian.com
ORCA	DFT Tool	HOMO–LUMO gap and electronic descriptors calculation	https://orcaforum.kofo.mpg.de/

5.1 Databases for Phytochemical Screening

Phytochemical discovery begins with structured data mining from curated databases. Resources such as PubChem, TCMSP (Traditional Chinese Medicine Systems Pharmacology Database), IMPPAT (Indian Medicinal Plants, Phytochemistry and Therapeutics), and NPASS provide comprehensive information on chemical structures, bioactivities, and traditional uses. These repositories are crucial for identifying lead candidates and standardizing compound information (Bultum et al. 2019; Ru et al. 2014; Mohanraj et al. 2018; Zeng et al. 2018).

5.2 Target Prediction Tools

To predict the molecular targets of phytochemicals, researchers commonly use tools such as SwissTargetPrediction and SuperPred. These platforms utilize data on structural similarities and bioactivity to forecast potential protein targets, aiding in the identification of therapeutic pathways and possible off-target interactions (Gfeller et al. 2014; Nickel et al. 2014).

5.3 Network Pharmacology

This approach examines phytochemicals across multiple targets and disease pathways at a systems level. By incorporating protein–protein interactions, gene expression data, and compound–target relationships, tools like Cytoscape, STRING, and others enable the visualization and formulation of hypotheses for complex herbal mixtures (Kohl et al. 2011; Szklarczyk et al. 2019).

5.4 Molecular Docking

Docking algorithms evaluate how phytochemicals interact with target proteins at the binding site level. Tools like AutoDock Vina, PyRx, and others are widely used for structure-based screening. Binding affinity scores and interaction residues help prioritize promising compounds for further validation (Trott and Olson 2010; Dallakyan and Olson 2015).

5.5 ADMET Profiling

ADMET (Absorption, Distribution, Metabolism, Excretion, and Toxicity) profiling predicts the pharmacokinetic behaviour and safety of compounds. Tools like SwissADME, pkCSM, and others evaluate factors such as oral bioavailability, blood–brain barrier (BBB) permeability, CYP inhibition, and toxicity risks, allowing for the early-stage elimination of unsuitable candidates (Daina et al. 2017; Pires et al. 2015).

5.6 5.6 Molecular Dynamics (MD) Simulation

MD simulation assesses the stability, conformational changes, and binding behaviour of protein–ligand complexes over time. Tools such as GROMACS, Desmond, and others simulate atomic interactions in a solvated environment, providing deeper insights that go beyond static docking poses (Abraham et al. 2015; Cole et al. 2015).

5.7 Density Functional Theory (DFT) Analysis

DFT is a quantum mechanical approach that predicts molecular reactivity, stability, and electronic behaviour. Tools such as Gaussian, ORCA, and others compute parameters like HOMO–LUMO gap, molecular electrostatic potential, and dipole moment, critical for understanding bioactivity at the electronic level (Volokhov et al. 2020; Neese 2022).

6 Conclusion and Future Perspectives

The renewed global interest in plant-based therapeutics has established phytoceuticals as an important bridge between traditional medicinal wisdom and modern pharmaceutical innovation. This chapter has highlighted how advancements in novel drug delivery systems, green extraction methods, in silico screening, and phytochemical profiling have contributed to improving the bioavailability, therapeutic precision, and standardization of phytoceuticals.

Despite these advancements, several challenges remain, most notably the limited availability of large-scale clinical trials, variability in raw material quality, and inconsistencies in regulatory standards across regions. Addressing these issues will require continued interdisciplinary collaboration and stronger integration of preclinical and clinical validation pathways.

Looking ahead, the incorporation of technologies such as 3D printing, advanced extraction techniques, metabolomic tools, and CRISPR-based plant optimization is expected to accelerate the development of next-generation phytoceuticals. These innovations hold the potential to enhance not only formulation stability and therapeutic efficacy but also scalability and personalization of treatment.

With growing consumer demand for natural and evidence-based interventions, phytoceuticals are well-positioned to become a central component of integrative and preventive healthcare in the years to come.

References

Abdullah A, Biswas P, Sahabuddin M et al (2023a) Molecular dynamics simulation and pharmacoinformatic integrated analysis of bioactive phytochemicals from Azadirachta indica (Neem) to treat diabetes mellitus. J Chem 2023:4170703. https://doi.org/10.1155/2023/4170703

Abdullah A, Khan F, Ali G et al (2023b) Phytonutrients standardization for effective therapeutic outcomes. In: Khan H, Aschner M, Mirzaei H (eds) Phytonutrients and neurological disorders. Academic, pp 19–31

Abraham MJ, Murtola T, Schulz R et al (2015) GROMACS: high performance molecular simulations through multi-level parallelism from laptops to supercomputers. SoftwareX 1:19–25

Adiki SK, Sangeetha S, Kamireddy S et al (2023) Phytosomes: a novel phytoconstituent delivery approach to improve the efficacy of obesity treatment. Curr Nutr Food Sci 19:229–237. https://doi.org/10.2174/1573401318666220901125859

Algahtani MS, Ahmad MZ, Shaikh IA et al (2021) Thymoquinone loaded topical nanoemulgel for wound healing: formulation design and in-vivo evaluation. Molecules 26:3863. https://doi.org/10.3390/molecules26133863

Alotaibi NM, Alotaibi MO, Alshammari N et al (2023) Network pharmacology combined with molecular docking, molecular dynamics, and in vitro experimental validation reveals the therapeutic potential of Thymus vulgaris L. essential oil (thyme oil) against human breast cancer. ACS Omega 8:48344–48359. https://doi.org/10.1021/acsomega.3c07782

Asokkumar K, Ramachandran S (2020) Herb-drug interactions: focus on adverse drug reactions and pharmacovigilance of herbal medicines. In: Sen S, Chakraborty R (eds) Herbal medicine in India: indigenous knowledge, practice, innovation and its value. Springer, Singapore, pp 547–571

Awasthi A, Kumar B, Gulati M et al (2022) Novel nanostructured lipid carriers co-loaded with mesalamine and curcumin: formulation, optimization and in vitro evaluation. Pharm Res 39:2817–2829. https://doi.org/10.1007/s11095-022-03401-z

BCC Research (2024) Global nutraceutical market: industry size & growth analysis. BCC Research. https://www.bccresearch.com/market-research/food-and-beverage/nutraceuticals-global-markets.html. Accessed 7 June 2025

Bultum LE, Woyessa AM, Lee D (2019) ETM-DB: integrated Ethiopian traditional herbal medicine and phytochemicals database. BMC Complement Altern Med 19:212. https://doi.org/10.1186/s12906-019-2634-1

Carrera C, Aliaño-González MJ, Rodríguez-López J et al (2021) Optimization of an ultrasound-assisted extraction method for the analysis of major anthocyanin content in Erica australis flowers. Molecules 26:2884. https://doi.org/10.3390/molecules26102884

Chakraborty K, Shivakumar A, Ramachandran S (2016) Nanotechnology in herbal medicines: a review. Int J Herb Med 4:21–27

Cole DJ, Tirado-Rives J, Jorgensen WL (2015) Molecular dynamics and Monte Carlo simulations for protein–ligand binding and inhibitor design. Biochim Biophys Acta 1850:966–971

Colombo R, Cavalloro V, Papetti A et al (2023) Evolving challenges and opportunities in plant-based drug discovery and development. In: Ethnobotany and ethnopharmacology of medicinal and aromatic plants. CRC Press

Dai L-X, Li J-C, Miao X-L et al (2021) Ultrasound-assisted extraction of five anthraquinones from Rheum palmatum water extract residues and the antimicrobial activities. Ind Crops Prod 162:113288. https://doi.org/10.1016/j.indcrop.2021.113288

Daina A, Michielin O, Zoete V (2017) SwissADME: a free web tool to evaluate pharmacokinetics, drug-likeness and medicinal chemistry friendliness of small molecules. Sci Rep 7:42717

Dallakyan S, Olson AJ (2015) Small-molecule library screening by docking with PyRx. In: Hempel JE, Williams CH, Hong CC (eds) Chemical biology. Springer, New York, NY, pp 243–250

de Barros GL, Silva FTS, Teixeira RS et al (2024) Anthocyanin extraction methods: synthesis of morpho-anatomical knowledge for decision-making based on decision-tree. Int J Food Prop 27:1315–1346. https://doi.org/10.1080/10942912.2024.2409893

De Rubis G, Paudel KR, Manandhar B et al (2023) Agarwood oil nanoemulsion attenuates cigarette smoke-induced inflammation and oxidative stress markers in BCi-NS1.1 airway epithelial cells. Nutrients 15:1019. https://doi.org/10.3390/nu15041019

Dima C, Assadpour E, Dima S, Jafari SM (2021) Nutraceutical nanodelivery: an insight into the bioaccessibility/bioavailability of different bioactive compounds loaded within nanocarriers. Crit Rev Food Sci Nutr 61:3031–3065. https://doi.org/10.1080/10408398.2020.1792409

Divakar M, Lakshmidevi S (2012) Wound healing activity of the leaves of Wrightia tinctoria (Roxb.) R. Br. Indian Drugs 49(3):40–46

dos Santos LF, Lopes ST, Nazari MT et al (2023) Fruit pomace as a promising source to obtain biocompounds with antibacterial activity. Crit Rev Food Sci Nutr 63:12597–12609. https://doi.org/10.1080/10408398.2022.2103510

Ernst E (2005) The efficacy of herbal medicine—an overview. Fundam Clin Pharmacol 19:405–409. https://doi.org/10.1111/j.1472-8206.2005.00335.x

Gfeller D, Grosdidier A, Wirth M et al (2014) SwissTargetPrediction: a web server for target prediction of bioactive small molecules. Nucleic Acids Res 42:W32–W38

Ghosh N, Ghosh RC, Kundu A, Mandal SC (2018) Herb and drug interaction. In: Natural products and drug discovery. Elsevier, pp 467–490

Grand View Research (2024) Herbal medicine market size to reach $328.72Bn by 2030. Grand View Research. https://www.grandviewresearch.com/press-release/global-herbal-medicine-market. Accessed 7 June 2025

Hart BL (2005) The evolution of herbal medicine: behavioural perspectives. Anim Behav 70:975–989. https://doi.org/10.1016/j.anbehav.2005.03.005

Kalita I, Bhattacharjee S, Saharia M (2025) Advancements in medicinal plant research: harnessing artificial intelligence, machine learning, deep learning, and bioinformatics. In: Biotechnology, multiple omics, and precision breeding in medicinal plants. CRC Press

Kareparamban JA, Nikam PH, Jadhav AP, Kadam VJ (2012) Phytosome: a novel revolution in herbal drugs. IJRPC 2:299–310

Khan S, Balick MJ (2001) Therapeutic plants of Ayurveda: a review of selected clinical and other studies for 166 species. J Altern Complement Med 7:405–515. https://doi.org/10.1089/10755530152639729

Kohl M, Wiese S, Warscheid B (2011) Cytoscape: software for visualization and analysis of biological networks. In: Hamacher M, Eisenacher M, Stephan C (eds) Data mining in proteomics. Humana Press, Totowa, pp 291–303

Konar N, Dalabasmaz S, Poyrazoglu ES et al (2014) The determination of the caffeic acid derivatives of Echinacea purpurea aerial parts under various extraction conditions by supercritical fluid extraction (SFE). J Supercrit Fluids 89:128–136. https://doi.org/10.1016/j.supflu.2014.02.014

Kumar M, Tomar M, Punia S et al (2020) Evaluation of cellulolytic enzyme-assisted microwave extraction of Punica granatum peel phenolics and antioxidant activity. Plant Foods Hum Nutr 75:614–620. https://doi.org/10.1007/s11130-020-00859-3

Lee S-Y, Shin YW, Hahm K-B (2008) Phytoceuticals: mighty but ignored weapons against helicobacter pylori infection. J Dig Dis 9:129–139. https://doi.org/10.1111/j.1751-2980.2008.00334.x

Li S, Zhang B (2013) Traditional Chinese medicine network pharmacology: theory, methodology and application. Chin J Nat Med 11:110–120. https://doi.org/10.1016/S1875-5364(13)60037-0

Li X, Liang S, Tan CH et al (2021) Nanocarriers in the enhancement of therapeutic efficacy of natural drugs. BIO Integr 2:40

Lin Y, Zhang Y, Wang D et al (2022) Computer especially AI-assisted drug virtual screening and design in traditional Chinese medicine. Phytomedicine 107:154481. https://doi.org/10.1016/j.phymed.2022.154481

Liu H, Li Y, Zhang X et al (2022) Chitosan-coated solid lipid nano-encapsulation improves the therapeutic antiairway inflammation effect of berberine against COPD in cigarette smoke-exposed rats. Can Respir J 2022:8509396. https://doi.org/10.1155/2022/8509396

Ma X, Sui X, Liu C et al (2023) Co-delivery of berberine and magnolol targeted liposomes for synergistic anti-lung cancer. Colloids Surf A Physicochem Eng Asp 673:131773. https://doi.org/10.1016/j.colsurfa.2023.131773

Madaan K, Lather V, Pandita D (2016) Evaluation of polyamidoamine dendrimers as potential carriers for quercetin, a versatile flavonoid. Drug Deliv 23:254–262. https://doi.org/10.3109/10717544.2014.910564

Malik R, Paudel KR, Manandhar B et al (2023) Agarwood oil nanoemulsion counteracts LPS-induced inflammation and oxidative stress in RAW264.7 mouse macrophages. Pathol Res Pract 251:154895. https://doi.org/10.1016/j.prp.2023.154895

Manach C, Scalbert A, Morand C et al (2004) Polyphenols: food sources and bioavailability. Am J Clin Nutr 79:727–747. https://doi.org/10.1093/ajcn/79.5.727

Mohanraj K, Karthikeyan BS, Vivek-Ananth RP et al (2018) IMPPAT: a curated database of Indian medicinal plants, phytochemistry and therapeutics. Sci Rep 8:4329

Neese F (2022) Software update: the ORCA program system—version 5.0. WIREs Comput Mol Sci 12:e1606. https://doi.org/10.1002/wcms.1606

Ng ZY, Wong J-Y, Panneerselvam J et al (2018) Assessing the potential of liposomes loaded with curcumin as a therapeutic intervention in asthma. Colloids Surf B Biointerfaces 172:51–59. https://doi.org/10.1016/j.colsurfb.2018.08.027

Nickel J, Gohlke B-O, Erehman J et al (2014) SuperPred: update on drug classification and target prediction. Nucleic Acids Res 42:W26–W31

Patra A, Abdullah S, Pradhan RC (2021) Microwave-assisted extraction of bioactive compounds from cashew apple (Anacardium occidentale L.) bagasse: modeling and optimization of the process using response surface methodology. Food Meas 15:4781–4793. https://doi.org/10.1007/s11694-021-01042-1

Paul SR, Ray S (2023) A critical analysis on 'Theory of Knowledge' (epistemology) of Charaka Samhita and its importance in clinical medicine. Int Res J Ayurveda Yoga. https://doi.org/10.48165/IRJAY.2023.6910

Petrini O (2002) Clinical development of phytopharmaceuticals. Wien Med Wochenschr 152:204–208

Pires DEV, Blundell TL, Ascher DB (2015) pkCSM: predicting small-molecule pharmacokinetic and toxicity properties using graph-based signatures. J Med Chem 58:4066–4072. https://doi.org/10.1021/acs.jmedchem.5b00104

Prajapati P, Pathan A, Prajapati D (2023) Phytopharmaceuticals regulatory requirements and licensing process. Int J Drug Regul Aff 11:43–52

Qadir R, Anwar F, Batool F et al (2019) Enzyme-assisted extraction of Momordica balsamina L. fruit phenolics: process optimized by response surface methodology. J Food Meas Charact 13:697–706. https://doi.org/10.1007/s11694-018-9982-2

Rizi HAY, Shin DH, Rizi SY (2022) Polymeric nanoparticles in cancer chemotherapy: a narrative review. Iran J Public Health 51:226

Rombolà L, Scuteri D, Marilisa S et al (2020) Pharmacokinetic interactions between herbal medicines and drugs: their mechanisms and clinical relevance. Life 10:106. https://doi.org/10.3390/life10070106

Ru J, Li P, Wang J et al (2014) TCMSP: a database of systems pharmacology for drug discovery from herbal medicines. J Cheminform 6:13. https://doi.org/10.1186/1758-2946-6-13

Saab M, Raafat K, El-Maradny H (2021) Transdermal delivery of capsaicin nanoemulgel: optimization, skin permeation and in vivo activity against diabetic neuropathy. Adv Pharm Bull 12:780–790. https://doi.org/10.34172/apb.2022.080

Singh H, Bharadvaja N (2021) Treasuring the computational approach in medicinal plant research. Prog Biophys Mol Biol 164:19–32. https://doi.org/10.1016/j.pbiomolbio.2021.05.004

Singh A, Kalaivani M, Chaudhary P et al (2019) Opportunities and challenges in development of phytopharmaceutical drug in India—a SWOT analysis. J Young Pharm 11:322

Singh K, Bhushan B, Chanchal DK et al (2023) Emerging therapeutic potential of cannabidiol (CBD) in neurological disorders: a comprehensive review. Behav Neurol 2023:8825358. https://doi.org/10.1155/2023/8825358

Singh M, De Rubis G, Kokkinis S et al (2024) Curcumin-loaded liposomes modulating the synergistic role of EpCAM and estrogen receptor alpha in lung cancer management. Pathol Res Pract 257:155317. https://doi.org/10.1016/j.prp.2024.155317

Subramoniam A (2014) Present scenario, challenges and future perspectives in plant-based medicine development. Ann Phytomed 3:31–36

Sultan MH, Javed S, Madkhali OA et al (2022) Development and optimization of methylcellulose-based nanoemulgel loaded with Nigella sativa oil for oral health management: quadratic model approach. Molecules 27:1796. https://doi.org/10.3390/molecules27061796

Suriya Prakaash KK, Narayansamy D (2025) Advancements in nanotechnology for targeted drug delivery in idiopathic pulmonary fibrosis: a focus on solid lipid nanoparticles and nanostructured lipid carriers. Drug Dev Ind Pharm 51:285–294. https://doi.org/10.1080/03639045.2025.2468811

Szklarczyk D, Gable AL, Lyon D et al (2019) STRING v11: protein–protein association networks with increased coverage, supporting functional discovery in genome-wide experimental datasets. Nucleic Acids Res 47:D607–D613

Tedesco D, Steidler S, Galletti S et al (2004) Efficacy of silymarin-phospholipid complex in reducing the toxicity of aflatoxin B1 in broiler chicks. Poult Sci 83:1839–1843. https://doi.org/10.1093/ps/83.11.1839

Trott O, Olson AJ (2010) AutoDock Vina: improving the speed and accuracy of docking with a new scoring function, efficient optimization, and multithreading. J Comput Chem 31:455–461. https://doi.org/10.1002/jcc.21334

Vázquez-Espinosa M, González de Peredo AV, Ferreiro-González M et al (2019) Optimizing and comparing ultrasound- and microwave-assisted extraction methods applied to the extraction of antioxidant capsinoids in peppers. Agronomy 9:633. https://doi.org/10.3390/agronomy9100633

Volokhov V, Zyubina T, Volokhov A et al (2020) Predictive quantum-chemical design of molecules of high-energy heterocyclic compounds. In: Voevodin V, Sobolev S (eds) Supercomputing. Springer, Cham, pp 310–319

Vrushabh MS, Atram DSC, Dipali BV et al (2025) Review on phytosome for topical drug delivery. Asian J Pharm Res Dev 13:131–137. https://doi.org/10.22270/ajprd.v13i3.1566

Wang W, Zhu R, Xie Q et al (2012) Enhanced bioavailability and efficiency of curcumin for the treatment of asthma by its formulation in solid lipid nanoparticles. Int J Nanomedicine 7:3667–3677. https://doi.org/10.2147/IJN.S30428

Williamson EM (2001) Synergy and other interactions in phytomedicines. Phytomedicine 8:401–409. https://doi.org/10.1078/0944-7113-00060

World Health Organization (2023) Integrating traditional medicine in health care. WHO Feature Story. https://www.who.int/southeastasia/news/feature-stories/detail/integrating-traditional-medicine. Accessed 7 June 2025

Yeung S, Paudel KR, Rubis GD et al (2024) Exploring the current advancements of quercetin nanoformulations alleviating respiratory diseases. Future Med Chem 16:925–928. https://doi.org/10.1080/17568919.2024.2347067

Yuan H, Ma Q, Ye L, Piao G (2016) The traditional medicine and modern medicine from natural products. Molecules 21:559. https://doi.org/10.3390/molecules21050559

Zeng X, Zhang P, He W et al (2018) NPASS: natural product activity and species source database for natural product research, discovery and tool development. Nucleic Acids Res 46:D1217–D1222

Zolotarskaya OY, Xu L, Valerie K, Yang H (2015) Click synthesis of a polyamidoamine dendrimer-based camptothecin prodrug. RSC Adv 5:58600–58608. https://doi.org/10.1039/C5RA07987J

Biotechnological and Quality Enhancements

Epigenetic Reprogramming by Endophytes: Unlocking Silent Biosynthetic Gene Clusters for Next-Generation Phytopharmaceuticals

Shraddha Patel, Chandrabhan Prajapati, Sachchida Nand Rai, Partha Palit, and Santosh Kumar Singh

Abstract Endophytes that live in plant tissues without causing any symptoms have become major sources of biologically active secondary metabolites that have important medicinal applications. These endophytic fungi and bacteria are capable of synthesizing a diverse range of compounds that are similar to their host plants' metabolites. Major classes of secondary metabolites created by endophytes include alkaloids, phenolics, flavonoids, terpenoids, and polyketides. Such metabolites display a broad range of biological activities, comprising antimicrobial, anticancer, antioxidant, anti-inflammatory, antidiabetic, cardioprotective, and neuroprotective effects. Notable compounds such as Taxol, huperzine A, resveratrol, pestacin, and vincristine have been identified from various endophytic species and are being explored for their role in the treatment of cancer, neurological disorders, cardiovascular diseases, and microbial infections. The ability of endophytes to express silent biosynthetic gene clusters and adapt metabolite production in response to host or environmental cues further enhances their biotechnological value. Advances in co-culture strategies and epigenetic modulation have improved metabolite yields and enabled the discovery of novel compounds. As sustainable alternatives to plant harvesting, endophytes hold immense promise for drug discovery and development, offering a renewable and eco-friendly source of pharmacologically active molecules. Continued exploration of endophytic diversity at different geographical locations may unlock new pathways for therapeutic innovation.

S. Patel · C. Prajapati · S. N. Rai · S. K. Singh (✉)
Centre of Experimental Medicine and Surgery, Institute of Medical Sciences, Banaras Hindu University, Varanasi, Uttar Pradesh, India
e-mail: shraddhapatel@bhu.ac.in; cbbhu.123@bhu.ac.in; snchaurasia@bhu.ac.in; santosh.singh01@bhu.ac.in

P. Palit
Drug Discovery Research Laboratory, Assam University, Silchar, Department of Pharmaceutical Sciences, Silchar, Assam, India

S. Kumar Tripathi et al. (eds.), *Phytoceuticals for Sustainable Medication*, Interdisciplinary Biotechnological Advances,
https://doi.org/10.1007/978-981-95-7588-6_4

Keywords Endophytes · Secondary metabolite · Fungi · Bacteria · Antioxidant · Anticancer

1 Introduction

Endophytes stand as a diverse group of microbes that exist asymptomatically inside the internal tissues of healthy plants, without causing any immediate disease symptoms. The word "endophyte" is derived from the Greek words *endon* (within) and *phyton* (plant), reflecting their ecological niche (Petrini 1991; Schulz and Boyle 2005). Common entry sites for endophytes include natural openings such as root hairs or lateral roots, stomata, wounds, and hydathodes on above-ground parts of the plant (Hardoim et al. 2015). Once inside, these endophytes primarily colonize the intercellular spaces across numerous plant parts, like root, stem, leaves, and flower (Kandel et al. 2017). They have been noted from plants thriving in various environments, including tropical, temperate, cold, hot, and even deep-sea regions (Ali et al. 2018; Calado et al. 2021; Janso and Carter 2010). Furthermore, seaweeds and marine algal species act as hosts (Lini et al. 2020). Based on the host genetic makeup, age, tissue variety, and atmospheric variables, these bacteria develop complicated relations with their hosts, which can range from beneficial and commensal to latent harmful associations (Agler et al. 2016; Coleman-Derr et al. 2016; Wagner et al. 2016). Endophytes are separated from various plant sections, including stems and roots, by employing appropriate sterilizing techniques. The bioactive metabolites of these microorganisms are then obtained by cultivating them on plates containing media. Several solvents are used to extract their secondary metabolites, which are then separated and chemically characterized using methods such as chromatography, nuclear magnetic resonance (NMR), and Fourier transform infrared spectroscopy (FTIR) (Fig. 1). These endophytes are well known to produce an extensive range of metabolites, involving those that were previously thought to be exclusive to higher plants (Nicoletti and Fiorentino 2015). Endophytes are essential to plant health because they increase plant development by generating phytohormones, increasing resistance to stress, and creating natural insecticides that provide herbivore protection; they also protect plants from pathogens by competing for colonization sites and nutrients and initiating plant resistance machineries (Abdelaziz et al. 2022; Badawy et al. 2021; Heydari and Pessarakli 2010). In recent years, the separation and study of endophytes and the exploration of their natural products have drawn a lot of interest from scientists. These endophytes possess remarkable potential for synthesizing a wide variety of chemically distinct secondary metabolites, like terpenes, alkaloids, phenols, isocoumarins, and steroids, offering valuable applications across pharmaceutical, agricultural, and other industrial sectors (Manganyi and Ateba 2020; Passari et al. 2017; Rai et al. 2014) (Fig. 2). Various studies have identified these bioactive compounds with broad therapeutic potential, exhibiting anti-inflammatory (Tan et al. 2020), antifungal (Abdou et al. 2020), antidiabetic (Al-Hosni et al. 2020), antiviral (Ding et al. 2010), anticancer,

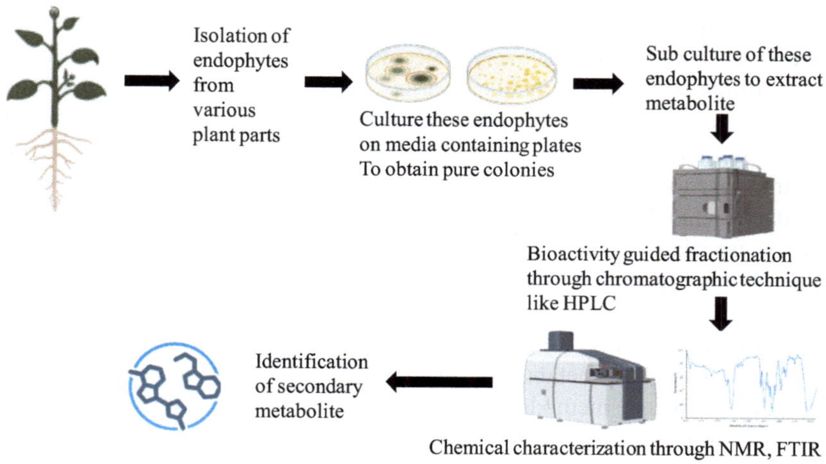

Fig. 1 Schematic representation of various steps involved in the isolation of endophytes from plants and the identification of secondary metabolites. Healthy fragments of plant from leaf, stem, and roots are used to isolate endophytes. To get rid of impurities, these tissues are cleansed, sliced into tiny pieces, and surface sterilized. After that, the pieces are put on nutrient plates to cultivate microorganisms, and subculturing is used to produce pure microbial strains. The species is identified with the use of molecular techniques. The microbes are cultured in media to produce metabolites, and the chemicals are extracted using organic solvents. The most promising extracts are identified by screening them for biological activity. Purification of the active ingredients is aided by methods such as column chromatography, HPTLC, and HPLC. Spectroscopic techniques like mass spectrometry, FT-IR, and NMR are used to study their structures. The purified chemicals are next examined for various kinds of bioactivity. (The drawing was created by using templates from biorender.com)

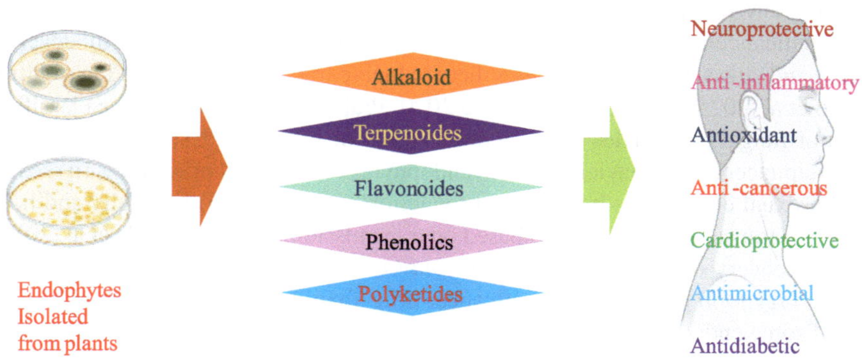

Fig. 2 The diagram illustrates different classes of secondary metabolites produced by endophytes and their application in various medical condition

and other biological activities (Hashem et al. 2023; Prajapati et al. 2024b, 2025b). Numerous pharmacological effects have been shown by these endophyte-derived metabolites, many of which have unique structures not present in other natural sources. Through symbiotic adaptation, endophytes can synthesize chemicals that are similar to plants or completely different from them, making them attractive substitutes for existing drug discovery processes that struggle with issues like resistance to drugs and minimal chemical variety. As a result, a detailed investigation of endophytic secondary metabolites is crucial for both finding novel lead compounds and creating environmentally friendly, sustainable supplies of therapeutic medicines that have the potential to transform contemporary medicine. The generation of secondary metabolites by endophytes and their importance in the pharmaceutical industry, especially in the treatment of various disease, are the main topics of this chapter. It draws attention to the extraordinary diversity of endophytic microorganisms, including bacteria and fungi as well as their ability to generate a broad range of bioactive compounds that may have therapeutic uses. The chapter also looks at the different ways these metabolites are used to treat different illnesses. Furthermore, it talks about effective methods that have been used to increase the yield and variety of metabolite production, such as cocultivation along with various cutting-edge techniques. The main objective of this chapter is to highlight the crucial role of endophytes specially bacteria and fungi as a sustainable and valuable source of secondary metabolites and to underline their growing importance in drug discovery and disease management.

2 Type and Diversity of Endophytes

2.1 Fungal Endophyte

Fungal endophytes are microorganisms that live symbiotically within plant tissues lacking any harm. They produce diverse secondary metabolites having antimicrobial, anticancer, and antioxidant properties. Endophytes also enhance plant development and stress resistance, making them valuable in both medicine and agriculture (Gao et al. 2025; Manganyi and Ateba 2020; Prajapati et al. 2025a). The classification of fungal endophytes is based on a variety of standards. Examples include (i) clavicipitaceous/nonclavicipitaceous endophytes on the basis of ecology, (ii) sexual and asexual endophytes based on reproduction mode, and (iii) vertically and horizontally transmitted endophytes based on transmission mode (Bamisile et al. 2018). The discovery of endophytic fungi *Taxomyces andreanae*, from the inner bark of *Taxus brevifolia* producing the anticancer drug Taxol has raised interest in the ability of some endophytic fungi to create chemicals linked to secondary metabolism in plants (Stierle et al. 1993). A number of research teams have since investigated endophytic fungi for the synthesis of related secondary metabolites. Fungal endophyte *Cochliobolus hawaiiensis* has been isolated from *Millingtonia hortensis* L.f. (Pandy et al. 2023). *Aspergillus, Trichoderma,* Fusarium, *Penicillium, Colletotrichum,* and *Chaetomium* are some of the endophytic fungal taxa that are most frequently reported. These fungi have the capacity to generate a wide range of chemically distinct secondary metabolites, including alkaloids, phenolics, terpenes, xanthone, quinones, coumarins, and flavonoids, which are known to have antiviral, antifungal, and antibacterial properties (Attia et al. 2022; Prajapati et al. 2024a). An endophytic fungus *Hormonema dematioides* isolated from *Juniperus communis* produced a range of cyclic dipeptides with potent antimicrobial activity (Kim and Cheng 2024). From *Lagopsis supine*, five endophytic fungus from the genera *Alternaria* and *Aspergillus* were isolated (Zhang et al. 2022). The endophytic fungus *Aspergillus niger* has been linked to *Ficus retusa* (Moglad et al. 2023). A total of 56 endophytes have been isolated from *Cyclocarya paliurus*. Exopolysaccharide, which exhibits antioxidant properties, has been isolated from *Aspergillus versicolor, Penicillium citrinum*, and *Monascus purpureus* (Tao et al. 2024). Endophytic fungi exhibit a remarkable variety in phylogeny and have been identified in nearly all land plants studied to date. Most commonly noted genera include *Penicillium*, *Alternaria*, and *Colletotrichum*, in addition to *Xylaria* and *Aspergillus*. Additional genera frequently reported are *Gibberella*, *Nigrospora, Glomerella*, *Phoma*, *Leptosphaerulina*, and *Phomopsis* (Zheng et al. 2016). The diversity and functional capabilities of these microorganisms are influenced by several factors. Notably, these endophytes generate a wide variety of biologically active metabolites with noteworthy pharmaceutical potential.

2.2 *Bacterial Endophytes*

Bacterial endophytes are a group of nonpathogenic, symbiotic bacteria living inside plant tissues and don't seem to be harmful. In medicinal plants, these endophytes play an essential role in plant growth, stress mitigation, and most notably, the biosynthesis and modulation of secondary metabolites that possess therapeutic potential (Kandel et al. 2017). They colonize intercellular or vascular tissues after entering the plant through a variety of natural openings or wounds and forming mutualistic relationships. While the bacteria obtain nutrition and shelter, the host plant gains improved metabolite profiles, increased tolerance to biotic and abiotic challenges, and increased growth (Santoyo et al. 2016). *Bacillus subtilis* and other *Bacillus* species are very common endophytes (Stein 2005). *Bacillus* spp., such as *B. thuringiensis* and *B. cereus*, were found to be associated with *Trigonella foenum* (Jasim et al. 2015). *Curtobacterium, Mycobacterium* sp., *Micrococcus*, *Brevibacterium,* species of *Kocuria, Nocardioides*, and *Kineococcus, Kytococcus, Marmoricola* sp., *Microbacterium,* and *Micromonospora* are the reported genera, and various others like *Agrococcus, Amnibacterium* species, *Brachybacterium, Citricoccus, Dermacoccus, Glutamicibacter, Gordonia, Isoptericola, Janibacter, Leucobacter, Nocardiopsis, Pseudokineococcus*, and *Verrucosispora* have been isolated as endophytes from various plants (Jiang et al. 2018). *Bacillus, Pseudomonas, Streptococcus, Paenibacillus, Acidomonas, Ralstonia, Alcaligenes, Staphylococcus*, and *Micrococcus* are other endophytes that have been isolated from other plants (Sharma and Mallubhotla 2022). Bacillales, Enterobacterales, and Pseudomonadales were common bacterial orders linked to these plants (Wu et al. 2021). Endophytic actinobacteria are well known for their capability to generate a wide variety of biologically active metabolites such as immunosuppressive, antibacterial, and antitumor compounds (Nimnoi et al. 2010). These days, endophytic actinobacteria derived from medicinal plants are crucial since there is a growing opportunity to explore new natural products (Castillo et al. 2003; Nimnoi et al. 2010). *Streptomyces* is one of the most common genera of actinobacteria within medicinal plants (Qin et al. 2012). *Micromonospora*, *Actinopolyspora*, and *Nocardia* genera *Saccharopolyspora*, *Promicromonospora*, *Streptosporangium*, and *Rhodococcus* are the next most common genera (Zhao et al. 2011). A number of uncommon genera, such as *Dietzia*, *Microtetraspora*, *Actinocorallia*, *Verrucocsispora*, *Isoptericola*, and *Kytococcus*, were also discovered in medicinal plants (Gohain et al. 2015; Qin et al. 2012). These diverse endophytic organisms represent an untapped resource for biotechnological and agricultural innovation.

3 Endophytes from Extreme Environment

Plants thriving in diverse environments are likely to host unique endophytes with exceptional bioactive properties. For example, endophytic bacteria from *Plectranthus tenuiflorus*, an important medicinal plant native to higher altitudes and dry regions, exhibited robust inhibitory activity against several human pathogenic microbes like *Proteus mirabilis*, *Escherichia coli*, *Streptococcus agalactiae*, and *Candida albicans* (El-Deeb et al. 2013). Members of the phyla Proteobacteria, Firmicutes, Actinobacteria, and Bacteroidetes have been reported in extreme environments, with Bacillaceae and Enterobacteriaceae identified as key taxa present in such conditions (Zhang et al. 2019). *Curvularia protuberata*, a fungal endophyte associated with *Dichanthelium lanuginosum*, is capable of surviving extreme thermal conditions in Yellowstone National Park (Márquez et al. 2007). Similarly, *Diplodia mutila*, an endophyte of *Iriartea deltoidea*, exhibits sensitivity toward light intensity. High illumination levels (408 ± 17.3 μmol m^{-2} s^{-1} ± SE) enhance the production of oxidative radicals like reactive oxygen species, leading to tissue necrosis and increased cell death, whereas lower light levels (208.2 ± 6.1 μmol m^{-2} s^{-1} ± SE) favor endosymbiotic proliferation (Alvarez-Loayza et al. 2011). Additionally, thermotolerant fungal endophytes obtained from a desert-adapted plant, *Cullen plicata Delile*, have been found to improve host plant resilience to drought and heat stress through ecophysiological adaptations, ultimately promoting plant growth (Ali et al. 2019).

4 Endophytes to Mimic the Host Plant's Metabolites

Over time, the intricate process of coevolution has driven both plants and endophytes to adopt their genetic composition, enabling them to coexist and survive in a mutually beneficial relationship (Usman et al. 2024). It is believed that endophyte has evolved along with the plant for a long time. This long-standing association allows fungal endophytes to influence plant metabolism while simultaneously boosting their own biosynthetic capabilities. Additionally, they can harness genetic information to produce bioactive metabolites that closely resemble those synthesized by their plant hosts (Singh et al. 2022). Increasing evidence indicates that entire gene clusters may be transferred from host plants to fungi via horizontal gene transfer. Concentrated gene sequences linked to certain plant metabolic pathways suggest that this mechanism helps fungi to establish new biosynthetic capabilities (Barreiro et al. 2019). Endophytes can therefore produce the same metabolite as their host by sharing the host genome.

5 Horizontal Gene Transfer (HGT) Between Plant and Endophyte

HGT is a biological process that gives new functional traits to the associated microbes and underlies the evolutionary flexibility of endophytes inside host plants. Despite being largely unexplored, research on endophytic bacteria has shown that HGT contributes to the biodegradation of toluene and lowers the incidence of illness in corn and Triticum durum (Wang et al. 2010). The term "horizontal gene transfer" describes the movement of genetic material between biological organisms' genomes through mechanisms other than fertilization. Bacterial, fungal, and eukaryotic genomes all exhibit HGT, a universal phenomenon (Bansal and Meyer 2002; Vos et al. 2015). Nevertheless, it is rare and only acts as a substitute mechanism for genetic material transfer across distantly related species (Tiwari and Bae 2020). The genetic gap between living species in the course of evolution is one more factor impacting HGT; gene transmission is more prevalent in closely associated species, while less frequent in far related species (Choi and Kim 2007). It is a common phenomenon that has been seen in endophytes and contributes to metabolite production.

6 Influence of Host Plant Genotype and Environmental Conditions

The creation and diversity of secondary metabolites by fungal endophytes are shaped by various environmental and host-related factors. Key influences include the time and season of sample collection, plant type, tissue source, and habitat, especially extreme environments like saline soils, high altitudes, deserts, rainforests, and swamps (Hashem et al. 2023). Abiotic conditions such as temperature, humidity, light, soil pH, and nutrient availability also play a critical role. Geographical location affects the abundance and composition of endophytes due to varying environmental pressures (U'ren et al. 2012). Additionally, intrinsic plant factors, species, growth stage, and genetic background significantly influence endophytic fungal communities (Juybari et al. 2019; Mishra et al. 2012). Endophyte isolation may be lessened by seasonal variations, especially in rainfall and moisture. This is probably because of host stress reactions such as increased storage of nonstructural carbohydrates (Mishra et al. 2012). Biosynthetic genes in fungi are frequently found in heterochromatic areas of the genomes close to the telomere (Brosch et al. 2008). Epigenetically, their expression is usually controlled by processes including DNA methylation as well as histone deacetylation (Pettit 2011). Both biotic and abiotic factors can alter chromatin structure. Endophytes are closely linked to their host, so any changes or unfavorable conditions affecting the host also impact them, ultimately influencing their diversity and metabolite production.

7 Signaling Molecules (Quorum Sensing) in Metabolite Expression

Signaling molecules such as those involved in quorum sensing play an essential regulatory part in the expression of secondary metabolites in microbial endophytes. Quorum sensing is a population density-dependent communication mechanism primarily observed in bacteria, where the accumulation of signaling molecules, commonly N-acyl homoserine lactones in Gram-negative bacteria and oligopeptides in Gram-positive species, trigger coordinated gene expression once a threshold concentration is reached (Joo et al. 2021; Thumpati et al. 2025; Williams 2007). In the context of endophytes, quorum sensing enables synchronized expression of genes responsible for metabolite biosynthesis, biofilm formation, virulence factor production, and stress responses. Bacterial endophytes such as *Pseudomonas aeruginosa* use QS to regulate phenazine biosynthesis, compounds known for antimicrobial and plant-growth-promoting activity (Higgins et al. 2018). In fungi, although classical QS systems are less well defined, molecules like farnesol and tyrosol in *Candida albicans* have been shown to influence morphogenesis and secondary metabolism, suggesting similar regulatory strategies (Barriuso 2015). Recent studies also show that chromatin-level regulation and epigenetic modifications can interact with environmental cues and QS molecules to activate silent biosynthetic gene clusters. Organic acids like citric, malic, fumaric, and salicylic acid serve as vital nutritional signals that facilitate the recruitment of endophytic bacteria and their metabolite expression (Wang et al. 2023b). These molecules also affect the synthesis of secondary metabolites.

8 Classes of Secondary Metabolite

Secondary metabolites are small molecules produced by organisms, typically encoded by groups of neighboring genes known as biosynthetic gene clusters. These clusters direct the step-by-step formation of complex bioactive compounds (Keller 2019). Several well-known secondary metabolites have been isolated from endophytes belonging to various classes.

8.1 Alkaloids

Alkaloids are a broad and structurally varied class of organic compounds found in nature that have at least a single nitrogen atom, usually in a heterocyclic ring, and exhibit significant bioactivities. These nitrogenous substances are usually made by plants from amino acids, but they are also present in bacteria, fungi, marine life, and most importantly, endophytic microorganisms like fungi and actinobacteria (Bribi 2018). Many alkaloids isolated from plants have already been investigated for their possible use in the production of drugs, and several of these compounds are also present in endophytes (Prajapati et al. 2025a). 3-Acetonylidene-7-prenylindolin-2--one, in addition to 6-prenylindole, has been obtained from *Streptomyces* species (Zhang et al. 2014). Lansai A-D were isolated from *Streptomyces* sp. SUC1, an endophytic microbe (Tuntiwachwuttikul et al. 2008), and gancidin W metabolite was reported from *Streptomyces* sp. SUK10 (Zin et al. 2017). The presence of alkaloids like ismine, homolycorine, tazettine, hippeastrine, lycorine, hemanthamine, and galanthamine in bacterium extracts underscores the significant place of endophytic bacteria in alkaloid production (Ptak et al. 2022). Variecolorin, the grand alkaloid E-7, and an alkaloid called Dioxopiperazine were found in *Eurotium rubrum* (Li et al. 2008). Several potent anticancer alkaloids like Mycoleptodiscin B from *Mycoleptodiscus* sp. (Ortega et al. 2013) and *Trichoderma gamsii* from *Panax notoginseng* produced trichoderons A and B (Ding et al. 2012). Several other alkaloids with their therapeutic properties are listed in Table 1.

8.2 Terpenoids

Terpenes and terpenoids, key components of essential oils from medicinal plants, are extensively used in perfumery and medicine. Besides plants, microbes, including endophytic actinobacteria, are also valuable sources (Liu et al. 2021). *Taxomyces andreanae*, an endophyte from *Taxus brevifolia*, produces Taxane in addition to Taxol (Stierle et al. 1993). *Paraconiothyrium* sp. MY-42 yields Sphaeropsidins A and D, showing moderate cytotoxicity against tumor cells (Shiono et al. 2011). Xiamycin is produced by *Streptomyces* species GT2002/1503 (Ding et al. 2010). Anticancerous metabolite paclitaxel, Podophyllotoxin camptothecin, Vinca alkaloids, and fusidic acid represent some natural terpenoid products (de Souza et al. 2011). Xylarenones A and B and xylarenic acid are also terpenes with anticancerous properties (Hu et al. 2008). *Xylarialean* sp. A45 produces triterpenes Xylariacin A–C, showing moderate cytotoxicity against HepG2 cells (Lin et al. 2011). *Periconia* sp., from *Annona muricata*, yields unique terpenoids (+)-(3S,6S,7R,8S)-periconone A and (−)-(1R,4R,6S,7S)-2-caren-4,8-olide with mild cytotoxicity against various human tumor cell lines (Ge et al. 2011). Various other compounds related to this group are listed in Table 1.

Table 1 A list of therapeutic metabolites generated from various endophytes

S.No	Class of metabolite	Secondary metabolite	Endophyte	Type	Host	Bioactivity	Reference
1.	Alkaloids	Vincristine, vinblastine,	*Botryosphaeria laricina* CRS1	Fungus	*Catharanthus roseus*	Anticancerous activity	Bandara et al. (2021)
2.	Alkaloid	Berberin	*Alternaria* sp.	Fungus	*Coptis chinensis*	Antibacterial, antidiabetic, antihypertensive,	Zhang et al. (2016)
3.	Alkaloid	Piperine	*Periconia* sp.	Fungus	*Piper longum L.*	Antimycobacterial and anticancerous	Verma et al. (2011)
4.	Alkaloids	Vincristine	*Cladosporium* sp.	Fungus	*Catharanthus roseus*	Anticancer	Nguyen et al. (2023)
5.	Alkaloid	Kakadumycin A	*Streptomyces* sp.	Bacteria	*Grevillea pteridifolia*	Antibacterial and antimalarial	Castillo et al. (2003)
6.	Alkaloid	2-Methyl-7-phenylindole	*Curvularia geniculata* L.	Fungus	*Phyllanthus niruri* L.	Antioxidative and cytotoxic activity	Kalimuthu et al. (2022)
7.	Alkaloid	Aconitine	*Acremonium alternatum*	Fungus	*Argemone mexicana*	Anti-inflammatory	Bhadra and Vasundhara (2024)
8.	Alkaloid	Sanguinarine	*Fusarium proliferatum* BLH51	Fungus	*Macleaya cordata*	Anti-inflammatory	Wang et al. (2014b)
9.	Alkaloid	Camptothecin and 10-hydroxycamptothecin	*Fusarium solani*	Fungus	*Apodytes dimidiata* E. Mey. ex Arn	Anticancerous	Shweta et al. (2010)
10.	Alkaloid	Dioxopiperazine	*Eurotium rubrum*	Fungus	*Hibiscus tiliaceus*	Antioxidant and cytotoxic	Li et al. (2008)
11.	Alkaloid	Rohitukine	*Fusarium proliferatum*	Fungus	*Dysoxylum binectariferum* Hook. f,	Anticancer activity	Mohana Kumara et al. (2012)
12.	Alkaloid	2-(Furan-2-yl)-6-(2S,3S,4 trihydroxybutyl)pyrazine	*Jishengella endophytica*	Bacteria	*Xylocarpus granatum*	Antiviral	Wang et al. (2014a)

13.	Alkaloid	Reserpine	*Bacillus* spp.	Bacteria	*Rauvolfia serpentina*	Antibacterial and antioxidant	Lata and Gond (2025)
14.	Alkaloid	Quinine quinidine, cinchonine, cinchonidine	*Fusarium incarnatum, F. solani, F. oxysporum*	Fungus	*Cinchona calisaya*	Antimalarial, antiarrhythmic, analgesic	Hidayat et al. (2016)
15.	Alkaloid	Munumbicins	*Streptomyces species*	Bacteria	*Kennedia nigriscans*	Antibacterial	Castillo et al. (2002)
16.	Sesquiterpene alkaloid	Huperzine A	*Fusarium* sp.	Fungus	*Huperzia serrata*	Treatment of Alzheimer's disease	Le et al. (2020)
17.	Alkaloid	Corynesidone D	*Corynespora cassiicola*	Fungus	*Gongronema latifolium*	Anti-inflammatory, anticancer agent	Okoye et al. (2013)
18.	Alkaloid	Capsaicin	*Alternaria alternata*	Fungus	*Capsicum annuum*	Anti-inflammatory and antiulcerative	Devari et al. (2014)
19.	Flavonoids	Silybin A and Silybin B	*Aspergillus iizukae*	Fungus	*Silybum marianum*	Neuroprotective property, anti-inflammatory	El-Elimat et al. (2014)
20.	Flavonoids	Kaempferol	*Fusarium chlamydosporum*	Fungus	*Tylophora indica*	Antimicrobial property	Chaturvedi et al. (2014)
21.	Flavonoids	Luteolin	*Aspergillus fumigatus*	Fungus	*Cajanus cajan (L.) Millsp.*	Anti-inflammatory, antioxidant	Zhao et al. (2014)
22.	Flavonoids	Rutin	*Aspergillus flavus*	Fungus	*Aegle marmelos*	Antioxidant and antimicrobial	Patil et al. (2015)
23.	Lignans	Podophyllotoxin	*Trametes hirsuta*	Fungus	*Podophyllum hexandrum*	Anticancerous	Puri et al. (2006)
24.	Lignan	Deoxypodophyllotoxin	*Aspergillus fumigatus* Fresenius	Fungus	*Juniperus communis* L. Horstmann	Antitumor and antiproliferative properties	Kusari et al. (2009a)
25.	Phenol	Gallic acid	*Phomopsis* sp.	Fungus	*Acer ginnala*	Antioxidant, anti-inflammatory, antimicrobial	Qi et al. (2009)

(continued)

Table 1 (continued)

S.No	Class of metabolite	Secondary metabolite	Endophyte	Type	Host	Bioactivity	Reference
26.	Phenol	Curcumin	*Penicilliumfrequen tans*	Fungus	*Curcuma wenyujin*	Antimicrobial, anticancerous properties, antioxidant along with anti-inflammatory	Yan et al. (2014)
27.	Phenolic glycosides	Tyrosol	*Colletotrichum coccodes*	Fungus	*Houttuynia cordata* Thunb	Antimicrobial	Talukdar et al. (2021)
28.	Polyphenols	Resveratrol	*Alternaria alternata* SK	Fungus	*Solanum melongena*	Anticancerous, antioxidant, and antistaphylococcal	Abdel-Hadi et al. (2022)
29.	Coumarin	Scopoletin, fraxetin	*Fusarium oxysporum* GU-7	Fungus	*Glycyrrhiza uralensis*	Antioxidant property	Sun et al. (2023)
30.	Tannin	Ellagic acid	*Xylaria acuta*	Fungus	*Millingtonia hortensis L.f.*	Antibacterial and antifungal properties	Sumanth et al. (2024)
31.	Terpenoids	Diosgenin	*Fusarium oxysporum*	Fungus	*Dioscorea zingiberensis*	Antitumor, anti-inflammatory	Biswas et al. (2020)
32.	Terpenoid	Azadirachtin A and B	*Eupenicillium parvum*	Fungus	*Azadirachta indica* A. Juss.	Insecticidal property	Kusari et al. (2012)
33.	Terpenoid	Ginkgolide B	*Fusarium oxysporum*	Fungus	*Ginkgo biloba*	Platelet activating factor	Cui et al. (2012)
34.	Terpenoid	Ophiobolin K, 6-epi-ophiobolin K	*Aspergillus calidoustus*	Fungus	*Acanthospermum australe*	Antifungal, trypanocidal, and cytotoxicity	Rodrigues de Carvalho et al. (2016)
35.	Terpenoid	Punctaporonin H	*Pestalotiopsis theae*	Fungus	*Camellia sinensis Theacea*	Antibacterial and cytotoxicity	Liu et al. (2021)
36.	Terpenoid	Taxol (paclitaxel)	*Taxomyces andreanae*	Fungud	*Taxus baccata*	Anticancerous	Stierle et al. (1993)

37.	Terpenoid	Scorpinone	*Lophiostoma* sp.	Fungus	*Eucalyptus exserta*	Antibacterial	Mao et al. (2021)
38.	Quinone	Hypericin and Emodin	*Thielavia subthermophila*	Fungus	*Hypericum perforatum*	Cytotoxic and anticancerous	Kusari et al. (2009b)
39.	Athraquinone	Physcion	*Aspergillus versicolor*	Fungus	*Juncus rigidus*	Antioxidant, anticholinesterase activity, anti-inflammatory	Elawady et al. (2023)
40.	Quinone	2-Methoxy-6-methyl-1,4-benzoquinone	*Aspergillus ochraceus*	Fungus	*Lagopsis supina*	Antimicrobial, cytotoxic	Zhang et al. (2022)
41.	Lactone	β-Resorcylic Acid	*Colletotrichum gloeosprioides* JS0419	Fungus	*Suaeda japonica*	Anti-inflammatory	Kim et al. (2023)
42.	Xanthones and benzophenones	Griseophen xanthone A, digriseophene A	*Penicillium* sp. ct-28	Fungus	*Corydlis tomentella*	Cytotoxic	Ming et al. (2022)
43.	Xanthones	Phomoxanthone A	*Paecilomyces* sp.	Fungus	*Schnella splendens*	Antimicrobial activity	Ramos et al. (2022)
44.	Cyclic peptide	Beauvericin	*Fusarium oxysporum*	Fungus	*Cinnamomum kanehirae*	Anticancerous	Wang et al. (2011)
45.	Polyketide	Sterigmatocystin	*Aspergillus nidulans*	Fungus	*Nyctanthes arbor-tristis* Linn	Antiproliferative activity	Sana et al. (2019)
46.	Polyketides	Trichodenoids A and B	*Trichoderma reesei*	Fungus	*Gastrodia elata* Blume	Cardioprotective effect	Jiang et al. (2025)
47.	Amino acid derivative	Myriocin	*Mycosphaerella* sp.	Fungus	*Eugenia bimarginata* DC.	Antifungal	Pereira et al. (2015)
48.	Amino acid derived group	Terezine E	*Mucor* sp.	Fungus	*Centaurea stoebe*	Antifungal and cytotoxicity	Abdou et al. (2020)
49.	Peptides	Ecomycins	*Pseudomonas viridiflava*	Bacteria	*Lactuca sativa*	Antifungal	Redgrave et al. (1998)
50.	Napthoquinone	Anhydrofusarubin dihydrojavanicin	*Fusarium* sp. and *Lasiodiplodia theobromae*	Fungus	*Avicennia lanata*	Antitrypanosomal	Mazlan et al. (2020)

8.3 Flavonoids

Flavonoids are a group of secondary metabolites characterized by a benzopyrone core structure, typically bearing mono- or polyphenolic groups. These bioactive compounds are widely distributed throughout various parts of plants (Roy et al. 2022). Flavonoids possess diverse medicinal properties, containing antioxidant, antitumor, antimicrobial, neuroprotective, and anti-inflammatory activities, along with the ability to modulate cellular enzyme functions. Quercetin-3-O-rutinoside and quercitrin are flavonoid glycosides derived from quercetin, with strong antioxidant activity (Negi and Dave 2010). Several flavonoids such as 7-methoxy-3,3′,4′,6-tetrahydroxyflavone, fisetin, and naringenin, in addition to xenognosin B, were obtained from *Streptomyces* sp. BT01, showing strong activity toward Gram-positive bacteria, including *Bacillus cereus, B. subtilis,* and *Staphylococcus aureus* (Taechowisan et al. 2014). Other flavonoids like kaempferol, isoscutellarin, umbelliferone, and cichoriin from *Streptomyces* sp. Tc052 exhibited antioxidant and nitric oxide inhibition activity (Taechowisan et al. 2009). Flavonoid like quercetin, hespertin, and naringin exhibit antiviral properties (Roy et al. 2022), and vitexin, along with their derivatives, apigenin, have been found very effective toward hepatitis C virus, herpes simplex virus 1(HSV-1), human hepatitis A, B, and C, rhesus rotavirus (RRV), and influenza viruses (Khachatoorian et al. 2012). These flavonoids have been isolated from various endophytes and show their enormous potential in drug development.

8.4 Phenolic Compound

Phenolics are a diverse group of secondary metabolites defined by one or more hydroxyl (-OH) groups attached to an aromatic (phenyl) ring. These metabolites are recognized for their antioxidant, antimicrobial, and anti-inflammatory properties. Microorganisms, including endophytic fungi and bacteria, are a significant and underexplored source of phenolic compounds. Graphislactone A, for example, is a phenolic compound isolated from certain endophytic fungi (Song et al. 2005). Gallic acid, a member of the phenolic compound group, has also been isolated from *Phomopsis* sp. (Qi et al. 2009). Resveratrol, isolated from *Alternaria alternata* SK, is another phenolic compound that exhibits broad pharmaceutical properties and holds significant potential for the management of various diseases (Abdel-Hadi et al. 2022). Evariquinone isolated from *Colletotrichum* sp. JS-0367 found in *Morus alba,* is another compound with potent neuroprotective properties (Song et al. 2018). β-Resorcylic acid isolated from *Colletotrichum gloeosprioides* JS0419 is also a type of phenolic compound with anti-inflammatory properties (Kim et al. 2023). Curcumin isolated from *Penicillium frequentans* also belongs to this category (Yan et al. 2014). Salvianolic acid C, identified from *Phoma glomerata* D14, an endophyte of *Salvia miltiorrhiza* Bunge, exhibited a strong antiplatelet aggregation effect (Li et al. 2016). Ellagic acid obtained from *Xylaria acuta* exhibited antimicrobial properties (Sumanth et al. 2024). A wide variety of these compounds have been isolated from diverse sources, showing enormous potential in research.

8.5 Polyketides

The chemically varied and physiologically active category of secondary metabolites known as polyketides is found in bacteria, fungi, plants, and animals. Polyketides can be created from basic acyl building blocks and have a wide variety of structural features (Miyanaga 2017). The widely recognized anticancer drug doxorubicin is a polyketide that is derived from fungi (Tacar et al. 2013). Xanthoquinodin B9 is a novel natural metabolite that was isolated from endophytic fungi *Chaetomium globosum* 7s-1, which is found in *Rhapis cochinchinensis* (Lour.) Mart. Its IC50 value is 7.04, 18.4, 0.98 μM for cancer cell lines (KB, MCF-7, and NCI-H187) and 1.78 μM for the noncancerous cell line, indicating cytotoxic potential (Tantapakul et al. 2020). *Bacillus subtilis* produces a variety of polyketide antibiotics, including bacillomycin, fengycin, iturin, lichenysin, mycosubtilin, plipastin, pumilacidin, and surfactin (Stein 2005). Clethramycin, formed by *Streptomyces hygroscopicus* TP-A0623, has been reported to prevent both spheroplast regeneration as well as germ tube creation in *Candida albicans* microbes (Furumai et al. 2003). Ansamitocin with potent cytotoxic activity has been isolated from various endophytes (Siyu-Mao et al. 2013). Another compound, pterocidin, obtained from *S. hygroscopicus* TP-A0451, exhibited cytotoxic effects against several human malignant cell lines (Igarashi et al. 2006). Additionally, linfuranone has demonstrated a notable antidiabetic effect along with an antiatherogenic property in mouse ST13 pre-adipocyte models (Indananda et al. 2013). Several endophytic fungi have yielded cytotoxic polyketides. Chaetoglobosin X, isolated from *Chaetomium globosum* (*Curcuma wenyujin*), exhibited potent cytotoxicity against MFC and H22 cancer cells (Wang et al. 2012).

8.6 Peptides and Other Derivatives

Streptomyces sp. TC022, reported in *Alpinia galangal*, produces actinomycin D, a potent polypeptide known for its antifungal and antitumor properties (Taechowisan et al. 2006). Saadamycin, a coumarin, has been isolated from *Streptomyces* sp. Hedaya 48 and acts as an antifungal agent (El-Gendy and El-Bondkly 2010). *Micromonospora* sp., isolated from *Pueraria candollei* roots, was reported for the first time to produce S-adenosyl-N-acetylhomocysteine (Boonsnongcheep et al. 2017). It has antibacterial and antioxidant properties. *Pseudomonas viridiflava* and *Pseudomonas syringae*, endophytic bacteria related to various plants, were found to produce novel lipopeptides called ecomycins, along with pseudomycins (Harrison et al. 1991; Redgrave et al. 1998). Beauvericin also belongs to this category of metabolite (Wang et al. 2011). Myriosin and Terezine E, listed in Table 1, are amino acid derivatives.

9 Pharmaceutical Applications of Endophytic Metabolites

9.1 Anticancerous Compound

Since the isolation of the anticancerous medication "Taxol" from *Taxomyces andreanae* at the beginning of the 1990s, the hunt for novel pharmaceutical goods and medications with microbial origins has begun. Fungi were the source of both of these medications. First, *Taxus brevifolia* and then *Taxus wallinchiana* were used to isolate Taxol. These two species contain endophytic fungi, specifically *Taxomyces andreanae* and *Pestalotiopsis microspore*, respectively (Stierle et al. 1993; Strobel et al. 1996). The finding of anticancer drugs from fungal endophytes has unlocked new avenues in drug development, showcasing their potential to produce effective compounds. Taxol is produced by numerous other endophytic organisms as well (Pandy et al. 2023). First obtained from *Camptotheca acuminata*, camptothecin is a crucial anticancer drug (Wall et al. 1966). Endophytes like *Paenibacillus polymyxa* LY214 and *Trichoderma atroviride* LY357 were both discovered to produce CPT in the screening process of endophytes within *Camptotheca acuminate* (Pu et al. 2013, 2015). It is a strong inhibitor of DNA topoisomerase I. Clinical derivatives that are often used as anticancer medicines, like 10-hydroxycamptothecin (Shweta et al. 2010), topotecan (Cormio et al. 2011), and irinotecan (Radajewska et al. 2023), were developed using CPT as their foundation (Prajapati et al. 2024a). *Buergenerula spartinae*, a novel isolate from the *Cymbidium orchid*, exhibited the maximum L-asparaginase action (1.736 unit/mL), making it very useful in tumor treatment (Chua et al. 2024). A metabolite obtained from WYJ-E14 strain of an endophyte in *Curcuma wenyujin* showed strong inhibition of melanoma and glioma cell proliferation (Huang et al. 2024). *Fusarium oxysporum* LHS-P1-3, from peanut roots, produced six anticancer compounds including beauvericin and various enniatins. Additionally, three endophytes from *Catharanthus roseus* were found to synthesize vincristine and vinblastine, helping address the limited availability of these vital anticancer alkaloids (Nguyen et al. 2023). Beauvericin, isolated from *Talaromyces* sp. SAF14, demonstrated strong cytotoxic action against A549, MCF-7, and KB cell lines, having IC_{50} values of 5.36 ± 2.49, 1.96 ± 1.09, and 4.46 ± 0.68 μM, respectively (Li et al. 2024). *Streptomyces* sp. reported from *Maytenus hookeri* gained attention for producing naphthomycin K along with two identified compounds, naphthomycins A and naphthomycins E, all of which exhibited cytotoxic activity contrary to P388 and A-549 cancer cell line (Lu and Shen 2007). Certain fungi, for example, *Botryosphaeria laricina* CRS1 obtained from *Catharanthus roseus*, can produce vinblastine and vincristine, with yields enhanced by host plant extract elicitors (Bandara et al. 2021). Nine new prenylated p-terphenyls prenylterphenyllins F–J (1, 2, 4–6) and prenylcandidusins D–G (3, 7–9) were reported from the *Aspergillus candidus* LDJ-5. Structural elucidation was done using NMR and MS analysis. Notably, compound 3 features a rare 6,5,6,6-fused ring system. Compounds 4–6 showed antimicrobial activity, while compounds 1, 4, 6, and 9 exhibited cytotoxicity (Zhou et al. 2020). Endophytes exhibit vast diversity and produce natural compounds with anticancer, antiproliferative, and proapoptotic properties, making them valuable resources for drug development and effective cancer treatment strategies.

9.2 Antimicrobials

A significant issue facing health services is the increase of dangerous bacteria and fungi that are unaffected by commercial medications. This is because microbes are increasing new defense mechanisms for antimicrobial medicines (Costelloe et al. 2010). Bioactive secondary metabolites from endophytes such as steroids, flavonoids, terpenoids, peptides, alkaloids, and phenolics exhibit strong antimicrobial activity and offer promising alternatives against antibiotic-resistant pathogens (Khalil et al. 2021; Osama et al. 2024). *Aspergillus cejpii* is an endophytic fungus separated from *Hedera helix* L. root and it exhibited strong antimicrobial properties against *E. coli*, *Acinetobacter baumannii*, *Pseudomonas aeruginosa*, *Staphylococcus aureus*, *Salmonella typhi*, *Serratia marcescens*, *Pseudomonas aeruginosa*, and *Acinetobacter baumannii*. Its active portion analysis results in the separation of compound spiculisporic acid (Osama et al. 2024). Seven metabolites were isolated from *Aspergillus* species linked with *Melia azedarach*. Notably, asperazine, asperpyrone A, and rubrofusarin B demonstrated inhibitory effects against the pathogen *Alternaria solani*. Additionally, asperpyrone A was reported to possess significant antibacterial properties (Mulyani et al. 2023). The inhibitory activity of phomoxanthone A from *Paecilomyces* sp. was higher against *Bacillus subtilis* (MIC of 7.81 $\mu g\ mL^{-1}$) and also had a strong inhibitory effect against *Trypanosoma cruzi* epimastigote forms and Leishmania amazonensis promastigote forms (Ramos et al. 2022). *Botryosphaeria mamane* CF2-13, isolated from *Arrabidaea chica*, showed strong antimicrobial activity against various pathogens, notably *S. aureus* (MIC = 0.312 mg/mL), along with *Escherichia coli*, *Serratia marcescens*, *Klebsiella pneumoniae*, *Salmonella enterica*, *Aspergillus brasiliensis*, and *Candida albicans* (Gurgel et al. 2023). *Chaetomium ovatoascomatis* NRC, isolated from *Euphorbia milii*, exhibited potent and broad-spectrum antimicrobial activity. Metabolite profiling through LC–MS/MS and GC–MS revealed several bioactive compounds, with grevilline B, aflatoxin G2, apigenin, and 9,12-octadecadienoic acid methyl ester as main constituents (Shaker et al. 2022). A streptomycete endophyte (NRRL 30562) isolated from *Kennedia nigriscans*. This strain produces a novel class of broad-spectrum peptide antibiotics known as munumbicins (Castillo et al. 2002). Two antifungal metabolites, 3-acetonylidene-7-prenylindolin-2 one and 6-Prenylindole, have been obtained from *Streptomyces* sp. from different host origins (Singh and Dubey 2018; Zhang et al. 2014). Gancidin W, obtained from *Streptomyces* sp. SUK10, shows a potent effect against *Plasmodium berghei* PZZ1/100 (Zin et al. 2017). It has antimalarial activity. Xiamycin, created by *Streptomyces* sp. GT2002/1503 and reported in *Bruguiera gymnorrhiza*, has been shown to specifically inhibit R5-tropic HIV infection (Ding et al. 2010). Numerous compounds with potent antimicrobial properties have been isolated from endophytes, highlighting their rich diversity and the discovery of novel strains.

9.3 Antioxidants

Antioxidant molecules help mitigate oxidative damage caused by free radicals and are also known to suppress harmful effects arising from oxidative chain reactions. Several studies have inspected the antioxidant potential of endophytes isolated from diverse medicinal plants (Sharaf et al. 2022). Following the finding of pestacin and isopestacin, potent antioxidants generated by *Pestalotiopsis microspora*, an endophyte form *Terminalia morobensis*, curiosity about antioxidant chemicals from fungal endophytes increased dramatically (Strobel et al. 2002). When endophytic fungi were isolated from *Cymbidium* orchid roots, they demonstrated significant antioxidant capability. The most active of them was *Lasiodiplodia theobromae*. High antioxidant properties were also shown by *Buergenerula spartinae, Fusarium fujikuroi*, and *Fusarium incarnatum* (Chua et al. 2024). Aspergillus flavus produces kojic acid, which showed DPPH free radical scavenging action with the IC50 value of 99.3 μg/ml (Shah et al. 2024). *Lasiodiplodia* sp., derived from *Handroanthus impetiginosus*, produces a variety of metabolites having antioxidant qualities (Silva Tironi et al. 2025). The *Arrabidaea chica*-isolated endophyte *Colletotrichum* sp. CG1-7 showed encouraging activity during the DPPH test, having an EC50 of 11 μg/mL (Gurgel et al. 2023). Quercetin, created by *Nigrospora oryzae* found in *Tinospora cordifolia*, exhibits notable neuroprotective and antioxidative effects (Vig et al. 2022). Additionally, *Fictibacillus phosphorivorans* P1U2 produces quercetin (Ashafani et al. 2023). *Pseudopestalotiopsis camelliae-sinensis* and *Didymella sinensis*, two endophytic fungi linked to *Camellia sinensis* (L.) Kuntze, have been found to contain catechin. These endophytes' remarkable antioxidative capability was attributed to their great capacity to generate catechin (Sidhu et al. 2024).

9.4 Anti-Inflammatory Compound

The capacity of endophytes in producing a diverse range of bioactive secondary metabolites is making them a promising source for anti-inflammatory medicines. These substances have the potential to be used therapeutically in inflammatory illnesses since they can alter important inflammatory processes like NF-κB and COX-2 (Koopklang et al. 2024). An endophytic fungi, called *Biscogniauxia petrensis*, was isolated in *Dendrobium* orchids and has been shown to produce sesquiterpenoids with significant anti-inflammatory qualities (Han et al. 2023). *Stagonosporopsis oculihominis* produces bioactive substances with anti-inflammatory properties, including p-hydroxybenzaldehyde, p-hydroxyphenylacetic acid, and (Z)-1-hydroxy-4-(2-nitroethenyl)-benzene (Yue and Yu 2022). Mechanistic studies revealed that ravenelin obtained from *Setosphaeria rostrate* suppresses the expression of iNOS and COX-2 enzymes (Koopklang et al. 2024). In addition, *Aspergillus niger*, isolated from *Elaeocarpus floribundus* Blume, showed significant inhibitory activity against the inflammatory response. The active fraction from *A. niger* was found to contain a diverse array of pharmacologically important compounds, comprising tensyuic acid, nigragillin, hexylitaconic acid, chlorogenic acid, TMC-256C1, fumaric acid, asnipyrone B, asperenone, and fusarubin (Mazumder et al. 2021). Demethylincisterol A3, isolated from the endophytic fungus *Aspergillus tennesseensis* 1022LEF, exhibited strong anti-inflammatory activity. It acts as a dual-function modulator by directly inhibiting acetylcholinesterase and upregulating α7nAChR expression (Su et al. 2022). Ethyl acetate extract of endophytic bacteria *Bacillus subtilis* strain MG 692780 from *Emilia sonchifolia* exhibited noteworthy anti-inflammatory property by suppressing the inflammation induced by carrageenan and formalin in mice (Urumbil and Anilkumar 2021). Epicatechin, which has been derived via *Curvularia australiensis* FC2AP, possesses anti-inflammatory and anticancer properties (Mani et al. 2021). Having an IC_{50} value of 2.61 μmol/L, preussomerin EG1, which was obtained from *Edenia gomezpompae*, demonstrated a potent inhibitory effect against nitric oxide generation (Tan et al. 2020). Thus, endophytes found in medicinal plants provide anti-inflammatory chemicals that show promise as substitutes for manufactured medications.

9.5 *Cardioprotective Compound*

The capacity of microorganisms to generate biologically active secondary metabolites including resveratrol, diosgenin, aspernolide F, and caffeic acid is making them powerful sources of cardioprotective compounds. In order to prevent or manage cardiovascular disorders, these substances are useful since they have potent anti-inflammatory, antihypertensive, antithrombotic, and antioxidative effects (Papikinou et al. 2024). By regulating lipid profiles and modifying vascular tone, endophyte-derived chemicals can shield heart cells against oxidative injury (Abdel-Hadi et al. 2022). Resveratrol, a widely used secondary metabolite, has shown promise in preventing strokes. It was obtained from *Alternaria alternata* SK, which is connected to *Solanum melongena*. It decreases blood cholesterol, increases the antioxidant capacity, and aids in controlling the metabolism of lipids (Abdel-Hadi et al. 2022). Resveratrol is known to have both preventive and therapeutic benefits for a number of illnesses, such as pneumonia, acute breathing distress syndrome, tumors, diabetes, and cardiovascular conditions (Filardo et al. 2020). Isolated from various sections of *Dioscorea zingiberensis*, *Fusarium* sp., *Curvularia lunata*, and *Aspergillus flavus* showed noticeably elevated diosgenin synthesis, which was confirmed by HPLC testing (Xiang et al. 2018). It exhibits cardioprotective effects by modulating the opening of potassium channels (Badalzadeh et al. 2015) and also protects against high glucose-induced myocardial injury, especially when used in combination with morroniside (Pi et al. 2017). Aspernolide F, a novel cardioprotective butyrolactone, was isolated from *Aspergillus terreus* found within *Carthamus lanatus* and has shown efficacy against doxorubicin-induced cardiotoxicity. The study highlights that the cardioprotective effects of Aspernolide F may be attributed to its strong antioxidant and anti-inflammatory properties (El-Agamy et al. 2019). The endophytic fungus *Muyocopron laterale* from *Tylophora ovata* yielded five new xanthones muyocoxanthones O–S, showed moderate protective effects with cell viabilities ranging from 54.8% to 62.4%. These metabolites show potential in protecting against oxidative cardiac injury (Cao et al. 2023). Numerous compounds with cardioprotective properties have been isolated from endophytes. These compounds often offer safer, more affordable alternatives with fewer side effects compared to conventional therapies.

9.6 Antidiabetic Compound

Diabetes mellitus is one of the most problematic health issues related to lifestyle disorders in the twenty-first century and the fastest-growing urban epidemic worldwide. Endophytic fungi related to medicinal plants represent a promising natural reserve for the finding of novel antidiabetic compounds (Agrawal et al. 2022). The endophytic fungus *Aureobasidium pullulans*, obtained from the bark of *Boswellia sacra*, was identified as a source of the fatty acid derivative methyl-5-docosenoate. This compound showed strong α-glucosidase inhibitory activity with an IC_{50} of 23.3 mM. Molecular docking studies indicated that it interacts via p-alkyl interactions with key catalytic residues Glu276 and Asp214 of α-glucosidase (Al-Hosni et al. 2020). An endophyte *Penicillium canescens* from *Juniperus polycarpos* fruits yielded one novel xanthone and two known xanthones, showing a strong inhibitory effect of α-glucosidase, with IC_{50} ranging from 38.80 to 75.20 μM (Malik et al. 2020). The ethyl acetate portion of *Penicillium oxalicum* has demonstrated possible antidiabetic as well as antioxidant qualities (Nagarajan et al. 2025). From *Alternaria* species, alternarienoic acid, altenuene, and altenusin were extracted; these substances exhibited potent inhibitory action on enzymes like lipase and α-glucosidase (Elbermawi et al. 2022). Various other compounds with antidiabetic properties are listed in Table 1.

9.7 Neuroprotective Compound

Exposure to natural or synthetic toxins can lead to neurotoxicity, damaging neurons and impairing nervous system function. It is often linked to mitochondrial damage, oxidative stress, and elevated ROS levels. Symptoms include memory loss, cognitive and behavioral changes, numbness, weakness, and sexual dysfunction. Older individuals and those with neurological disorders are particularly vulnerable. Endophytes can produce neuroprotective compounds, making them valuable in the treatment of neurodegenerative diseases (Prajapati et al. 2025c; Rai et al. 2025; Todkar et al. 2023). Evariquinone, isolated from *Colletotrichum* sp. JS-0367, found in *Morus alba* leaves, showed strong neuroprotective effects by reducing glutamate-induced apoptotic cytotoxicity in HT22 cells (Song et al. 2018). Chrysogenamide A, derived from *Penicillium chrysogenum* No. 005 living in roots of *Cistanche deserticola* (Y.C. Ma), demonstrated neuroprotective property in SH-SY5Y human neuroblastoma cells by reducing hydrogen peroxide-induced cell death and preserving cell viability under oxidative stress (Lin et al. 2008). *Fusarium* sp. Rsp5.2, reported from *Huperzia serrata*, produces huperzine A, a compound known for its acetylcholinesterase inhibitory activity (Le et al. 2020). Several other endophytic species also produce huperzine A and contribute significantly to the protection against neurodegenerative diseases.

10 Strategies to Enhance Metabolite Production

Various strategies have been developed to activate silent biosynthetic gene clusters and enhance metabolite production including coculturing, epigenetic modification, and genomics-based methods (Fig. 3). It has been discovered by genome sequencing that microbes contain a significantly greater number of gene clusters for secondary metabolite production than previously believed. Biosynthetic gene clusters (BGCs) are typically composed of these genes and can even be transferred from one organism to another. Researchers may more easily locate, examine, and contrast the genes that produce these useful molecules because of this grouping (Cimermancic et al. 2014). The production of known or predicted secondary metabolites is attributed to the approximately 20 gene clusters found in actinobacteria that participate in the synthesis of naturally occurring chemicals (Passari et al. 2017). The existence of BGCs, which include those generating polyketide synthase and nonribosomal peptide synthetase, has been discovered by genomic research of the genera *Bacillus* and *Streptomyces*, which are known to produce antimicrobial chemicals. Surfactins, iturins, and fengycins, which are NRPS-derived chemicals generated from *Bacillus* species, have been shown to have potent antimicrobial action (Jasim et al. 2016). These findings show that culturable endophytes have a high genetic capacity, making them desirable candidates for future research on the creation of pharmaceutical and natural products.

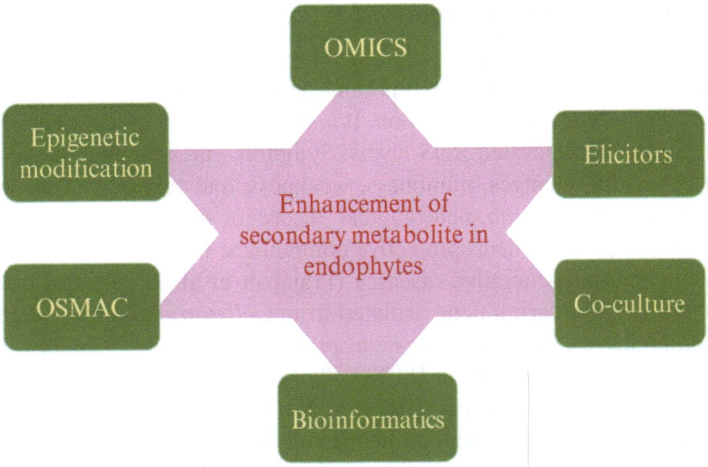

Fig. 3 Strategies to enhance secondary metabolite of endophytes

The coculture strategy involves growing two or greater than two microorganisms in the one medium to enhance secondary metabolite production, activate cryptic genes (Wakefield et al. 2017). The coculture study between *Armillaria* plus *Epicoccum* species yielded eight novel elements, one of which had anticancer properties (Li et al. 2020). When *Talaromyces pinophilus* and *Paraphaeosphaeria* sp. are cocultured, novel secondary metabolites are produced (Murakami et al. 2020). Coculturing of *Bacillus subtilis* and *Aspergillus sydowii* produces seven novel bioactive chemicals (Sun et al. 2021). Additionally, two new o-aminobenzoic acid compounds were generated by cocultivating Bionectria sp. together with either *Streptomyces lividans* or *B. subtilis* (Kamdem et al. 2018). In conjunction with the emergence of fresh metabolites that were not present axenic controls, the generation of constantly present fungal metabolic products increased by over 78 times when *Fusarium tricinctum* plus *Bacillus subtilis* had been cocultivated (Ola et al. 2013). This approach not only enhances the yield of known metabolites but also induces the production of novel bioactive compounds, which holds significant promise for advancing natural product discovery, particularly in the search for new therapeutic agents.

One of the processes that controls the manufacture of fungal secondary metabolites is thought to be the silencing or activation of genes via chromatin-level regulation (Keller 2019; Verma et al. 2023). The epigenetic modification approach involves using small molecules to modify the chromatin structure, thereby altering the secondary metabolite profile. This can enhance metabolite production or activate silent biosynthetic gene clusters (Pillay et al. 2022). Four novel compounds were discovered when 75% of the SM biosynthesis genes in *Calcarisporium arbuscular* NRRL3705 were activated by interrupting hdaA (Mao et al. 2015). When the endophytic fungus *Penicillium chrysogenum* Fes1701's hdaA gene was deleted, the functional meleagrin emerged and other associated clusters of biosynthesis genes became expressed (Ding et al. 2020). Furthermore, *Aspergillus fumigatus* produced ten times as much fumiquinazoline C when histone deacetylase was inhibited with valproic acid (Magotra et al. 2017) and *Diaporthe* sp. produced new compounds like xylarolide A, xylarolide B, and diportharine (Sharma et al. 2018). For example, 5-azacytidine-induced chemical epigenetic alteration of *Cochliobolus lunatus* produced novel metabolites, including α-pyrones, cochliobopyrones, isocoumarins, and chromones (Wu et al. 2019). *Bjerkandera adusta* HS-28 also produced tremulane sesquiterpenoids when trichostatin A was added to it (Huang et al. 2020a). Epigenetic modifiers may imitate plant-fungi genomic interactions necessary for metabolite manufacturing, as evidenced by their activation of quiet biosynthetic pathways in endophytic fungi. Genetic engineering techniques such as CRISPR/Cas9-based DNA editing have emerged as a key instrument for increasing the creation of secondary metabolites in endophytic fungi due to their accuracy, effectiveness, and capacity to incorporate transgenes, activate dormant biosynthetic routes, and remove unwanted alleles (Wang et al. 2023a). For example, lovastatin plus Taxol generation from filamentous fungus has been enhanced by CRISPR-mediated amplification of important enzymes and inhibition of competing paths (El-Sayed et al. 2017). whereas PEG-mediated CRISPR change in *Pestalotiopsis fici* increased metabolite production (Xu et al. 2021), likewise, dual-gRNA suppressing of the MAPK pathway gene in *Phomopsis liquidambaris* stimulated flavonoid synthesis (quercetin, naringenin, kaempferol), boosting stress tolerance (Huang et al. 2020b). Degenerate PCR can be used to find the matching genes in endophytes that produce the same substance (genome mining) (Challis 2008), when the biosynthesis pathway of a product in a certain plant species is known in part or in full (Van Lanen and Shen 2006). Alternative methods are provided for unculturable endophytes by methods such as environmental PCR, metagenomics, or structure-based gene targeting (Chiang et al. 2011; Kayser and Warzecha 2012). Additionally, bioinformatics platforms like Secondary Metabolite Unknown Regions Finder (SMURF) and Antibiotics and Secondary Metabolite Analysis Shell (antiSMASH), PRISM (PRediction Informatics for Secondary Metabolomes) are valuable for detecting specific gene clusters responsible for bioactive metabolite production (Kayser and Warzecha 2012; Miller et al. 2012). Genetic manipulation of fungal genomes remains a significant challenge, particularly for newly isolated or less-studied fungal species that lack comprehensive genomic information.

11 Challenges and Future Direction

Sustainable secondary metabolite production by endophytes often declines with repeated subculturing due to the loss of host-derived signals and microbial interactions that activate biosynthetic gene clusters. However, adding autoclaved host plant material to axenic cultures reactivated flavonolignan synthesis, highlighting the role of host cues in restoring silent pathways (El-Elimat et al. 2014). Bacterial endophyte also shows a reduction in secondary metabolite production after continuous subculturing (Pu Xiang et al. 2015). Low yield is an important obstacle in the bioproduction of bioactives from endophytic fungi. Many endophytes have very specific nutritional needs, such as trace elements or unusual carbon/nitrogen sources, which are uncommon in common laboratory media like PDA (potato dextrose agar) or malt extract agar. Fungal fermentations in artificially defined laboratory media often fail to replicate the natural endophytic environment, leading to the activation of only a limited number of biosynthetic pathways for secondary metabolite production (Verma et al. 2023). As a result, the full metabolic potential of endophytic fungi remains underutilized. Sustainable use of endophytes also helps protect medicinal plants from overharvesting, which threatens biodiversity and ecological balance. Ex situ cultivation of endophytes offers an eco-friendly alternative for metabolite production. Future approaches to the long-term cultivation of endophytes for the generation of secondary metabolites include host-mimicking conditions to activate dormant gene clusters, genomics, synthetic biology, and coculture techniques. Scalable bioreactors facilitate environmental friendly large-scale manufacturing, while the metabolomics method and CRISPR allow for fine pathway control. Innovation that is both lawful and responsible is ensured by combining conservation ethics with ABS agreements. All of these methods work together to fully realize endophytes' ability as a dependable, environmentally benign source of new bioactive chemicals for industrial and medicinal uses.

12 Conclusion

The unique bioresource status of endophytic microorganisms has made them a notable reservoir for the extraction of biologically active secondary metabolites. Endophytes like fungi have become a viable and sustainable source of new bioactive secondary metabolites in response to the increasing need for safe, efficient, and low-toxicity medicinal treatments (Prajapati et al. 2025a). They will play a crucial role in the discovery and creation of drugs in the coming years due to their extraordinary capacity to create a broad range of biologically active chemicals that frequently resemble those present within host plants. With a broad array of biological functions, including anticancer, antibacterial, antioxidant, and beneficial effects on inflammation, these metabolites, which include alkaloids, terpenoids with polyketides, are extremely desirable for use in the medicinal field. In addition to promoting plant safety and health, the mutually beneficial relationship between endophytes and the plants they colonize also illustrates the microorganisms' capacity for evolution to produce chemicals with medicinal value. There is an urgent need to learn more about the metabolic potential of endophytic fungi, as evidenced by the growing number of new compounds that are being found from these organisms. To identify the underlying processes and improve metabolite output, integrative methods combining genomes, metabolomics and bioinformatics are crucial. Therefore, through biology, pharmacodynamic, and preclinical research, the ongoing study of endophytic fungi holds enormous promise for discovering novel therapeutic candidates and comprehending their modes of action. Pharmaceutical studies can get closer to more creative, effective, and sustainable answers to the world's health problems by utilizing these microbial allies.

Acknowledgements SKS lab would like to acknowledge funding from the Institution of Eminence Incentive Grant Scheme, Trans-Disciplinary Research Scheme, Department of Science and Technology, SEED grant, New Delhi, and funding from the Institute of Medical Sciences intramural grant, Banaras Hindu University, Varanasi, India. SP would like to acknowledge CSIR (09/0013(19565)/2024-EMR-I) for providing fellowship assistance. CP & SNR would like to acknowledge CSIR (09/0013(12277)/ 2021-EMR-I) and ICMR (3/1/3/196/Neuro/2021-NCD-I) for providing fellowship assistance, respectively.

Conflict of Interest The authors declare there is no conflict of interest.

References

Abdelaziz AM, El-Wakil DA, Attia MS, Ali OM, AbdElgawad H, Hashem AH (2022) Inhibition of Aspergillus flavus growth and aflatoxin production in Zea mays L. using endophytic Aspergillus fumigatus. J Fungi 8(5):482

Abdel-Hadi A, Aloyuni S, Alharbi R, Jahan S, Darwish O, Senthilkumar S et al (2022) Stroke preventing effect of resveratrol isolated from fungi and in vivo activity in male albino rats. J King Saud Univ-Sci 34(5):102074

Abdou R, Shabana S, Rateb ME (2020) Terezine E, bioactive prenylated tryptophan analogue from an endophyte of Centaurea stoebe. Nat Prod Res 34(4):503–510

Agler MT, Ruhe J, Kroll S, Morhenn C, Kim S-T, Weigel D, Kemen EM (2016) Microbial hub taxa link host and abiotic factors to plant microbiome variation. PLoS Biol 14(1):e1002352

Agrawal S, Samanta S, Deshmukh SK (2022) The antidiabetic potential of endophytic fungi: future prospects as therapeutic agents. Biotechnol Appl Biochem 69(3):1159–1165

Al-Hosni S, Rizvi TS, Khan A, Ali L, Rehman NU, Rashid U et al (2020) Diketopeprazin and Methyl-5-docosenoate from endophytic fungi Aureobasidium pollulan BSS6 with α-Glucosidase inhibition and its validation through molecular docking. S Afr J Bot 134:322–328

Ali AH, Abdelrahman M, Radwan U, El-Zayat S, El-Sayed MA (2018) Effect of Thermomyces fungal endophyte isolated from extreme hot desert-adapted plant on heat stress tolerance of cucumber. Appl Soil Ecol 124:155–162

Ali AH, Radwan U, El-Zayat S, El-Sayed MA (2019) The role of the endophytic fungus, Thermomyces lanuginosus, on mitigation of heat stress to its host desert plant Cullen plicata. Biol Futur 70(1):1–7

Alvarez-Loayza P, White JF Jr, Torres MS, Balslev H, Kristiansen T, Svenning J-C, Gil N (2011) Light converts endosymbiotic fungus to pathogen, influencing seedling survival and niche-space filling of a common tropical tree, Iriartea deltoidea. PLoS One 6(1):e16386

Ashafani NF, Astuti RI, Listiyowati S, Batubara I (2023) Quercetin-containing extract from clove Syzygium aromaticum L. endophytic bacteria, Fictibacillus phosphorivorans P1U2, exhibits antimutagenic activity in yeast Saccharomyces cerevisiae. HAYATI J Biosci 30(4):734–742

Attia MS, Hashem AH, Badawy AA, Abdelaziz AM (2022) Biocontrol of early blight disease of eggplant using endophytic aspergillus terreus: improving plant immunological, physiological and antifungal activities. Bot Stud 63(1):26

Badalzadeh R, Yavari R, Chalabiani D (2015) Mitochondrial ATP-sensitive K+ channels mediate the antioxidative influence of diosgenin on myocardial reperfusion injury in rat hearts. Gen Physiol Biophys 34(3):323–329

Badawy AA, Alotaibi MO, Abdelaziz AM, Osman MS, Khalil AM, Saleh AM et al (2021) Enhancement of seawater stress tolerance in barley by the endophytic fungus Aspergillus ochraceus. Meta 11(7):428

Bamisile BS, Dash CK, Akutse KS, Keppanan R, Wang L (2018) Fungal endophytes: beyond herbivore management. Front Microbiol 9:544

Bandara CJ, Siriwardhana A, Karunaratne DN, Ratnayake Bandara BM, Wickramasinghe A, Krishnarajah SA, Karunaratne V (2021) Production of vincristine and vinblastine by the endophytic fungus Botryosphaeria laricina strain (CRS1) is dependent on stimulating factors present in Catharanthus roseus. Nat Prod J 11(2):221–230

Bansal AK, Meyer TE (2002) Evolutionary analysis by whole-genome comparisons. J Bacteriol 184(8):2260–2272

Barreiro C, Gutiérrez S, Olivera ER (2019) Fungal horizontal gene transfer: a history beyond the phylogenetic kingdoms. In: Horizontal gene transfer: breaking borders between living kingdoms. Springer, pp 315–336

Barriuso J (2015) Quorum sensing mechanisms in fungi. Aims Microbiol 1(1):37–47

Bhadra F, Vasundhara M (2024) Anti-inflammatory potential of aconitine produced by endophytic fungus Acremonium alternatum. World J Microbiol Biotechnol 40(9):274

Biswas D, Nazir R, Biswas P, Kumar V, Nandy S, Mukherjee A et al (2020) Endophytic sources of diosgenin, a natural steroid with multiple therapeutic values. S Afr J Bot 134:119–125

Boonsnongcheep P, Nakashima T, Takahashi Y, Prathanturarug S (2017) Diversity of endophytic actinomycetes isolated from roots and root nodules of Pueraria candollei Grah. ex Benth. and the analyses of their secondary metabolites. Chiang Mai J Sci 44(1):1–14

Bribi N (2018) Pharmacological activity of alkaloids: a review. Asian J Botany 1(1):1–6

Brosch G, Loidl P, Graessle S (2008) Histone modifications and chromatin dynamics: a focus on filamentous fungi. FEMS Microbiol Rev 32(3):409–439

Calado M d L, Silva J, Alves C, Susano P, Santos D, Alves J et al (2021) Marine endophytic fungi associated with Halopteris scoparia (Linnaeus) Sauvageau as producers of bioactive secondary metabolites with potential dermocosmetic application. PLoS One 16(5):e0250954

Cao H-Y, Sun S-f, Yi C, Yang C-y, Chen K-l, Zhang X-w, Liu Y-B (2023) Muyocoxanthones O–S: undescribed xanthones with antioxidative damage bioactivity to cardiomyocytes from the endophytic fungus Muyocopron laterale. Phytochemistry 209:113625

Castillo UF, Strobel GA, Ford EJ, Hess WM, Porter H, Jensen JB et al (2002) Munumbicins, wide-spectrum antibiotics produced by Streptomyces NRRL 30562, endophytic on Kennedia nigriscans. Microbiology 148(9):2675–2685

Castillo U, Harper JK, Strobel GA, Sears J, Alesi K, Ford E et al (2003) Kakadumycins, novel antibiotics from Streptomyces sp. NRRL 30566, an endophyte of Grevillea pteridifolia. FEMS Microbiol Lett 224(2):183–190

Challis GL (2008) Genome mining for novel natural product discovery. J Med Chem 51(9):2618–2628

Chaturvedi P, Gajbhiye S, Roy S, Dudhale R, Chowdhary A (2014) Determination of Kaempferol in extracts of Fusarium chlamydosporum, an endophytic fungi of Tylophora indica (Asclepeadaceae) and its anti-microbial activity. IOSR J Pharm Biol Sci 9(1):51

Chiang Y-M, Chang S-L, Oakley BR, Wang CC (2011) Recent advances in awakening silent biosynthetic gene clusters and linking orphan clusters to natural products in microorganisms. Curr Opin Chem Biol 15(1):137–143

Choi I-G, Kim S-H (2007) Global extent of horizontal gene transfer. Proc Natl Acad Sci 104(11):4489–4494

Chua RW, Song KP, Ting ASY (2024) Antioxidant properties and L-asparaginase activities of endophytic fungi from Cymbidium orchids. Folia Microbiol 69(4):713–722

Cimermancic P, Medema MH, Claesen J, Kurita K, Brown LCW, Mavrommatis K et al (2014) Insights into secondary metabolism from a global analysis of prokaryotic biosynthetic gene clusters. Cell 158(2):412–421

Coleman-Derr D, Desgarennes D, Fonseca-Garcia C, Gross S, Clingenpeel S, Woyke T et al (2016) Plant compartment and biogeography affect microbiome composition in cultivated and native agave species. New Phytol 209(2):798–811

Cormio G, Loizzi V, Gissi F, Camporeale A, De Mitri P, Leone L et al (2011) Long-term topotecan therapy in recurrent or persistent ovarian cancer. Eur J Gynaec Oncol-ISSN 32(2):153–155

Costelloe C, Metcalfe C, Lovering A, Mant D, Hay AD (2010) Effect of antibiotic prescribing in primary care on antimicrobial resistance in individual patients: systematic review and meta-analysis. BMJ 340

Cui Y, Yi D, Bai X, Sun B, Zhao Y, Zhang Y (2012) Ginkgolide B produced endophytic fungus (Fusarium oxysporum) isolated from Ginkgo biloba. Fitoterapia 83(5):913–920

Devari S, Jaglan S, Kumar M, Deshidi R, Guru S, Bhushan S et al (2014) Capsaicin production by Alternaria alternata, an endophytic fungus from Capsicum annum; LC–ESI–MS/MS analysis. Phytochemistry 98:183–189

Ding L, Münch J, Goerls H, Maier A, Fiebig H-H, Lin W-H, Hertweck C (2010) Xiamycin, a pentacyclic indolosesquiterpene with selective anti-HIV activity from a bacterial mangrove endophyte. Bioorg Med Chem Lett 20(22):6685–6687

Ding G, Wang H, Li L, Chen AJ, Chen L, Chen H et al (2012) Trichoderones A and B: two pentacyclic cytochalasans from the plant endophytic fungus Trichoderma gamsii. Eur J Org Chem 2012(13):2516–2519

Ding Z, Zhou H, Wang X, Huang H, Wang H, Zhang R et al (2020) Deletion of the histone deacetylase HdaA in endophytic fungus Penicillium chrysogenum Fes1701 induces the complex response of multiple bioactive secondary metabolite production and relevant gene cluster expression. Molecules 25(16):3657

El-Agamy DS, Ibrahim SR, Ahmed N, Khoshhal S, Abo-Haded HM, Elkablawy MA et al (2019) Aspernolide F, as a new cardioprotective butyrolactone against doxorubicin-induced cardiotoxicity. Int Immunopharmacol 72:429–436

Elawady ME, Hamed AA, Alsallami WM, Gabr EZ, Abdel-Monem MO, Hassan MG (2023) Bioactive metabolite from endophytic aspergillus versicolor SB5 with anti-acetylcholinesterase, anti-inflammatory and antioxidant activities: in vitro and in silico studies. Microorganisms 11(4):1062

Elbermawi A, Ali AR, Amen Y, Ashour A, Ahmad KF, Mansour E-SS, Halim AF (2022) Anti-diabetic activities of phenolic compounds of Alternaria sp., an endophyte isolated from the leaves of desert plants growing in Egypt. RSC Adv 12(38):24935–24945

El-Deeb B, Fayez K, Gherbawy Y (2013) Isolation and characterization of endophytic bacteria from Plectranthus tenuiflorus medicinal plant in Saudi Arabia desert and their antimicrobial activities. J Plant Interact 8(1):56–64

El-Elimat T, Raja HA, Graf TN, Faeth SH, Cech NB, Oberlies NH (2014) Flavonolignans from Aspergillus iizukae, a fungal endophyte of milk thistle (Silybum marianum). J Nat Prod 77(2):193–199

El-Gendy MM, El-Bondkly AM (2010) Production and genetic improvement of a novel antimycotic agent, saadamycin, against dermatophytes and other clinical fungi from endophytic Streptomyces sp. Hedaya48. J Ind Microbiol Biotechnol 37(8):831–841

El-Sayed AS, Abdel-Ghany SE, Ali GS (2017) Genome editing approaches: manipulating of lovastatin and taxol synthesis of filamentous fungi by CRISPR/Cas9 system. Appl Microbiol Biotechnol 101(10):3953–3976

Filardo S, Di Pietro M, Mastromarino P, Sessa R (2020) Therapeutic potential of resveratrol against emerging respiratory viral infections. Pharmacol Ther 214:107613

Furumai T, Yamakawa T, Yoshida R, Igarashi Y (2003) Clethramycin, a new inhibitor of pollen tube growth with antifungal activity from Streptomyces hygroscopicus TP-A0623 I. Screening, taxonomy, fermentation, isolation and biological properties. J Antibiot 56(8):700–704

Gao Y, Xu Y, Dong Z, Guo Y, Luo J, Wang F et al (2025) Endophytic fungal diversity and its interaction mechanism with medicinal plants. Molecules 30(5):1028

Ge H-L, Zhang D-W, Li L, Xie D, Zou J-H, Si Y-K, Dai J (2011) Two new terpenoids from endophytic fungus Periconia sp. F-31. Chem Pharm Bull 59(12):1541–1544

Gohain A, Gogoi A, Debnath R, Yadav A, Singh BP, Gupta VK et al (2015) Antimicrobial biosynthetic potential and genetic diversity of endophytic actinomycetes associated with medicinal plants. FEMS Microbiol Lett 362(19):fnv158

Gurgel RS, de Melo Pereira DÍ, Garcia AVF, Fernandes de Souza AT, Mendes da Silva T, de Andrade CP et al (2023) Antimicrobial and antioxidant activities of endophytic fungi associated with Arrabidaea chica (Bignoniaceae). J Fungi 9(8):864

Han L, Zheng W, Qian S-Y, Yang M-F, Lu Y-Z, He Z-J, Kang J-C (2023) New guaiane-Type Sesquiterpenoids biscogniauxiaols A–G with anti-fungal and anti-inflammatory activities from the endophytic fungus Biscogniauxia Petrensis. J Fungi 9(4):393

Hardoim PR, Van Overbeek LS, Berg G, Pirttilä AM, Compant S, Campisano A et al (2015) The hidden world within plants: ecological and evolutionary considerations for defining functioning of microbial endophytes. Microbiol Mol Biol Rev 79(3):293–320

Harrison L, Teplow DB, Rinaldi M, Strobel G (1991) Pseudomycins, a family of novel peptides from Pseudomonas syringae possessing broad-spectrum antifungal activity. Microbiology 137(12):2857–2865

Hashem AH, Attia MS, Kandil EK, Fawzi MM, Abdelrahman AS, Khader MS et al (2023) Bioactive compounds and biomedical applications of endophytic fungi: a recent review. Microb Cell Factories 22(1):107

Heydari A, Pessarakli M (2010) A review on biological control of fungal plant pathogens using microbial antagonists. J Biol Sci 10(4):273–290

Hidayat I, Radiastuti N, Rahayu G, Achmadi S, Okane I (2016) Three quinine and cinchonidine producing Fusarium species from Indonesia. Curr Res Environ Appl Mycol 6(1):20–34

Higgins S, Heeb S, Rampioni G, Fletcher MP, Williams P, Cámara M (2018) Differential regulation of the phenazine biosynthetic operons by quorum sensing in Pseudomonas aeruginosa PAO1-N. Front Cellular Infect Microbiol 8:252

Hu ZY, Li YY, Huang YJ, Su WJ, Shen YM (2008) Three new sesquiterpenoids from Xylaria sp. NCY2. Helv Chim Acta 91(1):46–52

Huang L, Wang S-L, Xu Y-L, Yu H-F, Zhan Z-J, Shan W-G et al (2020a) Induced production of tremulane sesquiterpenoids in Bjerkandera adusta by chemical epigenetic modification. Chem Nat Compd 56:754–756

Huang P-W, Yang Q, Zhu Y-L, Zhou J, Sun K, Mei Y-Z, Dai C-C (2020b) The construction of CRISPR-Cas9 system for endophytic Phomopsis liquidambaris and its PmkkA-deficient mutant revealing the effect on rice. Fungal Genet Biol 136:103301

Huang X, Chen Z, Wang L, Ran J, Wang J, Jiang J et al (2024) Metabolite profiling and genomic properties of an endophytic Bacillus siamensis strain with anti-tumor activity isolated from medicinal plant Curcuma Wenyujin. Plant Cell, Tissue Organ Culture 156(2):64

Igarashi Y, Miura S-S, Fujita T, Furumai T (2006) Pterocidin, a cytotoxic compound from the endophytic Streptomyces hygroscopicus. J Antibiot 59(3):193–195

Indananda C, Igarashi Y, Ikeda M, Oikawa T, Thamchaipenet A (2013) Linfuranone A, a new polyketide from plant-derived Microbispora sp. GMKU 363. J Antibiot 66(11):675–677

Janso JE, Carter GT (2010) Biosynthetic potential of phylogenetically unique endophytic actinomycetes from tropical plants. Appl Environ Microbiol 76(13):4377–4386

Jasim B, Geethu P, Mathew J, Radhakrishnan E (2015) Effect of endophytic Bacillus sp. from selected medicinal plants on growth promotion and diosgenin production in Trigonella foenum-graecum. Plant Cell, Tissue Organ Culture 122(3):565–572

Jasim B, Sreelakshmi K, Mathew J, Radhakrishnan E (2016) Surfactin, iturin, and fengycin biosynthesis by endophytic Bacillus sp. from Bacopa monnieri. Microb Ecol 72(1):106–119

Jiang Z-k, Tuo L, Huang D-l, Osterman IA, Tyurin AP, Liu S-w et al (2018) Diversity, novelty, and antimicrobial activity of endophytic actinobacteria from mangrove plants in Beilun Estuary National Nature Reserve of Guangxi, China. Front Microbiol 9:868

Jiang R, Guo J, Yang S, Zeng H, Wei J, Jin X et al (2025) Trichodenoids A and B, two skeletally unprecedented polyketides from Trichoderma reesei with cardioprotective effects against H2O2-induced injury. J Agric Food Chem 73(11):6736–6744

Joo H-S, Deyrup ST, Shim SH (2021) Endophyte-produced antimicrobials: a review of potential lead compounds with a focus on quorum-sensing disruptors. Phytochem Rev 20(3):543–568

Juybari HZ, Tajick Ghanbary MA, Rahimian H, Karimi K, Arzanlou M (2019) Seasonal, tissue and age influences on frequency and biodiversity of endophytic fungi of Citrus sinensis in Iran. Forensic Pathol 49(6):e12559

Kalimuthu AK, Parasuraman P, Sivakumar P, Murugesan S, Arunachalam S, Pandian SRK et al (2022) In silico, in vitro screening of antioxidant and anticancer potentials of bioactive secondary metabolites from an endophytic fungus (Curvularia sp.) from Phyllanthus niruri L. Environ Sci Pollut Res 29(32):48908–48925

Kamdem RS, Wang H, Wafo P, Ebrahim W, Özkaya FC, Makhloufi G et al (2018) Induction of new metabolites from the endophytic fungus Bionectria sp. through bacterial co-culture. Fitoterapia 124:132–136

Kandel SL, Joubert PM, Doty SL (2017) Bacterial endophyte colonization and distribution within plants. Microorganisms 5(4):77

Kayser O, Warzecha H (2012) Pharmaceutical biotechnology: drug discovery and clinical applications. John Wiley & Sons

Keller NP (2019) Fungal secondary metabolism: regulation, function and drug discovery. Nat Rev Microbiol 17(3):167–180

Khachatoorian R, Arumugaswami V, Raychaudhuri S, Yeh GK, Maloney EM, Wang J et al (2012) Divergent antiviral effects of bioflavonoids on the hepatitis C virus life cycle. Virology 433(2):346–355

Khalil A, Abdelaziz A, Khaleil M, Hashem A (2021) Fungal endophytes from leaves of Avicennia marina growing in semi-arid environment as a promising source for bioactive compounds. Lett Appl Microbiol 72(3):263–274

Kim MJ, Cheng Z (2024) Anti-bacterial cyclic dipeptides from Hormonema dematioides, an endophytic fungus of Juniperus communis. Nat Prod Res:1–6

Kim J, Baek JY, Bang S, Kim J-Y, Jin Y, Lee JW et al (2023) New anti-inflammatory β-resorcylic acid lactones derived from an endophytic fungus, Colletotrichum sp. ACS Omega 8(3):3530–3538

Koopklang K, Choodej S, Hantanong S, Intayot R, Jungsuttiwong S, Insumran Y et al (2024) Anti-inflammatory properties of oxygenated isocoumarins and xanthone from thai mangrove-associated endophytic fungus Setosphaeria rostrata. Molecules 29(3):603

Kusari S, Lamshöft M, Spiteller M (2009a) Aspergillus fumigatus Fresenius, an endophytic fungus from Juniperus communis L. Horstmann as a novel source of the anticancer pro-drug deoxypodophyllotoxin. J Appl Microbiol 107(3):1019–1030

Kusari S, Zühlke S, Kosuth J, Cellarova E, Spiteller M (2009b) Light-independent metabolomics of endophytic Thielavia subthermophila provides insight into microbial hypericin biosynthesis. J Nat Prod 72(10):1825–1835

Kusari S, Verma VC, Lamshoeft M, Spiteller M (2012) An endophytic fungus from Azadirachta indica A. Juss. that produces azadirachtin. World J Microbiol Biotechnol 28(3):1287–1294

Lata R, Gond SK (2025) Antibacterial and antioxidant potentials, detection of host origin compounds, and metabolic profiling of endophytic Bacillus spp. isolated from Rauvolfia serpentina (L.) Benth. ex Kurz. Sci Rep 15(1):2094

Le TTM, Hoang ATH, Nguyen NP, Le TTB, Trinh HTT, Vo TTB, Quyen DV (2020) A novel huperzine A-producing endophytic fungus Fusarium sp. Rsp5. 2 isolated from Huperzia serrate. Biotechnol Lett 42(6):987–995

Li DL, Li XM, Li TG, Dang HY, Wang BG (2008) Dioxopiperazine alkaloids produced by the marine mangrove derived endophytic fungus Eurotium rubrum. Helv Chim Acta 91(10):1888–1893

Li X, Zhai X, Shu Z, Dong R, Ming Q, Qin L, Zheng C (2016) Phoma glomerata D14: an endophytic fungus from Salvia miltiorrhiza that produces salvianolic acid C. Curr Microbiol 73(1):31–37

Li H-T, Tang L-H, Liu T, Yang R-N, Yang Y-B, Zhou H, Ding Z-T (2020) Protoilludane-type sesquiterpenoids from Armillaria sp. by co-culture with the endophytic fungus Epicoccum sp. associated with Gastrodia elata. Bioorg Chem 95:103503

Li H, Lin C, Chen K, Zhou Z, Chen Z, Ding B et al (2024) New polyketides and cytotoxic alkaloids from the mangrove endophytic fungus Talaromyces sp. SAF14. Nat Prod Res:1–5

Lin Z, Wen J, Zhu T, Fang Y, Gu Q, Zhu W (2008) Chrysogenamide A from an endophytic fungus associated with Cistanche deserticola and its neuroprotective effect on SH-SY5Y cells. J Antibiot 61(2):81–85

Lin T, Lin X, Lu CH, Shen YM (2011) Three new triterpenes from Xylarialean sp. A45, an endophytic fungus from Annona squamosa L. Helv Chim Acta 94(2):301–305

Lini IF, Afroz F, Begum N, Rony SR, Sharmin S, Moni F, Sohrab MH (2020) Identification and bioactive potential of endophytic fungi from marine weeds available in the coastal area of Bangladesh. Int J Pharm Sci Res 11(3):1249–1257

Liu G, Huo R, Zhai Y, Liu L (2021) New bioactive sesquiterpeniods from the plant endophytic fungus Pestalotiopsis theae. Front Microbiol 12:641504

Lu C, Shen Y (2007) A novel ansamycin, naphthomycin K from Streptomyces sp. J Antibiot 60(10):649–653

Magotra A, Kumar M, Kushwaha M, Awasthi P, Raina C, Gupta AP et al (2017) Epigenetic modifier induced enhancement of fumiquinazoline C production in Aspergillus fumigatus (GA-L7): an endophytic fungus from Grewia asiatica L. AMB Express 7:1–10

Malik A, Ardalani H, Anam S, McNair LM, Kromphardt KJ, Frandsen RJN et al (2020) Antidiabetic xanthones with α-glucosidase inhibitory activities from an endophytic Penicillium canescens. Fitoterapia 142:104522

Manganyi MC, Ateba CN (2020) Untapped potentials of endophytic fungi: a review of novel bioactive compounds with biological applications. Microorganisms 8(12):1934

Mani VM, Soundari AJPG, Balasubramanian B, Park S, Issara U, Preethi K, Liu W-C (2021) Evaluation of dimer of epicatechin from an endophytic fungus Curvularia australiensis FC2AP on acute toxicity levels, anti-inflammatory and anti-cervical cancer activity in animal models. Molecules 26(3):654

Mao XM, Xu W, Li D, Yin WB, Chooi YH, Li YQ et al (2015) Epigenetic genome mining of an endophytic fungus leads to the pleiotropic biosynthesis of natural products. Angew Chem Int Ed 54(26):7592–7596

Mao Z, Zhang W, Wu C, Feng H, Peng Y, Shahid H et al (2021) Diversity and antibacterial activity of fungal endophytes from Eucalyptus exserta. BMC Microbiol 21(1):155

Márquez LM, Redman RS, Rodriguez RJ, Roossinck MJ (2007) A virus in a fungus in a plant: three-way symbiosis required for thermal tolerance. Science 315(5811):513–515

Mazlan NW, Tate R, Yusoff YM, Clements C, Edrada-Ebel R (2020) Metabolomics-guided isolation of anti-trypanosomal compounds from endophytic fungi of the mangrove plant Avicennia lanata. Curr Med Chem 27(11):1815–1835

Mazumder K, Ruma YN, Akter R, Aktar A, Hossain MM, Shahina Z et al (2021) Identification of bioactive metabolites and evaluation of in vitro anti-inflammatory and in vivo antinociceptive and antiarthritic activities of endophyte fungi isolated from Elaeocarpus floribundus blume. J Ethnopharmacol 273:113975

Miller KI, Qing C, Sze DMY, Neilan BA (2012) Investigation of the biosynthetic potential of endophytes in traditional Chinese anticancer herbs. 7(5):e35953

Ming Q, Li Y, Jiang X, Huang X, He Y, Qin L et al (2022) Xanthones and benzophenones isolated from the endophytic fungus Penicillium sp. ct-28 of Corydlis tomentella and their cytotoxic activity. Fitoterapia 157:105127

Mishra A, Gond SK, Kumar A, Sharma VK, Verma SK, Kharwar RN, Sieber TN (2012) Season and tissue type affect fungal endophyte communities of the Indian medicinal plant Tinospora cordifolia more strongly than geographic location. Microb Ecol 64:388–398

Miyanaga A (2017) Structure and function of polyketide biosynthetic enzymes: various strategies for production of structurally diverse polyketides. Biosci Biotechnol Biochem 81(12):2227–2236

Moglad E, Elekhnawy E, Negm WA, Eliwa D, Sami Younis S, Mohamed Elmansory B et al (2023) Antibacterial and anti-toxoplasma activities of Aspergillus Niger endophytic fungus isolated from Ficus retusa: in vitro and in vivo approach. Artif Cells Nanomed Biotechnol 51(1):297–308

Mohana Kumara P, Zuehlke S, Priti V, Ramesha BT, Shweta S, Ravikanth G et al (2012) Fusarium proliferatum, an endophytic fungus from Dysoxylum binectariferum Hook. f, produces rohitukine, a chromane alkaloid possessing anti-cancer activity. Antonie Van Leeuwenhoek 101(2):323–329

Mulyani Y, Sinaga SE, Supratman U (2023) Phytochemistry and biological activities of endophytic fungi from the meliaceae family. Molecules 28(2):778

Murakami S, Hayashi N, Inomata T, Kato H, Hitora Y, Tsukamoto S (2020) Induction of secondary metabolite production by fungal co-culture of Talaromyces pinophilus and Paraphaeosphaeria sp. J Nat Med 74:545–549

Nagarajan K, Chelladurai MD, Mani S, Pavadai P, Theivendren P, Palanisamy P et al (2025) Unlocking antidiabetic potential: novel compounds from endophytic fungi isolated from Manihot esculenta Crantz tuberous roots. J Mol Struct 1337:142083

Negi BS, Dave BP (2010) In vitro antimicrobial activity of Acacia catechu and its phytochemical analysis. Indian J Microbiol 50:369–374

Nguyen D, Nguyen N, Nguyen V, Nguyen T, Do T, Nguyen T et al (2023) Isolation and identification of vincristine and vinblastine producing endophytic fungi from Catharanthus roseus (L.) G. Don. Russ J Plant Physiol 70(8):188

Nicoletti R, Fiorentino A (2015) Plant bioactive metabolites and drugs produced by endophytic fungi of Spermatophyta. Agriculture 5(4):918–970

Nimnoi P, Pongsilp N, Lumyong S (2010) Endophytic actinomycetes isolated from Aquilaria crassna Pierre ex Lec and screening of plant growth promoters production. World J Microbiol Biotechnol 26:193–203

Okoye FBC, Lu S, Nworu CS, Esimone CO, Proksch P, Chadli A, Debbab A (2013) Depsidone and diaryl ether derivatives from the fungus Corynespora cassiicola, an endophyte of Gongronema latifolium. Tetrahedron Lett 54(32):4210–4214

Ola A, Thomy D, Lai D, Brötz-Oesterhelt H, Proksch P (2013) Inducing secondary metabolite production by the endophytic fungus Fusarium tricinctum through coculture with Bacillus subtilis. J Nat Prod 76(20942099):31

Ortega HE, Graupner PR, Asai Y, TenDyke K, Qiu D, Shen YY et al (2013) Mycoleptodiscins A and B, cytotoxic alkaloids from the endophytic fungus Mycoleptodiscus sp. F0194. J Nat Prod 76(4):741–744

Osama S, El Sherei M, Al-Mahdy DA, Bishr M, Salama O, Raafat MM (2024) Antimicrobial activity of spiculisporic acid isolated from endophytic fungus Aspergillus cejpii of Hedera helix against MRSA. Braz J Microbiol 55(1):515–527

Pandy R, Kumar SS, Suresh P, Annaraj J, Pandi M, Vellasamy S, Sagadevan S (2023) Screening and characterization of fungal taxol-producing endophytic fungi for evaluation of antimicrobial and anticancer activities. Open Chem 21(1):20220344

Papikinou M-A, Pavlidis K, Cholidis P, Kranas D, Adamantidi T, Anastasiadou C, Tsoupras A (2024) Marine fungi bioactives with anti-inflammatory, antithrombotic and antioxidant health-promoting properties against inflammation-related chronic diseases. Mar Drugs 22(11):520

Passari AK, Mishra VK, Singh G, Singh P, Kumar B, Gupta VK et al (2017) Insights into the functionality of endophytic actinobacteria with a focus on their biosynthetic potential and secondary metabolites production. Sci Rep 7(1):11809

Patil M, Patil R, Maheshwari V (2015) Biological activities and identification of bioactive metabolite from endophytic Aspergillus flavus L7 isolated from Aegle marmelos. Curr Microbiol 71(1):39–48

Pereira CB, De Oliveira DM, Hughes AF, Kohlhoff M, La Vieira M, Martins Vaz AB et al (2015) Endophytic fungal compounds active against Cryptococcus neoformans and C. gattii. J Antibiot 68(7):436–444

Petrini O (1991) Fungal endophytes of tree leaves. In: Microbial ecology of leaves. Springer, pp 179–197

Pettit RK (2011) Small-molecule elicitation of microbial secondary metabolites. Microb Biotechnol 4(4):471–478

Pi W-X, Feng X-P, Ye L-H, Cai B-C (2017) Combination of morroniside and diosgenin prevents high glucose-induced cardiomyocytes apoptosis. Molecules 22(1):163

Pillay LC, Nekati L, Makhwitine PJ, Ndlovu SI (2022) Epigenetic activation of silent biosynthetic gene clusters in endophytic fungi using small molecular modifiers. Front Microbiol 13:815008

Prajapati C, Kumar D, Ambastha V, Singh SK (2024a) Fungal endophytes as potential anticancer candidate over synthetic drugs: latest development and future prospects. In: Endophytic fungi: the hidden sustainable jewels for the pharmaceutical and agricultural industries. Springer, pp 27–56

Prajapati C, Rai SN, Mishra SS, Singh SK, Singh AK (2024b) Natural sources of drugs for neurodegenerative diseases. In: Neurodegenerative diseases. CRC Press, pp 120–134

Prajapati C, Rai SN, Singh AK, Chopade BA, Singh Y, Singh SK et al (2025a) An update of fungal endophyte diversity and strategies for augmenting therapeutic potential of their potent metabolites: recent advancement. Appl Biochem Biotechnol 197(5):2799–2866

Prajapati C, Rai SN, Singh AK, Rajak N, Garg N, Singh SK (2025b) Untargeted metabolomics and bioactivities assessment of Xylaria ellisii, an endophytic fungus isolated from the leaf of the plant Acorus calamus Linn. Curr Pharm Des 31(22):1781–1799

Prajapati C, Tripathi PN, Sood S, Rai SN, Mishra SS, Singh SK, Tiwari AK (2025c) Intellectual property rights in neuroprotective biomaterials. In: Biomaterials and neurodegenerative disorders. Springer, pp 251–269

Ptak A, Morańska E, Warchoł M, Gurgul A, Skrzypek E, Dziurka M et al (2022) Endophytic bacteria from in vitro culture of Leucojum aestivum L. a new source of galanthamine and elicitor of alkaloid biosynthesis. Sci Rep 12(1):13700

Pu Xiang PX, Chen Fei CF, Yang Yun YY, Qu XiXing QX, Zhang GuoLin ZG, Luo YingGang LY (2015) Isolation and characterization of Paenibacillus polymyxa LY214, a camptothecin-producing endophytic bacterium from Camptotheca acuminata. J Ind Microbiol Biotechnol 42(8):1197–1202

Pu X, Qu X, Chen F, Bao J, Zhang G, Luo Y (2013) Camptothecin-producing endophytic fungus Trichoderma atroviride LY357: isolation, identification, and fermentation conditions optimization for camptothecin production. Appl Microbiol Biotechnol 97(21):9365–9375

Pu X, Chen F, Yang Y, Qu X, Zhang G, Luo Y (2015) Isolation and characterization of Paenibacillus polymyxa LY214, a camptothecin-producing endophytic bacterium from Camptotheca acuminata. J Indust Microbiol Biotechnol 42(8):1197–1202

Puri SC, Nazir A, Chawla R, Arora R, Riyaz-ul-Hasan S, Amna T et al (2006) The endophytic fungus Trametes hirsuta as a novel alternative source of podophyllotoxin and related aryl tetralin lignans. J Biotechnol 122(4):494–510

Qi FH, Jing TZ, Wang ZX, Zhan YG (2009) Fungal endophytes from Acer ginnala Maxim: isolation, identification and their yield of gallic acid. Lett Appl Microbiol 49(1):98–104

Qin S, Chen HH, Zhao GZ, Li J, Zhu WY, Xu LH et al (2012) Abundant and diverse endophytic actinobacteria associated with medicinal plant Maytenus austroyunnanensis in Xishuangbanna tropical rainforest revealed by culture-dependent and culture-independent methods. Environ Microbiol Rep 4(5):522–531

Radajewska A, Moreira H, Bęben D, Siwiela O, Szyjka A, Gębczak K et al (2023) Combination of irinotecan and melatonin with the natural compounds wogonin and celastrol for colon cancer treatment. Int J Mol Sci 24(11):9544

Rai M, Agarkar G, Rathod D (2014) Multiple applications of endophytic Colletotrichum species occurring in medicinal plants. In: Novel plant bioresources: applications in food, medicine cosmetics, pp 227–236

Rai SN, Singh P, Prajapati C, Tiwari N, Singh V, Patil RR et al (2025) Autophagy modulating potential of mucuna pruriens in Parkinson's disease. Curr Tradit Med 11:1–11

Ramos G d C, Silva-Silva JV, Watanabe LA, Siqueira JE d S, Almeida-Souza F, Calabrese KS et al (2022) Phomoxanthone A, compound of endophytic fungi Paecilomyces sp. and its potential antimicrobial and antiparasitic. Antibiotics 11(10):1332

Redgrave S, Condron T, Strobel. (1998) Ecomycins, unique antimycotics from Pseudomonas viridiflava. J Appl Microbiol 84(6):937–944

Rodrigues de Carvalho C, Vieira M d LA, Cantrell CL, Wedge DE, Alves TM, Zani CL et al (2016) Biological activities of ophiobolin K and 6-epi-ophiobolin K produced by the endophytic fungus Aspergillus calidoustus. Nat Prod Res 30(4):478–481

Roy A, Khan A, Ahmad I, Alghamdi S, Rajab BS, Babalghith AO et al (2022) Flavonoids a bioactive compound from medicinal plants and its therapeutic applications. Biomed Res Int 2022(1):5445291

Sana T, Siddiqui BS, Shahzad S, Farooq AD, Siddiqui F, Sattar S, Begum S (2019) Antiproliferative activity and characterization of metabolites of Aspergillus nidulans: an endophytic fungus from Nyctanthes arbor-tristis Linn. against three human cancer cell lines. Med Chem 15(4):352–359

Santoyo G, Moreno-Hagelsieb G, del Carmen Orozco-Mosqueda M, Glick BR (2016) Plant growth-promoting bacterial endophytes. Microbiol Res 183:92–99

Schulz B, Boyle C (2005) The endophytic continuum. Mycol Res 109(6):661–686

Shah WH, Khan W, Nisa S, Barfuss MH, Schinnerl J, Bacher M et al (2024) Hplc, nmr based characterization, antioxidant and anticancer activities of chemical constituents from therapeutically active fungal endophytes. J Microbiol Biotechnol 34(7):1452

Shaker KH, Zohair MM, Hassan AZ, Sweelam H-t M, Ashour WE (2022) LC–MS/MS and GC–MS based phytochemical perspectives and antimicrobial effects of endophytic fungus Chaetomium ovatoascomatis isolated from Euphorbia milii. Arch Microbiol 204(11):661

Sharaf MH, Abdelaziz AM, Kalaba MH, Radwan AA, Hashem AH (2022) Antimicrobial, antioxidant, cytotoxic activities and phytochemical analysis of fungal endophytes isolated from Ocimum basilicum. Appl Biochem Biotechnol:1–19

Sharma M, Mallubhotla S (2022) Diversity, antimicrobial activity, and antibiotic susceptibility pattern of endophytic bacteria sourced from Cordia dichotoma L. Front Microbiol 13:879386

Sharma V, Singamaneni V, Sharma N, Kumar A, Arora D, Kushwaha M et al (2018) Valproic acid induces three novel cytotoxic secondary metabolites in Diaporthe sp., an endophytic fungus from Datura inoxia Mill. Bioorg Med Chem Lett 28(12):2217–2221

Shiono Y, Kikuchi M, Koseki T, Murayama T, Kwon E, Aburai N, Kimura K-I (2011) Isopimarane diterpene glycosides, isolated from endophytic fungus Paraconiothyrium sp. MY-42. Phytochemistry 72(11–12):1400–1405

Shweta S, Zuehlke S, Ramesha B, Priti V, Kumar PM, Ravikanth G et al (2010) Endophytic fungal strains of Fusarium solani, from Apodytes dimidiata E. Mey. ex Arn (Icacinaceae) produce camptothecin, 10-hydroxycamptothecin and 9-methoxycamptothecin. Phytochemistry 71(1):117–122

Sidhu D, Vasundhara M, Dey P (2024) Chemical characterization, pathway enrichments and bioactive potentials of catechin-producing endophytic fungi isolated from tea leaves. RSC Adv 14(45):33034–33047

Silva Tironi L, Barbosa Moreira DM, Dias Bruzadelli RF, Gilberto Ferreira A, Schripsema J, Hortolan Luiz JH (2025) Antioxidant potential and chemical evaluation of extracts from endophytic fungus Lasiodiplodia sp. Chem Biodivers 22(1):e202401649

Singh R, Dubey AK (2018) Diversity and applications of endophytic actinobacteria of plants in special and other ecological niches. Front Microbiol 9:1767

Singh D, Thapa S, Mahawar H, Kumar D, Geat N, Singh S (2022) Prospecting potential of endophytes for modulation of biosynthesis of therapeutic bioactive secondary metabolites and plant growth promotion of medicinal and aromatic plants. Antonie Van Leeuwenhoek 115(6):699–730

Siyu-Mao, Hong-Chen, Li-Chen, Chuanxi-Wang, Wei-Jia, Xiaoming-Chen et al (2013) Two novel ansamitocin analogs from Actinosynnema pretiosum. Nat Prod Res 27(17):1532–1536

Song YC, Huang WY, Sun C, Wang FW, Tan RX (2005) Characterization of graphislactone A as the antioxidant and free radical-scavenging substance from the culture of Cephalosporium sp. IFB-E001, an endophytic fungus in Trachelospermum jasminoides. Biol Pharm Bull 28(3):506–509

Song JH, Lee C, Lee D, Kim S, Bang S, Shin M-S et al (2018) Neuroprotective compound from an endophytic fungus, Colletotrichum sp. JS-0367. J Nat Prod 81(6):1411–1416

de Souza JJ, Vieira IJC, Rodrigues-Filho E, Braz-Filho R (2011) Terpenoids from endophytic fungi. Molecules 16(12):10604–10618

Stein T (2005) Bacillus subtilis antibiotics: structures, syntheses and specific functions. Mol Microbiol 56(4):845–857

Stierle A, Strobel G, Stierle D (1993) Taxol and taxane production by Taxomyces andreanae, an endophytic fungus of Pacific yew. Science 260(5105):214–216

Strobel G, Yang X, Sears J, Kramer R, Sidhu RS, Hess W (1996) Taxol from Pestalotiopsis microspora, an endophytic fungus of Taxus wallachiana. Microbiology 142(2):435–440

Strobel G, Ford E, Worapong J, Harper JK, Arif AM, Grant DM et al (2002) Isopestacin, an isobenzofuranone from Pestalotiopsis microspora, possessing antifungal and antioxidant activities. Phytochemistry 60(2):179–183

Su J-C, Pan Q, Xu X, Wei X, Lei X, Zhang P (2022) Structurally diverse steroids from an endophyte of Aspergillus tennesseensis 1022LEF attenuates LPS-induced inflammatory response through the cholinergic anti-inflammatory pathway. Chem Biol Interact 362:109998

Sumanth B, Uzma F, Konappa N, Ali D, Alarifi S, Srinivas C, Jogaiah S (2024) Isolation of antimicrobial ellagic acid from endophytic fungi and their target-specific drug design through computational docking. Biomass Conversion Biorefinery 14(19):24867–24888

Sun Y, Liu W-C, Shi X, Zheng H-Z, Zheng Z-H, Lu X-H et al (2021) Inducing secondary metabolite production of Aspergillus sydowii through microbial co-culture with Bacillus subtilis. Microb Cell Factories 20:1–16

Sun Y, Ren G, Shi Q, Zhu H, Zhou N, Kong X et al (2023) Identification of a novel coumarins biosynthetic pathway in the endophytic fungus Fusarium oxysporum GU-7 with antioxidant activity. Appl Environ Microbiol 89(1):e01601–e01622

Tacar O, Sriamornsak P, Dass CR (2013) Doxorubicin: an update on anticancer molecular action, toxicity and novel drug delivery systems. J Pharm Pharmacol 65(2):157–170

Taechowisan T, Wanbanjob A, Tuntiwachwuttikul P, Taylor WC (2006) Identification of Streptomyces sp. Tc022, an endophyte in Alpinia galanga, and the isolation of actinomycin D. Ann Microbiol 56(2):113–117

Taechowisan T, Chuaychot N, Chanaphat S, Shen YJ (2009) Antioxidative and inhibitory activity on nitric oxide production of flavonoids from Streptomyces sp. *Tc052*. J Pharm Res 2:313–316

Taechowisan T, Chanaphat S, Ruensamran W, Phutdhawong WS (2014) Antibacterial activity of new flavonoids from Streptomyces sp. BT01; an endophyte in Boesenbergia rotunda (L.) Mansf. J Appl Pharma Sci 4(4):008–013

Talukdar R, Padhi S, Rai AK, Masi M, Evidente A, Jha DK et al (2021) Isolation and characterization of an endophytic fungus Colletotrichum coccodes producing tyrosol from Houttuynia cordata Thunb. using ITS2 RNA secondary structure and molecular docking study. Front Bioeng Biotechnol 9:650247

Tan Y, Guo Z, Zhu M, Shi J, Li W, Jiao R et al (2020) Anti-inflammatory spirobisnaphthalene natural products from a plant-derived endophytic fungus Edenia gomezpompae. Chin Chem Lett 31(6):1406–1409

Tantapakul C, Promgool T, Kanokmedhakul K, Soytong K, Song J, Hadsadee S et al (2020) Bioactive xanthoquinodins and epipolythiodioxopiperazines from Chaetomium globosum 7s-1, an endophytic fungus isolated from Rhapis cochinchinensis (Lour.) Mart. Nat Prod Res 34(4):494–502

Tao X, Chen X, Dong R, Wang G, Xu X, Yu Q et al (2024) Characterization and antioxidant properties of three exopolysaccharides produced by the Cyclocarya paliurus endophytic fungus. Int J Biol Macromol 271:132110

Thumpati P, Rai SN, Prajapati C, Ramakrishna K, Singh SK (2025) Targeting c-MYC G-quadruplexes for cancer treatment with small molecules. Sci Pharm 93(1):6

Tiwari P, Bae H (2020) Horizontal gene transfer and endophytes: an implication for the acquisition of novel traits. Plants 9(3):305

Todkar V, Habbu P, Kulkarni V, Madagundi S (2023) Neuroprotective metabolites from endophytic microbes: a review. RGUHS J Pharma Sci 13(3)

Tuntiwachwuttikul P, Taechowisan T, Wanbanjob A, Thadaniti S, Taylor WC (2008) Lansai A–D, secondary metabolites from Streptomyces sp. SUC1. Tetrahedron 64(32):7583–7586

U'ren JM, Lutzoni F, Miadlikowska J, Laetsch AD, Arnold AE (2012) Host and geographic structure of endophytic and endolichenic fungi at a continental scale. Am J Bot 99(5):898–914

Urumbil SK, Anilkumar MN (2021) Anti-inflammatory activity of endophytic bacterial isolates from Emilia sonchifolia (Linn.) DC. J Ethnopharmacol 281:114517

Usman M, Shah IH, Sabir IA, Malik MS, Rehman A, Murtaza G et al (2024) Synergistic partnerships of endophytic fungi for bioactive compound production and biotic stress management in medicinal plants. Plant Stress 11:100425

Van Lanen SG, Shen B (2006) Microbial genomics for the improvement of natural product discovery. Curr Opin Microbiol 9(3):252–260

Verma VC, Lobkovsky E, Gange AC, Singh SK, Prakash S (2011) Piperine production by endophytic fungus Periconia sp. isolated from Piper longum L. J Antibiot 64(6):427–431

Verma A, Tiwari H, Singh S, Gupta P, Rai N, Kumar Singh S et al (2023) Epigenetic manipulation for secondary metabolite activation in endophytic fungi: current progress and future directions. Mycology 14(4):275–291

Vig R, Bhadra F, Gupta SK, Sairam K, Vasundhara M (2022) Neuroprotective effects of quercetin produced by an endophytic fungus Nigrospora oryzae isolated from Tinospora cordifolia. J Appl Microbiol 132(1):365–380

Vos M, Hesselman MC, Te Beek TA, van Passel MW, Eyre-Walker A (2015) Rates of lateral gene transfer in prokaryotes: high but why? Trends Microbiol 23(10):598–605

Wagner MR, Lundberg DS, Del Rio TG, Tringe SG, Dangl JL, Mitchell-Olds T (2016) Host genotype and age shape the leaf and root microbiomes of a wild perennial plant. Nat Commun 7(1):12151

Wakefield J, Hassan HM, Jaspars M, Ebel R, Rateb ME (2017) Dual induction of new microbial secondary metabolites by fungal bacterial co-cultivation. Front Microbiol 8:1284

Wall ME, Wani MC, Cook CA, Palmer KH, McPhail AA, Sim G (1966) Plant antitumor agents. I. The isolation and structure of camptothecin, a novel alkaloidal leukemia and tumor inhibitor from camptotheca acuminata1, 2. J Am Chem Soc 88(16):3888–3890

Wang Y, Li H, Zhao W, He X, Chen J, Geng X, Xiao M (2010) Induction of toluene degradation and growth promotion in corn and wheat by horizontal gene transfer within endophytic bacteria. Soil Biol Biochem 42(7):1051–1057

Wang Q-X, Li S-F, Zhao F, Dai H-Q, Bao L, Ding R et al (2011) Chemical constituents from endophytic fungus Fusarium oxysporum. Fitoterapia 82(5):777–781

Wang Y, Xu L, Ren W, Zhao D, Zhu Y, Wu X (2012) Bioactive metabolites from Chaetomium globosum L18, an endophytic fungus in the medicinal plant Curcuma wenyujin. Phytomedicine 19(3–4):364–368

Wang P, Kong F, Wei J, Wang Y, Wang W, Hong K, Zhu W (2014a) Alkaloids from the mangrove-derived actinomycete Jishengella endophytica 161111. Mar Drugs 12(1):477–490

Wang X-J, Min C-L, Ge M, Zuo R-H (2014b) An endophytic sanguinarine-producing fungus from Macleaya cordata, Fusarium proliferatum BLH51. Curr Microbiol 68(3):336–341

Wang D, Jin S, Lu Q, Chen Y (2023a) Advances and challenges in CRISPR/Cas-based fungal genome engineering for secondary metabolite production: a review. J Fungi 9(3):362

Wang Y, Li Z, Xu M, Xiao Z, Liu C, Du B et al (2023b) Signal molecules regulate the synthesis of secondary metabolites in the interaction between endophytes and medicinal plants. Processes 11(3):849

Williams P (2007) Quorum sensing, communication and cross-kingdom signalling in the bacterial world. Microbiology 153(12):3923–3938

Wu J-S, Shi X-H, Zhang Y-H, Yu J-Y, Fu X-M, Li X et al (2019) Co-cultivation with 5-azacytidine induced new metabolites from the zoanthid-derived fungus Cochliobolus lunatus. Front Chem 7:763

Wu W, Chen W, Liu S, Wu J, Zhu Y, Qin L, Zhu B (2021) Beneficial relationships between endophytic bacteria and medicinal plants. Front Plant Sci 12:646146

Xiang H, Zhang T, Pang X, Wei Y, Liu H, Zhang Y et al (2018) Isolation of endophytic fungi from Dioscorea zingiberensis CH Wright and application for diosgenin production by solid-state fermentation. Appl Microbiol Biotechnol 102(13):5519–5532

Xu X, Huang R, Yin W-B (2021) An optimized and efficient CRISPR/Cas9 system for the endophytic fungus Pestalotiopsis fici. J Fungi 7(10):809

Yan J, Qi N, Wang S, Gadhave K, Yang S (2014) Characterization of secondary metabolites of an endophytic fungus from Curcuma wenyujin. Curr Microbiol 69(5):740–744

Yue J-Y, Yu Y (2022) Isolation and identification of endophytic fungi from Dendrobium huoshanense with their antibacterial and anti-inflammatory activities. Pak J Pharm Sci 35(4)

Zhang J, Wang J-D, Liu C-X, Yuan J-H, Wang X-J, Xiang W-S (2014) A new prenylated indole derivative from endophytic actinobacteria Streptomyces sp. neau-D50. Nat Prod Res 28(7):431–437

Zhang F-H, Xiang J-H, Cui W-X, Yu J, Wang Y, Li Q-F (2016) Isolation and identification of berberine from endophytic fungi HL-Y-3. Zhongguo Zhong Yao Za Zhi 41(16):2998–3001

Zhang Q, Acuña JJ, Inostroza NG, Mora ML, Radic S, Sadowsky MJ, Jorquera MA (2019) Endophytic bacterial communities associated with roots and leaves of plants growing in Chilean extreme environments. Sci Rep 9(1):4950

Zhang D, Sun W, Xu W, Ji C, Zhou Y, Sun J et al (2022) Antimicrobial and cytotoxic activity of endophytic fungi from Lagopsis supina. J Microbiol Biotechnol 33(4):543

Zhao K, Penttinen P, Guan T, Xiao J, Chen Q, Xu J et al (2011) The diversity and anti-microbial activity of endophytic actinomycetes isolated from medicinal plants in Panxi plateau, China. Curr Microbiol 62:182–190

Zhao J, Ma D, Luo M, Wang W, Zhao C, Zu Y et al (2014) In vitro antioxidant activities and antioxidant enzyme activities in HepG2 cells and main active compounds of endophytic fungus from pigeon pea [Cajanus cajan (L.) Millsp.]. Food Res Int 56:243–251

Zheng Y-K, Qiao X-G, Miao C-P, Liu K, Chen Y-W, Xu L-H, Zhao L-X (2016) Diversity, distribution and biotechnological potential of endophytic fungi. Ann Microbiol 66(2):529–542

Zhou G, Chen X, Zhang X, Che Q, Zhang G, Zhu T et al (2020) Prenylated p-terphenyls from a mangrove endophytic fungus, Aspergillus candidus LDJ-5. J Nat Prod 83(1):8–13

Zin NM, Baba MS, Zainal-Abidin AH, Latip J, Mazlan NW, Edrada-Ebel R (2017) Gancidin W, a potential low-toxicity antimalarial agent isolated from an endophytic Streptomyces SUK10. Drug Des Develop Ther:351–363

Endophyte-Mediated Biosynthesis of Valuable Secondary Metabolites

Ramkumar Muthu, Rajkumar Prabhakaran, Eldho Paul, Sivaprakasam Chinnarasu, and Maruthanayagam Veerabadhran

Abstract Despite being a little-known group of microorganisms that live inconspicuously within plant tissues, endophytes are gaining recognition as possible contributors to the natural synthesis of secondary metabolites. The bioactivity and biology of natural products were not given enough attention in the past, but a recent surge in interest seems to indicate that these microbial partners should be taken seriously due to the possibility that they produce bioactive compounds in amounts that are on par with or greater than those of their host plants. From alkaloids and terpenoids to flavonoids and phenolics, the endophyte metabolites display exceptional and diverse biological activities and limitless potential for use in pharmaceutical, agricultural, and industrial functions. The core idea of this chapter stresses the important concept of endophytes as ubiquitous regulators of host metabolism and biochemistry, activating clusters of biosynthetic genes to cospeciate advanced mechanisms of chemical defense. This chapter presents the dynamic nature of plant–endophyte crosstalk, ecological and evolutionary selective pressures generating diversity of metabolites, new methods of exploration like metagenomics, metabolomics, and synthetic biology, and together these advances represent enormous

R. Muthu
Department of Biotechnology, Sri Kaliswari College (Autonomous), Sivakasi, Tamil Nadu, India

R. Prabhakaran
Department of Biochemistry, Karpagam Academy of Higher Education, Deemed to be University, Coimbatore, Tamil Nadu, India

E. Paul
One Clinical Research, Mentor Education, Perth, WA, Australia

S. Chinnarasu
Division of Endocrinology, Diabetes and Metabolism, Ohio State University Wexner Medical Center, Columbus, OH, USA

M. Veerabadhran (✉)
Bioprospecting Research Unit, Department of General Surgery, Saveetha Medical College and Hospital, Saveetha Institute of Medical and Technical Sciences (SIMATS), Thandalam, Chennai, Tamil Nadu, India

S. Kumar Tripathi et al. (eds.), *Phytoceuticals for Sustainable Medication*, Interdisciplinary Biotechnological Advances,
https://doi.org/10.1007/978-981-95-7588-6_5

potential toward opening microbial treasure troves. In this chapter, it is illustrated that endophytes and their metabolites are offering unique new advances and potential for growth. Therefore, endophytes and their metabolites can be viewed as progressive biofactories and potential game-changers for the future of sustainable bioprospecting and green innovations.

Keywords Endophyte · Secondary metabolites · Molecular mechanisms · Fungi · Bioactivity

1 Introduction

The rising global need for environmentally compatible and bio-based alternatives in health care, agriculture, and biotechnology has resulted in interest in alternative sources of high-value bioactive chemicals. The most promising candidates are endophytes, which are microorganisms that live in plant tissues without causing damage. Endophytes are mainly bacteria and fungi. Endophytes possess an extraordinary ability to biosynthesize secondary compounds that often equal or exceed the medicinal capabilities of those produced by their host plants, which is more than just a colonization role (Kusari et al. 2023). Metabolites such as alkaloids, terpenoids, flavonoids, and polyketides exhibit a wide range of bioactivities such as antimicrobial, anticancer, antioxidant, anti-inflammatory, and immunomodulatory activities, making them potential candidates for pharmaceutical, nutraceutical, and agro-industrial use (Singh and Dubey 2024). The adaptive co-evolution of endophytes in symbiosis with host plants provides important characteristics that enable endophytes to occupy numerous ecological niches, which enhance chemical diversity and specificity of metabolites. The symbiosis creates an opportunity for occasionally sharing biosynthetic pathways or horizontal biosynthetic transfer, resulting in the production of metabolites that are structurally similar or identical to the host plant. Preliminary, endophyte-mediated production offers a more reliable, controllable, sustainable, and scalable strategy to plant-based extraction methods that are often burdened by low yields; long crop cycles; or ambiguity or sensitivities to growing conditions. Endophytic biosynthetic potential has been discovered and harnessed much more directly because of sophisticated tools such as metagenomics, metabolomics, genome editing, and synthetic biology, particularly for extracting new metabolites from rare or unculturable groups of microbes (Kumar and Radhakrishnan 2020). It is notable that the limits of sourcing natural products have been broadened with the discovery of endophytes producing key plant-derived bioactive compounds such as taxol, camptothecin, vinblastine, and podophyllotoxin (Jiang et al. 2023). At the same time, biotechnological innovations in applying endophytic biosynthetic processes for global industrial scale-up of metabolite production with relevant improvements in using pathway engineering, expression of heterologous genes, and CRISPR/Cas9-based genome editing (Ma et al. 2025). Additionally, it is now understood that their relationships with host plants cause intricate signaling and epigenetic reprogramming that modifies the regulation of biosynthetic gene clusters, as well as plant health and stress mitigation. Unfortunately, there are still large gaps in our knowledge of the production of secondary metabolites in fungal sources. Many uncultured and uncharacterized taxa are still unaccounted for because the bulk of current knowledge exists surrounding known culturable endophytes. In addition, molecular mechanisms underpinning biosynthesis, regulation, and host endophyte specificity of metabolites are completely unknown (Singh and Dubey 2024). To ensure that endophytes can develop their maximum potential, they will need to close these gaps, potentially using interdisciplinary approaches. Endophytes represent a diverse yet underutilized source of metabolic diversity that offers sustainable options for growing secondary metabolites and opportunities in drug discovery, agriculture, and biotechnology. Advances in genomics, transcriptomics, metabolomics, and synthetic biology are making it possible to identify unique bioactive compounds of considerable therapeutic and commercial value. Therefore, this chapter reveals the biology, biochemistry, and other secondary metabolic biosyntheses mediated by endophytes, discusses recent mechanistic findings, and explores potential methods and emerging approaches to advance endophyte applications to resolve challenges, contributing to the future opportunities available to health and industry.

2 Diversity and Ecology of Endophytes: Exploring Their Natural Habitats and Symbiotic Relationships

This interesting group of plant micro-biomes comprises entophytic microorganisms that live within plant tissues without causing symptoms. Symbiotic organisms comprise fungi, bacteria, and actinomycetes, and they are incredibly diverse across many species of plants that contribute to the health of the plant and stability within ecosystems (Fazeli 2024). The ecological roles of endophytes are complicated and can affect all aspects of plant growth, stress load, and resistance to pathogens. Endophytes have been identified in an array of natural habitats, from tropical rainforests to dry desert ecosystems. These environments, no matter if the partnership is classified as beneficial or harmful, allow for mutualistic relationships in which the endophytes interact with their host plants in intricate and nuanced ways. A possible example of this in relation to drought conditions is present in forest ecosystems in which fungal endophytes that associate with tropical trees can enhance drought resistance, possibly by stimulating the production of bioactive metabolites, which in turn, transform and alter a plant's physiological responses to water stress (Roy and Banerjee 2018). In an agricultural setting, the presence of endophytes associated with cereal crops may offer benefits related to improvements in the uptake of nutrients, deterrence of pest insects, or aiding in what seems to be systemic resistance responses to pathogens (Watts et al. 2023). The world of endophytes has become more recognized as ecologically complex and diverse with advances in high-throughput sequencing and culture-centered microbial characterization. Endophytes are also of interest for natural product discoveries and potential agricultural applications (Tiwari and Bae 2022). In addition, endophytes often have affiliations with plants in ways that go beyond the normal plant–microbe association whereby endophytes mediate, or have a role, in how plants respond to environmental stresses, and their role in ecosystem function (Najjar 2025). The ecology and diversity of endophytes continues to be a rapidly evolving field of study that possesses substantial potential to guide sustainable agriculture and biotechnology. Future research on the ecological interactions of these organisms in their native surroundings is necessary to gain ecological and agricultural benefits. The increasing demand in the world for sustainable and bio-based products in health care, agriculture, and biotechnology has inspired research to find alternative sources of higher-value bioactive compounds.

3 Current Status of Entophytes Fungi

Although current estimates reveal that there are over 1.20 million fungal endophytes worldwide, only about 16% have been described, and sufficient detailed studies have been conducted that illustrate a substantial, extensive, and largely unexplored source of fascinating bioactive products that are waiting to be discovered, which could lead to a major impact in pharmaceutical-related research. Fungal endophytes collectively rely on a complex interaction of molecular pathways to help coordinate the creation and release of bioactive products while producing and releasing metabolites via fermentation, coordinating regulatory, enzymatic, and genetic elements in their structure (Deepika et al. 2016). Recent research studies have shown the many roles of mycelial interactions with the host plant in terms of uptake of nutrients, producing phytohormones, and producing metabolites that are antimicrobial or anticancer. However, new technologies in omics, such as genomics, transcriptomics, and metabolomics, allow for more clear-cut and clearer explorations of their bioactive synthesis interactions and the biosynthetic pathways compared to their host plants. Although there is a broad diversity of endophytic fungi, only a very small portion has been investigated and characterized, there remains an enormous amount of potential in that field. The cultivation stage of fungi still has hurdles to deal with, and thus, a reliable, universally repeatable source of metabolites, which needs further study regarding its genetic and metabolic potential. With the combination of epigenetic and advanced genome editing methods such as CRISPR-Cas9, there are promising prospects to stimulate the production of secondary metabolites and discover new therapeutic agents. As the world is drawing attention to the serious challenges of antibiotic resistance, the need for more sustainable agriculture, and potentially a way to tap into more sustainable options and new compounds with biologically active properties, endophytic fungi may be at the forefront of biotechnological research in the near future. To utilize the potential of these microbes for biotechnology, medicine, and agriculture, we will need to continue to learn more, understand more, and explore them more (Liao et al. 2025).

3.1 Global Perspectives on Endophytic Fungi

Endophytic fungi, in general, have value worldwide in discovering new antimicrobial compounds, which are essential in the fight against antimicrobial resistance (AMR). Endophytic fungi can produce antimicrobial secondary metabolites like polyketides and peptides through the polyketide synthase (PKS) and non-ribosomal peptide synthetase (NRPS) pathways (Nazir et al. 2024), which have the opportunity to exhibit antibacterial and antifungal/transdermal activities toward multidrug-resistant pathogens. Endophytes may be capable of affecting sustainable agriculture by improving nutrient uptake, producing phytohormones (auxins, gibberellic acid), and enhancing plant tolerance to stresses. They may also possess enzymatic bioremediation capabilities to break down pollutants in the environment. Currently, the Genomic studies of endophytic fungi have expanded our understanding of their metabolic pathways. For instance, Rana and Singh (2023) completed a genomic analysis on a novel *Fusarium* endophyte isolated from India to look into the biosynthetic gene clusters responsible for the metabolism of secondary metabolites, and discovered several unique biosynthetic gene clusters. The clarity that the genomic analysis of the endophytic fungus provides illuminates the uncharted wealth of bioactive compounds and metabolites that remain to be discovered by endophyte fungi, and emphasizes the need to continue both investigation and bioprospecting.

3.2 Indian Context of Endophytic Fungi

India's vast biodiversity and climatic zones create a great environment for many endophytic fungus communities. An emerging understanding of endophytic fungi in terms of distribution, diversity, and biochemical potential is developing on the Indian subcontinent. Kushwaha et al. (2024) provided documentation on endophytic and pathogenic fungal communities highly associated with pea roots in the sub-humid and dry temperate regions of Himachal Pradesh. The surveys reported a high occurrence of endophytic fungi on the pea root and in the surrounding rhizosphere, with the greatest presence occurring in the Kangra zone, suggesting that endophytic fungi can help with nutrition and disease resistance. Similarly, Nongthombam et al. (2024) carried out a research assessment on the endophytic fungi associated with *Chromolaena odorata*, which is used medicinally, from Manipur. The study found many endophytic fungi, where some provided significant antibacterial, antifungal, and antioxidative capacity, showing the potential of this plant-based for contribution as medicinal contributions. Moreover, finding *Pestalotiopsis pauciseta*, an endophytic fungus that can produce paclitaxel, an antitumor agent, demonstrates the massive medicinal horizons of India's endophytic fungi diversity. This symbiosis is important for India because entophytes can leverage India's biological resources for potential technology (e.g., environmental management, agriculture, and health). Continued research into these symbiotic organisms is warranted to determine what endophytes can do for society.

4 Molecular Mechanisms of Endophyte-Mediated Secondary Metabolite Biosynthesis

Endophytes are microorganisms that reside within plant tissues without causing harm. Endophytes and their ability to stimulate the biosynthesis of secondary metabolites (SM) related to plant defense and pharmaceuticals are important aspects of plant–microbe interactions. Elicitation of SM biosynthesis occurs by various molecular mechanisms, one of which is the initiation or activation of "silent" biosynthetic gene clusters (BGCs) through epigenetic medications (Fig. 1). Further, evidence has shown that epigenetic elicitors like DNA methyl transferase inhibitors (5-azacytidine) and histone deacetylase inhibitors (trichostatin A) can reactivate

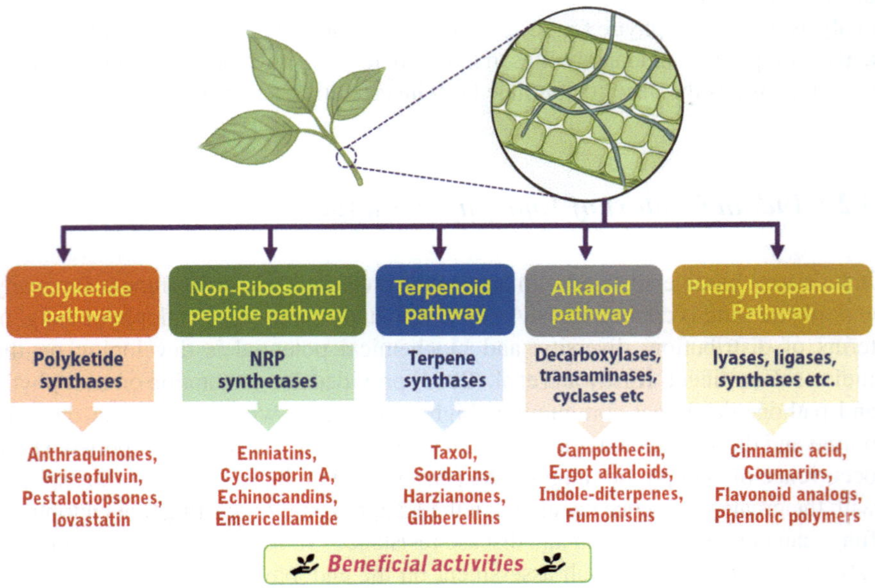

Fig. 1 Schematic illustration of the major biosynthetic pathways involved in secondary metabolite production. Polyketides, non-ribosomal peptides, terpenoids, alkaloids, and phenylpropanoids are synthesized through their respective pathways, utilizing precursor molecules derived from central carbon metabolism (e.g., glycolysis and the TCA cycle). The resulting metabolites are subsequently transported to the host, where they exert beneficial biological activities

silent BGCs and produce new bioactive compounds. In addition to epigenetic regulation, there is an array of signaling molecules that mediate plant–endophyte communications to elicit endophyte-induced SM biosynthesis by activating hexokinase signaling pathways and transcriptional cascades of SM biosynthesis-related protein-coding genes. Examining the genetic coordination of SM production more closely, we can take the example of loline alkaloids produced by Epichloe endophytes infecting grasses. The LOL gene cluster consists of at least eleven genes, and these co-regulated genes were the basis for the insecticidal loline alkaloids published in Spiering et al. (2005). Consequently, there have been a number of molecular approaches using empirical omics technologies (such as genomics, transcriptomics, proteomics, and metabolomics) that have provided us with some insight into the molecular networks that regulate SM biosynthesis by endophytes. The references above have shown that endophytes can enhance the production of some SMs which were already being produced by the host, and can also induce the de novo synthesis of SMs that would not ordinarily be produced in the host plant. Consequently, they will only increase the number of compounds that can be used for pharmaceutical R&D. Manipulating such mechanisms would provide a sustainable and efficient means of producing commercially relevant SMs while potentially limiting supply and variability issues as related to plant sources. As characterized by the myriads of plant–endophyte interactions, the potential for endophytes in SM biosynthesis is still in its infancy (including optimization of culture conditions, genetic engineering the endophyte, and an understanding of plant–endophyte signaling networks). Nevertheless, all these examples present a pathway for innovation in agriculture, medicine, and biotechnology based on tapping into the potential symbiosis of endophytes and their host plants to promote plant resilience to stress and higher-value secondary metabolites.

5 Bioactive Secondary Metabolites Produced by Endophytes: Structures, Functions, and Potential Applications

Now, endophytic microorganisms, such as bacteria and fungi, can be an enormous source of bioactive compounds exhibiting many pharmacological properties, which have been recognized extensively. Endophytic microorganisms reside in the plant tissue and do not cause damage, which shows their unique biosynthetic pathway of secondary metabolites with antimicrobial, cytotoxic, and therapeutic effects. Research work has recently underscored emerging bioactive compound potential for endophytes as a pool for novel bioactive compounds. The bioactive compounds include alkaloids, polyketides, and terpenoids. Newer studies have documented the bioactive alkaloids of endophytic Aspergillus species. According to Liu et al. (2023a), the 13 secondary metabolites isolated from the desert plant endophyte *Neocamarosporium betae* included four new polyketides. Some of the isolated compounds were notably cytotoxic to HepG2 cells. *Pestalotiopsis pauciseta* isolated from medicinal plants is reported to produce taxol, a prominent anticancer compound. The bioactivity of the fungal-derived taxol is similar to that of which is already in use as a standard drug. The trade of bacterial endophytes, specifically those belonging to the *Streptomyces* genus, has been identified as a producer of bioactive compounds. Zotchev (2024) described several metabolites having antibacterial and cytotoxic effects, including piericidins and aureothin. With the aid of advanced metabolomic approaches, endophyte-derived compounds can now be identified. Vigneshwari et al. (2019) were able to demonstrate hypericin production from *Epicoccum nigrum*, using HPLC-UV and LC-HRMS/MS methodologies. Similarly, Lu et al. (2019) employed RT-PCR to identify the starvation-induced production of phenylpropanoids in *Alternaria* sp. MG1 using GC-TOF-MS-based metabolomics. Many of the biosynthetic gene clusters (BGCs) from endophytes are silent or non-expressible in lab conditions. The identification of new compounds from endophytes and other sources requires methods for promoting not only the expression of a BGC, but also the ability to activate it to produce a metabolite of economic significance. Co-cultivation, epigenetic modifiers, and genetic engineering techniques are some of the approaches commonly used to activate BGCs. Methods for awakening and harnessing BGC have been reviewed recently. There is a great diversity of 27 bioactive metabolites from endophytic fungi, with many exhibiting multiple biological activities, including, but not limited to, antimicrobial, antioxidant, anticancer, antidiabetic, neuroprotector, and anti-hypercholesterolemic. Endophytes include an array of microorganisms, particularly fungi and bacteria, which all produce secondary metabolites as endophytically growing organisms produce a unique secondary metabolite profile. A compiled submitted list of endophytes and bioactive compounds is shown in Table 1 and Fig. 2.

5.1 Structures, Functions, and Potential Applications of Endophyte Fungi

Endophytic fungi are a unique and diverse group of microorganisms that colonize inside the tissue of plants without causing visible damage or disease of the host plant. Because endophytes have bioactive secondary metabolites, promote plant growth, and environmental stress tolerances (Rodriguez et al. 2009), they have gained much attention. As mutualistic symbionts, endophytes are important in regulating plant health and productivity, therefore being possible modifiers of sustainable agricultural systems.

Table 1 List of Potent Bioactive Metabolites from Fungal Endophytes

S. No	Compound Name	Bioactivity	Potential Role
1	Danthron	Antimicrobial, Anticancer	Exhibits cytotoxic and antimicrobial properties.
2	Xanthomycin	Antioxidant, Anticancer	Known for its free radical scavenging activity.
3	Fusarithioamide A	Antimicrobial, Antidiabetic	Shows promising antimicrobial effects.
4	Phomoenamide	Anticancer, Antioxidant	Displays anticancer potential.
5	Altersolanol A	Antioxidant, Antimicrobial	Notable for its strong antioxidant properties.
6	Emodin	Anticancer, Antidiabetic	Widely studied for its antitumor properties.
7	Epoxydon	Antimicrobial	Recognized for its antibacterial properties.
8	Piperine	Antioxidant, Antidiabetic	A well-known bioenhancer and antioxidant.
9	Chaetominine	Anticancer, Antimicrobial	Effective against various cancer cell lines.
10	Chrysin	Antioxidant, Anticancer	Exhibits strong free radical scavenging abilities.
11	Epicocconigrone A	Antimicrobial	Known for its potent antibacterial properties.
12	Scequinadoline D	Neuroprotective	Provides neuroprotective effects.
13	Asperpyridone A	Antimicrobial	Shows significant antibacterial effects.
14	Herbarin	Antioxidant	Exhibits strong antioxidant properties.
15	Neglectine A	Antimicrobial	Demonstrates potent antimicrobial activity.
16	Epoxycytochalasin H	Anticancer	Noted for its cytotoxic activity against cancer cells.
17	Monocerin	Antimicrobial	Displays strong antifungal properties.
18	Viridiol	Anticancer	Known for its cytotoxic properties.
19	Phomoarcherin B	Antioxidant, Anticancer	Exhibits antioxidant and anticancer effects.
20	Codinaeopsin	Antimicrobial	Displays significant antimicrobial effects.
21	Evariquinone	Anticancer, Antimicrobial	Known for its dual activity against microbes and cancer.
22	Quercetin	Antioxidant, Anticancer	Widely recognized for its antioxidant properties.
23	Fischerin	Antimicrobial	Effective against various microbial strains.
24	Fusarubin	Antimicrobial	Demonstrates strong antibacterial properties.
25	Colletotrichamide C	Anticancer	Known for its anticancer potential.
26	Lovastatin	Anti-hypercholesterolemic	Widely used as a cholesterol-lowering agent.
27	Diaporthin E	Anticancer	Cytotoxic activity.

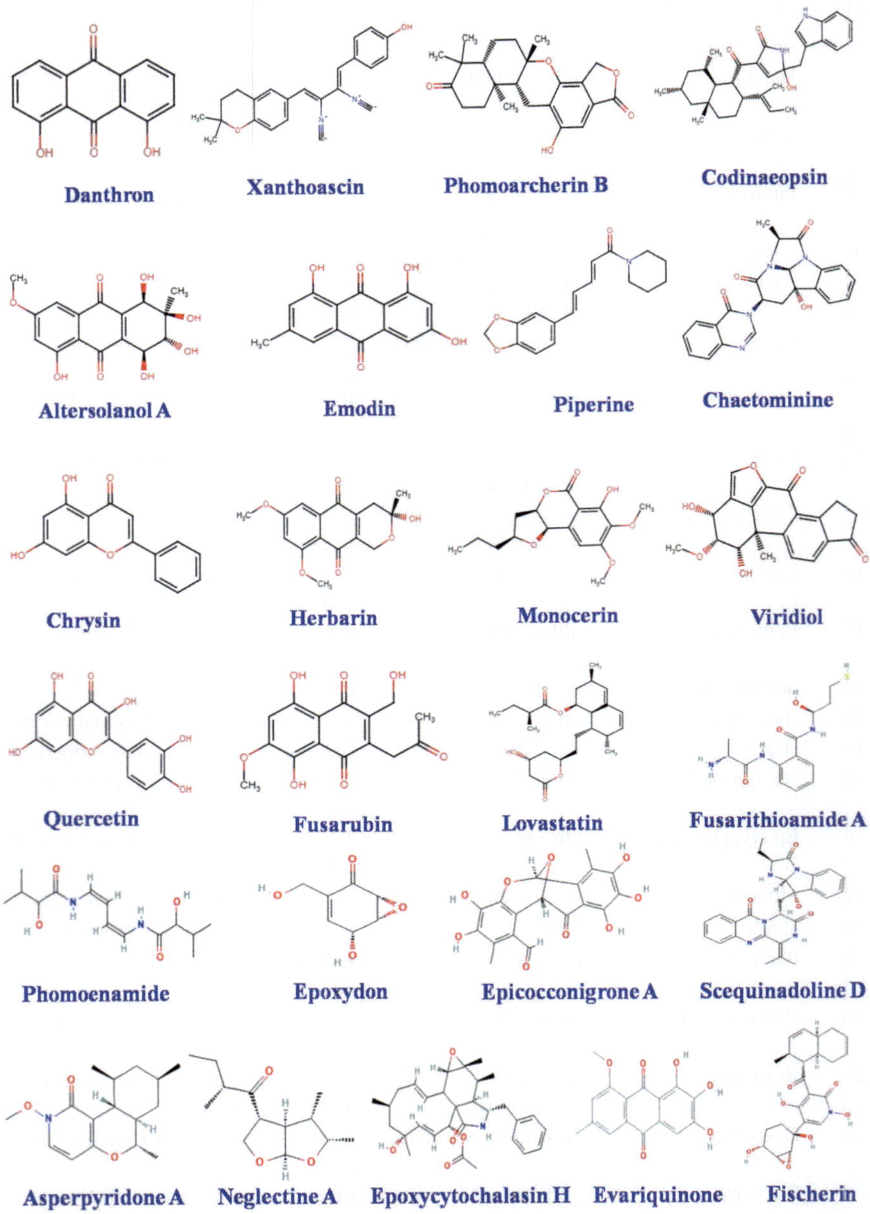

Fig. 2 List of the molecular structures of strong bioactive metabolites from fungal endophytes

5.2 Structural Adaptations

Endophytic fungi exhibit adaptations that enable them to colonize plant tissues. Portions of the mycelium grow into the intercellular spaces of host cells as hyphae and are also capable of producing appressoria, specialized infection structures (Rodriguez et al. 2009). The ability of endophytes to produce a hyphal or appressorial presence differs with host plant physiology and environmental conditions, which illustrates the complication of the endophyte and host associations.

5.3 Functional Roles and Secondary Metabolite Production

One of the most fascinating features of endophytic fungi is their ability to produce a myriad of different secondary metabolites like alkaloids, terpenes, polyketides, peptides, etc. For example, the endophyte *Taxomyces andreanae* produces paclitaxel (taxol), an exceptionally potent and significant anticancer compound. These bioactive compounds even exhibit antimicrobial, antiviral, antioxidant, and anticancer activity, implying that endophytes have the potential to be a new source for pharmaceuticals (Gouda et al. 2016). Many of the plant growth-promoting characteristics are linked to endophytes producing phytohormones such as indole-3-acetic acid (IAA), gibberellins, and cytokinins (Khan et al. 2017). Endophytes aid in obtaining nutrients through solubilizing phosphorus and producing siderophores to chelate iron, thus increasing the amount of iron that is available to the plant. Because all these traits are growth-promoting, endophytes have been investigated for potential applications in sustainable agriculture.

Endophytes enhance the resilience of plants against abiotic stress, including drought, salinity, and heavy metal toxicity. They accomplish this by altering the signal transduction pathways that control stress-related gene expression and producing antioxidants for the cellular oxidative damage response. For example, Epichloë species protect their host grass from herbivory and the effects of environmental stresses (Rodriguez et al. 2009). With their capacity to inhibit plant pathogens and promote crop growth, endophytic fungi have been more widely accepted as biocontrol agents in sustainable agriculture. For example, species from the *Trichoderma* and *Penicillium* genera have both demonstrated efficacious effects on preventing soil-borne diseases (Gouda et al. 2016). By functioning as biocontrol agents, it reduces the dependency on chemical pesticides, enabling agriculture to become more sustainable. Given the vast amount of bioactive compounds produced by endophytic fungi, they have a vast resource for drug discovery. For example, flavipin produced from *Chaetomium globosum* has been suggested to have additional anticancer activity. The area of pharmaceuticals using endophytes for the discovery of novel therapeutics is a developing area of translational pharmaceutical research. Endophytic fungi have enzymes that degrade environmental pollutants such as heavy metals and hydrocarbons (Khan et al. 2017). This asset has been researched as a bioremediation source for contaminated soils and water bodies, laying the path for sustainable bioremediation of environmental contamination. Endophytic fungi are an astonishing group of microorganisms that are diverse but possess a very defined structure, function, and applications. Since endophytes can improve plant growth, produce bioactive natural products, and withstand environmental stresses, they are well suited for agriculture, pharmaceuticals, and environmental remediation or management processes. As research continues, it is becoming ever more apparent that endophytic fungi can have significant potential to alleviate global issues.

6 Case Studies Highlighting Endophyte-Derived Bioactive Compounds

Endophytic fungi represent an abundant and largely unexplored source of secondary metabolites displaying a variety of bioactivity (Singh et al. 2021). Interest in natural products derived from endophytes surged after the first report of taxol production in an endophyte, *Taxomyces andreanae*, and has led to the discovery of many new chemical entities (Nongthombam et al. 2024). Endophytes are closely associated with their plant hosts; they provide metabolites that help the host plant defend itself (Mengistu 2020; Li et al. 2022). *Taxomyces andreanae* was first isolated from the inner bark of *Taxus brevifolia* and was subsequently discovered to be the first non-plant organism capable of producing the anticancer compound taxol (paclitaxel). Cheng et al. (2013) used comparative genomics to reclassify *Taxomyces andreanae* and determine that it belongs to the phlebioid clade of the *Basidiomycota* and is closely related to *Ceriporiopsis gilvescens* and others, although its ability to produce taxol has yet to be determined. Taxol, a complicated diterpenoid, inhibits cell division; apoptosis in rapidly growing cells is achieved through the stabilization of microtubules and prevention of depolymerization during division, leading to M-phase arrest. The significance of this observation was that there was biotechnological potential to be made, as we could synthesize taxol by fermentation, and this would sustain production rates beyond the slow-growing. Not only was taxol clinically important, but it remains so today in the treatment of cancers such as ovarian cancer, breast cancer, and non-small-cell lung cancer, in which its biosynthesis from fungi is appealing due to fermentation and scalability. *Fusarium solani* has been identified as an endophytic fungus from a medicinal plant, *Nothapodytes foetida*, and is of increasing significance as a microbial producer of camptothecin (Fig. 2), a very potent anticancer monoterpene indole alkaloid. Venugopalan et al. (2016) were able to increase the production of camptothecin from *F. solani* by a up to 152 times with optimal fermentation conditions (pH 6.0, 32 °C, 80 rpm) in their experiment with the addition of ethanol was also successful, as was the addition of tryptamine and BSA in producing extracts that demonstrated bioactivity with strong cytotoxicity against colon and breast cancer cells. Camptothecin has selective inhibition of the DNA topoisomerase I, causing stabilization of the cleavable enzyme-DNA complex, leading to DNA damage and ultimately apoptosis in rapidly growing cancer cells. The semi-synthetic derivatives of camptothecin, topotecan and irinotecan, are routinely used in the treatment of colorectal, ovarian, and small-cell lung cancers. The microbial production of camptothecin using *F.solani* proposes a sustainable source of camptothecin for use in research and to mitigate ecological and supply constraints on this chemical obtained from plants. *Phialocephala fortinii* is an endophytic fungus cultivated from the rhizome of *Podophyllum peltatum*, which is a microbial source of the lignan podophyllotoxin (which is best known for its antimitotic properties). Podophyllotoxin exerts its activity through binding to tubulin and preventing polymerization into microtubules, disrupting the mitotic spindle, leading to metaphase cell-cycle arrest in rapidly dividing cancer cells. In a direct clinical capacity, podophyllotoxin is limited by its toxicity, podophyllotoxin is a relative precursor for the semi-synthetic development of chemotherapeutic agents such as etoposide and teniposide, which are commonly used therapies against testicular cancer, small-cell lung carcinoma, and lymphomas. *P. fortinii* represents an alternative source of podophyllotoxin that is both sustainable and scalable. This chapter presents notable case studies to show the importance of endophytic fungi's role in natural product chemistry and pharmacognosy (Table 2).

7 Genetic and Metabolic Engineering Strategies for Enhanced Endophyte-Derived Secondary Metabolite Production

Metabolic engineering has been characterized as a disruptive technology for increasing the production of bioactive compounds from endophytes (living within plant tissues without causing harm), an ongoing and sustainable producer of biocontrolled chemical substances that can be used in agriculture, medicines and industry (Fig. 3). The overarching aim of metabolic engineering is to modify and enhance specific metabolic pathways in endophytes, enabling increase in the yield efficiency and diversity of secondary metabolites. This chapter is a compilation of selected case studies that concentrate on the genetic and metabolic engineering of endophytes to improve levels of functional secondary metabolite production, where we highlight not only the role of endophytes but also important roles (see Table 3) *Mycoendophytes* (endophytes synonymous with fungi). Recently, there have been rapid advances in areas such as genetic manipulation and synthetic biology that have extended the overall scope for metabolic engineering in endophytes and enabled far more precise engineering of their metabolic networks. One of the more traditional strategies for metabolic engineering is overexpression of rate-limiting enzymes in structural/functional biochemical pathways. The overexpression of a rate-limiting enzyme, for example, acetyl-CoA carboxylase (ACC), in projects with fungal endophytes has improved fatty acid production, an important structural element to many secondary

Table 2 Notable Case Studies of Bioactive Compounds from Endophytic Fungi

Endophytic Fungus	Host Plant	Bioactive Compound	Compound Class	Bioactivity	Reference
Taxomyces andreanae	*Taxus brevifolia*	Taxol (Paclitaxel)	Diterpenoid	Anticancer (ovarian, breast, lung cancers)	El-Sayed et al. (2020)
Fusarium solani	*Nothapodytes foetida*	Camptothecin	Quinoline alkaloid	Anticancer (topoisomerase I inhibitor)	Venugopalan and Srivastava (2015)
Arcopilus aureus	*Vitis vinifera*	Resveratrol; Sclerotiorin	Stilbenoid; Azaphilone	Neuroprotective, Cardioprotective; Anticancer	Dwibedi and Saxena (2018)
Mucor fragilis	*Salvia miltiorrhiza*	Podophyllotoxin; Kaempferol	Lignan; Flavonoid	Anticancer; Antioxidant	Gupta et al. (2023)
Macrophomina phaseolina	*Gynura procumbens*	Isoelemicin, Terpinen-4-ol, Eucalyptol, Oleic acid, β-Pinene	Phenylpropanoid, Terpenoids, Fatty acids	Antioxidant, Antimicrobial	Abdulhadi et al. (2020)
Trichoderma harzianum	*Rosmarinus officinalis*	Gliotoxin	Various	Antimicrobial	Leylaie and Zafari (2018)

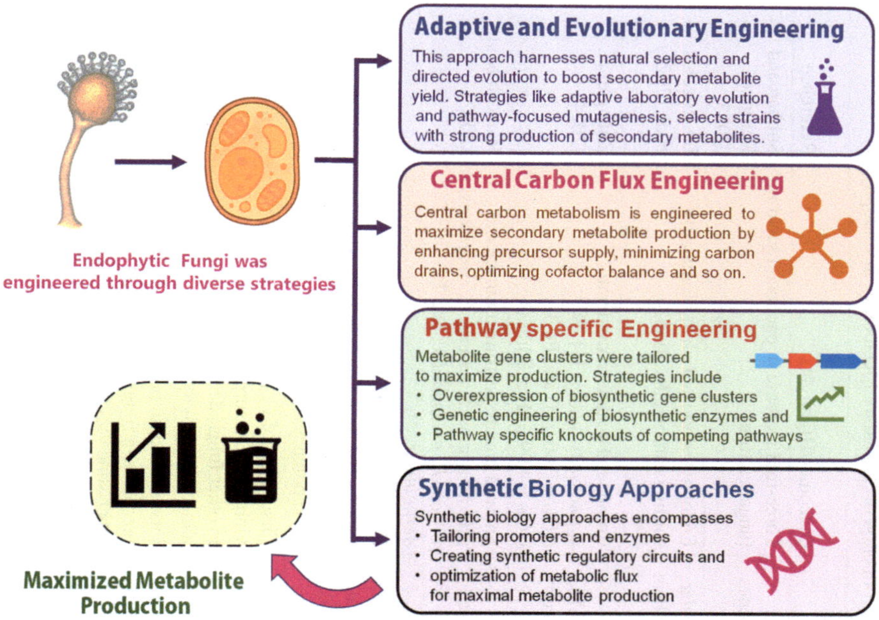

Fig. 3 Schematic illustration of diverse strategies employed to enhance secondary metabolite production in endophytic fungi. Adaptive and evolutionary engineering exploit natural selection under simulated conditions to generate efficient, high-yielding strains. Central carbon flux engineering redirects primary metabolic pathways to increase precursor availability, thereby boosting metabolite synthesis. Pathway-specific engineering, like gene overexpression, can also increase production several-fold. More novel and effective approaches, such as those used in synthetic biology through modifications to promoters and enzyme engineering, provide alternative approaches to optimize biosynthetic pathways. In addition, high-throughput screening applications enable rapid identification and selection of better producer strains

metabolites. In the same way, clothing key enzymes in shikimic and polyketide pathways produce higher levels of antimicrobial products and phytohormones, which show the advantages of enhancement of biochemical productivity when targeting specific enzymes (Liu et al. 2023a, b). Another important strategy is pathway rerouting, where current metabolic pathways are altered to increase production of desired metabolites using either gene knockouts of competing pathways or heterologous pathways from other microorganisms. For example, a microbial phenylpropanoid pathway was introduced into the endophytic fungus *Phomopsis* sp. leading to the production of flavonoids, a group of bioactive compounds with important pharmaceutical potential (Kumar et al. 2023). This approach not only increased target product yield but also minimized unwanted intermediates. Furthermore, the development of CRISPR-Cas9 technology is beginning to alter endophyte metabolic engineering and offers a more accurate and successful route for genome editing.

Through the modification of regulator genes, researchers can create new, faster strategies to realize useful metabolites. A more recent example, using

Table 3 Recent Studies have explored Metabolic Engineering Strategies to Enhance the Production of Secondary Metabolites in Endophytes

Endophyte Species	Host Plant/ Source	Targeted Secondary Metabolites	Genetic/Metabolic Engineering Strategy	Outcomes/Highlights	Reference
Fusarium oxysporum	*Taxus chinensis*	Paclitaxel (taxol)	Overexpression of key paclitaxel biosynthesis genes	Three-fold increase in paclitaxel yield in fungal culture	Subban and Kempken (2023)
Serendipita indica and Serendipita herbamans	*Solanum lycopersicum*	Carbohydrate metabolism	Physiological and molecular analyses of sugar metabolism	Endophytes boosted plant biomass by shifting carbon allocation.	De Rocchis et al. (2022)
Fusarium concentricum	*Anoectochilus roxburghii*	Fusaconate A	Isolation and structural elucidation via HR-ESI-MS, 1D & 2D NMR spectroscopy	Compound 4 showed moderate cytotoxicity against HT29 (IC_{50} = 7.60 μM) and PC3 (IC_{50} = 4.99 μM) cell lines;	Zhang et al. (2024)
Aspergillus niger	*Dodonaea viscosa*	4a-methyl-dodecahydro-1H-pyrrolo[3,4-b] quinoline-6-one	Optimization of culture parameters using response surface methodology	Showed broad-spectrum antibacterial activity against *S. aureus*, *B. coagulans*, *E. coli*, *K. pneumoniae*, and *P. aeruginosa*.	Ramesh et al. (2022)
Endophytic fungi (unspecified isolates)	*Bauhinia guianensis*	Fumigaclavine C and Pseurotin A (alkaloids)	Isolation by column chromatography, identification via 1D/2D NMR, and mass spectrometry	First report of these alkaloids from endophytes of *B. guianensis* showing broad-spectrum antibacterial activity with good potency	Pinheiro et al. (2013)
Curvularia verruculosa	*Catharanthus roseus (leaves)*	Vinblastine	HPLC quantification; Cytotoxicity assay on HeLa cells	First report of *C. verruculosa* producing vinblastine in surplus amounts compared to other fungi; demonstrated strong anticancer activity	Parthasarathy et al. (2020)
Nigrospora zimmermanii	*Catharanthus roseus*	Vincristine	Synthetic biology approach to reconstruct partial vincristine pathway	First successful production of vincristine precursor in fungus, Maximum vincristine yield of 5.344 μg/mL in parent culture;	Birat et al. (2022)

Burkholderia seminalis	*Musa* spp.	Pyrroloquinoline quinone	Multi-omics approaches	PQQ enhanced banana growth and conferred resistance to Fusarium wilt	Hung et al. (2024)
Bacillus cereus and Bacillus mycoides	*Urtica dioica L*	Biosurfactants and polyphenols	Isolation of endophytes; identification by biochemical tests & 16S rRNA sequencing; culture extract analysis	All isolates produced biosurfactants & polyphenols; *B. cereus* and *B. mycoides* had the greatest capacity; extracts showed polyphenol concentration of 1.633 mol L^{-1} (9.691 mg L^{-1})	Marchut-Mikołajczyk et al. (2023)

CRISPR-Cas9 technology, shows how one could knock out a repressor gene in the endophyte *Colletotrichum gloeosporioides*, then increase production of the anticancer product called taxol by 10 times with more taxol produced (Zhang et al. 2023). All in all, this method illustrates a new method of genome editing that can be used to diversify the biosynthetic capacity of entophytes. Beyond genome editing, co-culturing has also become an increasing and exciting way to maximize the metabolite production of endophytes. Specifically, co-culturing endophytes with other microorganisms can stimulate, or as some say induce, dormancy, or sometimes referred to as cryptic biosynthetic gene clusters that may not have had the opportunity to be stimulated under traditional laboratory culture. For example, with an endophytic fungus like *Alternaria* sp., the co-cultivation with *Bacillus subtilis* was shown to induce new polyketide biosynthesis, which had excellent antibacterial activity (Sun et al. 2022). This demonstrates the importance of a microbe-microbe interaction to induce metabolic pathways. Co-cultivation not only stimulates an often dormant gene cluster that relates to metabolism, but it is also something that has been applied in the agricultural area. CRISPR-Cas9 helps to represent a new age in metabolic engineering with endophytes and provides many advantages from that access to genome editing, as it has never been done before. CRISPR-Cas9 allows manipulation of a repressor (a key regulator gene), which may increase bioproduction of commercially valuable metabolites. For example, CRISPR-Cas9 was used to knock out a repressor gene in the endophytic fungus *Colletotrichum gloeosporioides* to receive a ten-fold increase in production of the anticancer product-taxol (Zhang et al. 2023). Generally, this supports the use of genome editing opportunities to obtain the full biosynthetic potential of endophytes. Along with genome editing, co-culture techniques have been a popular strategy to enhance the production of metabolites from endophytes. Starting co-cultures with endophytes alongside another microorganism can result in functional biosynthetic gene cluster up-regulation that is quiescent under standard laboratory conditions. For example, the co-culture of the endophyte *Alternaria* sp. with the bacterium *Bacillus subtilis* emerged via activated pathways that neither of them could access alone and biosynthetically produced a new polyketide with antibacterial activity (Sun et al. 2022). This commensal interaction demonstrated that the interaction between microbes can very much influence the modulation of metabolic pathways. Also, adaptive laboratory evolution (ALE) has been used to optimize endophytes for enhanced metabolite production. Endophytes that were maintained in suboptimal conditions can acquire beneficial mutations that can increase biosynthesis with protracted exposure to selective pressures. Overall, computational modeling and omics technologies are now increasingly prevalent in the practice of metabolic engineering and contribute to the understanding of metabolic flux, gene expression, and gene regulatory networks of endophytes. Multi-omics has added additional detail to research, including genomics, transcriptomics, proteomics, and metabolomics, and their ability to identify regulatory nodes and rate-limiting steps in metabolic pathways will facilitate directed genetic activity. The combination of these techniques now allows for greater rational design of endophytes with improved biosynthetic capacity (Chen et al. 2022a). Hence, advances in synthetic biology and genome editing, combined with computational biology, have allowed for the rapid evolution of metabolic engineering practices that result in improved endophyte-derived metabolite synthesis costs. The use of directed genetic techniques, as opposed to trial and error, allows researchers to understand endophytes as microbial factories that are capable of synthesizing a wide range of metabolites important to the pharmaceutical, agricultural, and industrial sectors.

8 Challenges and Limitations in Harnessing Endophytes for Metabolite Production

Endophytes have become the focus of interest as possible sources of bioactive secondary metabolites due to their diverse groups of microorganisms that can live in plant tissues, causing no apparent disease injury to the plant. Secondary metabolites are prized for their potential bioactivity for uses ranging from pharmaceuticals to agriculture and biotechnology. However, there are significant difficulties for the successful use of endophytes as a source for the production of metabolites. An important consideration is the variability in yields of bioactive metabolites, and there are a large number of environmental parameters (for example, temperature, humidity, the plant species in which the endophyte is found) that contribute to environmental variation in the production of bioactive metabolites by endophytes. This is evident in the variability of the same endophytic strain yields due to different cultivation conditions, which makes it difficult to standardize the conditions of production (Zakariyah et al. 2024). Another key issue with growing endophytes relates specifically to growing endophytes in vitro. Many endophytes are either unable to be cultured away from host plants, or when cultured, they lose their biosynthetic potential on isolation. Traditional axenic (pure) culture methods often cannot duplicate the extensive integration of biochemical interactions that are present in the host environment, leading to inactivation of important biosynthetic gene clusters that allow for metabolite production (Somjaipeng et al. 2016). While co-cultivating with other microorganisms has been examined as a method for activating these dormant biosynthetic pathways, this method adds further complexity and unpredictability. The complexity of endophyte biosynthetic pathways must be considered. These biosynthetic pathways are often controlled by cryptic gene clusters, which are not well characterized and whose function is poorly understood. The limitations of genomic data will also limit the goals of manipulating/enhancing biosynthetic pathways for more metabolite production (Medema and Fischbach 2015). Also, many factors can affect the expression of these biosynthetic genes, so the more variables there are, the more challenging it becomes to achieve consistent yields of a metabolite. Finally, scaling up production of endophyte-derived metabolites from a lab environment to an industrial production level is an especially resistant problem. Not only are there generally low yields of metabolites, complex extraction processes, and additional capital costs for specialized cultivation facilities, but it is often prohibitively expensive to consider production (Ganeshan et al. 2021). The endophytes themselves tend to lose their metabolite-yielding capacity or severely limit their potential after only several rounds of making subcultures (Singh and Kumar 2023). The regulatory and safety issues surrounding endophyte-derived metabolites complicate the utilization of endophyte-derived metabolites in pharmaceuticals and agriculture. More specifically, endophyte-derived compounds must be thoroughly assessed for toxicity, allergenicity, and persistence in the environment before commercialization. Some endophyte-derived metabolites have been shown to be hepatotoxic or nephrotoxic, which should be tested for toxicity via toxicology testing even after having a historical record of being safe for human consumption (Wijesekara and Xu 2023). There are also ecological and ethical issues associated with endophyte utilization. The assessment and characterization of endophytes typically involve their isolation from host plants, and further host plant diversity may include endophytic exploitation or utilization that may eventually deplete host populations and degrade their environments. Similarly, the use of non-specific endophyte-derived compounds may possibly raise ethical considerations for irresponsible harvesting or implementation. An additional example may be polycultures of non-target species having resultant resistant outcomes to the endophyte-derived compound. Some of the alternative strategies explored by some researchers regarding endophytes as a source of metabolites; however, there are very limited measures for addressing and dealing with them, and certainly, no adequate alternatives for ensuring procurement utilization through beneficial production. Future studies will aim to develop optimal cultivation protocols, elucidate complex biosynthetic pathways with improved understanding, and develop scalable production systems that are also cost-effective. Further, it is also very important to address regulatory, safety, and ethical obstacles in future studies for the responsible exploitation of endophytes in many sectors.

9 Industrial Applications and Commercial Potential of Endophyte-Derived Metabolites

Endophytes are microorganisms that live asymptomatically within plant tissues and have become a highly productive source of new bioactive metabolites with major industrial and commercial implications. Endophyte metabolites fall into a wide range of chemical classes such as alkaloids, flavonoids, terpenoids, and polyketides that have been applied successfully to the pharmaceutical, agriculture, cosmetics, and food industrial sectors (Singh et al. 2022; Li et al. 2023). The pharmaceutical industry has utilized and benefited from a select number of endophytic (algal and fungal) compounds with prospective antimicrobial, anticancer, anti-inflammatory, and antioxidant characteristics. Endophytes derived from medicinal plants and their potent secondary metabolites can biosynthesize compounds similar or identical to those of their host plant. For example, taxol, a very popular anticancer drug from the

Pacific yew tree, has been isolated from endophytic fungi, thus creating an alternate and sustainable supply (El-Sayed et al. 2020). More recently, anticancer agents as endophytes have expanded, with endophytic fungi reporting novel compounds that showed efficacy toward a multi-drug resistant cancer cell line. The possibilities of scalable fermentation of these microbes offer a commercially feasible alternative to extraction from plants, and can ameliorate a multitude of issues associated with low yield, slow growth, and environmental sustainability. In addition, endophyte-derived metabolites have enormous potential to be used in sustainable agriculture in the form of biofertilizers, biopesticides, and plant growth promoters. A portion of endophytes also produce natural insecticides and fungicides to reduce the over-reliance on synthetic agrochemicals that are detrimental to the health of humans and the environment. For example, volatile organic compounds (VOCs) produced from bacterial endophytes have demonstrated biocontrol activity against crop pathogens, where higher resilience and yield were shown in plants (Yousefvand et al. 2023). In addition to this, the metabolites endophytes can secrete to the plant include siderophores and phytohormones that can contribute to nutrient uptake from the plant as well as influence growth, which means they could be potential eco-friendly agricultural formulations (Singh et al. 2022). The food industry is more frequently using endophyte-derived metabolites as natural preservatives and nutraceutical additives. Endophytic microorganisms are useful to produce antioxidants and antimicrobial peptides that help extend food product durability while ensuring safety and high-quality (Mishra et al. 2020). Additionally, these metabolites, which are frequently abundant in bioactive compounds, help create functional foods that offer health advantages beyond simple sustenance. Indeed, endophytes from edible plants used as dietary supplements have been the focus of recent studies that have found new compounds that could modify gut microbiota to influence human health (Chen et al. 2022a). Endophytes have now (because of their anti-aging, moisturizing, and anti-inflammatory compounds, among others) made their way into the cosmetic industry. This means that in response to oxidative and environmental stress, cosmetic companies could use natural antioxidants and UV-protective compounds derived from the endophytes. Of all industries, the cosmetics industry has arguably expanded the most in these areas (sustainable/product line) market in reaction to the increasing demand for "greener," environmentally benign products. With this growth, cosmetic companies have more opportunities than ever to utilize endophytes in their new product developments. Although the potential applications are exciting, the commercial realization of metabolites from endophytic organisms faces hurdles, including strain stability, metabolite yield, and downstream processing issues. However, metabolic engineering and fermentation technology are dealing with these impediments while improving the production systems to be optimized. In biosciences, biochemistry and natural products share a close affiliation and influence one another; likewise, synthetic biology and genomic mining can identify and improve pathways allowing them to be scaled for industrial use (Seshadri et al. 2025).

10 Future Directions: Emerging Trends and Prospects in Endophyte Research

Explosive growth is an appropriate description for the endophyte research area which has taken enormous advantage of the vast potential of these microorganisms in many disciplines such as agriculture, medicine, and biotechnology in the last few decades. New technologies and interdisciplinary research are allowing researchers to expand their boundaries of endophyte research that we believe will be transformative from both scientific and practical perspectives. In this chapter, we have presented some key emerging and potential trends that we expect will influence the future directions in endophyte research. One of the major drivers of change will be the ability to use multi-omics technologies such as genomics, transcriptomics, proteomics, and metabolomics to provide detailed molecular perspectives on the mutual interactions between the endophyte and the host plants and to know how to leverage the biosynthesis of key secondary metabolites (Subudhi et al. 2018). High-throughput sequencing and metabolite profiling will continue to be combined to find new biosynthetic gene clusters that will lead to the discovery of new bioactive molecules for novel pharmaceutical or sustainable agricultural products (Mishra et al. 2022). Our knowledge of microbial heterogeneity in plant tissues will be improved by the developing field of single-cell omics, which will provide cellular resolution of endophytic functions that were previously unachievable. Synthetic biology is another avenue supporting exciting developments in endophytes. Currently, gene editing technologies such as CRISPR-Cas9 systems are widely used to manipulate biosynthetic pathways, improve symbiont effectiveness, and increase persistence in the host plants (Verma et al. 2023). Metabolic engineering systems are being utilized to alter endophytes to optimize them for use in producing rare and high-value natural products that can be scaled to commercial levels in the pharmaceutical and agrochemical sectors. In addition, engineered endophytes may also provide a source for bioremediation of environmental pollutants. Concurrently, research on the ecological role of endophytes in the plant microbiome is also emerging. A focus will need to be placed on the complex interactions of endophytes with other microbes and pathogens, exploring potential synergistic and antagonistic relationships so as to select and design microbial consortia for suppressing pathogens and encouraging plant health and productivity (Vishwakarma et al. 2020). Developments regarding in situ imaging and spatial metagenomics will lead to dynamic monitoring of microbial colonization and communication in plant tissues that will enhance our understanding of endophyte host inter-relations (Kandel et al. 2017). As climate change poses new and worsening challenges, endophytes are increasingly recognized as a potential means of enhancing crop resilience. Some endophytes are able to provide increases in tolerance to abiotic stresses such as drought, salinity, and nutrient deficiencies, and allow plants to better adapt to these conditions (Chitnis et al. 2020). As a consequence, the establishment and implementation of endophyte-based bioinoculants across a variety of agro ecosystems may increase rapidly as they assist in reducing the reliance on chemical fertilizers and pesticides while moving toward sustainable agriculture (Sharma et al. 2023).

There will be substantive issues in relation to safety, regulation, and intellectual property (IP) to contend with before endophyte-based products are ready for commercialization. Before commercialization can occur, researchers, entrepreneurs, and manufacturers must develop standardized protocols concerning which endophytes are isolated, characterized, and the decision of your choice of quality control (QC) measures, to comply with regulations and gain market acceptance (Chandra et al. 2024). It will be important to establish frameworks for collaboration among academic institutions, businesses, and policymakers in order to ensure the responsible growth of endophyte research into actionable outcomes. There is increasing evidence that endophytes have even greater biotechnological potential than the benefits of the plants themselves. Endophytes can produce novel antibiotics, immunomodulators, and bioactive metabolites with antiviral and anticancer properties; some are currently being subjected to clinical trials (Falade et al. 2021). Future studies will also assess endophyte-derived enzymes and biomolecules as feedstock for important industrial processes (e.g., biocatalysts, biosensors, etc.).

11 Conclusions

Endophyte-mediated biosynthesis that utilizes valuable secondary metabolites signifies a paradigm shift in biotechnology and the discovery of natural products. Endophytes have potential agency between a large array of microorganisms, as a means to produce sustainable relationships for industrial bioproducts, agrochemicals, and drugs due to their remarkable and diverse abilities to produce bioactive compounds. As we elucidate the complexity of biology and metabolic pathways, these symbiotic partners will continue to provide innovative answers to challenging issues in human health, agriculture, and eco-sustainable development. In order to leverage the capabilities of endophytes, a multi-faceted strategy that incorporates current omics technologies, synthetic biology, and ecological parameters is required. An integrated model expedites the discovery of new metabolites and, more specifically, optimizes the directed evolution of endophytes for metabolite tractability and performance. These early discoveries have the potential to be environmentally sustainable, economically viable, and scalable bioprocesses to replace damaging synthetics and extraction. Additionally, the fundamental role endophytes play in phytometabolism in response to stress conditions shows their importance to sustainable climate-resilient solutions in agriculture. Prioritizing the commercializing of endophyte-derived metabolites and bioinoculants may provide a path to reduce dependencies on synthetic agrochemicals while enabling better environmental stewardship, and promoting food security at the global level. To conclude, endophytes present a diverse and rapidly progressing platform for continuing discoveries in natural product biosynthesis across several sectors. To maximize the potential for endophyte metabolites as long-term solutions for social good, more resources are necessary for more fundamental research and technology development, and an enabling regulatory environment.

References

Abdulhadi SY, Hasan GQ, Gergees RN (2020) Molecular detection and antimicrobial activity of endophytic fungi isolated from a medical plant *Rosmarinusofficinalis*. arXiv 2303:05242

Birat K, Binsuwaidan R, Siddiqi T et al (2022) Report on vincristine-producing endophytic fungus *Nigrospora zimmermanii* from leaves of *Catharanthus roseus*. Metabolites 12(11):1119

Chandra H, Yadav A, Prasad R et al (2024) Fungal endophytes from medicinal plants acting as natural therapeutic reservoir. The Microbe 3:100073

Chen W, Yu L, Zhu B et al (2022a) *Dendrobium officinale* endophytes may colonize the intestinal tract and regulate gut microbiota in mice. Evid Based Complement Alternat Med 2022:2607506

Chen X, Sun Y, Chong Y et al (2022b) Transcriptomic and metabolomic approaches deepen our knowledge of plant-endophyte interactions. Front Plant Sci 13:819

Cheng Y, Wang Y, Liu Y (2013) A re-assessment of *Taxomycesandreanae*, the alleged taxol-producing fungus, using comparative genomics. IMA Fungus 4(1):27–33

Chitnis VR, Suryanarayanan TS, Nataraja KN et al (2020) Fungalendophyte-mediated crop improvement: the way ahead. Front Plant Sci 11:561007

De Rocchis V, Jammer A, Camehl et al (2022) Tomato growth promotion by the fungal endophytes Serendipita indica and Serendipita herbamans is associated with sucrose de-novo synthesis in roots and differential local and systemic effects on carbohydrate metabolisms and gene expression. J Plant Physiol 276:153755

Deepika VB, Murali TS, Satyamoorthy K (2016) Modulation of genetic clusters for synthesis of bioactive molecules in fungal endophytes: a review. Microbiol Res 182:125–114

Dwibedi V, Saxena S (2018) *Arcopilusaureus*, a resveratrol-producing endophyte from *Vitisvinifera*. Appl Biochem Biotechnol 186:476–495

El-Sayed AS, El-Sayed MT, Rady AM et al (2020) Exploiting the biosynthetic potency of taxol from fungal endophytes of conifers plants; genome mining and metabolic manipulation. Molecules 25(13):3000

Falade O, Adewole KE, Ekundayo et al (2021) Therapeutic potentials of endophytes for healthcare sustainability. Egypt J Basic Appl Sci 8(1):117–135

Fazeli M (2024) Theendophytes: a new resource for vulnerable plant bioactive compounds. In: de Oliveira MS, Andrade EHA, Kumar R, Mali SN (eds) Medicinal plants - chemical, biochemical, and pharmacological approaches. IntechOpen, pp 1–20

Ganeshan S, Kim SH, Vujanovic V (2021) Scaling-up production of plant endophytes in bioreactors: concepts, challenges and perspectives. Bioresour Bioprocess 8:1–16

Gouda S, Das G, Sen SK et al (2016) Endophytes: a treasure house of bioactive compounds of medicinal importance. Front Microbiol 7:1538

Gupta A, Meshram V, Gupta M et al (2023) Fungal endophytes: microfactories of novel bioactive compounds with therapeutic interventions; a comprehensive review on the biotechnological developments in the field of fungal endophytic biology over the last decade. Biomolecules 13(7):1038

Hung SHW, Yu MY, Liu CH et al (2024) Endophytic pyrroloquinoline quinone enhances banana growth and immunity against *Fusarium wilt* for plant-microbe mutualisms. bioRxiv, 2024–08

Jiang H, Chen L, Zhao Q (2023) Endophytes as alternative producers of plant-derived pharmaceuticals. In: Endophytic microorganisms: potential applications. Springer Nature, pp 133–157

Kandel SL, Joubert PM, Doty SL (2017) Bacterial endophyte colonization and distribution within plants. Microorganisms 5(4):77

Khan AL, Shahzad R, Al-Harrasi A et al (2017) Endophytic microbes: a resource for producing extracellular enzymes. In: Endophytes: crop productivity and protection, vol 2. Springer, pp 95–110

Kumar A, Radhakrishnan EK (eds) (2020) Microbial endophytes: functional biology and applications. Woodhead Publishing

Kumar AP, Bhasker K, Nikhil BSK et al (2023) Role of phenylpropanoids and flavonoids in plant defense mechanism. Int J Environ Clim Change 13(9):2951–2960

Kusari S, Hertweck C, Spiteller M (2023) Chemical ecology of endophytic fungi: origins of secondary metabolites. In: Endophytes and secondary metabolites. Springer Nature, pp 1–25
Kushwaha K, Pal J, Banyal D (2024) Endophytic and pathogenic fungal root communities associated with pea in sub-humid and dry temperate regions of Himachal Pradesh. HJAR 50(1):88–95
Leylaie S, Zafari D (2018) Antiproliferative and antimicrobial activities of secondary metabolites and phylogenetic study of endophytic Trichoderma species from Vincaplants. Front Microbiol 9:1484
Li Z, Wen W, Qin M et al (2022) Biosynthetic mechanisms of secondary metabolites promoted by the interaction between endophytes and plant hosts. Front Microbiol 13:928967
Li Z, Xiong K, Wen W et al (2023) Functional endophytes regulating plant secondary metabolism: current status, prospects and applications. Int J Mol Sci 24(2):1153
Liao C, Doilom M, Jeewon R et al (2025) Challenges and update on fungal endophytes: classification, definition, diversity, ecology, evolution and functions. Fungal Divers 131:301–367
Liu P, Tan Y, Yang J et al (2023a) Bioactive secondary metabolites from endophytic strains of *Neocamarosporiumbetae* collected from desert plants. Front Plant Sci 14:1142212
Liu S, Wang BB, Xu JZ et al (2023b) Engineering of shikimate pathway and terminal branch for efficient production of L-tryptophan in Escherichia coli. Int J Mol Sci 24(14):11866
Lu Y, Che J, Xu X et al (2019) Metabolomics reveals the response of the phenylpropanoid biosynthesis pathway to starvation treatment in the grape endophyte *Alternaria* sp. MG1. J Agric Food Chem 68(4):1126–1135
Ma B, Li Y, Wang et al (2025) Advances in CRISPR/Cas9-based gene editing in filamentous fungi. J Fungi 11(5):350
Marchut-Mikołajczyk O, Chlebicz M, Kawecka M et al (2023) Endophytic bacteria isolated from Urtica dioica L.-preliminary screening for enzyme and polyphenols production. Microb Cell Fact 22(1):169
Medema MH, Fischbach MA (2015) Computational approaches to natural product discovery. Nat Chem Biol 11(9):639–648
Mengistu AA (2020) Endophytes: colonization, behaviour, and their role in defense mechanism. Int J Microbiol 2020(1):6927219
Mishra RC, Goel M, Barrow CJ et al (2020) Endophytic fungi-an untapped source of potential antioxidants. Curr Bioact Compd 16(7):944–964
Mishra S, Priyanka, Sharma S (2022) Metabolomic insights into endophyte-derived bioactive compounds. Front Microbiol 13:835931
Najjar AA (2025) Therapeutic potential of endophytic microbes: emphasizing both fungal and bacterial endophytes. Appl Microbiol (2673-8007) 5(1)
Nazir A, Puthuveettil AR, Hussain FHN et al (2024) Endophytic fungi: nature's solution for antimicrobial resistance and sustainable agriculture. Front Microbiol 15:1461504
Nongthombam KS, Mutum SS, Pandey RR (2024) Distribution, diversity and biochemical analysis of endophytic fungi associated with chromolaena odorata. J Appl Life Sci Int 27(1):17–29. https://doi.org/10.9734/jalsi/2024/v27i1634
Parthasarathy R, Shanmuganathan R, Pugazhendhi A (2020) Vinblastine production by the endophytic fungus *Curvularia verruculosa* from the leaves of *Catharanthus roseus* and its *in vitro* cytotoxicity against HeLa cell line. Anal Biochem 593:113530
Patel V, Sharma N, Mehta R (2024) Synthetic biology and metabolic engineering of endophytes for drug discovery. In: Emerging trends in synthetic biology. Springer Nature, pp 201–225
Pinheiro E, Carvalho J, Santos et al (2013) Antibacterial activity of alkaloids produced by endophytic fungus *Aspergillus* sp. EJC08 isolated from medical plant *Bauhinia guianensis*. Nat Prod Res 27(18):1633–1638
Ramesh M, Kavitha K, Rajalakshmi A et al (2022) 4a-methyl-dodecahydro-1H-pyrrolo [3, 4-b] quinoline-6-one produced by Endophytic fungi Aspergillus Niger E12 obtained from Dodonaea viscosa plant leaves as a novel antibacterial compound. Appl Biochem Biotechnol 194(11):5132–5150

Rana S, Singh SK (2023) Insights into the genomic architecture of a newly discovered endophytic *Fusarium* species belonging to the *Fusariumconcolor* complex from India. Front Microbiol 14:1266620

Rodriguez RJ, White JF, Arnold AE et al (2009) Fungal endophytes: diversity and functional roles. New Phytol 182(2):314–330

Roy S, Banerjee D (2018) Diversity of endophytes in tropical forests. In: Pirttilä A, Frank A (eds) Endophytes of forest trees, Forestry Sciences, vol 86. Springer, Cham

Seshadri K, Abad AN, Nagasawa KK et al (2025) Synthetic biology in natural product biosynthesis. Chem Rev 125(7):3814–3931

Sharma I, Raina A, Choudhary M et al (2023) Fungal endophyte bioinoculants as a green alternative towards sustainable agriculture. Heliyon 9(9):e19487

Singh R, Dubey A (2024) Microbial biotechnology in natural product synthesis. In: Advances in microbial biotechnology. Springer Nature, pp 45–68

Singh VK, Kumar A (2023) Secondary metabolites from endophytic fungi: production, methods of analysis, and diverse pharmaceutical potential. Symbiosis 90(2):111–125

Singh A, Singh DK, Kharwar RN et al (2021) Fungalendophytes as efficient sources of plant derived bioactive compounds and their prospective applications in natural product drug discovery: insights, avenues, and challenges. Microorganisms 9(1):197

Singh D, Thapa S, Mahawar H et al (2022) Prospecting potential of endophytes for modulation of biosynthesis of therapeutic bioactive secondary metabolites and plant growth promotion of medicinal and aromatic plants. Antonie Van Leeuwenhoek 115(6):699–730

Somjaipeng S, Medina A, Magan N (2016) Environmental stress and elicitors enhance taxol production by endophytic strains of *Paraconiothyrium variabile* and *Epicoccumnigrum*. Enzyme Microb Technol 90:69–75

Spiering M, Moon CD et al (2005) Gene clusters for insecticidal loline alkaloids in the grass-endophytic fungus *Neotyphodium uncinatum*. Genetics 169(3):1403–1414

Subban K, Kempken F (2023) Insights into Taxol® biosynthesis by endophytic fungi. Appl Microbiol Biotechnol 107(20):6151–6162

Subudhi E, Sahoo RK, Dey S et al (2018) Unraveling plant-endophyte interactions: an omics insight. In: Endophytes and secondary metabolites. Springer, pp 1–19

Sun Y, Shi X, Xing Y et al (2022) Co-culture of *Aspergillussydowii* and *Bacillus subtilis* induces the production of antibacterial metabolites. Fungal Biol 126(4):320–332

Tiwari P, Bae H (2022) Endophytic fungi: key insights, emerging prospects, and challenges in natural product drug discovery. Microorganisms 10(2):360

Venugopalan A, Srivastava S (2015) Endophytes as in vitro production platforms of high value plant secondary metabolites. Biotechnol Adv 33(6):873–887

Venugopalan AV, Potunuru UR, Madhulika Dixit MD, Smita Srivastava SS (2016) Effect of fermentation parameters, elicitors and precursors on camptothecin production from the endophyte Fusarium solani. Bioresour Technol 206:104–111. https://doi.org/10.1016/j.biortech.2016.01.079

Verma V, Batta A, Singh HB et al (2023) Bioengineering of fungal endophytes through the CRISPR/Cas9 system. Front Microbiol 14:1146650

Vigneshwari A, Rakk D, Németh A et al (2019) Host metabolite producing endophytic fungi isolated from Hypericumperforatum. PLoS One 14(5):e0217060

Vishwakarma K, Kumar N, Shandilya C et al (2020) Revisiting plant–microbe interactions and microbial consortia application for enhancing sustainable agriculture: a review. Front Microbiol 11:560406

Watts D, Palombo EA, Castillo AJ et al (2023) Endophytes in agriculture: potential to improve yields and tolerances of agricultural crops. Microorganisms 11(5):1276

Wenderoth M, Pinecker C, Voss B et al (2017) Establishment of CRISPR/Cas9 in *Alternariaalternata*. Fungal Genet Biol 101:55–60

Wijesekara T, Xu B (2023) Health-promoting effects of bioactive compounds from plant endophytic fungi. J Fungi 9(10):997

Yousefvand M, Harighi B, Azizi A (2023) Volatile compounds produced by endophytic bacteria adversely affect the virulence traits of *Ralstoniasolanacearum*. Biol Control 178:105145

Zakariyah RF, Ajijolakewu KA, Ayodele AJ et al (2024) Progress in endophytic fungi secondary metabolites: biosynthetic gene cluster reactivation and advances in metabolomics. Bull Natl Res Cent 48(1):44

Zhang H, Xia YQ, Xia Y et al (2023) A CRISPR/Cas9-based study of CgloRPCYG, a gene that regulates pathogenicity, conidial yield, and germination in *Colletotrichumgloeosporioides*. Agronomy 13(7):1681

Zhang X, L L, Bai J et al (2024) Alkaloids isolated from the endophytic fungus Fusarium concentricum. Nat Prod Res 38(9):1517–1523

Zhou J, Li X, Chen Y et al (2017) De novo transcriptome assembly of *Phomopsisliquidambari* provides insights into genes associated with different lifestyles in rice (Oryza sativa L.). Front Plant Sci 8:121

Zotchev SB (2024) Unlocking the potential of bacterial endophytes from medicinal plants for drug discovery. Microb Biotechnol 17(2):e14382

The Role of PGPRs in Enhancing the Quality and Production of Medicinally Important Plants

Younes Rezaee Danesh and Marika Pellegrini

Abstract Plant growth-promoting rhizobacteria (PGPRs) are essential for improving the growth, yield, and quality of medically important plants. These beneficial bacteria colonize plant roots and act through several channels using nitrogen fixation, phosphate solubilization, phytohormone generation, and the induction of systemic resistance. PGPRs enhance plant health and the biosynthesis of secondary metabolites, basic determinants of the medicinal value of plants. The increasing worldwide need for herbal treatments demands environmentally friendly approaches to optimizing the output of medicinal plants. PGPRs offer a good substitute for chemical fertilizers and pesticides by motivating plant resilience against biotic and abiotic pressures and reducing environmental impact. PGPRs have been found in many studies to help the accumulation of bioactive compounds, including phenolics, flavonoids, and alkaloids, supporting the therapeutic effects of the medicinal plants. This chapter reviews the mechanisms by which PGPRs influence medicinal plants' metabolic pathways and development. Emphasizing their contribution to raising phytochemical enrichment, stress tolerance, and plant productivity, it draws attention to recent PGPR applications. Furthermore, the chapter covers problems and future directions in commercializing PGPR-based bioformulations for the mass production of medicinal plants. By including PGPRs in systems for manufacturing medicinal plants, we can open the road for sustainable agriculture and guarantee premium plant-based medicines. This material will be very helpful for researchers, agronomists, and practitioners seeking original ideas to enhance the growth and quality of medicinally important plants.

Y. R. Danesh (✉)
Department of Plant Protection, Faculty of Agriculture, Van Yuzuncu Yil University, Van, Türkiye

M. Pellegrini
Department of Life, Health and Environmental Sciences, University of L'Aquila, L'Aquila, Italy
e-mail: marika.pellegrini@univaq.it

S. Kumar Tripathi et al. (eds.), *Phytoceuticals for Sustainable Medication*, Interdisciplinary Biotechnological Advances,
https://doi.org/10.1007/978-981-95-7588-6_6

Keywords Plant Growth-Promoting Rhizobacteria (PGPR) · Medicinal plants · Secondary metabolites · Biofertilizers · Plant stress tolerance · Sustainable agriculture

1 Introduction

1.1 Importance of Medicinal Plants

Long the cornerstone of traditional medicine, medicinal plants remain extremely valuable in modern pharmacology. In underdeveloped countries, over 80% of people depend on traditional remedies, mostly from plant sources worldwide (Ghorbani 2005). Phytochemicals, including alkaloids, terpenoids, flavonoids, and phenolics, pique more interest in the pharmaceutical, nutraceutical, and cosmetic sectors. Thus, medical plants are in more demand there (Atanasov et al. 2015). Moreover, the trend for natural products mixed with concerns about synthetic drug side effects has significantly expanded the global herbal medicine market during the past 10 years (Ekor 2014). Still, given the growing demand, the sustainable production of medicinal herbs offers a major challenge. Problems including habitat destruction, overharvesting, soil damage, and climate change compromise medical plant availability and quality (Sharma et al. 2023). Therefore, innovative, eco-friendly solutions for better farming and preserving these valuable resources are much sought after.

1.2 Challenges in Production and Quality Maintenance

The yield of medicinal plants is much influenced by environmental elements, including soil fertility, water availability, and biotic and abiotic pressures. These elements affect the synthesis and accumulation of main metabolites and plant development (Afzal et al. 2023). Though some conventional agricultural methods rely on chemical fertilizers and pesticides to boost output, these approaches can compromise the quality of bioactive compounds, harm soil health, and pollute ecosystems (Pahalvi et al. 2021). Maintaining consistency and standardization of medicinal plants-derived products presents a great difficulty. Phytochemical profiles produced by environmental stresses or agricultural techniques can affect the therapeutic efficacy (Raudone and Savickiene 2024). Thus, sustainable and biologically based solutions are essential for maximum yield and quality and for lowering environmental impact.

1.3 Emerging Role of Plant-Associated Microbiomes

Based on recent developments in plant microbiome research, plant-associated microbial communities promote plant growth, health, and resilience (Compant et al. 2019). Especially the microbiome found in the rhizosphere—the root-associated area—interacts extensively with plants for disease resistance, stress tolerance, and nutrient acquisition (Berg et al. 2016). The microbiome influences not only development and health but also secondary metabolism in medicinal plants, thus affecting the concentration and composition of therapeutic molecules (Pang et al. 2021). Knowing and applying these favorable interactions provides a future direction for medicinal herbs' effective and environmentally friendly growth.

1.4 Introduction to PGPRs

Among the several plant-associated bacteria, plant growth-promoting rhizobacteria (PGPRs) have attracted special interest for their several benefits (Backer et al. 2018). PGPRs are a class of free-living, soil-bound bacteria that colonize plant roots and promote development in several ways. They increase nutrient availability by nitrogen fixing, phosphate solubilization, and siderophore synthesis; by synthesis of phytohormones including auxins, cytokinins, and gibberellins, they affect plant development (Lugtenberg and Kamilova 2009). PGPRs also help plant stress tolerance by producing stress-alleviating enzymes and inducing Induced Systemic Resistance (ISR), enabling plants to fight against diseases (Pieterse et al. 2012). The accumulating significant molecules, including phenolic acids, alkaloids, and flavonoids (Rizvi et al. 2022), can be greatly changed by the growing data showing PGPRs on the biosynthesis of secondary metabolites in medicinal plants. PGPRs show great potential as the main biotechnological tools to increase the quantity and quality of medicinal plant output. Including PGPR-based technologies into medicinal plant production could help support sustainable development, lower dependency on chemical inputs, and enhance the homogeneity and efficacy of herbal remedies. This chapter thus explores the processes by which PGPRs affect the secondary metabolite synthesis, stress tolerance, and growth in medicinal plants. It stresses the most recent scientific achievements, examines present issues, and explores future directions for PGPR application in medicinal plant agriculture.

2 PGPRs and Their Mechanisms of Action

PGPRs and their modes of action via a spectrum of direct and indirect channels enhance plant performance. These comprise phytohormone synthesis, nutrient acquisition facilitation, abiotic stress reduction, systemic resistance against pathogens, and modification of secondary metabolites. Understanding these mechanisms helps one to include PGPRs into sustainable agricultural systems, particularly for the growing medical plants. Figure 1 summarizes the primary mechanisms by which PGPRs enhance plant growth.

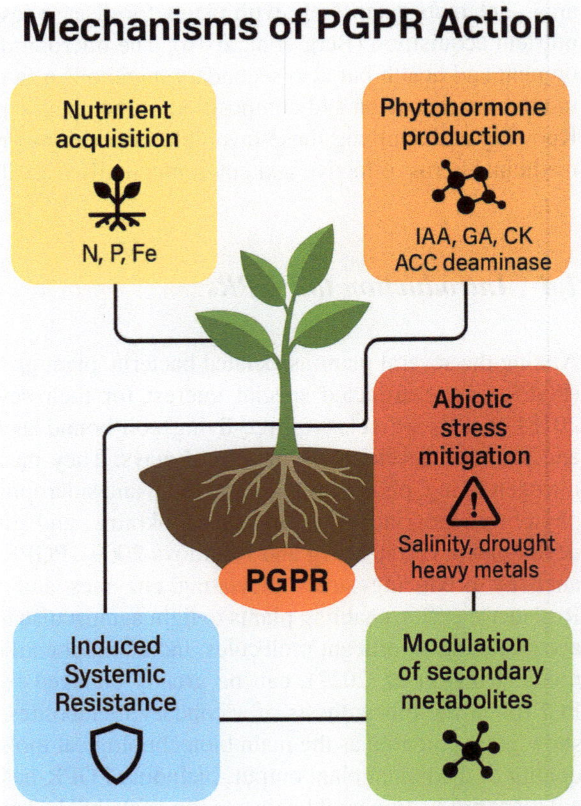

Fig. 1 Mechanisms of action of plant growth-promoting rhizobacteria (PGPRs). PGPRs promote plant growth and resilience through five main pathways: nutrient acquisition (e.g., nitrogen, phosphorus, iron), phytohormone production (e.g., IAA, gibberellins, cytokinins), mitigation of abiotic stresses (e.g., salinity, drought, heavy metals), induction of systemic resistance (ISR), and modulation of secondary metabolite biosynthesis

2.1 Getting Nutrients (N, P, K, Fe)

By increasing the availability and absorption of essential nutrients, including nitrogen (N), phosphorus (P), potassium (K), and iron (Fe), PGPRs mostly help plants grow. PGPRs that fix nitrogen—that is, *Azospirillum*, *Azotobacter*, and *Gluconacetobacter*—turn atmospheric nitrogen into ammonia, which plants most rapidly consume (Bhattacharyya and Jha 2012). Reducing reliance on synthetic nitrogen fertilizers helps to support sustainable farming systems. Phosphorus is often found in insoluble forms in the soil. PGPRs, including species of *Pseudomonas* and *Bacillus*, secrete organic acids (e.g., gluconic acid, citric acid) and phosphatases that solubilize bound phosphates, so rendering them available to plants (Sharma et al. 2013). Potassium-solubilizing bacteria, such as *Frateuria aurantia*, function similarly by releasing potassium from silicate minerals. Siderophore synthesis mediated by PGPRs helps plants acquire iron. Siderophores are tiny, high-affinity iron-chelating molecules secreted by bacteria under iron-limited conditions. These molecules bind Fe^{3+} and assist the host plants and bacteria to absorb it, indirectly increasing plant growth and limiting pathogen spread (Saha et al. 2016).

2.2 Phytohormone Synthesis

Auxins (e.g., indole-3-acetic acid, IAA), cytokinins, gibberellins, and ethylene modulators—which control plant development and growth—are among the phytohormones PGPRs synthesize (Glick 2014). The IAA is produced by strains including *Azospirillum*, *Pseudomonas*, and *Bacillus*, which stimulate root elongation, root hair development, and lateral root development (Spaepen and Vanderleyden 2011). The gibberellin-producing bacteria alter stem elongation and seed germination, while cytokinin-producing PGPRs affect cell division and shoot development (Kudoyarova et al. 2014). Some PGPRs can also generate ACC deaminase, an enzyme that breaks down 1-aminocyclopropane-1-carboxylate (ACC), the precursor of ethylene, a hormone that, at high levels, stunts plant development under stress conditions (Shahid et al. 2023). Thus, by lowering ethylene levels, PGPRs help plants retain growth under less than ideal conditions.

2.3 Mitigation of Stresses (Drought, Salinity, Heavy Metals)

Environmental stresses, including salinity, drought, and heavy metal contamination, greatly limit plant growth and productivity. PGPRs can reduce these stresses using several channels. PGPR-induced production of exopolysaccharides, which help preserve soil moisture around roots, can, for example, increase drought tolerance (Vurukonda et al. 2016). Some PGPRs also upregulate plant antioxidant systems, lowering oxidative damage under water shortage. PGPRs promote the accumulation of osmolytes like proline and glycine betaine in plant tissues and control Na^{+}/K^{+} ratios, helping preserve ion homeostasis in saline environments (Etesami and Beattie 2018). In saline soils, PGPRs can generate ACC deaminase, which is beneficial since it reduces the ethylene-mediated inhibition of root development. Likewise, in soils contaminated with heavy metals, including cadmium, lead, and arsenic, some PGPRs show metal-tolerant properties, including biosorption, bioaccumulation, and sequestration, thus lowering metal toxicity to plants (Yan et al. 2020). Furthermore, the PGPR-induced antioxidant enzyme activity enhances the detoxification of reactive oxygen species produced under heavy metal stress.

2.4 Induced Systemic Resistance

PGPRs also greatly help plants to develop systemic resistance (ISR) against a wide spectrum of pathogens. Unlike pathogen infection-induced systemic acquired resistance (SAR), ISR is started by nonpathogenic bacteria and is independent of salicylic acid signaling (Pieterse et al. 2012). Rather, it is linked to the ethylene and jasmonic acid signaling system pathways. PGPRs, including *Bacillus subtilis* and

Pseudomonas fluorescens, can prime plant defense systems, so accelerating and strengthening activation of defense responses upon pathogen attack (Berendsen et al. 2012). Among these priming activities are cell wall reinforcement, accumulation of antimicrobial secondary metabolites, and upregulation of pathogenesis-related proteins. PGPRs application in agriculture offers protection against bacterial, fungal, and viral pathogens and increases tolerance to some abiotic stresses, highlighting the several advantages of PGPRs use.

2.5 Modulation of Secondary Metabolites

The evidence shows that PGPRs directly or indirectly control the biosynthesis of secondary metabolites in medicinal plants. Medicinal plants' therapeutic effects depend on secondary metabolites, including alkaloids, flavonoids, terpenoids, and phenolic compounds (Tungmunnithum et al. 2018). Using several pathways, PGPRs affect secondary metabolism: enhancement of nutrient and water availability, modification of hormonal balances, and generation of mild stress responses that initiate secondary metabolite pathways (Narayanan and Glick 2022). The synthesis of valuable compounds, including artemisinin in *Artemisia annua* and withanolides in *Withania somnifera*, has been demonstrated to improve after inoculation with *Bacillus* and *Pseudomonas* strains (Semenzato and Fani 2024). Therefore, PGPRs not only help to improve growth and stress tolerance but also greatly contribute to the qualitative enhancement of medicinal plants by providing an environmentally friendly approach to increase the synthesis of plant-derived metabolites. Figure 2 summarizes the modulation of secondary metabolite pathways in medicinal plants.

3 How PGPRs Affect the Yield and Growth of Medicinal Plants

PGPRs are significant since they promote medicinal plants' growth, development, biomass, and secondary metabolites. They colonize the internal plant tissues and create interactions that greatly affect medicinal plant species' phytochemical properties and growth. Their application offers a practical approach to raising the quality and yield of medicinal plants in sustainable agriculture and pharmaceutical sectors.

3.1 Specific Plant Examples (e.g., Artemisia, Withania, Ocimum, Curcuma)

The PGPR inoculation has significant effects on different medicinal plants. *Artemisia annua* is well-known for producing the antimalarial chemical artemisinin. Inoculation with *Azospirillum brasilense* and *Pseudomonas fluorescens* has

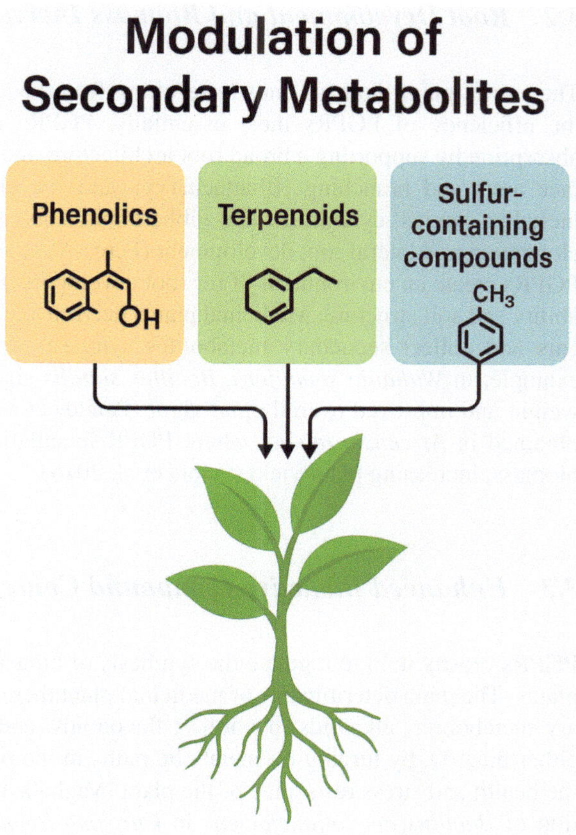

Fig. 2 PGPR-mediated modulation of secondary metabolite pathways in medicinal plants. PGPRs influence key metabolic routes responsible for the synthesis of bioactive compounds such as phenolics, terpenoids, and sulfur-containing molecules. These interactions enhance the therapeutic value of medicinal plants by stimulating secondary metabolite accumulation

increased biomass and artemisinin content (Gupta et al. 2016). Similarly, extensively used in Ayurvedic medicine, *Withania somnifera* (Ashwagandha) has shown amazing growth-promoting effects when treated with *Bacillus subtilis* and *Pseudomonas putida*, increasing root biomass and raising levels of withanolides, the main bioactive constituent of this plant (Pandey et al. 2018). Respected for their pharmacological properties, *Ocimum sanctum*—holy basil—responds especially to PGPR treatments. Results on inoculating *Bacillus megaterium* and *Pseudomonas aeruginosa* show that it increases plant height and essential oil content (Rizvi et al. 2022). Suggesting that microbial inoculants can be a main tool in improving the pharmacological efficacy of plant-derived products, the treatment with PGPRs such as *Azotobacter chroococcum* and *Bacillus amyloliquefaciens* has been reported to increase rhizome yield and curcumin concentration in *Curcuma longa* (turmeric) (Khan et al. 2023).

3.2 Root Development and Biomass Increase

The rise in plant biomass, mostly resulting from better root development, defines the efficiency of PGPRs most essentially. PGPRs increase nutrient and water absorption by supporting a broad root architecture, including more root length, surface area, and branching (Bhattacharyya and Jha 2012). Using phytohormones including auxins, cytokinins, and gibberellins, these bacteria directly induce root elongation and lateral root development (Pérez-Montaño et al. 2014). Furthermore, PGPRs create an environment fit for root development by enhancing nutrient availability and soil structure. Medicinal plants need strong root systems to absorb nutrients and collect secondary metabolites synthesized or stored in the roots. For example, in *Withania somnifera*, *Bacillus subtilis* significantly increased root dry weight and improved overall plant vigor (Pandey et al. 2018). Similar results were obtained in *Artemisia annua*, where PGPR inoculation increased shoot and root biomass, increasing plant yield (Gupta et al. 2016).

3.3 Enhanced Bioactive Compound Content

PGPRs mostly help to regulate the synthesis of bioactive compounds in medicinal plants. The main determinants of medicinal plant therapeutic effects are the secondary metabolites, alkaloids, phenolics, flavonoids, and terpenoids. PGPRs can act either directly, by turning on metabolic paths in the plant, or indirectly, by raising the health and stress resistance of the plant (Vaghela and Gohel 2023). An inoculation of *Bacillus amyloliquefaciens* in *Curcuma longa* raises curcumin content, a chemical with anti-inflammatory and antioxidant properties (Khan et al. 2023). In *Ocimum sanctum* (Rizvi et al. 2022), PGPR treatment similarly increased the eugenol- and other valuable terpenoid-rich essential oil accumulation. PGPRs, through complex interactions, can boost secondary metabolite synthesis. Following increasing secondary metabolism (Pérez-Montaño et al. 2014), some PGPRs generate elicitor molecules that weaken the plant defense systems. The other groups priming the host plant to generate more secondary metabolites connected to its defense mechanism cause systemic resistance (Vaghela and Gohel 2023). Moreover, PGPRs can help plants cope with abiotic stresses, including salinity and drought, under which secondary metabolite synthesis usually results as part of the stress response (Bhattacharyya and Jha 2012). Through stress reduction, PGPRs thus indirectly help to produce medicinally significant compounds. PGPRs' positive effects on medicinal plants offer a practical means of bioaugmentation techniques to boost the quantity and quality of plant drugs. Future research should optimize formulations for field use, clarify the molecular dialogues between PGPRs and their host plants, and gain knowledge of PGPR long-term effects.

4 PGPRs and Secondary Metabolite Production

PGPRs are rather well-known for enabling the growth and development of plants. Apart from these benefits, more and more studies show their importance in controlling the synthesis of secondary metabolites in medicinal plants. Often, secondary metabolites define their pharmacological value, including phenolics, alkaloids, and terpenoids. They are basic for the therapeutic action of the medicinal plants. PGPRs directly boost metabolism or induce plant defense reactions that upregulate secondary metabolite synthesis, influencing the biosynthesis routes generating these molecules. Table 1 summarizes the primary scientific evidence on the Modulation of Secondary Metabolite Pathways in Medicinal Plants by PGPRs.

4.1 Modulation of Alkaloids, Terpenoids, Phenolics Key Pathways

The secondary metabolite synthesis of plants follows complex, highly regulated routes. PGPRs change these systems via several avenues. In plants, they can generate phytohormones, elicitors, or volatile organic compounds (VOCs), among other signaling molecules. These signaling molecules activate particular transcription factors, raising biosynthetic gene expression (Vaishnav et al. 2019). Among the most well-investigated secondary metabolites impacted by PGPRs are phenolics, including lignins, tannins, and flavonoids. Usually, PGPR inoculation increases the phenylpropanoid pathway, which produces these molecules. For instance, plants treated with beneficial bacteria have shown notably higher expression of phenylalanine ammonia-lyase (PAL), an enzyme essential to the biosynthesis of phenolics (Vaghela and Gohel 2023). PGPRs can similarly influence the synthesis of different

Table 1 PGPR-mediated modulation of secondary metabolite pathways in medicinal plants and associated scientific evidence

Secondary metabolite type	PGPR mode of action	Example medicinal plants	References
Phenolics	Induction of the phenylpropanoid pathway; upregulation of PAL enzyme	*Ocimum basilicum* (sweet basil)	Tamayo-Aguilar et al. (2021)
Alkaloids	Activation of biosynthetic enzymes like TDC and STR via hormonal modulation (e.g., JA, SA)	*Catharanthus roseus* (Madagascar periwinkle)	Sharma et al. (2018)
Terpenoids	Stimulation of MVA and MEP pathways, triggered by PGPR-produced VOCs (e.g., acetoin)	*Curcuma longa* (turmeric)	Khan et al. (2023)
Mixed/other (e.g., essential oils, saponins)	General enhancement via stress priming, nutrient availability, and elicitor signaling	*Glycyrrhiza glabra* (licorice)	Tshikhudo et al. (2023)

pharmacologically active nitrogen-containing compounds, including alkaloids. The modulation of alkaloid pathways often consists of upregulating enzymes such as tropinone reductase or strictosidine synthase, depending on the plant species. Under stress, known to regulate alkaloid biosynthesis, some PGPRs can copy or change plant hormone levels, including jasmonic and salicylic acid (Egamberdieva et al. 2017). Still other crucial classes of secondary metabolites under PGPR influence are terpenoids. The mevalonate (MVA) and methylerythritol phosphate (MEP) pathways help plants to perform terpenoid biosynthesis. PGPR-induced activation of these pathways follows from improved synthesis of carotenoids, saponins, and essential oils. For example, changing gene expression in the MVA and MEP pathways has shown that bacteria producing VOCs such as acetoin and 2,3-butanediol induce terpenoid biosynthesis (Bitas et al. 2013).

4.2 Especially Selected Examples

Medicinal plants abound in many examples of PGPRs enhancing secondary metabolite synthesis. In *Ocimum basilicum* (sweet basil), *Bacillus subtilis* greatly increased the synthesis of phenolic compounds and essential oils rich in linalool and eugenol, so improving the antioxidant properties of the plant (Tamayo-Aguilar et al. 2021). Renowned for their strong alkaloids, vincristine and vinblastine, inoculation with *Pseudomonas fluorescens* strains enhanced the accumulation of these anticancer compounds. In Madagascar periwinkle, *Catharanthus roseus*, crucially for the pathway of alkaloid biosynthesis, the PGPR treatment increased the expression of important genes, including tryptophan decarboxylase (TDC) and strictosidine synthase (STR) (Sharma et al. 2018). Likewise, in *Curcuma longa* (turmeric), *Bacillus amyloliquefaciens* improved plant development and raised the concentration of curcumin, a secondary metabolite with anti-inflammatory and anticancer effects (Khan et al. 2023). These results imply that PGPRs can be focused on biofortifying medicinal plants for better pharmacological impact. Another remarkable example is *Glycyrrhiza glabra* (liquorice), in which co-inoculation with *Azospirillum brasilense* and *Pseudomonas putida* greatly raised the glycyrrhizin content, a triterpenoid saponin in charge of the plant's anti-inflammatory effect (Tshikhudo et al. 2023). Usually, PGPR-mediated stress priming underlies the processes behind these changes, which start secondary metabolic pathways as part of the plant's adaptive response. Moreover, changes in nutrient absorption, particularly nitrogen and phosphorus, indirectly support higher secondary metabolite biosynthesis, since many of these molecules are nitrogen- and carbon-rich (Chen et al. 2024). Given these benefits, including PGPRs inoculants into the techniques of cultivating medicinal plants, one finds a sustainable and ecologically friendly approach to raise output and quality. Future research should further investigate the identification of specific bacterial metabolites and signaling pathways engaged in secondary metabolite modulation to provide new directions for developing precision bioinoculants.

5 Strategies for PGPR Application in Medicinal Plant Cultivation

Choosing suitable application strategies is only one aspect of PGPR success in medicinal plant development; another is the choice of suitable microbial strains. In order to best use PGPRs, several methods—including inoculating seeds, soil treatment, spraying foliage, and using consortia—have been under study. These methods have particular benefits; their success will depend on the plant type, the bacterial strains used, and the surroundings.

5.1 *Seed Treatment*

Seed inoculation is among the easiest and most often used methods for introducing PGPRs to plants. Under this method, good bacteria are suspended over seeds before they are planted. This guarantees early protection and growth promotion by ensuring the bacteria colonize the rhizosphere as soon as the seed germinates (Vejan et al. 2016). Several studies have found success with seed inoculation in medicinal plants. In *Ocimum sanctum*, or holy basil, *Bacillus subtilis* seed treatment raised germination rates, seedling vigor, and biomass (Rizvi et al. 2022). Similarly, seed coating with *Pseudomonas fluorescens* improved seedling emergence and growth parameters in *Withania somnifera* (ashwagandha), helping to establish better plants and produce more secondary metabolites (Pandey et al. 2018). The seed inoculation provides simplicity of application, advantage, and cost economy, especially for large-scale operations (Backer et al. 2018), since the carrier-based formulations will help maintain bacterial viability during storage and guarantee homogeneous application.

5.2 *Soil Treatment*

Soil treatment directly applies PGPRs into the soil by mixing microbial inoculants into the soil medium or by irrigation systems. This method seeks to increase the rhizosphere's microbial population, improving nutrient cycling, stress tolerance, and disease suppression (Aloo et al. 2019). The plant growth, curcumin content, and nutrient absorption were enhanced by soil amendment with *Azospirillum brasilense* and *Bacillus megaterium* in *Curcuma longa* (turmeric) (Khan et al. 2023). Similarly, in *Artemisia annua* (sweet wormwood), the application PGPRs increased artemisinin concentration in combination with plant biomass (Gouda et al. 2018). One main benefit of soil amendment is its capacity to improve soil health and sustain a larger microbial population. The other parameters, like soil type, moisture content, and competing native bacteria, could affect the success of this approach (Compant et al. 2019).

5.3 Foliar Sprays

PGPRs are applied in foliar parts, straight onto the leaves. This approach offers endophytic colonization and can set off a systematic plant response, improving resistance against biotic and abiotic stresses (Kloepper and Ryu 2006). Essential oil yield and menthol content were much improved by foliar spraying with *Bacillus pumilus* in *Mentha arvensis* (Japanese mint) (Meena et al. 2017). Moreover, foliar application of *Pseudomonas* spp. enhanced the accumulation of phenolic compounds in *Echinacea purpurea*, improving antioxidant properties (Saharan and Nehra 2011). The foliar spraying is successful and can be used as a supplementary technique along with root inoculation. Environmental factors such as humidity, temperature, and UV exposure on leaf surfaces can affect bacterial survival (Pereira et al. 2014).

5.4 Consortia Applications

Recent developments show how well consortia—combining several PGPR strains—achieve synergistic effects. Such consortia can simultaneously target several plant growth and defense pathways, producing more consistent and strong results (Singh et al. 2011). In *Glycyrrhiza glabra* (liquorice), a consortium of *Azospirillum, Pseudomonas*, and *Bacillus* species produced notably higher root biomass and glycyrrhizin content than single-strain treatments (Tshikhudo et al. 2023). Similarly, in *Withania somnifera*, multistrain inoculation improved root yield and withanolide accumulation (Pandey et al. 2018). Consortia have advantages, including improved colonization efficiency, a wider range of disease suppression, and greater resilience to environmental stresses. However, to fully maximize the benefits, issues such as microbial compatibility, competition, and formulation stability must be carefully controlled (Timmusk et al. 2017).

Finally, selecting appropriate delivery techniques for specific crops and environmental conditions is most important for effectively using PGPRS in medicinal plant production. PGPRs could be further improved by combining techniques, such as seed inoculation and soil or foliar treatments. Future studies should focus on developing precision agriculture technologies and smart formulations to maximize the use of PGPRs and promote sustainable medicinal plant production.

6 Challenges and Limitations

PGPRs show great potential for improving the synthesis of secondary metabolites, the extension of medicinal plants, and the general crop yield. Still, as summarized in Table 2, there are several reasons that hinder their general acceptance in commercial farming. Such problems include environmental variance, host specificity, marketing difficulties, and legal questions. Overcoming these obstacles will enable PGPRs to realize their full potential in manufacturing medicinal plants.

Table 2 Key challenges and limitations in the application of plant growth-promoting rhizobacteria (PGPRs) for medicinal plant production

Challenge	Description	Impact	Proposed solution
Environmental variability	Soil type, pH, moisture, and climate influence PGPR viability and effectiveness	Inconsistent results across environments	Develop robust, climate-resilient PGPR formulations
Host specificity	PGPR effectiveness is often species-specific due to host-microbe compatibility	Limits the broad application across different medicinal plants	Screen and match PGPR strains to specific plant species
Legal and regulatory issues	Complex, varying regulatory frameworks govern PGPR product approval	Delays in commercialization and product deployment	Harmonize and simplify regulatory protocols
Commercialization barriers	Issues with production cost, formulation stability, and scalability	Low market competitiveness compared to chemical alternatives	Improve cost-effective production and stabilize formulations for storage and delivery

6.1 Environmental Variability

Environmental variability is among the main challenges to PGPRs' appropriate application. Thus, soil characteristics, climate, and other environmental factors greatly affect PGPR performance. With temperature, humidity, soil pH, nutrient availability, and moisture content, PGPR viability, activity, and efficacy change (Vejan et al. 2016). For example, some PGPR strains may perform poorly but benefit under less ideal conditions (Ehinmitan et al. 2024). Moreover, affecting PGPRs' rhizosphere colonizing ability is the type of soil and microbial community composition. Native microorganisms in different environments could affect PGPRs, compromising their efficacy (Compant et al. 2019). The unequal performance of PGPRs under evolving environmental conditions calls for the development of stronger and more flexible microbial formulations able to operate over a spectrum of climates and soil types (Shah et al. 2021).

6.2 Host Specificity

Host specificity is another restriction influencing PGPRs' use in the production of medicinal plants. Not every PGPR is equally successful among the several plant species. PGPRs have occasionally plant-specific benefits; some strains may only boost development or increase secondary metabolite synthesis in specific host plants (Saeed et al. 2021). The physiology of the plant, the root exudates, and the plant's capacity for positive interactions with some strains of bacteria create this specificity.

For example, the inoculation of *Withania somnifera* (ashwagandha) by *Bacillus subtilis* has been shown to improve growth and secondary metabolites, but this may not be effective on other plants, such as *Curcuma longa* (turmeric) (Pandey et al. 2018; Khan et al. 2023). The host specificity of many medicinal plants reduces the general significance of PGPRs. Therefore, thorough screening and identification of plant-specific PGPR strains are essential to overcome this and maximize their use in different medicinal plant species (Ehinmitan et al. 2024).

6.3 Legal Issues

The legal surroundings around PGPRs constitute still another major obstacle to be overcome. Though PGPRs have great potential to support environmentally friendly farming practices and increase agricultural output, their commercial use is sometimes quite strictly under control. Policies vary from country to country or region to region; some require thorough safety and efficacy testing before a product is approved for agricultural use (Lugtenberg and Kamilova 2009). This regulatory complexity can delay the commercialization of PGPR-based products and limit their availability in some markets. Since they must undergo extensive field trials to demonstrate safety and efficacy, small-scale manufacturers and researchers find great challenge in PGPR formulations (Neuhoff et al. 2024). Moreover, the difficulty of getting regulatory permission results from inconsistent approaches for evaluating PGPRs' efficacy and safety (Basu et al. 2021). Standardized testing approaches and regulatory process simplification help accelerate the PGPR-based product approval process, enabling their broad application in agriculture.

6.4 Challenges in Commercialization

Among the several obstacles to PGPRs' commercialization are cost, scalability, and product stability. One main challenge is the stability of PGPR formulations over time, particularly under different environmental conditions. When used on plants, the PGPRs can be compromised in transportation or storage, affecting their viability and efficacy (Zhang et al. 2025). Furthermore, the quality of PGPR-based products is much influenced by UV light exposure and temperature fluctuations. A further major obstacle to PGPR commercialization is price. Commercial PGPR manufacture calls for enormous quantities of costly microbial inoculants. Apart from manufacturing expenses, PGPR formulation and packaging are expensive. In regions where traditional agricultural practices predominate, these criteria especially help PGPR-based products to be less competitive than conventional chemical fertilizers and pesticides (de Andrade et al. 2023). Scalability presents yet another challenge for PGPRs' general acceptance in the manufacturing of medicinal plants. Mass PGPR production in enough quantities for widespread agricultural application requires specific resources and infrastructure. Maintaining constant quality and ensuring PGPRs are used at the required dosage will also help to produce the expected results. Particularly in underdeveloped regions where infrastructure could be limited, these logistical difficulties can compromise the commercial success of PGPR products (Kloepper and Ryu 2006).

7 Future Prospective

PGPRs offer amazing chances for sustainable development. Future developments in synthetic biology, microbiome engineering, formulation technologies, and field-scale validation will be important. These novel methods could solve present constraints related to PGPR applications, increase commercial viability, and improve PGPRs' efficacy.

7.1 Synthetic Approaches in Biological Sciences

Synthetic biology is one of the most interesting directions PGPR can take. Synthetic biology is the design and building of new biological parts, devices, and systems free from natural occurrences in the surroundings. In the PGPRs framework, synthetic biology can generate bacterial strains with improved features supporting plant development, stress tolerance, and secondary metabolite synthesis (Backer et al. 2018). Scientists have successfully altered PGPR strains to produce either exopolysaccharides or more phytohormones, including indole-3-acetic acid (IAA), which can increase plant root development and stress tolerance. Moreover, the PGPRs were changed by synthetic biology to increase their resilience in different environments. The PGPRs can survive in extreme temperatures, drought, or saline soils with stress-responsive genes (Giannelli et al. 2023). Synthetic biology techniques will help researchers increase the synthesis of bioactive compounds from medicinal plants by PGPRs.

7.2 Microbiome Engineering

Another futuristic approach that might change PGPR application in the manufacturing of medicinal plants is microbiome engineering. Microbial populations abound in plants' rhizosphere and endosphere by nature. The development and health of plants depend on these microbial populations. Still, many factors can influence these populations, including environmental conditions, type of soil, and plant species. By changing the plant-associated microbiome, researchers can maximize the microbial populations, thereby enhancing the benefits of PGPRs. Microbiome engineering aims to design and control microbial populations so that specific plant health benefits follow. For example, rhizosphere-introduced beneficial bacteria can increase nutrient uptake, control disease, or produce valuable secondary metabolites (Chepsergon and Moleleki 2023). Important microbial strains that influence specific plant traits have been identified through developments in metagenomics and bioinformatics. The inoculation of PGPRs in combination with these technologies can generate powerful, plant-specific microbiomes that enhance the synthesis of secondary metabolites and the growth of medicinal plants (de Andrade et al. 2023). As microbiome engineering continues to evolve, a new avenue for maximizing the efficacy of PGPRs and tailoring microbial populations for different medicinal plants may be opening up.

7.3 Technologies for Formulation

The effective formulation technologies are closely linked to the PGPRs' commercialization. The PGPR-based products must survive the conditions in which they are stored, transported, and applied while maintaining their beneficial effects on crops. The stability, shelf life, and efficacy of PGPR products depend on the development of formulation technologies. In order to improve the performance of PGPR, several formulation methods are being introduced. For example, microencapsulation and nanoencapsulation methods can help protect PGPRs from environmental stresses, including UV, drying, and high temperatures (Yang et al. 2024). These techniques encapsulate PGPRs in a protective matrix to regulate their release and increase their persistence in the soil. Also, choosing liquid formulations, alginate-based beads, or biodegradable polymers ensures that PGPRs reach the plant rhizosphere, where they are most effective, thus improving their delivery and efficacy (Moradipour et al. 2019). Furthermore, the general efficacy of PGPR applications can be raised by developing consortia-based formulations or co-inoculants combining several beneficial bacteria. Targeting specific PGPR mechanisms, such as disease suppression, stress reduction, or nutrient acquisition, these consortia can be customized (Yang et al. 2024). Such multistrain formulations can also reduce the possibility for microbial competition, thus improving the general success of PGPR inoculation in many agricultural environments.

7.4 Validation Using Field-Scale Tools

Research on PGPRs in the laboratory and greenhouse has made great strides. However, field-scale validation is required for the practical application of PGPRs. Field-scale validation is essential to evaluate PGPR-based products under real agricultural conditions, where environmental factors and microbial interactions are much more complicated. Field studies are necessary to determine the long-term benefits and practical feasibility of PGPRs application in the production of medicinal plants. These field studies also help with environmental variability, plant-microbe interactions, and scalability, which greatly affect the efficacy of PGPR treatments (Alzate Zuluaga et al. 2024). For example, PGPR performance in the field can be influenced by soil microbial communities, climatic conditions, and management practices; therefore, it is critical to evaluate PGPR efficacy under a range of field conditions. Large-scale studies will also provide important information on the financial feasibility of PGPR-based products and their potential to replace or complement conventional pesticides and fertilizers (Shah et al. 2021). To understand the ecological impact of PGPRs, field-scale validation is essential in evaluating their performance. Questions about potential ecological disruption or unintended spread of modified strains arise when introducing nonnative microorganisms into agricultural ecosystems. Field trials must include a comprehensive assessment of the ecological impacts of PGPRs, including those on soil health, biodiversity, and the surrounding environment (Neuhoff et al. 2024). Effective validation at the field scale will provide evidence to support the widespread commercialization of PGPR-based products and their incorporation into sustainable agricultural practices.

8 Conclusion

Particularly in the manufacturing of medicinal plants, the use of PGPRs in agricultural techniques has shown great potential to improve plant development, yield, and synthesis of important bioactive molecules. Given their several main benefits, PGPRs are a sustainable and effective tool for enhancing the supply and quality of medicinal plants. These benefits include better plant health, lowering environmental stresses, and producing secondary metabolites through increased nutrient absorption. PGPRs also improve soil condition by helping to increase microbial diversity and reduce reliance on chemical fertilizers and pesticides.

8.1 Benefits

One of PGPRs' main advantages is their ability to increase nutrient acquisition, particularly nitrogen, phosphorus, potassium, and iron. In nutrient-deficient soils or under stress, PGPRs allow plants access to vital nutrients more efficiently by solubilizing nutrients or fixing nitrogen. Auxins, cytokinins, and gibberellins are among the phytohormones that PGPRs also produce that stimulate root development, increase water and nutrient absorption, raise general plant vigor, and promote plant growth. PGPRs also quite effectively lower salinity, drought, and heavy metal toxicity, among other environmental stresses. Under these stress conditions, PGPRs activate plant defense systems, including synthesizing osmolytes, antioxidants, and stress-related proteins, allowing plants to negotiate negative environmental elements. Moreover, they induce systemic resistance (ISR) in plants, providing enhanced defense against various diseases. This ISR response increases plant resilience even more. Thus, PGPRs are a good tool for preserving plant health without synthetic chemical inputs. Apart from these effects on development, PGPRs are crucial in boosting medicinal plants' secondary metabolite synthesis. The secondary metabolites, including alkaloids, terpenoids, flavonoids, and phenolic compounds, have medicinal action. Higher bioactive molecule concentrations in treated plants result from PGPRs shown to regulate the biosynthesis of these molecules. For medicinal plants, the concentration of bioactive compounds directly determines the plant's therapeutic value, which is particularly crucial. Several studies have shown that PGPR inoculation increases the yield of important secondary metabolites in *Withania somnifera*, *Artemisia annua*, and *Curcuma longa*, providing PGPRs a possible means of improving the quality and efficacy of medicinal crops.

8.2 Directions of Future Orientation

Several fascinating research directions have great potential to increase the efficacy and widen their scope of use as PGPR-based applications keep growing in popularity in agricultural activities. Among important areas is the development of more effective and concentrated PGPR formulations. Synthetic biology and microbiome engineering could help PGPR strains with desired traits, such as enhanced stress resistance, better fit with particular plant species, or best production of beneficial metabolites, be designed. These generated strains would be more suited for many environmental conditions, thus PGPRs become more important in the production of medicinal plants. Still another interesting avenue for future study is the combination of PGPRs with contemporary agricultural technologies, including precision farming and nanotechnology. Under field conditions, developed PGPR formulations kept in nanoparticles or microcapsules would increase their stability, bioavailability, and potency. Furthermore, precision farming methods, including soil moisture and nutrient monitoring, could be applied to change PGPR treatments, ensuring they are used at the best times and dosages. Another area of great need for research is the function of the plant microbiome in PGPR interactions. Understanding the intricate interactions among PGPRs, plant species, and the native soil microbiome will enable one to know how PGPRs produce their positive effects. Plant-associated microbial communities able to improve plant health and secondary metabolite synthesis could be produced using microbiome engineering. This approach could lead to more sustainable farming methods and less demand for outside inputs like chemical fertilizers and pesticides. Long-term studies and field-scale trials will assist in validating PGPR's efficacy in practical agricultural environments. Laboratory and greenhouse studies have shown their advantages, even if field trials are required to evaluate PGPRs' performance under different environmental settings. These studies will enable formulations to be maximized, application methods to be improved, and how PGPR-based treatments would, over time, affect soil condition and plant output. PGPRs offer a reasonable and environmentally friendly approach to raise the content of bioactive compounds, growth, and yield of medicinal plants. Using improved nutrient acquisition, environmental stress reduction, and encouragement of secondary metabolite synthesis, PGPRs can greatly contribute to producing valuable medicinal plants. Targeting formulations, microbiome engineering, and field-scale validation as research develops will help PGPRs even more to transform medical plant production and support more sustainable agricultural practices all around.

References

Afzal I, Habiba U, Yasmeen H (2023) Review on the therapeutic potential of phytochemicals from medicinal plants. J Bioresour Manage 10(4):7

Aloo BN, Makumba BA, Mbega ER (2019) The potential of Bacilli rhizobacteria for sustainable crop production and environmental sustainability. Microbiol Res 219:26–39

Alzate Zuluaga MY, Fattorini R, Cesco S, Pii Y (2024) Plant-microbe interactions in the rhizosphere for smarter and more sustainable crop fertilisation: the case of PGPR-based biofertilizers. Front Microbiol 15:1440978

Atanasov AG, Waltenberger B, Pferschy-Wenzig EM, Linder T, Wawrosch C, Uhrin P, Temml V, Wang L, Schwaiger S, Heiss EH, Rollinger JM, Schuster D, Breuss JM, Bochkov V, Mihovilovic MD, Kopp B, Bauer R, Dirsch VM, Stuppner H (2015) Discovery and resupply of pharmacologically active plant-derived natural products: a review. Biotechnol Adv 33(8):1582–1614

Backer R, Rokem JS, Ilangumaran G, Lamont J, Praslickova D, Ricci E, Subramanian S, Smith DL (2018) Plant growth-promoting rhizobacteria: context, mechanisms of action, and roadmap to commercialisation of biostimulants for sustainable agriculture. Front Plant Sci 9:1473

Basu A, Prasad P, Das SN, Kalam S, Sayyed RZ, Reddy MS, El Enshasy H (2021) Plant growth-promoting rhizobacteria (PGPR) as green bioinoculants: Recent developments, constraints, and prospects. Sustainability 13(3):1140

Berendsen RL, Pieterse CMJ, Bakker PAHM (2012) The rhizosphere microbiome and plant health. Trends Plant Sci 17(8):478–486

Berg G, Rybakova D, Fischer D, Cernava T (2016) The plant microbiome explored: implications for experimental botany. J Exp Bot 67(4):995–1002

Bhattacharyya PN, Jha DK (2012) Plant Growth-Promoting Rhizobacteria (PGPR): emergence in agriculture. World J Microbiol Biotechnol 28(4):1327–1350

Bitas V, Kim HS, Bennett JW, Kang S (2013) Sniffing on microbes: diverse roles of microbial volatile organic compounds in plant health. Mol Plant-Microbe Interact 26(8):835–843

Chen Q, Song Y, An Y, Lu Y, Zhong G (2024) Soil microorganisms: their role in enhancing crop nutrition and health. Diversity 16(12):734

Chepsergon J, Moleleki LN (2023) Rhizosphere bacterial interactions and impact on plant health. Curr Opin Microbiol 73:102297

Compant S, Samad A, Faist H, Sessitsch A (2019) A review on the plant microbiome: ecology, functions, and emerging trends in microbial application. J Adv Res 19:29–37

de Andrade LA, Santos CHB, Frezarin ET, Sales LR, Rigobelo EC (2023) Plant growth-promoting rhizobacteria for sustainable agricultural production. Microorganisms 11(4):1088

Egamberdieva D, Wirth SJ, Alqarawi AA, Abd Allah EF, Hashem A (2017) Phytohormones and beneficial microbes: essential components for plants to balance stress and fitness. Front Microbiol 8:2104

Ehinmitan E, Losenge T, Mamati E, Ngumi V, Juma P, Siamalube B (2024) BioSolutions for green agriculture: unveiling the diverse roles of plant growth-promoting rhizobacteria. Int J Microbiol 2024:6181491

Ekor M (2014) The growing use of herbal medicines: issues relating to adverse reactions and challenges in monitoring safety. Front Pharmacol 4:177

Etesami H, Beattie GA (2018) Mining halophytes for plant growth-promoting halotolerant bacteria to enhance the salinity tolerance of non-halophytic crops. Front Microbiol 9:148

Ghorbani A (2005) Studies on pharmaceutical ethnobotany in the region of Turkmen Sahra, north of Iran (Part 1): general results. J Ethnopharmacol 102(1):58–68

Giannelli G, Potestio S, Visioli G (2023) The contribution of PGPR in salt stress tolerance in crops: unravelling the molecular mechanisms of cross-talk between plant and bacteria. Plants 12(11):2197

Glick BR (2014) Bacteria with ACC deaminase can promote plant growth and help to feed the world. Microbiol Res 169(1):30–39

Gouda S, Kerry RG, Das G, Paramithiotis S, Shin HS, Patra JK (2018) Revitalization of plant growth-promoting rhizobacteria for sustainable development in agriculture. Microbiol Res 206:131–140

Gupta R, Singh A, Gupta MM, Pandey R (2016) Cumulative role of bioinoculants on growth, antioxidant potential and artemisinin content in Artemisia annua L. under organic field conditions. World J Microbiol Biotechnol 32:167

Khan S, Ambika R, Rani K, Sharma S, Kumar A, Singh S, Thapliyal M, Rawat P, Thakur A, Pandey S, Thapliyal A, Pal M, Singh Y (2023) Rhizobacterial-mediated interactions in Curcuma longa for plant growth and enhanced crop productivity: a systematic review. Front Plant Sci 14:1231676

Kloepper JW, Ryu CM (2006) Bacterial endophytes as elicitors of induced systemic resistance. In: Schulz BJE, Boyle CJC, Sieber TN (eds) Microbial root endophytes, Soil biology, vol 9. Springer, pp 33–52

Kudoyarova GR, Melentiev AI, Martynenko EV, Timergalina LN, Arkhipova TN, Shendel GV, Kuz'mina LY, Dodd IC, Veselov SY (2014) Cytokinin producing bacteria stimulate amino acid deposition by wheat roots. Plant Physiol Biochem 83:285–291

Lugtenberg B, Kamilova F (2009) Plant-growth-promoting rhizobacteria. Ann Rev Microbiol 63:541–556

Meena KK, Sorty AM, Bitla UM, Choudhary K, Gupta P, Pareek A, Singh DP, Prabha R, Sahu PK, Gupta VK, Singh HB, Krishanani KK, Minhas PS (2017) Abiotic stress responses and microbe-mediated mitigation in plants: the omics strategies. Front Plant Sci 8:172

Moradipour M, Riseh RS, Mohammadinejad R, Hosseini A (2019) Nano-encapsulation of plant growth-promoting rhizobacteria and their metabolites using alginate-silica nanoparticles and carbon nanotube improves UCB1 pistachio micropropagation. J Microbiol Biotechnol 29:1096–1103

Narayanan Z, Glick BR (2022) Secondary metabolites produced by plant growth-promoting bacterial endophytes. Microorganisms 10(10):2008

Neuhoff D, Neumann G, Weinmann M (2024) Testing plant growth-promoting microorganisms in the field—a proposal for standards. Front Plant Sci 14:1324665

Pahalvi HN, Rafiya L, Rashid S, Nisar B, Kamili AN (2021) Chemical fertilizers and their impact on soil health. In: Dar GH, Bhat RA, Mehmood MA, Hakeem KR (eds) Microbiota and biofertilizers, vol 2. Springer, pp 55–81

Pandey SS, Singh S, Pandey H, Srivastava M, Ray T, Soni S, Pandey A, Shanker K, Babu CSV, Banerjee S, Gupta MM, Kalra A (2018) Endophytes of Withania somnifera modulate in planta content and the site of withanolide biosynthesis. Sci Rep 8:5450

Pang Z, Chen J, Wang T, Gao C, Li Z, Guo L, Xu J, Cheng Y (2021) Linking plant secondary metabolites and plant microbiomes: A review. Front Plant Sci 12:621276

Pereira RV, Bicalho ML, Machado VS, Lima S, Teixeira AG, Warnick LD, Bicalho RC (2014) Evaluation of the effects of ultraviolet light on bacterial contaminants inoculated into whole milk and colostrum, and on colostrum immunoglobulin G. J Dairy Sci 97(5):2866–2875

Pérez-Montaño F, Alías-Villegas C, Bellogín RA, del Cerro P, Espuny MR, Jiménez-Guerrero I, López-Baena FJ, Ollero FJ, Cubo T (2014) Plant growth promotion in cereal and leguminous agricultural important plants: from microorganism capacities to crop production. Microbiol Res 169(5–6):325–336

Pieterse CMJ, Van der Does D, Zamioudis C, Leon-Reyes A, Van Wees SCM (2012) Hormonal modulation of plant immunity. Annu Rev Cell Dev Biol 28:489–521

Raudone L, Savickiene N (2024) Phytochemical profiles of plant materials: from extracts to added-value ingredients. Plants 13(7):964

Rizvi A, Ahmed B, Khan MS, El-Beltagi HS, Umar S, Lee J (2022) Bioprospecting plant growth-promoting rhizobacteria for enhancing the biological properties and phytochemical composition of medicinally important crops. Molecules 27(4):1407

Saeed Q, Xiukang W, Haider FU, Kučerik J, Mumtaz MZ, Holatko J, Naseem M, Kintl A, Ejaz M, Naveed M, Brtnicky M, Mustafa A (2021) Rhizosphere bacteria in plant growth promotion, biocontrol, and bioremediation of contaminated sites: A comprehensive review of effects and mechanisms. Int J Mol Sci 22(19):10529

Saha M, Sarkar S, Sarkar B, Sharma BK, Bhattacharjee S, Tribedi P (2016) Microbial siderophores and their potential applications: a review. Environ Sci Pollut Res 23(5):3984–3999

Saharan BS, Nehra V (2011) Plant growth-promoting rhizobacteria: a critical review. Life Sci Med Res 21:1–30

Semenzato G, Fani R (2024) Endophytic bacteria: A sustainable strategy for enhancing medicinal plant cultivation and preserving microbial diversity. Front Microbiol 15:1477465

Shah A, Nazari M, Antar M, Msimbira LA, Naamala J, Lyu D, Rabileh M, Zajonc J, Smith DL (2021) PGPR in agriculture: a sustainable approach to increasing climate change resilience. Front Sustain Food Syst 5:667546

Shahid M, Singh UB, Khan MS, Singh P, Kumar R, Singh RN, Kumar A, Singh HV (2023) Bacterial ACC deaminase: insights into enzymology, biochemistry, genetics, and potential role in amelioration of environmental stress in crop plants. Front Microbiol 14:1132770

Sharma SB, Sayyed RZ, Trivedi MH, Gobi TA (2013) Phosphate solubilizing microbes: sustainable approach for managing phosphorus deficiency in agricultural soils. Springerplus 2:587

Sharma A, Verma P, Mathur A, Mathur AK (2018) Overexpression of tryptophan decarboxylase and strictosidine synthase enhanced terpenoid indole alkaloid pathway activity and antineoplastic vinblastine biosynthesis in Catharanthus roseus. Protoplasma 255(5):1281–1294

Sharma M, Saini L, Kumar P, Panigrahi S, Dwivedi P (2023) Strategies for conservation and sustainable use of medicinal plants. In: Jha S, Halder M (eds) Medicinal plants: biodiversity, biotechnology and conservation, vol 33. Springer

Singh JS, Pandey VC, Singh DP (2011) Efficient soil microorganisms: a new dimension for sustainable agriculture and environmental development. Agric Ecosyst Environ 140(3–4):339–353

Spaepen S, Vanderleyden J (2011) Auxin and plant-microbe interactions. Cold Spring Harb Perspect Biol 3:a001438

Tamayo-Aguilar Y, Juarez-Lopez P, Chavez-Garcia JA, Alia-Tejacal I, Guillen-Sanchez D, Perez-Gonzalez JO, Lopez-Martinez V, Rueda-Barrientos MC, Baque-Fuentes O (2021) Beneficial microorganisms enhance the growth of basil (Ocimum basilicum L.) under greenhouse conditions. Notulae Botanicae Horti Agrobotanici Cluj-Napoca 49(4):12452

Timmusk S, Behers L, Muthoni J, Muraya A, Aronsson A-C (2017) Perspectives and challenges of microbial application for crop improvement. Front Plant Sci 8:49

Tshikhudo PP, Ntushelo K, Mudau FN (2023) Sustainable applications of endophytic bacteria and their physiological/biochemical roles on medicinal and herbal plants: review. Microorganisms 11(2):453

Tungmunnithum D, Thongboonyou A, Pholboon A, Yangsabai A (2018) Flavonoids and other phenolic compounds from medicinal plants for pharmaceutical and medical aspects: an overview. Medicines (Basel) 5(3):93

Vaghela N, Gohel S (2023) Medicinal plant-associated rhizobacteria enhance the production of pharmaceutically important bioactive compounds under abiotic stress conditions. J Basic Microbiol 63(3–4):308–325

Vaishnav A, Shukla AK, Sharma A, Kumar R, Choudhary DK (2019) Endophytic bacteria in plant salt stress tolerance: current and future prospects. J Plant Growth Regul 38:650–668
Vejan P, Abdullah R, Khadiran T, Ismail S, Boyce AN (2016) Role of plant growth-promoting rhizobacteria in agricultural sustainability: a review. Molecules 21(5):573
Vurukonda SSKP, Vardharajula S, Shrivastava M, SkZ A (2016) Enhancement of drought stress tolerance in crops by plant growth-promoting rhizobacteria. Microbiol Res 184:13–24
Yan A, Wang Y, Tan SN, Mohd Yusof ML, Ghosh S, Chen Z (2020) Phytoremediation: a promising approach for revegetation of heavy metal-polluted land. Front Plant Sci 11:359
Yang P, Condrich A, Scranton S, Hebner C, Lu L, Ali MA (2024) Utilizing plant growth-promoting rhizobacteria (PGPR) to advance sustainable agriculture. Bacteria 3(4):434–451
Zhang S, Li F, Chang L, Zhang Q, Zhang Z, Wu T, Wu Y, Wang Z, Su Y, Yang X, Gao W, Li M, Wu Y, Jiang Y (2025) Broad-spectrum applications of plant growth-promoting rhizobacteria (PGPR) across diverse crops and intricate planting systems. Microbiol Spectrum 13(3):e0187924

Quality Approaches for Phytochemicals

Anshita Gupta, Deependra Soni, Durgesh Nandini Chauhan, Mayank Krishna Kulshrestha, and Nagendra Singh Chauhan

Abstract This chapter explores the quality approaches for phytochemicals, focusing on their significance in enhancing human health and their role in disease prevention. It delves into various extraction methods, purification techniques, and analytical assessments that ensure the integrity and potency of these bioactive compounds. By examining traditional and modern quality control strategies, the chapter emphasizes the importance of standardization, reproducibility, and regulatory compliance in phytochemical research. Furthermore, it highlights emerging trends in phytochemical applications, including their potential in nutraceuticals and pharmaceuticals, ultimately advocating for a comprehensive framework to enhance the quality and efficacy of phytochemicals in diverse applications.

Keywords Quality standardization · Metabolomics · Quality by design · High-Performance Liquid Chromatography (HPLC) · Mass Spectrometry (MS) · Nuclear Magnetic Resonance (NMR)

A. Gupta
Department of Pharmacy, Guru Ghasidas Vishwavidyalaya, Bilaspur, Chhattisgarh, India

D. Soni
School of Pharmacy, MATS University, Aarang, Chhattisgarh, India

D. N. Chauhan
Columbia Institute of Pharmacy, Raipur, Chhattisgarh, India

M. K. Kulshrestha
Shri Narayan Prasad Awasthi Govt. Ayurved College, Raipur, Chhattisgarh, India

N. S. Chauhan (✉)
Drugs Testing Laboratory Avam Anusandhan, Raipur, Chhattisgarh, India

S. Kumar Tripathi et al. (eds.), *Phytoceuticals for Sustainable Medication*, Interdisciplinary Biotechnological Advances,
https://doi.org/10.1007/978-981-95-7588-6_7

1 Introduction

In the evolving landscape of medicine and health, phytochemicals have emerged as pivotal compounds derived from plants, revered not only for their therapeutic potentials but also for their roles in enhancing human health (Alam et al. 2025). These bioactive molecules encompassing a vast array of chemical compounds such as flavonoids, alkaloids, polyphenols, and terpenes are recognized for their diverse biological activities, including anti-inflammatory, antioxidant, antimicrobial, and anticancer effects. Phytochemicals are integral to traditional herbal medicine systems, yet their relevance has surged within contemporary biomedical research, underpinning the necessity for a deeper understanding and rigorous application of quality approaches in their development (Balogun et al. 2023).

1.1 Overview of Phytochemicals and Their Importance

Phytochemicals, often termed the "hidden chemicals" of plants, constitute a complex group of naturally occurring compounds synthesized by plants as secondary metabolites. They serve various ecological functions, including plant defense against pathogens, herbivores, and environmental stressors. For humans, phytochemicals hold significant importance as they contribute substantially to the nutritional and medicinal properties of many fruits, vegetables, herbs, and spices. The consumption of phytochemical-rich foods has been associated with a lower risk of chronic diseases, including cancer, cardiovascular ailments, and neurodegenerative disorders (Devi 2025). Research has increasingly demonstrated that these compounds can modulate cellular processes and signaling pathways, leading to their potential as preventive and therapeutic agents. As the scientific community explores the molecular foundations of phytochemicals, substantial evidence has emerged regarding their efficacy. However, the translation of this knowledge into clinical applications necessitates a stringent focus on quality (Fig. 1). The complexity of plant materials, coupled with the variability in climatic conditions, cultivation practices, and harvesting methods, raises significant concerns about the consistency and potency of phytochemicals. Thus, the establishment of reliable quality assurance frameworks becomes imperative to ensure that herbal medicines are safe, effective, and reproducible (Balogun et al. 2023).

1.2 Need for Quality Approaches in Herbal Drug Development

The burgeoning interest in phytochemicals has sparked a renaissance in herbal medicine and the development of botanical dietary supplements. Nonetheless, the lack of standardization in herbal preparations poses challenges to both researchers and

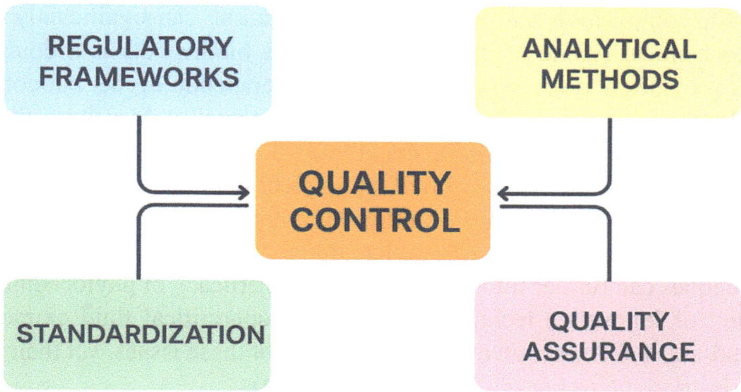

Fig. 1 Different quality control approaches for phytochemicals

consumers. Unlike conventional pharmaceuticals, where active ingredients and dosages can be precisely controlled through synthetic processes, herbal products often contain a multitude of phytochemical constituents with varying degrees of bioactivity. Therefore, ensuring quality in the context of herbal drug development is fundamentally different and significantly more complex. Quality approaches encompass a broad spectrum of strategies aimed at optimizing the development, formulation, and production of phytochemicals. This includes rigorous methodologies such as Good Manufacturing Practices (GMP), validation of analytical methods, and adherence to pharmacopoeial standards. It is crucial to establish standardized extraction processes that enhance the yield and stability of key phytochemicals while minimizing degradation or loss of bioactivity. Furthermore, the use of advanced analytical techniques such as high-performance liquid chromatography (HPLC), mass spectrometry (MS), and nuclear magnetic resonance (NMR) is vital for the accurate profiling of phytochemicals, allowing for the identification and quantification of active components in herbal formulations. In addition to ensuring the quality of phytochemicals, it is equally essential to foster transparency and traceability throughout the supply chain (Alam et al. 2025). Consumers must be assured of the authenticity and integrity of the herbal products they consume, requiring producers to implement stringent quality control measures right from raw material sourcing to final product distribution. Regulatory bodies worldwide are increasingly recognizing the need for such quality approaches, prompting discussions and initiatives aimed at establishing guidelines for acceptable standards in herbal drug development.

1.3 Challenges in Ensuring Consistent Quality of Phytochemicals

Despite the critical importance of quality approaches, numerous challenges persist in the quest for consistent quality of phytochemicals. One primary obstacle lies in the inherent variability of plant sources. Factors such as geographical location, climate, soil composition, and even seasonal fluctuations can significantly influence the phytochemical profile of plant materials. This biodiversity is a double-edged sword; it provides a vast reservoir of potential therapeutic agents but complicates the standardization process necessary for consistent quality. Moreover, there exists a profound challenge related to the extraction and processing of phytochemicals. Conventional extraction methods often fail to yield optimal results across different plant species, leading to variations in the concentration and activity of the desired compounds. Additionally, postharvest handling, storage conditions, and formulation techniques can further impact the stability and efficacy of phytochemicals. The integration of innovative technologies such as supercritical fluid extraction and ultrasound-assisted extraction may mitigate some of these issues, yet their adoption in the industry remains uneven (Shareef et al. 2024).

Finally, regulatory challenges add another layer of complexity. The regulatory landscape surrounding phytochemicals and herbal products varies widely between countries, with differing degrees of scrutiny applied to their development and market entry. Achieving compliance with local and international regulations necessitates an understanding of both the evolving scientific paradigms and the existing legal frameworks, which can often be daunting for manufacturers. The integration of robust quality approaches in the realm of phytochemicals is vital to harnessing their full potential as therapeutic agents. The intersection of scientific research, regulatory compliance, and consumer safety must align to foster the development of high-quality herbal medicines that meet the needs of modern society (Devi 2025). As we delve deeper into this exploration, it becomes evident that a multidisciplinary approach that encompasses chemistry, biology, environmental science, and pharmacology is essential to address the myriad challenges faced by the field. Ultimately, advancing our collective understanding of phytochemicals and committing to quality-centric practices will pave the way for the innovation and reliability necessary for the successful integration of these natural compounds into mainstream healthcare (Pathrikar et al. 2025a, b).

2 Regulatory Perspectives on Phytochemicals

The regulatory approaches to phytochemicals are rather complex, representing a dynamic interplay between different global frameworks and guidelines and standardization attempts. Some of the key global regulatory organizations that play strategic roles in defining the landscape for regulating herbal medicines and nutraceuticals include the World Health Organization (WHO), US Food and Drug Administration (USFDA), European Medicines Agency (EMA), and India's AYUSH. Each organization offers proprietary protocols specific to its regional interests while also pushing for compliance with safety and efficacy regulations. As an example, the WHO's strategy for traditional medicine focuses on ensuring quality in herbal products, promoting standardized definitions and evaluation, which are reflected in USFDA and EMA policies demanding stringent premarket testing for safety and efficacy (Alam et al. 2025). Further, the standards set for herbal medicinal products and nutraceuticals highlight the need for thorough safety information and efficacy support, in relation to contemporary scientific expectations as well as traditional consumption. Such guidelines seek to improve consumer trust and reduce risk due to misuse of herbal materials. In addition, standards of quality as defined in the pharmacopoeias like the Indian Pharmacopoeia, European Pharmacopoeia, Chinese Pharmacopoeia, and the United States Pharmacopeia (USP) are important in setting parameters for phytochemical products' identity, purity, and strength. They make sure that companies maintain rigid quality control guidelines, including procurement, processing, and assay of raw materials (Kagawad et al. 2021). The harmonization process through organizations like the International Organization for Standardization (ISO) is imperative in supporting international trade as well as having herbal medicines conform to globally accepted safety and quality standards. Country collaboration programs have led to research findings and regulatory procedures being shared among the nations, ultimately bringing about an integrated approach in regulating the phytochemical industry (Cai et al. 2019).

3 Quality by Design (QbD) for Phytochemicals

Quality by Design (QbD) is an innovative and systematic approach within the pharmaceutical and nutraceutical industries, aiming to enhance product quality through a structured and well-defined development process. At its core, QbD emphasizes understanding the product and its manufacturing processes, focusing on predefined objectives, known as Critical Quality Attributes (CQAs). In the context of phytochemicals, CQAs are inherent characteristics that must be controlled to ensure safety, efficacy, and stability. These attributes can include potency, purity, and profile of active compounds derived from herbal sources. By identifying these attributes early in the formulation process, researchers can align their design efforts toward achieving consistent product quality. A pivotal element of QbD is the Design of Experiments (DoE), which facilitates the systematic exploration of how various formulation and processing variables impact CQAs. Using statistical methods, DoE allows for the optimization of extraction methods, solvent selection, and formulation parameters, ultimately contributing to the standardization of herbal products. Case studies have illustrated the successful application of QbD principles to herbal formulations, showcasing how targeted experiments have led to improved consistency and quality of phytochemical extracts. For instance, one study demonstrated how QbD frameworks helped to refine the extraction process of flavonoids from a specific herb, resulting in higher yields and better quality profiles. As the industry continues to move toward more rigorous quality standards and regulatory compliance, the implementation of QbD principles in the development of phytochemicals represents not just a methodological shift but a necessary evolution toward achieving reliable and efficacious herbal products.

The evolving landscape of herbal medicine emphasizes the necessity for robust methodologies to ensure the quality and efficacy of phytochemicals. As herbal products continue to gain popularity, the concept of Critical Quality Attributes (CQAs) becomes imperative in maintaining consistent product quality and safety. CQAs are defined characteristics or properties that must be controlled within specific limits throughout the manufacturing process to ensure that the final product meets its intended quality standards. This essay will explore the importance of CQAs in phytochemical analysis, the application of Design of Experiments (DoE) in herbal standardization, and relevant case studies that highlight the successful application of Quality by Design (QbD) principles in developing herbal formulations.

3.1 Understanding Critical Quality Attributes (CQAs)

CQAs are pivotal for any product, particularly those derived from natural sources like plants. For phytochemicals, these attributes typically include aspects such as potency, purity, stability, and bioavailability. Potency refers to the degree of activity exerted by a compound, which is crucial in determining its efficacy. Purity encompasses the presence of active components devoid of contaminants, including heavy metals, pesticides, and microbial load. Stability pertains to the retention of chemical integrity over time, while bioavailability denotes the extent and rate at which the active ingredient or active moiety is absorbed and becomes available at the site of action. To define CQAs for phytochemicals, a systematic approach integrating scientific knowledge and regulatory guidelines is essential. This process begins with identifying the desired therapeutic outcomes and linking them to specific physicochemical properties of the phytochemicals. For instance, in the case of curcumin, a well-known phytochemical derived from turmeric, CQAs would include its concentration, the presence of curcuminoids, and solvent residues left after extraction. Moreover, understanding the mechanism of action and pharmacokinetics of herbs can aid in defining specific CQAs that ensure therapeutic effectiveness (Park et al. 2025).

3.2 Design of Experiments (DoE) in Herbal Standardization

Herbal standardization aims to bring consistency to herbal products by ensuring that they achieve predetermined quality benchmarks. DoE offers a structured methodology to assess the relationships between multiple factors affecting the quality, thereby enabling the optimization of formulations. By systematically varying parameters such as temperature, extraction time, solvent type, and particle size, researchers can identify the optimal conditions for maximizing yield and maintaining the integrity of bioactive compounds (Roselló-Soto et al. 2022). The application of DoE often involves two main types of designs: factorial designs and response surface methodology (RSM) (Bertani et al. 2020). Factorial designs allow researchers to evaluate the impact of several independent variables simultaneously, providing insights into interactions that might not be evident when one variable is changed at a time. RSM, on the other hand, is particularly useful in exploring the optimal conditions for maximum output while minimizing undesirable effects, such as degradation of sensitive compounds in an herbal extract (Tianjin et al. 2024). For example, in the standardization of ginseng extracts, a 23 factorial design could be employed to assess the effects of extraction time, ethanol concentration, and temperature on the yield of ginsenosides, the principal active components of ginseng. By analyzing the data obtained through such experiments, researchers can generate models that predict the quality of the extract under various conditions, facilitating more consistent production processes and ensuring compliance with defined CQAs.

3.3 *Quality by Design (QbD) in Herbal Formulations*

Quality by Design (QbD) is a systematic approach to pharmaceutical development that emphasizes understanding the product and process, allowing for improved control over CQAs. The QbD framework can be particularly advantageous when applied to herbal formulations. It integrates the principles of risk management, process analytical technology, and continuous improvement, ensuring that every step from the selection of raw materials to manufacturing processes is based on sound scientific principles (Chen et al. 2024a, b). A fundamental aspect of QbD is the use of prior knowledge to inform design decisions. In the formulation of herbal medicines, an extensive literature review, along with empirical data from previous studies, can guide the selection of excipients, packaging materials, and stability testing protocols. This knowledge base aids in anticipating challenges and developing strategies to mitigate risks associated with variability in raw plant materials, which can be influenced by factors such as geographical location, harvest time, and postharvest processing. Case studies provide tangible examples of how QbD can enhance herbal formulation development. For instance, a study focusing on the formulation of a herbal cough syrup utilizing honey and thyme demonstrated the application of QbD principles (Chen et al. 2024a, b). The researchers employed risk assessment tools to identify potential variabilities in raw material quality. By implementing DoE to optimize the proportions of active ingredients and vehicle, they achieved a formulation that consistently met established CQAs for taste, viscosity, and efficacy. Moreover, the integration of in vitro models during the formulation process has strengthened this approach. Using methods such as cellular assays to evaluate bioactivity helps confirm that the formulated product aligns with the intended therapeutic outcomes. Applying QbD in this context not only enhances product quality but also streamlines regulatory submissions by providing comprehensive documentation of the development process.

While the adoption of CQAs, DoE, and QbD principles represents a significant advancement in the field of herbal formulation, several challenges remain. One prominent issue is the inherent variability in the composition of herbal materials, influenced by both biological and environmental factors (Naznin et al. 2024). Standardization efforts must therefore account for this variability in a manner that ensures consistent product quality. Robust supply chain management and thorough quality assurance measures are essential to address these issues. Furthermore, the integration of advanced technologies, such as high-performance liquid chromatography (HPLC) and mass spectrometry (MS), into quality control processes can provide deeper insights into the composition of herbal products. These technologies not only facilitate accurate quantification of active components but also help identify impurities that could affect product safety and efficacy. In the future, increased collaboration between academia, industry, and regulatory bodies will be critical in advancing the standardization of herbal products (Mahboubifar et al. 2024). Developing clear guidelines regarding the implementation of QbD in herbal medicine will promote consistent practices across the industry and enhance consumer confidence in herbal remedies. Additionally, ongoing research aimed at elucidating the pharmacodynamics and pharmacokinetics of herbal formulations will further support the establishment of CQAs, ultimately leading to safer and more effective therapeutic products.

Critical Quality Attributes play an integral role in the standardization of herbal products, ensuring that they meet safety and efficacy requirements. By adopting Design of Experiments methodologies, researchers can systematically optimize formulation processes, thereby enhancing the quality of phytochemicals (Nahar et al. 2024). The principles of Quality by Design offer a valuable framework for developing herbal formulations that meet predetermined quality standards, ensuring product integrity from development through to manufacturing (Table 1). As the demand for herbal medicines continues to grow, so too must the commitment to

Table 1 Case studies involving different approaches to attain the quality of phytochemicals

Case study	Focus area	Key quality approaches used	Outcome/significance
Quality standardization of curcumin products	Standardization of turmeric-derived curcumin	HPLC quantification of curcuminoids, FTIR fingerprinting, contaminant screening, stability testing	Ensured batch-to-batch consistency, compliance with pharmacopoeial standards, and improved product marketability
QbD approach for ginseng formulations	Quality by design application in ginseng capsules/ extracts	Identification of critical quality attributes (CQAs), design of experiments (DoE), optimization of extraction parameters, LC-MS/MS profiling	Achieved optimized extraction yield, enhanced bioactive content, and reproducible product quality
Metabolomics-based authentication of green tea	Authentication and quality verification of green tea varieties	Untargeted metabolomics using LC-MS and NMR, multivariate statistical analysis, and chemometric modeling	Differentiated authentic vs. adulterated samples, identified key metabolite markers, and supported origin traceability

understanding and controlling the variables that impact their quality. Through rigorous scientific approaches and collaborative efforts, the potential of herbal formulations can be realized to the fullest, benefiting consumers and practitioners alike.

4 Phytochemical Profiling and Standardization

Phytochemical profiling and standardization play a profound role in the fields of pharmacognosy and phytotherapy. They not only provide insights into the chemical constituents of plant materials but also ensure consistency, quality, and efficacy in herbal products. This essay explores various aspects of phytochemical profiling and standardization, focusing on botanical identification and authentication, macroscopic, microscopic, and organoleptic evaluation, physicochemical parameters, phytochemical screening, and chemotaxonomy, along with marker-based standardization (Zou et al. 2024).

4.1 Botanical Identification and Authentication

Botanical identification and authentication are essential steps in the utilization of plants for medicinal purposes. The correct identification of plant species is paramount to prevent the use of adulterated or misidentified materials that may pose health risks. Techniques such as morphological identification, DNA barcoding, and chemical fingerprinting play central roles in this process. Morphological identification relies on distinctive attributes such as leaf shape, flower structure, and growth habit, which are observable without advanced technology. However, this method can be subjective and sometimes misleading due to phenotypic plasticity in response to environmental factors (Pathrikar et al. 2025a, b). Therefore, DNA barcoding has emerged as a reliable technique, utilizing segments of the chloroplast or nuclear genome to confirm species identity. By comparing genetic sequences to established databases, researchers can accurately identify and authenticate plant specimens. Additionally, chemical fingerprinting utilizes chromatographic techniques like High-Performance Liquid Chromatography (HPLC) or Gas Chromatography-Mass Spectrometry (GC-MS) to analyze the unique chemical profiles of specific plants. Each plant species possesses a characteristic profile, enabling systematic differentiation from adulterants or closely related species. It serves as a robust complement to morphological and genetic methods, ensuring high confidence in botanical identification.

4.2 Macroscopic, Microscopic, and Organoleptic Evaluation

Once botanical identification is confirmed, macroscopic, microscopic, and organoleptic evaluations further enhance the understanding of the plant material's quality. Macroscopic evaluation involves examining the physical characteristics of the plant, including size, color, and texture (Kumar et al. 2023). These parameters can indicate the plant's age, cultivation conditions, and potential contamination. Microscopic evaluation examines plant tissues' internal structures, providing insights into their cellular composition and organization. Techniques such as thin sectioning and staining highlight specific cellular features, allowing differentiation between various plant species or subspecies. For instance, the presence of certain types of stomata, trichomes, or vascular bundles can be indicative of plant identity and authenticity. Organoleptic evaluation encompasses sensory assessment, including taste, smell, and texture (Li et al. 2022). This evaluation helps establish the plant's freshness and quality while contributing to its pharmacological efficacy. Such assessments are crucial in identifying herbal remedies, where flavor and aroma significantly influence therapeutic properties.

4.3 Physicochemical Parameters (Moisture, Ash Values, Extractives)

Physicochemical parameters are critical indicators of the quality and stability of herbal materials. Moisture content affects the shelf life and potency of plant materials, where excessive moisture can promote microbial growth and degradation (Patel et al. 2021). Standardized methods, such as oven drying and Karl Fischer titration, are employed to determine moisture content, ensuring the preservation of active constituents. Ash values represent the inorganic residue remaining after combustion, which reflects the mineral content and purity of the sample. Total ash provides insight into the total inorganic content, while acid-insoluble ash indicates the presence of siliceous impurities that may compromise the quality of herbal materials. Extractives refer to the soluble constituents that can be extracted using various solvents, highlighting the bioactive compounds present in the plant material. The determination of extractives via different solvent systems (water, alcohol, hexane) allows for the evaluation of the phytochemical diversity within the plant. The findings help in formulating dosage forms and establishing the optimal extraction conditions for therapeutic applications (Singh et al. 2023).

4.4 Phytochemical Screening (Qualitative and Quantitative)

Phytochemical screening is an essential process in characterizing the bioactive components of medicinal plants. Qualitative screening aims to detect the presence of various classes of phytochemicals, including alkaloids, flavonoids, terpenoids, tannins, and saponins. Common methods include color reactions and precipitation tests, where specific reagents indicate the presence of these compounds through observable color changes or precipitate formation. Quantitative phytochemical analysis measures the concentration of active compounds within plant extracts, providing vital information for standardization and dosage recommendations (Huang et al. 2020). Techniques such as spectrophotometry, HPLC, and LC-MS are frequently employed to quantify phytochemicals accurately. For example, determining the levels of flavonoids in a herbal extract can guide the development of standardized formulations for therapeutic use. Phytochemical screening is not solely focused on identifying active constituents; it also provides insights into the relationship between these compounds and the biological effects exhibited by the plant. Understanding the quantity and nature of phytochemicals can help predict the pharmacological potential of herbal remedies based on traditional medicinal knowledge.

4.5 Chemotaxonomy and Marker-Based Standardization

Chemotaxonomy is the classification of plants based on their chemical constituents, which often reflects their evolutionary relationships. This approach enables researchers to group related species according to shared phytochemical traits, enhancing our understanding of plant taxonomy and biodiversity (Bian et al. 2022). For example, specific alkaloids might be unique to particular genera or families, consequently guiding the identification and authentication of herbal materials (Zhao et al. 2021).

Marker-based standardization focuses on the quantification of specific bioactive markers known to correlate with therapeutic efficacy (González-Ruiz et al. 2019). Identifying and validating these markers ensures that herbal products maintain consistent quality and efficacy across batches. Marker compounds can serve as benchmarks for the standardization of complex herbal mixtures, facilitating regulatory approval and consumer safety. With increasing interest in phytotherapeutics, the importance of marker-based standardization cannot be overstated (Wu et al. 2024). Thoroughly characterized plant extracts with defined marker profiles support pharmaceutical development and clinical research, providing transparency and reproducibility in herbal medicine. Phytochemical profiling and standardization are indispensable components of modern herbal medicine and biopharmaceutical research (Kim et al. 2025). The integration of botanical identification and authentication, macroscopic and microscopic evaluation, physicochemical parameters, phytochemical screening, and chemotaxonomy contributes to a comprehensive understanding of plant materials. This multifaceted approach not only ensures quality and efficacy in herbal products but also promotes sustainable practices in the utilization of plant resources. As the demand for herbal remedies continues to grow, the commitment to rigorous profiling and standardization will be essential in safeguarding public health and advancing scientific knowledge in pharmacognosy.

5 Quality Assessment of Phytochemicals Using Analytical Techniques

Phytochemicals are plant-derived bioactive compounds that have received considerable attention in nutrition and medicine for their assumed health benefits. Identification, quantitation, and quality determination of such compounds are essential to ensure their safety and effectiveness. The essay entails a description of the different analysis methods utilized for quality determination of phytochemicals, including their principles, applications, and implications in quality and consistency assurance of plant-based products.

One of the major analytical methods applied in the analysis of phytochemicals is chromatography, including methods like thin-layer chromatography (TLC), high-performance liquid chromatography (HPLC), and gas chromatography (GC). TLC, being a cheap and easy method, is mainly applied in initial screening and identification of phytochemicals. HPLC, especially when combined with mass spectrometry (MS), provides high resolution and sensitivity and can be used to separate, identify, and quantify a wide variety of phytochemicals in multicomponent mixtures. GC, usually combined with MS, is especially ideal for volatile and semi-volatile substances. The selection of a chromatographic method is based on the characteristics of the target phytochemicals and the sample matrix complexity. Spectroscopic methods, including ultraviolet-visible (UV-Vis) spectroscopy, infrared (IR) spectroscopy, and nuclear magnetic resonance (NMR) spectroscopy, are instrumental in the structural elucidation and quality evaluation of phytochemicals (Martínez-Martínez et al. 2020).

UV-Vis spectroscopy is applied to identify the presence and amount of compounds containing UV-Vis absorbing chromophore, whereas IR spectroscopy gives information regarding the functional groups present within the molecule (Jain et al. 2022). NMR spectroscopy is a sensitive method for structure elucidation of the entire structure of phytochemicals, giving complete details about the connectivity and stereochemistry of the atoms within the molecule (Sharma et al. 2023). Mass spectrometry (MS) is frequently used in combination with chromatographic methods to give reliable mass measurements as well as structural details of phytochemicals (Li et al. 2024). Various ionization methods, including electrospray ionization (ESI) and matrix-assisted laser desorption/ionization (MALDI), are employed based on the nature of the analyte (Chen et al. 2023).

MS/MS experiments, which include fragmentation of preselected ions, offer further structural information and can be used for the identification of unknown compounds. Chromatography coupled with mass spectrometry offers a very sensitive and selective method for the identification and quantification of phytochemicals in complex matrices (Norouzi-Aliabad et al. 2021). In addition to these fundamental techniques, other analytical techniques also play a part in the quality assessment of phytochemicals. Capillary electrophoresis (CE) provides high-resolution separation of charged molecules and is especially suited to the analysis of polar phytochemicals like flavonoids and phenolic acids (Zhang et al. 2022). Electrochemical techniques like cyclic voltammetry may be employed to evaluate the antioxidant activity of phytochemicals.

X-ray crystallography is used to establish the three-dimensional structure of crystalline compounds with important information regarding their conformation and interaction with other molecules. The quality evaluation of phytochemicals includes not just the identification and quantitation of individual phytochemicals but also their purity and stability evaluation (Al-Motawa et al. 2020). Purity evaluation is generally carried out by chromatographic and spectroscopic methods to identify and quantify any impurities in the sample. Stability studies are done to assess the degradation of phytochemicals when stored under various conditions, which gives insights into their shelf life and ideal storage conditions (Silva et al. 2024). These researches are vital in order to guarantee the quality and effectiveness of phytochemical-derived products (Roberts et al. 2023).

Standardization of analytical procedures for analysis of phytochemicals is important in order to provide comparability of results from various laboratories and research. The International Organization for Standardization (ISO) and the United States Pharmacopeia (USP) have also established standardized procedures for the analysis of a number of phytochemicals. Such procedures give a step-by-step protocol for the sample preparation, analysis, and data interpretation that ensures accuracy and reliability of results. In the last few years, interest in the application of sophisticated analytical methods toward quality assessment of phytochemicals has increased (Lee et al. 2021). These methods include high-resolution mass spectrometry (HRMS), which allows precise mass measurements with high accuracy, making it possible to identify unknown compounds and detect small variations in molecular structure. Metabolomics strategies, which entail the global analysis of all the metabolites present in a biological sample, are being employed to investigate how phytochemicals act on metabolic pathways and to discover biomarkers for their activity. The evolution and utilization of analytical methods for the quality evaluation of phytochemicals have been shaped to a great extent by many scientists and researchers. Some of the notable scientists include Dr. Varro E. Tyler, who was famous for his research in pharmacognosy, and Dr. Norman R. Farnsworth, who made significant contributions in the field of ethnopharmacology and phytochemistry, and has paved the path for contemporary phytochemical analysis (Zhao et al. 2022).

Their work has stimulated the establishment of advanced analytical techniques and has led to greater insight into plant-derived compounds' chemical diversity and therapeutic potential. In the future, advances in analytical methods for phytochemical analysis will probably target elevating the sensitivity, throughput, and automation of these methods. Miniaturization of analytical tools, e.g., microfluidic systems, will allow the analysis of reduced sample volumes and enable the design of point-of-care diagnostics for phytochemicals. The combination of artificial intelligence and machine learning codes will allow for the automated analysis of difficult-to-handle data sets and the prediction of phytochemical properties (Navarro et al. 2019). These developments will additionally boost our capacity to evaluate the quality and effectiveness of phytochemicals and to tap their potential for enhancing human well-being. Phytochemical quality measurement is based on a wide range of analytical methods, such as chromatography, spectroscopy, and mass spectrometry. Such methods deliver useful information concerning the identity, amount, purity, and stability of phytochemicals, making certain that the plant-based product quality and uniformity are guaranteed.

The continued evolution of new and better analytical techniques will serve to continue to advance our capability for investigating these vital compounds and for realizing their full potential in bringing about health and well-being.

6 Quality Control of Raw Materials in Botanical Products: Ensuring Efficacy and Safety

The quality of raw materials is paramount in the production of botanical products. Good agricultural and collection practices (GACP), geographical origin and seasonal variation, adulteration prevention, and proper handling, storage, and preservation are key factors that influence the quality of raw materials (Tan et al. 2025). These elements, when meticulously managed, contribute to the safety and efficacy of the final botanical product.

6.1 Good Agricultural and Collection Practices (GACP)

Good Agricultural and Collection Practices (GACP) are a set of guidelines that ensure the consistent production of high-quality medicinal plants. These practices cover all stages of the plant's life cycle, from seed selection and cultivation to harvesting and initial processing. Adhering to GACP helps minimize contamination, ensures reproducibility, and preserves the inherent properties of the plant (Ramasamy et al. 2023). The implementation of GACP involves several critical steps. The first step involves selecting appropriate plant varieties and ensuring the seeds or propagules are of high quality. Crop management techniques, including proper irrigation, fertilization, and pest control, play a crucial role in plant growth. Harvesting at the right time, when the plant's active constituents are at their peak concentration, is essential. Postharvest handling, such as cleaning, drying, and sorting, must be carried out carefully to prevent degradation and contamination (Mohammed et al. 2022). Organizations such as the World Health Organization (WHO) and the European Medicines Agency (EMA) have developed GACP guidelines to promote standardization. These guidelines emphasize the importance of documentation, traceability, and quality assurance throughout the entire production process.

6.2 *Influence of Geographical Origin and Seasonal Variation*

The geographical origin and seasonal variation significantly influence the chemical composition of medicinal plants. Environmental factors such as climate, soil type, altitude, and sunlight exposure affect plant metabolism, leading to variations in the concentration of active compounds. Plants grown in different geographical regions may exhibit distinct chemical profiles (Yadav et al. 2023). For example, the concentration of certain alkaloids in a medicinal plant may vary depending on the soil composition and climate of the region where it is grown. Seasonal changes also play a role, as the levels of active constituents fluctuate throughout the year, influenced by factors like temperature, rainfall, and photoperiod. Understanding the impact of geographical origin and seasonal variation is crucial for ensuring the consistent quality of raw materials. Sourcing plants from specific regions known for their high quality and harvesting them at the optimal time of year can help maximize the concentration of desired compounds (Xu et al. 2024).

6.3 *Prevention of Adulteration and Substitution*

Adulteration and substitution are major concerns in the botanical industry. These practices involve intentionally or unintentionally replacing authentic plant material with inferior or unrelated species. Adulteration can compromise the safety and efficacy of botanical products and pose serious health risks to consumers.

Common methods of adulteration include substituting expensive herbs with cheaper alternatives, adding fillers to increase volume, and using plant material of lower quality or from different geographical origins. Microscopic analysis, chemical fingerprinting, and DNA barcoding are used to detect adulteration and ensure the authenticity of raw materials (Das et al. 2021).

Stringent quality control measures are necessary to prevent adulteration and substitution. These measures include thorough botanical identification, macroscopic and microscopic examination, chemical analysis, and DNA testing. Suppliers should be carefully vetted and required to provide certificates of analysis and other documentation to verify the authenticity and quality of their products.

6.4 Handling, Storage, and Preservation of Raw Botanicals

Proper handling, storage, and preservation are essential for maintaining the quality and stability of raw botanicals. These practices prevent degradation, microbial contamination, and loss of active constituents.

After harvesting, raw botanicals must be dried to reduce moisture content, which inhibits microbial growth and enzymatic activity. Drying methods include sun drying, air drying, and freeze drying. The choice of drying method depends on the plant material and the desired quality of the final product (Brenes-Belmont et al. 2023). Dried botanicals should be stored in a cool, dry, and dark place to prevent degradation. Proper packaging, such as airtight containers or moisture-proof bags, protects the material from environmental factors. Regular monitoring of storage conditions and periodic testing of the material can help detect any signs of deterioration.

Preservation techniques, such as extraction and stabilization, are used to maintain the quality of raw botanicals over extended periods. Extraction involves separating the active constituents from the plant material using solvents. Stabilization involves adding preservatives or antioxidants to prevent degradation and maintain the stability of the extract (Nguyen et al. 2022). By implementing GACP, considering the influence of geographical origin and seasonal variation, preventing adulteration and substitution, and employing proper handling, storage, and preservation techniques, manufacturers can produce high-quality botanical products that meet the needs of consumers and healthcare professionals. Continuous research and development in quality control methods will further enhance the reliability and consistency of botanical products in the future (Fig. 2).

7 Safety and Contaminant Evaluation of Phytochemicals

Phytochemicals, naturally occurring compounds in plants, are increasingly recognized for their potential health benefits. However, the safety and presence of contaminants in these compounds are critical considerations for their widespread use in dietary supplements, functional foods, and pharmaceuticals. This essay will examine the safety aspects of phytochemicals, focusing on potential toxicities and interactions, and will also address the evaluation of contaminants, including heavy metals, pesticides, and microbial agents (Sharma et al. 2025). The interest in phytochemicals has grown substantially in recent decades, driven by epidemiological studies linking plant-rich diets with reduced risks of chronic diseases (Jafari et al. 2021). This has led to the isolation, identification, and characterization of numerous compounds, such as flavonoids, terpenoids, alkaloids, and phenolic acids, each with unique biological activities. While many phytochemicals exhibit promising health-promoting properties, it is essential to recognize that they are not uniformly safe.

One of the primary concerns regarding the safety of phytochemicals is their potential toxicity. Some compounds, even at relatively low concentrations, can exert

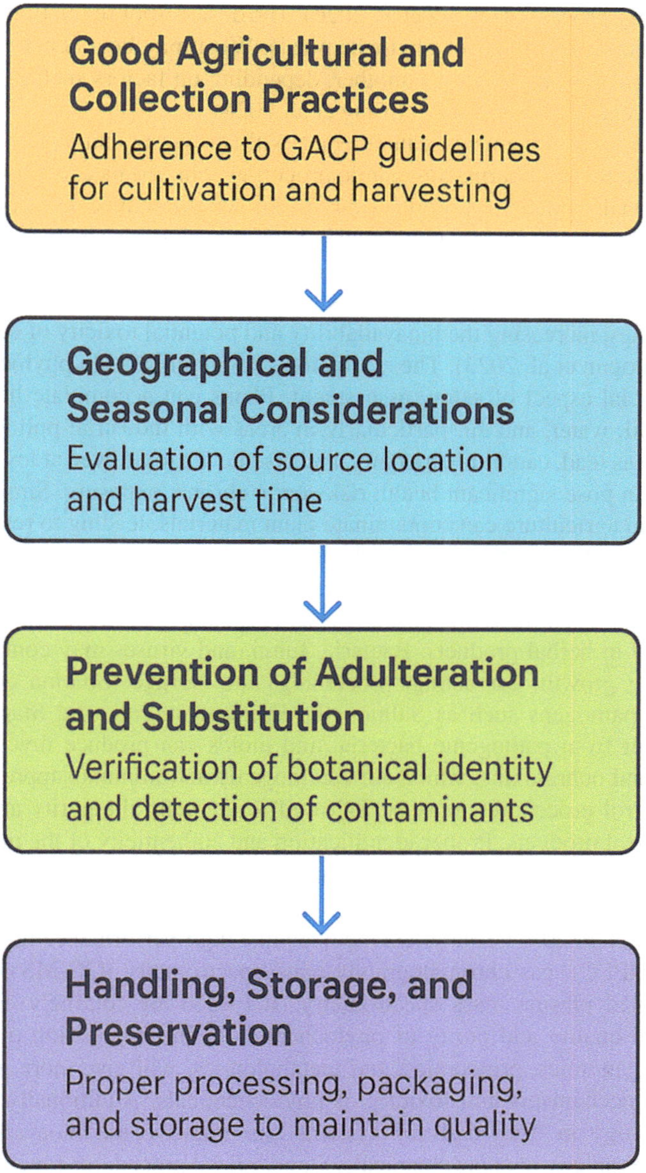

Fig. 2 Quality control of raw materials, which are critical for ensuring the safety and efficacy of botanical products

adverse effects on human health. For example, pyrrolizidine alkaloids, found in plants like comfrey and borage, are hepatotoxic and can cause liver damage with chronic exposure. Similarly, certain cyanogenic glycosides, present in foods like cassava and almonds, can release cyanide upon ingestion, leading to acute toxicity if not properly processed (Wang et al. 2020). The dose-response relationship is critical in evaluating the safety of phytochemicals. What may be a beneficial dose for one individual could be toxic to another, depending on factors such as age, health status, and genetic predisposition (Yang et al. 2024).

Moreover, phytochemicals can interact with drugs, potentially altering their pharmacokinetic and pharmacodynamic properties. For instance, St. John's Wort, a popular herbal remedy for depression, is known to induce cytochrome P450 enzymes, which can accelerate the metabolism of various drugs, including anticoagulants, oral contraceptives, and immunosuppressants, reducing their effectiveness. Similarly, grapefruit juice contains furanocoumarins that inhibit cytochrome P450 enzymes, increasing the bioavailability and potential toxicity of certain medications (Balogun et al. 2023). The evaluation of contaminants in phytochemicals is another crucial aspect of safety assessment. Plants can accumulate heavy metals from the soil, water, and air, particularly in areas with industrial pollution. Heavy metals such as lead, cadmium, mercury, and arsenic are toxic even at low concentrations and can pose significant health risks upon chronic exposure. Similarly, pesticides used in agriculture can contaminate plant materials, leading to residues in the final products. Organophosphates, carbamates, and pyrethroids are commonly used pesticides that can have neurotoxic effects (Palma et al. 2022).

Microbial contamination is also an issue, particularly in raw plant material that is employed in herbal products. Bacteria, fungi, and viruses may contaminate the plant during growth, harvesting, processing, and storage (Sharma et al. 2022). Foodborne pathogens such as Salmonella, Escherichia coli, and Staphylococcus aureus result from pathogenic bacteria, and molds can produce mycotoxins like aflatoxins and ochratoxins, which are carcinogenic and immunosuppressive. Strict quality control procedures must be followed to maintain the purity and safety of phytochemical products. Proper identification and authenticity of the plant species, heavy metal and pesticide residue testing, microbial contamination testing, and standardization of the concentration of active compounds must be performed (Choudhary et al. 2021). Analytical methods like high-performance liquid chromatography (HPLC), gas chromatography-mass spectrometry (GC-MS), and inductively coupled plasma mass spectrometry (ICP-MS) are routinely employed to evaluate the quality and purity of phytochemicals. The application of omics sciences, i.e., genomics, proteomics, and metabolomics, will give more insights into the action mechanisms and toxicity of phytochemicals. Additionally, the use of nanotechnology in drug delivery systems can improve the bioavailability and decrease the toxicity of some chemicals. Standardized procedures for extraction and purification will ensure consistency and quality of phytochemical products (Wu and Tang 2024). Although phytochemicals provide great potential benefits to health, their safety and quality with respect to the presence of contaminants need to be appropriately assessed. Possible toxicities, drug interactions, and heavy metal, pesticide, and microbial contamination are major concerns. Stringent quality control procedures, regulatory control, and ongoing research are necessary to validate the safe and effective application of phytochemicals in enhancing human health (Khatib et al. 2019) (Table 2).

Table 2 Stability protocols for herbal products

Parameters	Factors	Focus area	Key approaches/ methods	Outcome/ significance
Safety and contaminant evaluation	**Microbial load and pathogen testing**	Detection of microbial contamination in herbal materials	Total viable count (TVC), yeast & mold count, pathogen-specific tests (*E. coli, Salmonella, S. aureus*), rapid microbiological methods	Ensures microbiological safety, prevents product spoilage, and complies with regulatory limits
	Heavy metals, pesticide residues, and mycotoxins	Detection of toxic contaminants	Atomic Absorption Spectroscopy (AAS), Inductively Coupled Plasma–Mass Spectrometry (ICP-MS) for metals; GC-MS/LC-MS for pesticides; ELISA/ HPLC for mycotoxins	Prevents exposure to toxic substances, ensures compliance with pharmacopeial and food safety standards
	Allergenicity and toxicity concerns	Assessment of allergic and toxic responses	In vitro assays, animal toxicity studies, skin sensitization tests, allergen protein profiling	Minimizes risk of adverse reactions, supports product safety claims
	Methods for contaminant detection	Comprehensive detection techniques	Chromatography, spectroscopy, PCR-based assays, immunoassays	Enhances detection accuracy, supports traceability and recall processes
Stability and shelf-life studies	**Stability protocols for herbal products**	Standardized testing to determine product stability	ICH guidelines, real-time and accelerated stability studies, storage condition simulation	Determines product shelf life, establishes storage recommendations
	Influence of environmental factors	Impact of temperature, humidity, and light	Controlled chamber studies, photostability tests, hygroscopicity analysis	Identifies optimal storage conditions, prevents degradation of actives
	Accelerated stability testing for phytochemicals	Rapid prediction of shelf life	Elevated temperature/ humidity exposure (e.g., 40 °C/75% RH), chemical degradation kinetics analysis	Speeds up stability evaluation, predicts long-term quality and potency

8 Conclusion

Phytochemicals, bioactive compounds found in plants, are recognized for their potential health benefits and roles in disease prevention. As scientific research progresses, the importance of quality approaches in the study, extraction, and application of phytochemicals has become increasingly evident. Variability in plant sources poses a significant challenge to the consistency of phytochemical quality. Factors such as geographic location, climatic conditions, genetic diversity, and cultivation practices influence the production of phytochemicals in plants. Consequently, establishing standardized protocols for phytochemical extraction and analysis becomes imperative. These standards not only enhance reproducibility in experimental research but also ensure that products derived from these compounds meet regulatory requirements and consumer expectations.

Numerous studies have underscored the need for improved analytical techniques to assess the purity and potency of phytochemicals effectively. Traditional approaches often fall short of providing comprehensive insights into the complex interplay of phytochemicals and their biological activities. Modern techniques such as high-performance liquid chromatography (HPLC), mass spectrometry (MS), and nuclear magnetic resonance (NMR) spectroscopy offer enhanced specificity and sensitivity in identifying phytochemicals. Implementing these advanced methods across the board can reduce discrepancies in data reporting and facilitate more accurate comparisons between different studies. Furthermore, understanding synergistic effects among phytochemicals is paramount. Research has revealed that the combined action of multiple phytochemicals can lead to enhanced therapeutic effects compared to isolated compounds. However, this knowledge necessitates a thorough exploration of the interactions between various phytochemical constituents. Future studies must prioritize the investigation of these relationships through multifaceted approaches that encompass both in vitro and in vivo models. Quality assurance extends beyond analytical techniques; it encompasses sustainable sourcing and ethical practices surrounding the use of plant materials. Deforestation, overharvesting, and unsustainable agricultural practices threaten the availability of many plants rich in phytochemicals. The integration of sustainable practices into the phytochemical industry is not merely an ecological imperative but also a strategic advantage. In terms of regulatory frameworks, policymakers must establish clear guidelines governing the safety, efficacy, and marketing of phytochemical products. Current regulations often lag behind scientific advancements, creating uncertainties for manufacturers and consumers alike. By fostering collaboration between researchers, industry stakeholders, and government agencies, we can create a robust regulatory environment that encourages innovation while safeguarding public health. Establishing a transparent framework for the evaluation of phytochemical products will not only enhance consumer confidence but also drive market growth. Looking forward, the future of phytochemical research holds immense promise, contingent upon our commitment to implementing high-quality approaches. The evolving landscape requires a multidisciplinary focus, rigorous adherence to quality standards, and a dedication to sustainability. Additionally, embracing innovative technologies and fostering collaborative networks will be critical in unlocking the full potential of phytochemicals as health-promoting agents.

Conflict of Interest The authors have no financial conflict of interest.

References

Alam S, Khan MI, B B, Akhtar J, Ahmad M, Ahmad MD (2025) Standardization and GC-MS analysis of phytochemicals in Coccinia indica (Wight & Arn.) fruits. Pharm Res 17(2):507–518. https://doi.org/10.5530/pres.20251942. phcogres.com

Al-Motawa AA, Al-Jomah N, Al-Mashaan O, Hashem KM (2020) Validation of GC-MS method for quantification of essential oils in *Nigella sativa* seeds for quality control purposes. Pharm Biol 58(1):839–846. https://doi.org/10.1080/13880209.2020.1784388

Balogun FA, Oinesikhoo FT, Odusote AH (2023) Quality evaluation of traditional herbal teas using UV–Vis fingerprinting and principal component analysis. J Taibah Univ Sci 17(1):120–128. https://doi.org/10.1080/16583655.2022.2154771

Bertani FR, Businaro L, Gambacorta L et al (2020) Optical detection of Aflatoxins B in almonds using fluorescence spectroscopy and machine learning. Preprint [Internet]. arXiv. arXiv

Bian W, Yang Q, Zhang J, Liu J, Wu Z (2022) Metabolomic profiling combined with multivariate analysis to evaluate quality of *Camellia sinensis*. Food Chem 392:133–140. https://doi.org/10.1016/j.foodchem.2022.133140

Brenes-Belmont A, Reyes CID, Gómez-Zermeño MA, Salazar-Sabino CN (2023) Herbal matrix fingerprinting and chemometric discrimination of *Passiflora* spp. extracts. J Pharm Biomed Anal 222:115019. https://doi.org/10.1016/j.jpba.2023.115019

Cai Z, Wang C, Chen C, Zou L, Chai C, Chen J et al (2019) Chemometrics in quality control and evaluation of herbal medicines: UFLC-QTRAP-MS/MS profiling and multivariate statistics. Phytochem Anal 32(2):129–140. https://doi.org/10.1002/pca.2865. Analytical Science Journals

Chen L, Li Z, Luo X, Guo H (2023) Quality evaluation of *Ganoderma lucidum* spore powder using HPLC fingerprint and chemometric methods. J Pharm Biomed Anal 230:115246. https://doi.org/10.1016/j.jpba.2023.115246

Chen Y, Zhang J, Feng J, Chen W, Liu W, Chen J et al (2024a) A comprehensive evaluation strategy for assessing Chrysanthemi flos quality using HPLC, FT-NIR and chemometrics. Phytochem Anal 35(4):754–770. (First published 28 Jan 2024) Analytical Science Journals

Chen Y, Zhang J, Feng J, Chen W, Liu W, Chen J et al (2024b) Holistic quality evaluation method of Epimedii Folium based on NIR spectroscopy and chemometrics. Phytochem Anal 35(4):771–785. (First published 25 Jan 2024) Analytical Science Journals

Choudhary P, Malhotra S, Kumar V (2021) Authentication of *Boswellia serrata* oleo-gum resin via phytocannabinoid profiling and chemometric clustering. J Anal Methods Chem 2021:1–9. https://doi.org/10.1155/2021/6637712

Das A, Mahanta A, Thakur N, Sharma D (2021) Optimization of extraction of phenolic compounds from Indian medicinal plant using microwave-assisted extraction and QbD. Phytochem Lett 42:102–110. https://doi.org/10.1016/j.phytol.2020.11.010

Devi S (2025) Advancements in quantitative and qualitative methods for quality control of herbal drugs: a comprehensive review. Pharm Res 17(2):411–415. https://doi.org/10.5530/pres.20252077. phcogres.com

González-Ruiz V, Romero-Garcia J, García-Mendoza CM, Köck M (2019) FTIR-ATR spectroscopy combined with chemometrics for authentication of Mexican oregano essential oil. Food Control 98:263–271. https://doi.org/10.1016/j.foodcont.2018.11.028

Huang R, Chen X, Li S, Ye M (2020) Chemometric tools for authentication of *Panax ginseng* and its processed products. J Sep Sci 43(4):780–789. https://doi.org/10.1002/jssc.201900813

Jafari MR, Farajzadeh MA, Zandi-Khazal S (2021) Quality assessment of *Lavandula angustifolia* essential oil using UV–visible spectroscopy and chemometric pattern recognition. Ind Crop Prod 166:113502. https://doi.org/10.1016/j.indcrop.2021.113502

Jain S, Prasad S, Singh M (2022) Standardization and stability-indicating HPLC–UV assay method for rutin in herbal dosage forms. J Pharm Anal 12(3):320–327. https://doi.org/10.1016/j.jpha.2022.02.013

Kagawad P, Gharge S, Jivaje K, Hiremath SI, Suryawanshi SS (2021) Quality control and standardization of quercetin in herbal medicines by spectroscopic and chromatographic techniques. Future J Pharm Sci 7:176. https://doi.org/10.1186/s43094-021-00327-y. SpringerOpen

Khatib A, Kaabi M, Jaber N (2019) Simple and rapid UV spectrophotometric quality control method for safflower yellow in *Carthamus tinctorius* extracts. Anal Methods 11(45):6301–6306. https://doi.org/10.1039/C9AY01725A

Kim S-Y, Kim SY, Huh J, Lee SH (2025) Artificial intelligence-driven prediction of bioactive phytochemical yields in *Panax ginseng* cell cultures. Biotechnol Bioeng 122(6):789–801. https://doi.org/10.1002/bit.28290

Kumar S, Jaiswal AK, Aggarwal M, Ekbbal R, Gaurav (2023) A review on quality control aspects of Indian medicinal plants. Pharmacogn Rev 17(34):276–286. https://doi.org/10.5530/phrev.2023.17.7. Pharmacognosy Reviews

Lee J-H, Lim H, Lee S-H, Yoon M-S (2021) Rapid quality indexing of herbal teas by NMR metabolomics and multivariate data analysis. J Agric Food Chem 69(46):13810–13818. https://doi.org/10.1021/acs.jafc.1c05231

Li H, Shi R, Wang Q, Chen X, Zhang J (2024) Quantitative quality assessment of *Schisandra chinensis* by near-infrared hyperspectral imaging. Talanta 261:124490. https://doi.org/10.1016/j.talanta.2024.124490

Li J, Zhang Y, Sun Y, Liu X, Zhao S, Wang Y (2022) Application of UHPLC-QTOF-MS and network pharmacology for quality evaluation of *salvia miltiorrhiza*. J Chromatogr B Analyt Technol Biomed Life Sci 1202:122–133. https://doi.org/10.1016/j.jchromb.2022.123456

Mahboubifar M, Zidorn C, Farag MA, Zayed A, Jassbi AR (2024) Chemometric-based drug discovery from natural origins using hyphenated chromatographic techniques. Phytochem Anal 35(5):990–1016. (First published 28 May 2024) Analytical Science Journals

Martínez-Martínez L, González-Tovar I, Ruiz-Rejón C, Fernández-Gutiérrez A, Moreno-Marquez M (2020) Fast simultaneous determination of flavonoids and phenolic acids in *Rosmarinus officinalis* extracts using micro-extraction and UPLC–MS/MS. Anal Bioanal Chem 412(25):7093–7110. https://doi.org/10.1007/s00216-020-02680-w

Mohammed S, Hisam A, Ah Meh N, Inai SM (2022) Authentication and quality control of *Nigella sativa* oil using FTIR combined with pattern recognition. J Oleo Sci 71(1):47–59. https://doi.org/10.5650/jos.ess21032

Nahar L, Chaiwut P, Sangthong S, Theansungnoen T, Sarker SDS (2024) Progress in analysis of phytocannabinoids by HPLC and UPLC/UHPLC from 2020 to 2023. Phytochem Anal 35(5):927–989. (First published 04 June 2024) Analytical Science Journals

Navarro P, Pérez-Álvarez JA, Fernández-López J (2019) Spectroscopic fingerprinting and chemometric classification of saffron adulteration. Food Chem 295:470–477. https://doi.org/10.1016/j.foodchem.2019.02.128

Naznin M, Alam R, Alam MB, Jung MJ, Lee S-H, Kim S (2024) Biological activities and method development for polyphenolic compounds in Nymphaea rubra by UHPLC-Q-cIM-TOF-MS and UHPLC-TQ-MS. Phytochem Anal 35(4):786–798. (First published 26 Jan 2024) Analytical Science Journals

Nguyen TX, Le VH, Pham QD (2022) Quality control of *Centella asiatica* extracts: simultaneous determination of triterpenoids and antioxidant potency assessment. Phcog Mag 18(Suppl 2):S242–S249. https://doi.org/10.5530/phcog.2022.18.2s.44

Norouzī-Alīabad R, Farzādeh-Asl F, Amini-Manesh S, Mirjalili MH, Sonboli A (2021) Essential oil profiling and multivariate analysis of *Thymus daenensis* ecotypes for quality characterization. Ind Crops Prod 171:113913. https://doi.org/10.1016/j.indcrop.2021.113913

Palma E, Raposo F, Plaza M (2022) Quality control of microalgal phytochemicals using FTIR, GC–MS and chemometric tools. Algal Res 60:102551. https://doi.org/10.1016/j.algal.2021.102551

Park M, Somborn A, Schlehuber D, Lim HJ, Keuter V (2025) Non-destructive carotenoid quantification in leaves via Raman spectroscopy: optimizing treatment for LDA. Preprint [Internet]. arXiv. arXiv

Patel M, Rana K, Rathore RS, Dhutia HV (2021) Quality assurance in herbal formulations: validation of taraxerol in *Taraxacum officinale* by HPTLC. J Planar Chromatogr 34(2):112–119. https://doi.org/10.1556/1006.2021.34.2.4

Pathrikar SY, Mukhmale VS, Deshmukh NB, Deshmukh SP (2025a) Standardization extraction and phytochemical screening for herbal drugs. GSC Adv Res Rev 22(1):84–91. https://doi.org/10.30574/gscarr.2025.22.1.0518. GSC Online Press

Pathrikar SY, Mukhmale VS, Deshmukh NB, Deshmukh SP (2025b) Standardization, extraction and phytochemical screening for herbal drugs. GSC Adv Res Rev 22(1):84–91. https://doi.org/10.30574/gscarr.2025.22.1.0518. ResearchGate

Ramasamy R, Annamalai T, Sampath KS (2023) Rapid on-site detection of plant alkaloids using surface-enhanced Raman spectroscopy (SERS) and machine learning. Talanta 256:124321. https://doi.org/10.1016/j.talanta.2023.124321

Roberts E, Guntuku PD, Spicer L (2023) Quality-by-design (QbD) approach in extraction of alkaloids from *Cinchona officinalis*: process optimization using response surface methodology. Ind Crop Prod 198:116946. https://doi.org/10.1016/j.indcrop.2023.116946

Roselló-Soto R, Zia MF, et al (2022) Emerging advanced extraction technologies for phytochemicals: supercritical fluid extraction, HVED, PEF, etc. Procedures to evaluate potential of plants as natural food preservatives (review). PMC

Shareef THMA, Navabshan I, Masood MMD, Yuvaraj TE, Sherif A (2024) Investigation of phytochemicals, spectral properties, anticancer, antidiabetic, and antimicrobial activities of chosen Ayurvedic remedies. Preprint [Internet]. arXiv. arXiv

Sharma A, Agarwal S, Kuchhal N (2023) Evaluation of adulteration and quality control of turmeric powders using FT-IR spectroscopy. Food Res Int 164:112065. https://doi.org/10.1016/j.foodres.2023.112065

Sharma K, Kumar M, Yadav S, Bhat ZA, Rana K (2022) Simultaneous HPTLC analysis of multiple markers in Ayurvedic formulation: optimization and validation. BMC Complement Med Ther 22(1):54. https://doi.org/10.1186/s12906-022-03524-x

Sharma P, Mishra A, Khullar N (2025) Voice as a non-destructive quality marker: herbal powder classification via acoustic signatures and machine learning. Comput Electron Agric 206:107713. https://doi.org/10.1016/j.compag.2024.107713

Silva NR, Costa RGA, Naves AHP, Lima JC, Braz-Filho R, Braga FC (2024) Green and sustainable extraction methods for bioactive phytochemicals: supercritical CO_2, PEF, microwave-assisted. J Clean Prod 420:137564. https://doi.org/10.1016/j.jclepro.2023.137564

Singh A, Dhiman A, Kaur T, Mishra AK (2023) Real-time monitoring of essential oil composition using portable Raman spectroscopy plus chemometric analysis. Talanta 255:124078. https://doi.org/10.1016/j.talanta.2023.124078

Tan Z, Li L, Mei S (2025) Quality assessment of *Huperzia serrata* extracts by multiplex PCR and chemical profiling. Phytochem Anal 36(1):120–133. https://doi.org/10.1002/pca.3100

Tianjin Press of Chinese Herbal Medicines (2024) Phytochemistry, quality control and biosynthesis in ginseng research from 2021 to 2023: A state-of-the-art review concerning advances and challenges. Chinese Herbal Medicines 16(4):505–520. https://doi.org/10.1016/j.chmed.2024.08.002. ScienceDirect

Wang T, Zhao L, Meng X (2020) Quantitative method validation for glycoalkaloids in *Solanum tuberosum* using LC-MS/MS. Food Chem 315:126267. https://doi.org/10.1016/j.foodchem.2020.126267

Wu D, Sun C, Che C, Yang S (2024) Exploring the quality consistency of *Astragali radix* in commercial preparations using LC–MS fingerprinting and multivariate statistical analysis. Phytomedicine 100:154065. https://doi.org/10.1016/j.phymed.2024.154065

Wu H, Tang W (2024) Quality evaluation of *Echinacea purpurea* extracts using 1H-NMR-based metabonomics and multivariate statistics. J Pharm Biomed Anal 217:114831. https://doi.org/10.1016/j.jpba.2022.114831

Xu L, Li Y, Chen G, Wang J, Sun J (2024) Real-time monitoring of alkaloid extraction process using near-infrared spectroscopy and chemometrics. Anal Chim Acta 1148:338–347. https://doi.org/10.1016/j.aca.2020.338347

Yadav P, Singh R, Gupta SK (2023) High-throughput quality screening of phytochemicals in herbal raw materials using ambient mass spectrometry. Phytochem Anal 34(8):969–981. https://doi.org/10.1002/pca.3155

Yang Y, Ding N, Yang X (2024) Phytochemical fingerprinting of *Cuscuta reflexa* extracts via UHPLC–QTOF–MS and multivariate classification methods. Phytochem Anal 35(2):298–312. https://doi.org/10.1002/pca.3128

Zhang Q, Wu Z, Yu J, Wang J (2022) Comparative study on quality consistency of *Scutellaria baicalensis* by HPLC fingerprint, quantitative determination and chemometrics. Fitoterapia 155:105065. https://doi.org/10.1016/j.fitote.2021.105065

Zhao L, Huang Y, Zhao S, Li R, Cheng Q (2022) Standardized extraction of catechins from *Camellia sinensis* using ultrasound-assisted extraction coupled with factor analysis. Ultrason Sonochem 86:106032. https://doi.org/10.1016/j.ultsonch.2022.106032

Zhao Y, Wu F, Li J, Zhao G, Li X (2021) Development of an HPLC fingerprint combined with quantitative analysis for quality control of *Polygonum multiflorum*. J Pharm Biomed Anal 194:113726. https://doi.org/10.1016/j.jpba.2020.113726

Zou H, Zhang Z, Zhang H, Chen Y, Zhang H, Yan J (2024) Prediction of key quality attributes in salvia miltiorrhiza standard decoction using Gaussian process regression. Phytochem Anal 35(6):1345–1357. (First published 30 April 2024) Analytical Science Journals

Therapeutic Applications by Disease Category

Phytochemicals Potentially Applied to Noncommunicable Diseases

Haixia Chen, Wen Zhang, Siyu Wang, Yiping Li, and Lim Eng Keat

Abstract Noncommunicable diseases (NCDs) are characterized by their prolonged duration and slow progression. Cardiovascular disease, cancer, respiratory disease, and diabetes are principal NCDs occurring in modern world. Conventional pharmacological treatments for NCDs are not universally suitable across all patient demographics and are often associated with a range of adverse effects, which lead to usage of phytoceuticals for alleviating NCDs, due to their high safety profile. Various phytochemicals like curcumin, resveratrol, quercetin, berberine, and celastrol, belonging to numerous phytochemical classes like alkaloids, flavonoids, terpenoids, steroids, and so on, have been proven extensively crucial in benefacting patient health rejuvenation during any NCDs. Potential use of phytochemicals for treating diseases is due to various reasons, namely, the diversity of phytochemicals offering a wealth of candidate molecules for precision medicine. Second, the widely sourced phytochemicals can serve as a cost-effective means of disease prevention and control in resource-limited areas, facilitating low-cost intervention strategies. Furthermore, the global expansion of phytochemical-derived drugs, coupled with the principles of a green economy, has fostered sustainable development. Therefore, the study of phytochemicals serves as a vital link between traditional knowledge and modern science, representing a significant breakthrough in addressing the global challenges posed by NCDs. Through mechanistic analysis, technological innovation, and interdisciplinary collaboration, the application of phytochemicals is expected to facilitate a shift from disease treatment to health management, thereby providing scientific support for "Healthy China 2030 and the United Nations Sustainable Development Goals" (SDG 3).

H. Chen (✉) · W. Zhang · S. Wang · Y. Li · L. E. Keat
Tianjin Key Laboratory for Modern Drug Delivery & High-Efficiency, School of Pharmaceutical Science and Technology, Faculty of Medicine, Tianjin University, Tianjin, People's Republic of China
e-mail: chenhx@tju.edu.cn; zhang_wen9@tju.edu.cn; tjuwangsiyu2022@163.com; yli145@kent.edu

S. Kumar Tripathi et al. (eds.), *Phytoceuticals for Sustainable Medication*, Interdisciplinary Biotechnological Advances,
https://doi.org/10.1007/978-981-95-7588-6_8

Keywords Phytochemicals · Noncommunicable diseases · Mechanistic approach · Novel approaches

1 Introduction

1.1 Noncommunicable Diseases

Noncommunicable diseases (NCDs) are characterized by their prolonged duration and slow progression. The human body sustains redox homeostasis through a balance between pro-oxidant species produced during cellular metabolism and endogenous antioxidant defense systems. Nevertheless, when the levels of free radicals and reactive oxygen species exceed the neutralizing capacity of antioxidant mechanisms, oxidative stress ensues, resulting in cellular damage and potentially cell death. This physiological and pathological process is fundamental to the pathogenesis of numerous diseases, including NCDs (Carlos Kusano Bucalen et al. 2016; Liochev 2013; Poljsak et al. 2013).

Cardiovascular disease, cancer, respiratory disease, and diabetes are principal NCDs and serve as predominant factors contributing to complications associated with clinical manifestations (Budreviciute et al. 2020). Although these diseases significantly affect global health, other NCDs constitute an even greater proportion—55%—of the worldwide NCD burden. This category includes conditions such as musculoskeletal disorders, depression, and congenital immune disorders (Bhattacharya et al. 2023).

The global burden of NCDs has increasingly become a critical public health concern. The etiology of NCDs involves a complex interaction of genetic, physiological, behavioral, and environmental factors. In recent years, NCDs have been consistently recognized as among the top five leading causes of mortality worldwide. According to data from the World Health Organization (WHO), NCDs account for approximately 71% of all annual deaths globally. The WHO further projects that, in the absence of effective interventions, mortality attributable to NCDs is expected to rise to 55 million by 2030. Currently, numerous nations have developed comprehensive national strategies aimed at the prevention and management of NCDs, with the goal of improving patient outcomes and reducing the overall prevalence of these diseases.

Conventional pharmacological treatments for NCDs are not universally suitable across all patient demographics and are often associated with a range of adverse effects, including gastrointestinal disturbances, musculoskeletal pain, and persistent fatigue. In response to these limitations, there is a concerted global initiative aimed at discovering therapeutic agents for NCDs that demonstrate enhanced efficacy coupled with a reduced side effect profile. Natural products and phytochemicals represent valuable reservoirs for the development of therapeutic interventions across various pathological conditions. Specifically, phytochemicals derived from a wide array of botanical sources have garnered considerable scientific interest as complementary therapies in the prevention and management of NCDs, attributable to their potential safety, therapeutic effectiveness, and unique chemical and structural characteristics (Fan et al. 2022).

1.2 Phytochemicals

For thousands of years, around 25% of the pharmaceuticals utilized in the treatment of human diseases have been derived from plants. Plants exhibit medicinal properties and synthesize both primary and secondary metabolites. Primary metabolites are essential for plant growth and metabolic functions and also constitute significant nutritional components for human intake. Secondary metabolites, commonly referred to as phytochemicals, originate from primary metabolites through respiratory processes and fulfill diverse functions such as mediating competition, facilitating interspecies interactions, and providing defense against diseases (Pichersky and Gang 2000; Shin et al. 2018). The first phytochemical, morphine, was isolated in 1804 (Pooja and Kaid Johar 2019). Numerous phytochemicals have been identified, exhibiting diverse structural characteristics and biological activities. The molecular structures of several representative phytochemicals, including curcumin, quercetin, celastrol, resveratrol, and berberine, are illustrated in Fig. 1. The therapeutic efficacy of these phytochemicals is influenced by multiple factors, among which their concentration in human body fluids is paramount. Due to limited intestinal permeability and poor absorption, the bioavailability of phytochemicals can vary substantially, posing significant challenges for accurate quantification. Insufficient plasma

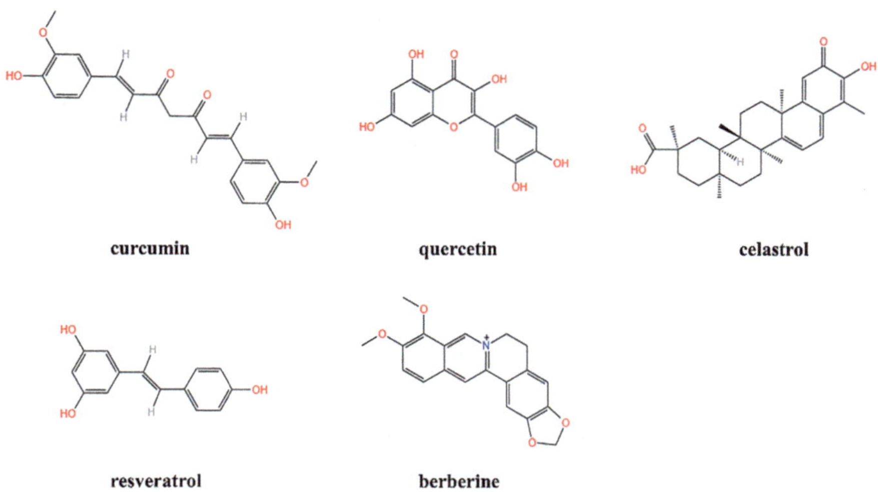

Fig. 1 The structures of several representative phytochemicals

concentrations may hinder the realization of their pharmacological potential, whereas excessively high concentrations may induce toxic effects (Pooja and Kaid Johar 2019).

Phytochemicals are extensively present in numerous edible plants and plant-derived products, such as fruits, vegetables, legumes, grains, bark, and spices. To date, more than 5000 distinct phytochemicals have been identified and characterized from a wide range of plant sources (Liu 2004). According to phytochemicals' biosynthetic origins, phytochemicals may be classified into three primary groups: phenolic compounds, terpenoids, and nitrogen-containing alkaloids or sulfur-containing compounds (Pooja and Kaid Johar 2019).

Phenolic compounds represent the largest and most widely distributed class of phytochemicals, encompassing flavonoids, non-flavonoids, and phenolic acids. A characteristic attribute of these compounds is their abundant phenolic hydroxyl groups, which are fundamental to their antioxidant, anti-inflammatory, antidiabetic, and various pharmacological activities. Dietary polyphenols have the capacity to modulate the growth of particular microbial communities through their interactions with the gut microbiota, thereby playing a significant role in the preservation and regulation of intestinal health.

Terpenoids are polycyclic compounds defined by the presence of a five-carbon isoprene structural unit. These compounds can be further categorized into monoterpenes, sesquiterpenes, and additional subclasses. Saponins include glycosylated steroids, triterpenoids, and steroidal alkaloids.

Alkaloids represent a class of phytochemicals characterized by the presence of heterocyclic nitrogen atoms and the exhibition of basic (alkaline) properties. Their classification is primarily based on the core carbon-nitrogen frameworks, which encompass structures such as pyrrolidine, pyridine, quinoline, and isoquinoline, among others. The biological activities of alkaloids are determined by the interactions between their functional groups and specific molecular targets. To date, approximately 2700 distinct alkaloid derivatives with a wide range of pharmacological effects have been isolated from diverse plant species (Pooja and Kaid Johar 2019).

Phytochemicals have the capacity to modulate multiple molecular pathways concurrently, thereby influencing disease progression through synergistic or complementary mechanisms. Moreover, based on their distinct modes of action, different phytochemicals can be strategically combined to maximize therapeutic efficacy.

1.3 The Biological Activity of Phytochemicals

Due to the diversity and complexity of phytochemicals, they serve as valuable resources for drug development. Currently, approximately 4000 different phytochemicals have been identified as having potential activity in combating various diseases, including immune regulation, cancer prevention, and metabolic regulation (Kadakol et al. 2016). Hence, undertaking comprehensive investigations into the pharmacological mechanisms of phytochemicals involved in the management of various NCDs holds substantial importance for clinical medicine.

Phytochemicals exhibit a wide range of biological activities in modulating immune system function, notably affecting inflammatory and autoimmune processes through the regulation of key signaling pathways such as NF-κB and JAK-STAT. Furthermore, they play a significant role in maintaining immune homeostasis by modulating the balance among various immune cell populations, including Th17/Treg subsets and macrophage polarization. Moreover, polyphenols have been shown to impact protein expression and immune regulation, thereby contributing to the prevention of disease (Chu 2022).

At the same time, phytochemicals regulate key metabolic pathways through multiple targets, such as AMPK, PPAR-γ, and interactions with intestinal flora. They exhibit unique biological activity in glucose and lipid metabolism disorder, hypertension, atherosclerosis, and other diseases (Agustín et al. 2018; Chu 2022; López-Alarcón and Denicola 2013). The research focuses on the molecular mechanisms by which phytochemicals improve insulin sensitivity, inhibit fat production, and regulate oxidative stress (de Bock et al. 2013; Kadakol et al. 2016; Lin et al. 2005). Additionally, when combined with structural optimization strategies, these compounds significantly enhance their bioavailability. Phytochemicals, characterized by their natural origin, low toxicity, and capacity for multifaceted intervention, present a potential avenue for the management of metabolic disorders.

Numerous phytochemicals demonstrate biological activity relevant to cancer prevention and therapy, presenting the possibility of improving clinical outcomes for individuals diagnosed with cancer while minimizing adverse side effects (Choudhari et al. 2020). They suppress cellular proliferation, induce programmed cell death, and regulate the cell cycle, apoptosis signaling, and the tumor microenvironment through multi-target mechanisms. These mechanisms entail the modulation of the PI3K/AKT/mTOR and additional signaling pathways, thereby exhibiting substantial antitumor efficacy (Chow et al. 2007; Kadakol et al. 2016; Karar and Maity 2011; Marchiani et al. 2014; Wang et al. 2014). Furthermore, these phytochemicals have demonstrated considerable efficacy in the prevention of early cancer development as well as in the suppression of cancer progression, encompassing processes such as cellular invasion and metastasis (Koh et al. 2020). Although tumor heterogeneity and drug resistance remain challenges, phytochemicals offer promising new research directions for the advancement of innovative anticancer agents and adjunctive therapies as a result of their low toxicity, high efficacy, and synergistic effects with radiotherapy and chemotherapy.

2 Phytochemicals in Immune Diseases

2.1 *Overview of the Pathogenesis of Immune Diseases*

2.1.1 Autoimmune Diseases

To date, approximately 150 distinct autoimmune disease types have been identified by researchers, alongside the development of various therapeutic approaches. The heterogeneity and increasing incidence of autoimmune disorders present considerable challenges to both healthcare systems and the pharmaceutical industry. Current pharmacological interventions for autoimmune diseases often lack specificity and are frequently accompanied by adverse effects such as infections, allergic reactions, and malignancies. In contrast, antigen-specific immunotherapies aim to induce immune tolerance to autoantigens while maintaining the integrity of systemic immune function (Song et al. 2024).

Autoimmune diseases cause a variety of patterns of inflammation and organ dysfunction (Pisetsky 2023) through complex mechanisms involving immune dysregulation, molecular mimicry, and systemic interactions. Rheumatoid arthritis (RA) and systemic lupus erythematosus (SLE) are exemplary autoimmune disorders characterized by chronic inflammatory responses targeting synovial joints and multiple organ systems, respectively. These conditions are commonly linked to aberrant activation of T and B lymphocytes, which leads to the generation of autoantibodies and subsequent tissue injury. In RA, inflammation of the synovium culminates in cartilage degradation and bone damage, whereas SLE manifests through clinical features such as nephritis, dermatological lesions, and neurological dysfunction, primarily due to immune complex deposition. Likewise, multiple sclerosis (MS) and type 1 diabetes mellitus (T1DM) develop as a consequence of hyperactivation of autoreactive T and B cells, which are recruited to inflict damage upon host tissues (Davidson and Diamond 2001; Pisetsky 2023).

Autoantibodies function as significant biomarkers for diagnostic purposes, categorization, and assessment of disease activity (Pisetsky 2023). Substantial research has demonstrated the clinical significance of autoantibodies in systemic autoimmune disorders. For example, anti-dsDNA antibodies are recognized as highly specific biomarkers for systemic lupus erythematosus (SLE), with their concentrations correlating with renal involvement. Similarly, anti-cyclic citrullinated peptide (anti-CCP) antibodies are instrumental in the diagnosis of RA and provide valuable prognostic information regarding disease progression. Recent developments in multiplex assay technologies have enabled the concurrent detection of multiple autoantibody profiles, thereby improving diagnostic accuracy and supporting the implementation of personalized therapeutic approaches.

Although T cells play a pivotal role in the pathogenesis of diseases, their evaluation continues to present significant challenges (Pisetsky 2023). The heterogeneity and dynamic functional states of T cells pose considerable challenges for their characterization in autoimmune diseases. Although flow cytometry facilitates the identification of CD4+ T cell subsets, such as Th17 cells and Tregs, this method often falls short in revealing the spatial interactions that take place within tissue microenvironments (Zhang et al. 2021). Single-cell RNA sequencing has revealed the clonal expansion of autoreactive T cells within lesions typical of multiple sclerosis. Furthermore, the transient nature of activation patterns and the expression of tissue-specific homing receptors necessitate longitudinal sampling, which presents practical challenges for clinical monitoring.

Autoimmune diseases result from the complex interplay between genetic predispositions and environmental factors. Genome-wide association studies (GWAS) have identified more than 100 genetic loci associated with susceptibility to SLE, with a substantial proportion involving HLA class II genes. Environmental triggers, such as Epstein-Barr virus infection, may promote molecular mimicry by viral proteins that possess epitopes homologous to self-antigens (Davidson and Diamond 2001). Ultraviolet radiation intensifies cutaneous lupus by inducing apoptosis and revealing intracellular antigens. Importantly, twin studies demonstrate discordance rates greater than 50%, highlighting the substantial influence of environmental and nongenetic factors in the pathogenesis of the disease.

Preclinical autoimmune disease offers a critical window for early intervention or preventive treatment (Pisetsky 2023). In type 1 diabetes, the detection of multiple islet autoantibodies occurs several years prior to the development of symptomatic hyperglycemia. Evidence from the TrialNet consortium demonstrates that teplizumab, an anti-CD3 monoclonal antibody, significantly delays the clinical onset of type 1 diabetes in individuals identified as high risk. Similarly, patients diagnosed with RA who present with anti-CCP antibodies and subclinical synovitis derive therapeutic benefits from the early initiation of methotrexate treatment (Klareskog et al. 2006). These results highlight the potential effectiveness of targeted immunomodulation during the asymptomatic phase in modifying the progression of the disease.

Rheumatoid Arthritis (RA)

Rheumatoid arthritis (RA) is an autoimmune disorder characterized by a variety of systemic manifestations. It affects approximately 1% of the global population. The prevalence of RA is projected to rise, driven by demographic changes, particularly within certain geographic regions. The disease typically manifests clinically between the ages of 35 and 60, although juvenile RA may occur in individuals younger than 16 years. Clinical features commonly include persistent joint stiffness, pain, and, in advanced cases, joint deformities. Current therapeutic approaches involve the use of disease-modifying antirheumatic drugs (DMARDs), biologic agents, and glucocorticoids, with the objectives of symptom alleviation and slowing disease progression. Nevertheless, these treatments are frequently limited by adverse side effects and variable patient responses (Shakeel et al. 2025).

Genetic determinants are fundamentally influential during the initial phase, severity, and advancement of RA. Among these, the class II MHC locus constitutes the most significant genetic risk factor. Specifically, the HLA-DR4 allele is found in approximately 70% of individuals with RA, in contrast to 30% of unaffected controls. The shared susceptibility epitope (SE) is situated at amino acid residues 70 to 74 in the third hypervariable region of the DRβ chain (Weyand et al. 1992). Beyond the SE, variations in amino acid residues within the DRβ chain significantly account for the relationship between the MHC and seropositive RA, as these variations affect the binding affinity for pro-arthritogenic antigens. Within this genetic context, posttranslational modifications of various auto-proteins—particularly citrullination—generate altered autoantigens that clearly trigger autoimmune responses mediated by CD4+ T lymphocytes in patients with AMPA and seropositive RA.

RA is categorized as two primary subtypes grounded in the detection or non-detection of anti-citrullinated protein antibodies (ACPAs). Citrullination is a biochemical modification characterized by the enzymatic conversion of arginine residues into citrulline, a reaction catalyzed by the enzyme peptidylarginine deiminase (PAD). This process occurs under physiological conditions commonly observed in mammals and may be elicited by environmental influences, including tobacco smoke (Klareskog et al. 2006). Tobacco use constitutes the primary determinant of risk associated with the onset of RA (Malmstrom et al. 2017). Cigarette smoking, functioning as an epigenetic factor and a regulator of the mucosal microbiota, predominantly influences RA in individuals possessing the HLA-SE allele (Ishikawa et al. 2019). HLA-SE and cigarette smoking seem to affect distinct preclinical phases of RA. In particular, cigarette smoking is associated with an increased probability of producing ACPA, whereas the presence of HLA-SE does not demonstrate a significant correlation with ACPA positivity in the general population. Conversely, HLA-SE is associated with a heightened risk of progressing to inflammatory arthritis. The risks associated with smoking have stimulated further research into the involvement of mucosal processes, especially within the pulmonary system, in the pathogenesis of RA (Alivernini et al. 2022). ACPAs are detectable in roughly two-thirds of patients with RA and may represent an essential diagnostic biomarker for individuals during the initial phases of the disorder (Weyand et al. 1992). The subset of RA patients exhibiting positivity for ACPA demonstrates a more severe clinical presentation relative to those who are ACPA-negative (Klareskog et al. 2006). Studies have indicated that ACPA-negative RA demonstrates a unique profile of genetic associations, and immune cells in this subgroup exhibit differential responses to citrullinated antigens relative to ACPA-positive patients. In terms of therapeutic outcomes, diminished efficacy of methotrexate (MTX) and rituximab has been documented among individuals with ACPA-negative RA. These findings highlight the need for further investigation into the underlying pathophysiological differences between these two subgroups.

RA is initiated through a complex, multiphase immunopathogenic process influenced by both genetic predisposition and environmental determinants (Guo et al. 2018). The initiating stage is characterized by molecular changes, such as the citrullination of arginine residues mediated by peptidyl-arginine deiminases (PADs), which is triggered by environmental factors including smoking, microbial pathogens (e.g., Porphyromonas gingivalis), and airborne pollutants. Genetic predisposition, particularly the expression of certain HLA-DR alleles including HLA-DR1 and HLA-DR4, enhances the ability of antigen-presenting cells to recognize citrullinated proteins, thereby promoting the generation of ACPAs. In the preclinical stage, a breakdown in immune tolerance occurs, as evidenced by the detection of ACPAs several years prior to the onset of clinical manifestations.

The maturation phase is characterized by systemic immune dysregulation, marked by epitope spreading and the activation of autoreactive lymphocytes. The migration of T lymphocytes, B cells, and macrophages within the synovial tissue facilitates interactions with fibroblast-like synoviocytes (FLSs), thereby enhancing pro-inflammatory cytokine networks, including TNF-α and IL-6. Simultaneously, impaired regulatory T-cell function and abnormal B-cell maturation contribute to the diversification of autoantibodies, such as rheumatoid factor (RF) and ACPA. This stage represents the progression from localized autoimmunity to established synovitis, as evidenced histopathologically by synovial hyperplasia and leukocyte infiltration.

During the targeting phase, persistent inflammation induces structural damage to the joints via cytokine-driven activation of osteoclasts and subsequent cartilage degradation. FLSs and macrophages exhibit elevated expression of matrix metalloproteinases (MMPs), which contribute to the breakdown of extracellular matrix components. Concurrently, receptor activator of nuclear factor κ-B ligand (RANKL) signaling enhances osteoclast differentiation, thereby disrupting normal bone remodeling processes. Additionally, angiogenesis within the hypertrophic synovium supports ongoing leukocyte infiltration, establishing a self-perpetuating inflammatory cycle. Clinically, these pathological mechanisms manifest as progressive joint swelling, pain, and radiographic evidence of erosive changes.

The fulminant phase is characterized by the destruction of end organs alongside systemic complications. The development of synovial pannus leads to the invasion of cartilage and subchondral bone, whereas persistent inflammation promotes oxidative stress and endothelial dysfunction, consequently elevating the risk of cardiovascular disease. Additionally, extra-articular manifestations, including pulmonary fibrosis and osteoporosis, indicate extensive immune system dysregulation. Therapeutic strategies targeting early-stage mechanisms (e.g., ACPA suppression, TLR inhibition) may help mitigate disease progression, underscoring the importance of stage-specific interventions in RA management.

Recent advancements in pharmacotherapy, particularly the introduction of JAK inhibitors and biologic DMARDs, represent a significant advancement in the management of RA through their more targeted modulation of specific inflammatory pathways. These therapeutic options offer alternatives for patients who demonstrate suboptimal responses to conventional treatment strategies. However, several challenges remain, including the substantial economic costs associated with biologic therapies, treatment-related adverse effects, and issues related to patient adherence. Concurrently, technological progress, especially the integration of artificial intelligence, is revolutionizing RA management by facilitating earlier diagnosis, enhanced risk stratification, and the development of personalized treatment regimens. These technological innovations hold the potential to fundamentally transform clinical practice by enabling healthcare professionals to implement proactive, individualized care tailored to the unique clinical profiles of patients.

The future management of RA is expected to adopt a more integrated and personalized approach that incorporates genetic data, emerging pharmacological therapies, and lifestyle modifications. This multifaceted strategy holds significant potential for enhancing therapeutic outcomes, slowing disease progression, and improving patients' long-term quality of life. However, several critical areas warrant further investigation, including the validation of genetic markers for early diagnosis and individualized treatment, the refinement of lifestyle interventions alongside evaluation of their long-term impact on disease trajectory, and the identification and resolution of barriers to the widespread adoption of artificial intelligence and advanced digital health technologies in clinical practice. It is essential that researchers and clinicians collaborate closely to explore these domains, ensuring that innovative treatments and technologies are both feasible and accessible, while addressing the diverse needs of individuals living with RA. Continued progress in research and clinical innovation has the potential to markedly improve the quality of care and patient outcomes for those affected by RA worldwide (Shakeel et al. 2025).

Systemic Lupus Erythematosus (SLE)

Systemic lupus erythematosus (SLE) impacts individuals across all age groups, ethnic origins, and gender identities. Nevertheless, more than 90% of newly confirmed diagnoses are observed in women of reproductive age (Doria et al. 2008). SLE is a persistent autoimmune disorder marked by inflammation of the microvasculature, involving multiple organ systems, and is linked to the generation of diverse autoantibodies, notably ANA. Historical records trace the recognition of this disease back to medieval times, with the term "lupus" first coined by the twelfth-century physician Rogerius. The systemic nature of the condition was later established by Moric Kaposi in 1872 (Cervera et al. 2003).

SLE induces dysregulation of the immune system, thereby impairing the organism's capacity to suppress and effectively respond to infectious agents. Individuals with SLE demonstrate heightened vulnerability to opportunistic pathogens, notably Salmonella, herpes zoster, and Candida species, as a consequence of altered immune function. Nutritional management in patients with lupus necessitates careful consideration due to disease-associated complications, including steroid-induced osteoporosis, diabetes mellitus, cardiovascular diseases, and renal dysfunction. Both the progression of the disease and its therapeutic interventions may lead to severe and potentially life-threatening complications (Hahn 2003).

Clinical manifestations of SLE exhibit considerable heterogeneity. Common constitutional symptoms include fever, malaise, arthralgia, myalgia, headache, anorexia, and weight fluctuations. Fatigue, pyrexia, joint pain, and changes in body mass are the most frequent presenting symptoms in both new cases and disease flares (Petri 2007). Fatigue is the most common constitutional symptom and may result from active disease processes, pharmacotherapy, lifestyle factors, or comorbid conditions such as fibromyalgia and mood disorders. Fatigue associated with disease activity typically correlates with other clinical and laboratory markers of active SLE. Febrile episodes, although common, require careful differential diagnosis to distinguish between disease activity, infections, and drug-induced hyperthermia. Weight loss may serve as an indicator of active disease, while weight gain might result from corticosteroid treatment or complications such as anasarca associated with nephrotic syndrome. These nonspecific clinical manifestations frequently overlap with symptoms observed in other autoimmune conditions, infectious diseases, endocrine disorders, and chronic pain syndromes (Greco et al. 2003).

SLE is typified by the generation of autoantibodies, such as ANA, anti-Sm, anti-dsDNA, aPL, and aβ2GPI antibodies, which may be identifiable several years before the clinical onset of the disease. These autoantibodies serve as principal agents in mediating inflammation and tissue injury in SLE through the formation of ICs that accumulate within multiple organs, comprising the kidneys, skin, and central nervous system, thereby initiating localized inflammatory processes. The synthesis of these antibodies is performed by plasma cells (PCs) and their immediate precursors, plasmablasts, which correspond to terminally differentiated B lymphocytes. Furthermore, B cells, as antecedents to plasma cells and effective APCs, demonstrate defective tolerance to self-antigens and may be involved in the development of SLE by displaying autoantigens to T cells, subsequently resulting in the initiation of Th cells (Iwata and Tanaka 2015).

Activated T cells reciprocally promote B cell proliferation and differentiation through CD40L/CD40 interactions. Activated B cells, supported by Tfh cells and FDCs, migrate to germinal centers (GCs), where antigen-specific clones undergo affinity maturation. Within these GCs, high-affinity autoreactive B cells proliferate and undergo differentiation to become MBCs and antibody-secreting PCs.

Intracellular signaling pathways that regulate the expression of type I interferons (IFNs), including those mediated by Toll-like receptors (TLRs), are activated upon the recognition of nucleic acids. The binding of type I IFNs to their cognate receptors triggers an intracellular signal transduction cascade predominantly involving the JAK/STAT pathway. This activation subsequently enhances the functional responses of both the innate and adaptive immune systems (Greth et al. 2017; Ramaswamy et al. 2021; Ronnblom and Leonard 2019). A well-documented positive correlation exists between type I IFNs and SLE. Notably, elevated systemic concentrations of type I IFNs have been observed in approximately half of individuals diagnosed with SLE (Xu et al. 2024). A greater proportion of patients with SLE were estimated to demonstrate upregulation of genes associated with type I IFNs signal transduction mediated within peripheral blood cells (Postal et al. 2020; Vanpouille-Box et al. 2019).

The synthesis of type I IFNs is predominantly initiated by pattern recognition receptors that detect nucleic acids. These receptors include endosomal TLRs, cGAS, and RIG-I RLRs which are linked to the mitochondrial antiviral-signaling protein (MAVS) (Wolf et al. 2024). These detection mechanisms exhibit persistent hyperactivity in SLE patients, with TLR7's pathogenic contributions to disease development being particularly well-documented (Hu et al. 2022). Notably, dysregulated initiation of the cGAS-STING axis has been identified as a critical driver of autoimmune responses and the progression of SLE (Schlee and Hartmann 2016; Vanpouille-Box et al. 2019).

Moreover, disruptions in nucleic acid homeostasis serve as a significant trigger for type I IFNs responses. The role of cytoplasmic nucleic acid sensing mechanisms in the pathogenesis of SLE has been thoroughly substantiated (Crowl et al. 2017; Skopelja-Gardner et al. 2020). Empirical and clinical research has demonstrated that ultraviolet (UV) radiation amplifies type I IFN signaling at both local and systemic scales (Alvarez-Rodriguez et al. 2019).

Type I IFNs are pivotal in orchestrating the initiation of both inherent and acquired immune responses. Upon binding to their specific receptors, type I IFNs trigger intracellular signaling pathways via the JAK/STAT pathway, resulting in the transcriptional activation of IFN-responsive genes that collectively define the "IFN signature" characteristic of an engaged immune system. Furthermore, type I IFNs directly stimulate dendritic cells (DCs), thereby augmenting their antigen-presenting capacity to T lymphocytes. This activation and subsequent polarization of T cells are essential for the effective priming of B cell differentiation. The resultant activated B cells produce autoantibodies, which, when produced excessively and inadequately cleared, may accumulate within tissues and organs, leading to pathological damage. This deleterious process is further mediated by interactions between CD40 and its ligand CD40L.

The pathogenesis of SLE is primarily linked to a dysregulation between pro-inflammatory Th17 cells and immunosuppressive Tregs (Chen et al. 2018; Talaat et al. 2015). Patients with SLE exhibit elevated proportions of Th17 cells, which show positive correlations with disease severity (Zhu et al. 2019). Conversely, Tregs, which are critical for maintaining immune tolerance, exhibit reduced levels or impaired functionality, strongly associated with disease initiation and progression (La Cava 2018; Ohl and Tenbrock 2015).

Distinct metabolic pathways define these T cell subsets: Th17 cell differentiation is primarily supported by glycolytic metabolism, while the development of Tregs depends on fatty acid oxidation (FAO) and oxidative phosphorylation (Kono et al. 2018). Empirical evidence indicates that the inhibition of glycolysis specifically suppresses the differentiation of Th17 cells, concurrently facilitating the expansion of Tregs (Cluxton et al. 2019; Kalim et al. 2018). Notably, impaired FAO correlates with enhanced Th17 responses and compromised Treg generation (Huang et al. 2017). These metabolic differences suggest therapeutic potential in modulating energy substrate utilization. Dietary interventions that favor lipid metabolism over carbohydrate dependence, such as low-carbohydrate or ketogenic regimens, may represent viable nutritional strategies for managing SLE.

Multiple Sclerosis (MS)

Multiple sclerosis (MS) is a neurodegenerative disorder characterized by immune-mediated damage to the myelin sheath that insulates nerve fibers. The precise etiology of MS remains unresolved. A prevailing hypothesis suggests that MS is an autoimmune condition involving the migration of autoreactive T lymphocytes from the peripheral immune system into the central nervous system (CNS) during the initial stages of lesion formation, a concept commonly referred to as the outside-in hypothesis. Alternatively, MS pathogenesis may originate from an intrinsic event within the CNS itself. Following infiltration into the CNS, self-reactive effector CD4+ T lymphocytes undergo local reactivation facilitated by APCs, which subsequently promotes the recruitment of additional T lymphocytes and macrophages, leading to the development of inflammatory lesions. Histopathological studies demonstrate a distinct spatial distribution within MS plaques, with CD8+ T cells predominantly localized at the lesion periphery, whereas CD4+ T cells are primarily concentrated in the deeper regions (Hauser et al. 2013). These infiltrating immune mediators initiate pathogenic cascades involving demyelination, oligodendrocyte apoptosis, and axonal injury, ultimately resulting in neurological deficits. Simultaneously, endogenous immunoregulatory mechanisms are activated to limit inflammation and promote tissue repair, processes associated with partial remyelination and clinical remission. However, if left untreated, disease progression typically presents as recurrent inflammatory episodes that eventually transition into progressive forms of MS. The subsequent discussion will systematically investigate the underlying mechanisms governing the functional roles of effector CD4+ and CD8+ T cell subsets within these pathological processes. Of particular significance, CD8+ T cells are observed to predominate relative to other T cell subsets, as well as B cells and plasma cells. It is postulated that the disease initiates with an inflammation-driven lesion predominantly constituted by CD8+ and CD4+ T cells, which in turn activate microglia and macrophages. This pathological process disrupts neural communication between the brain and peripheral systems, clinically manifesting as sensory disturbances, such as hypoesthesia, motor impairments, such as muscular weakness and instability in gait patterns, visual impairments, and a range of heterogeneous neurological symptoms.

Disease progression in MS exhibits considerable interindividual variability; however, irreversible axonal damage generally accumulates progressively, with symptom severity closely associated with lesion localization and the degree of disruption to neural pathways. At disease onset, approximately 85–90% of patients present with relapsing-remitting MS (RRMS), characterized by episodic neurological exacerbations lasting from days to weeks, followed by partial or complete recovery and variable remission intervals. Within a period of 10 to 40 years post-onset, 20–40% of RRMS cases evolve into secondary progressive MS (SPMS), which is typified by a continuous neurological decline often accompanied by progressive impairment in mobility. A distinct subset, comprising 10–15% of cases, manifests primary progressive MS (PPMS), defined by a gradual onset of symptoms and steady functional deterioration in the absence of acute relapses. Current therapeutic strategies, while not curative, focus on three primary goals: reducing the severity of relapses, delaying disease progression, and alleviating symptom burden. The preclinical phases of MS include clinically isolated syndrome (CIS), representing an initial demyelinating event necessitating differential diagnosis, and radiologically isolated syndrome (RIS), characterized by the presence of MS-typical neuroimaging abnormalities in asymptomatic individuals. The pathogenesis of MS is attributed to a complex interplay among genetic susceptibility, environmental factors, and immune dysregulation, although the precise mechanistic pathways remain incompletely understood. Importantly, active immunomodulatory treatments have demonstrated efficacy not only in reducing relapse frequency but also in decelerating the progression of sustained disability, underscoring the significant role of inflammation, particularly during the early stages of the disease.

The pathophysiological mechanisms underlying MS encompass various elements, such as oxidative stress imbalances, inflammatory and autoimmune responses, vascular contributions, and neurodegenerative processes (Miljkovic and Spasojevic 2013). In patients with early-stage MS, active white matter lesions are associated with inflammatory activity and disruption of the BBB. This relationship differs in progressive MS subtypes, where perivascular and parenchymal inflammation can occur in affected blood vessels without detectable serum protein extravasation. This finding indicates that inflammatory responses of this nature may not manifest as contrast enhancement on MRI scans, suggesting that therapeutic interventions aimed at modulating this inflammation should ideally be capable of crossing the intact BBB to effectively reach the CNS.

The compartmentalization of inflammatory processes within the CNS is further substantiated by the presence of meningeal inflammatory aggregates, which are particularly common in patients with early-onset progressive multiple sclerosis. Multiple studies have identified these aggregates as lymphoid follicle-like structures containing infiltrates of B lymphocytes and plasma cells. Moreover, cells expressing markers indicative of follicular dendritic cells have been detected in approximately 40% of progressive multiple sclerosis cases (Choi et al. 2012; Magliozzi et al. 2007; Serafini et al. 2004). The comparatively elevated prevalence observed may be attributable to study cohorts comprising a higher proportion of patients experiencing rapid disease progression and consequently shorter disease durations. Importantly, the degree and severity of active subpial cortical demyelination and neurodegeneration have been found to correlate with the magnitude of meningeal inflammation in both PPMS and SPMS. Comparative analyses reveal significantly greater cortical demyelination and neuronal loss in patients exhibiting meningeal lymphoid follicle-like aggregates compared to those with diffuse meningeal inflammation lacking organized structures (Choi et al. 2012; Magliozzi et al. 2007). These results characterize B-cell follicle-like aggregates within the meningeal layers of individuals diagnosed with progressive multiple sclerosis as indicators of pronounced inflammatory pathology.

Although these findings demonstrate associations between inflammatory activity and continuous tissue damage in progressive multiple sclerosis, they do not exclude the potential that inflammatory responses may occur as a consequence of primary neurodegenerative mechanisms during the course of disease progression.

B lymphocytes display functional heterogeneity in the course of their production of both pro-inflammatory cytokines and cytokines with anti-inflammatory properties. Notably, the STAT5 and STAT6 signaling pathways independently stimulate the production of GM-CSF in B lymphocytes. Compared to B cells from healthy individuals, those derived from MS patients exhibit increased GM-CSF secretion alongside decreased IL-10 production. GM-CSF produced by B cells augments the secretion of the T cell-stimulating cytokines IL-12 and IL-6 by myeloid cells, thereby collectively facilitating the differentiation of Th1 and Th17 cells (Li et al. 2015). Notably, anti-CD20 therapy in patients with MS is correlated with a reduction in GM-CSF production alongside an elevation in IL-10 levels within reconstituted B-cell populations. Given that GM-CSF and IL-10 production appear to be mutually exclusive within individual B cells, it remains uncertain whether individual B cells are subject to differential regulatory mechanisms governing their production of either pro-inflammatory or anti-inflammatory cytokines, or if distinct B-cell subsets are specialized to secrete specific cytokine profiles. Nevertheless, the prolonged clinical efficacy of therapeutic intervention targeting the CD20 antigen is probably due to the reduction in the population of MBCs and the consequent reduction in the secretion of pro-inflammatory cytokines by the residual B cell population (Hauser et al. 2013).

Variations in the frequencies and activation statuses of mature B cells are linked to disease activity and treatment outcomes in MS. Unlike RA or type 1 diabetes (T1D), MS does not exhibit abnormal persistence of autoreactive B cells during transitional developmental stages. However, despite apparently normal checkpoint regulation, mature naïve B cells in MS display aberrant activation and proliferative responses (Kinnunen et al. 2013). Moreover, MBCs originating from individuals diagnosed with MS demonstrate elevated levels of the co-stimulatory molecules CD80 and CD86 (Bar-Or et al. 2001). The atacicept clinical trial, which aimed to inhibit the activation of mature B cells mediated by BAFF, was unsuccessful and paradoxically intensified CNS inflammation. This adverse effect may have resulted from the enhanced activation of memory B cells, potentially mediated by IL-15-related pathways (Sergott et al. 2015). The enhanced stimulation of B lymphocytes may explain the initiation of multiple sclerosis observed following anti-TNFα treatment among individuals diagnosed with RA or CD, as such treatment leads to an expansion of memory B-cell populations. Furthermore, IL-21 produced by pathogenic Th17 cells may contribute to the advancement of the increased proliferation and survival of MBCs (Gharibi et al. 2016). Collectively, these findings highlight the enhanced pro-inflammatory properties of memory B cells in MS, including their capacity to drive T-cell activation and perpetuate neuroinflammation.

2.1.2 Chronic Inflammation

Inflammatory bowel disease (IBD), encompassing ulcerative colitis (UC) and Crohn's disease (CD), impacts an estimated between six and eight million individuals globally (Hauser et al. 1986). The clinical presentations of both UC and CD commonly encompass abdominal pain, diarrhea, and severe fatigue. In certain cases, IBD manifests as a mild disorder; however, for others, it can result in substantial disability and may precipitate life-threatening complications. Intestinal fibrosis constitutes a significant and frequent complication associated with IBD, affecting more than 30% of patients diagnosed with CD and approximately 5% of those with UC. This pathological condition can lead to intestinal obstruction, often necessitating surgical intervention. Intestinal fibrosis is characterized by persistent or unresolved inflammation within the intestinal tissue, which promotes excessive accumulation of extracellular matrix (ECM) components and consequently disrupts normal intestinal function. Despite notable progress in understanding the pathogenesis of IBD, the specific cellular and molecular mechanisms underlying fibrosis remain incompletely elucidated. IBD is a chronic, progressive disorder characterized by alternating periods of exacerbation and remission, which substantially impairs patients' quality of life and daily functioning, while also contributing to increased healthcare costs. Although it is widely accepted that IBD results from aberrant immune responses to microbial antigens in genetically susceptible individuals, the precise pathogenic pathways have yet to be fully defined.

A growing number of studies suggest that individuals diagnosed with IBD exhibit compositional changes in their gut microbiota (Frank et al. 2007; Manichanh et al. 2006). Parent and colleagues identified gut microbial dysbiosis in patients with IBD, characterized by the presence of Pseudomonas-like bacterial species in CD tissue samples (Parent and Mitchell 1978). Notably, pathogenic Escherichia coli exhibits intestinal expansion in IBD, demonstrating enhanced macrophage survival and the ability to stimulate TNF-α secretion and inflammatory responses (Chervy et al. 2020). In contrast, the probiotic bacterium *Faecalibacterium prausnitzii* enhances dendritic cell secretion of the anti-inflammatory cytokine IL-10 and concurrently inhibits the production of pro-inflammatory cytokines, specifically IL-12 and IFN-γ. Notably, the concentrations of these pro-inflammatory cytokines are markedly diminished within the intestinal environment of individuals with IBD (Lloyd-Price et al. 2019). Although these observations cannot establish causality between microbial dysbiosis and the pathogenesis of IBD, they suggest potential therapeutic targets. Experimental validation using germ-free mouse models colonized with microbiota from healthy donors versus those from IBD patients revealed increased susceptibility to colitis in recipients of IBD-associated microbial communities (Britton et al. 2019). The therapeutic efficacy of fecal microbiota transplantation (FMT) for IBD remains to be definitively demonstrated through clinical trials, primarily due to the absence of identification of critical compositional elements within the donor microbiota (Costello et al. 2019; Paramsothy et al. 2017; Rossen et al. 2015).

The intestinal microenvironment in IBD exhibits specific metabolic changes, including reduced tryptophan catabolism, diminished synthesis of SCFAs, and elevated levels of nicotinic acid derivatives and acylcarnitines (Liu et al. 2021). These metabolic alterations may play a direct role in promoting intestinal inflammation. SCFAs, notably butyrate, acetate, and propionate, modulate various biological functions and facilitate the expansion of Tregs within the intestinal environment (Brown et al. 2019; Dalile et al. 2019). Butyrate specifically maintains epithelial barrier integrity by inducing synaptopodin (SYNPO) and serves as the principal energy substrate for colonic epithelial cells (Li et al. 2020). The bidirectional interaction between bile acids and the gut microbiota is of significant importance, as a deficiency in bile acids facilitates small intestinal bacterial overgrowth, epithelial damage, and the activation of inflammatory responses, thereby highlighting their critical function in antimicrobial defense mechanisms (Banfi et al. 2021).

IL-6 is predominantly produced by macrophages and dendritic cells within the intestinal lamina propria. Elevated concentrations of IL-6 have been observed in the serum and intestinal tissues of patients with CD. These increased levels have been associated with clinical disease activity, relapse frequency, and the extent of inflammatory severity (Atreya and Neurath 2008). Following its interaction with the receptor, IL-6 initiates the activation of T lymphocytes expressing gp130, resulting in the translocation of the signal transducer and STAT3 into the nucleus. This process subsequently facilitates the transcriptional activation of antiapoptotic genes. This mechanistic understanding has informed the development of therapeutic interventions, exemplified by tocilizumab, a humanized monoclonal antibody directed against the IL-6 receptor, which will be examined in subsequent sections.

The IL-12 cytokine family plays a pivotal role in the pathogenesis of chronic inflammatory diseases. These cytokines are produced by DCs and contribute to the induction of pathogenic T-cell responses in experimental models of colitis (Leppkes and Neurath 2020; Roda et al. 2016). IL-12, a heterodimer consisting of the p40 and IL-12p35 subunits, exerts its biological effects via binding to the IL-12 receptor components IL-12Rβ1 and IL-12Rβ2. This cytokine facilitates the differentiation of naïve CD4+ T lymphocytes into Th1 cells characterized by the production of IFN-γ. Additionally, IL-12 augments the effector functions of NK cells, NKT cells, and cytotoxic T lymphocytes (Trinchieri 2003). Conversely, IL-23, a heterodimer consisting of the IL-23p19 and p40 subunits, initiates signaling via the IL-12Rβ1 and IL-23R receptors. This activation enhances Th17 cell responses and concurrently inhibits the anti-inflammatory functions mediated by Foxp3-positive Treg cells, ultimately contributing to the exacerbation of intestinal inflammation (Schiering et al. 2014; Teng et al. 2015). The following sections offer a detailed examination of the pathogenic roles of IL-17 cytokines, specifically IL-17A and IL-17F, in IBD.

IL-10, a principal anti-inflammatory cytokine, is synthesized by a diverse range of immune cell types, such as Tregs, macrophages, and DCs (Saraiva and O'Garra 2010). The receptor for IL-10, which consists of the IL-10Rα and IL-10Rβ subunits, is extensively expressed throughout various immune cell types, thereby enabling IL-10 to regulate both innate and adaptive immune responses (Wei et al. 2019). Genetic alterations in the IL-10 and IL-10R signaling pathways have been implicated in early-onset IBD, which is marked by exaggerated inflammatory responses within the intestinal mucosa. This association is further corroborated by experimental studies demonstrating that mice lacking either IL-10 or the IL-10R spontaneously develop colitis (Mas-Orea et al. 2021; Saha et al. 2021). Mechanistically, IL-10 inhibits Th1-mediated IFN-γ production in CD45RBhi CD4+ T-cell transfer models, attenuates Th17 cell responses in DSS-induced colitis, and facilitates Treg-mediated inhibition of pathogenic Th17 activity (Powrie et al. 1994). Additionally, IL-10 regulates macrophage redox balance through the ROS-NO pathway in DSS-induced colitis.

IL-1β, a macrophage-derived cytokine, synergizes with TNF-α and IL-6 to amplify intestinal inflammation in IBD. Preclinical investigations have demonstrated that elevated secretion of IL-1β is observed preceding the onset of colitis in murine models deficient in IL-10. The genetic deletion of inflammasome constituents, including caspase-1, results in a reduction of IL-1β and IL-18 release, consequently attenuating the severity of DSS-induced colitis. Moreover, both pharmacological and genetic suppression of IL-1β and IL-18 signaling pathways have been shown to ameliorate experimental colitis, underscoring their potential as therapeutic targets.

2.2 *Key Phytochemicals and Their Roles*

2.2.1 Curcumin

Curcumin is a bioactive compound extracted from the rhizome of *Curcuma longa*, commonly known as the turmeric plant. Native to South Asia, including regions such as China, turmeric is predominantly cultivated for its use in traditional medicinal practices (Govindarajan 1980). Curcumin is a yellow-orange crystalline substance with a molecular weight of 368 g/mol and a melting point of 183 °C. Chemically, it is classified as a polyphenolic compound featuring two aromatic rings, each substituted with hydroxyl and methoxy groups. These aromatic rings are connected by a seven-carbon linker that contains two α, β-unsaturated carbonyl moieties capable of reversible isomerization. Commercial curcumin formulations primarily comprise three main constituents, among which diferuloylmethane is the most abundant and biologically active, constituting approximately 82% of turmeric. Collectively, these compounds are referred to as "curcumin analogs" (Aggarwal et al. 2003; Bharti et al. 2003). Curcumin analogs demonstrate therapeutic efficacy in various diseases by modulating molecular signaling pathways. These compounds modulate critical transcription factors, for example, NF-κB, β-catenin, and peroxisome proliferator-activated receptors, as well as enzymatic targets including COX-2 and iNOS. Additionally, they modulate the expression levels of pro-inflammatory cytokines, notably TNF-α and IL-6 (Bharti and Aggarwal 2002; Bharti et al. 2003; Buhrmann et al. 2020; Mukhopadhyay et al. 2001; Shakibaei et al. 2007, 2015).

The biological and physiological properties of curcumin have been extensively examined and systematically studied, with particular emphasis on its relevance to neurodegenerative and inflammatory conditions, including Alzheimer's disease and dementia. Curcumin exhibits notable antioxidant activity through mechanisms such as the inhibition of lipid peroxidation and the scavenging of ROS (Ak and Gulcin 2008). The compound exhibits anti-inflammatory properties in experimental models of both acute and chronic inflammation (Srimal and Dhawan 1973). Beyond these roles, curcumin has been extensively studied for its potential as an anticancer agent. Clinical trials have assessed the oral administration of curcumin, both as a standalone treatment and in conjunction with standard chemotherapeutic drugs, in patients diagnosed with pancreatic and prostate cancers (Bayet-Robert et al. 2010; Dhillon et al. 2008; Mahammedi et al. 2016). Curcumin inhibits tumor growth and angiogenesis in mouse glioblastoma xenografts, and prolongs animal survival time. In addition, the combination therapy of curcumin and 5-fluorouracil has a significant inhibitory effect on cancer cells, providing a more effective treatment strategy for chemotherapy resistant colon cancer cells (Perry et al. 2010; Shakibaei et al. 2013, 2014, 2015).

Despite curcumin exhibiting a broad spectrum of advantageous health properties, its clinical utility is often constrained by its limited bioavailability, which results from inadequate absorption and rapid metabolic breakdown. However, the bioavailability of curcumin can be substantially increased through coadministration with certain adjuvants. Notably, piperine, a bioactive compound found in black pepper, has been shown to significantly augment the bioavailability of curcumin (Hewlings and Kalman 2017; Kaur et al. 2018; Patel et al. 2020). It is important to emphasize that, despite the considerable body of research investigating the anticancer properties of curcumin, the precise mechanism underlying its translocation across cellular membranes remains unclear. Investigations utilizing molecular dynamics simulations in conjunction with solid-state NMR experiments have demonstrated that curcumin can be incorporated into the plasma membrane (Barry et al. 2009). Nonetheless, the particular mechanisms of transport operating within the nervous system and neuroblastoma cells remain to be fully elucidated.

Despite these limitations, curcumin remains a major constituent of various spices and foods commonly consumed in the daily diet and is generally well tolerated even at relatively high doses without significant adverse effects. Therefore, it holds substantial potential as an agent for chemopreventive or therapeutic applications.

Inhibition of the NF-κB Pathway

NF-κB functions as a key transcriptional activator that modulates the expression of a broad spectrum of pro-inflammatory genes, thereby serving critical functions in the processes of both inherent and acquired immune responses, as well as in the regulation of inflammatory responses (Taniguchi and Karin 2018). Populations of innate immune cells, for example, DCs and neutrophils, depend on NF-κB-driven production of inflammatory mediators. Concurrently, they employ negative feedback mechanisms to preserve homeostasis and inhibit the initiation of chronic inflammatory processes (Barnabei et al. 2021). The stimulation of PRRs on these cells triggers NF-κB-dependent transcriptional activation of pro-inflammatory cytokines, in addition to type I IFN, chemokines, and antimicrobial proteins. This molecular response facilitates the coordinated processes of pathogen clearance and tissue repair (Gong et al. 2020; Takeuchi and Akira 2010). Canonical NF-κB signaling, initiated through PRR activation, drives the production of these inflammatory molecules (Hayden and Ghosh 2011; Mogensen 2009). Beyond its function in regulating inflammatory responses, NF-κB is essential for regulating signaling pathways mediated by GM-CSF and coordinating the differentiation processes of myeloid progenitor cells (Ebner et al. 2003). The differentiation pathway of innate immune cells originating from myeloid progenitor cells demonstrates a selective reliance on particular constituents of the NF-κB transcription factor family (Gerondakis et al. 1999).

Experimental evidence identifies that curcumin, a potent inhibitor of NF-κB, demonstrated anti-inflammatory and antineoplastic properties. Structural modifications of curcumin have led to the development of synthetic analogs exhibiting enhanced inhibitory effects on NF-κB and associated inflammatory signaling pathways, notably including EF24. Although the NF-κB inhibitory capacity of its structural analog, EF31, had not been previously characterized, a comparative pharmacological evaluation was conducted using murine RAW264.7 macrophage cells. These cells were pretreated for one hour with EF31, EF24, curcumin (at concentrations ranging from 1 to 100 μM), or vehicle control prior to stimulation with LPS to assess modulation of the NF-κB signaling pathway. Quantitative analyses demonstrated that EF31 significantly more effectively suppressed LPS-induced NF-κB DNA binding, with an IC50 of approximately 5 μM, in comparison to EF24 (IC50 ~ 35 μM) and curcumin (IC50 > 50 μM). Additionally, EF31 demonstrated enhanced inhibitory capacity of NF-κB nuclear translocation and reduced expression of downstream inflammatory mediators, including both transcriptional and protein levels of TNF-α and IL-6. Mechanistic investigations revealed that EF31 potently inhibited IκB kinase β (IKKβ) activity, with an IC50 of approximately 1.92 μM, markedly outperforming EF24 (IC50 ~ 131 μM). Importantly, EF31 displayed selective cytotoxicity toward NF-κB-dependent cancer cell lines while causing minimal and reversible cytotoxic effects in RAW264.7 macrophage cells. These findings establish EF31 as a pharmacologically optimized curcumin analog with superior NF-κB suppression and dual anti-inflammatory and anticancer activities compared to both EF24 and the parent compound. The improved therapeutic index positions EF31 as a promising candidate for further preclinical development.

Regulates Th17/Treg Balance

CD4+ helper T (Th) lymphocytes serve as central regulators of immune homeostasis, orchestrating the delicate balance between immunological tolerance and defensive responses. These cells achieve this through functional specialization into distinct effector subsets that maintain self-tolerance while enabling pathogen clearance. Dysregulation of Th cell differentiation and function underlies various pathological conditions, including autoimmune disorders, chronic inflammation, oncogenesis, and impaired antimicrobial immunity. Within the subsets of Th cells, Treg cells and Th17 cells assume notably pivotal but contrasting functions in immune regulation. Specifically, Treg cells predominantly facilitate immunosuppression and the maintenance of tissue homeostasis, whereas Th17 cells promote proinflammatory responses targeting pathogens and possess the capacity to contribute to the advancement of autoimmune diseases. Cytokine signaling networks precisely coordinate this functional counterbalance. The evolutionarily conserved TGF-β superfamily emerges as a pivotal regulatory axis, simultaneously governing the differentiation of immunosuppressive Tregs and the development of proinflammatory and immunomodulatory Th17 populations through context-dependent signaling mechanisms (Wang et al. 2023).

Experimental investigations employing DSS-induced ulcerative colitis (UC) models in diabetic db/db mice have demonstrated the therapeutic efficacy of curcumin administered at a concentration of 100 mg/kg/day for the treatment of diabetes-associated colitis. Curcumin intervention significantly alleviated diabetes-related colitic phenotypes, as evidenced by improved insulin sensitivity, reduced reduction in body weight, increased measurements of colon length and mass parameters, and reduced mucosal ulceration with diminished inflammatory cell infiltration compared to untreated controls. Immunological profiling revealed that curcumin administration rebalanced Th17/Treg responses by suppressing pro-inflammatory Th17 activation while enhancing immunosuppressive Treg functionality. Microbiome analysis further indicated curcumin-mediated modulation of gut microbial diversity and taxonomic composition across multiple classification levels (phylum, class, order, family, and genus) in diabetic colitis models. Collectively, these findings suggest that curcumin ameliorates type 2 diabetes-associated colitis through dual mechanisms: restoration of Th17/Treg homeostasis and structural reorganization of the intestinal microbiota. The compound's capacity to simultaneously address metabolic dysregulation, mucosal inflammation, and microbial dysbiosis positions it as a multifunctional therapeutic candidate for diabetes-complicated inflammatory bowel disorders (Xiao et al. 2022).

2.2.2 Quercetin

Quercetin, a naturally occurring flavonoid pigment widely distributed among numerous plant species, is found in high concentrations within fruits, beverages, and various plant tissues such as leaves, flowers, bark, stems, and rhizomes. Significant dietary sources of this phytochemical include species of *Rumex* (dock), *Nasturtium officinale* (watercress), *Ipomoea batatas* (sweet potato), *Allium cepa* (onion), *Vitis vinifera* (grapes), *multiple berry genera* (Rubus spp., Fragaria spp.), *Prunus avium* (cherry), and *Brassica oleracea* (broccoli).

This polyphenolic compound demonstrates a wide range of pharmacological properties, including chemopreventive, antiviral, anti-inflammatory, and antioxidant effects. A growing body of preclinical research identifies quercetin as a promising antineoplastic agent with multi-targeted therapeutic potential. This review offers a thorough analysis of the prospective clinical applications of quercetin in the treatment of diverse cancer types. The malignancies examined include, but are not limited to, colorectal cancer, lung adenocarcinoma, prostate cancer, urothelial bladder carcinoma, osteosarcoma, hematological cancers such as leukemia and lymphoma, glioblastoma multiforme, cervical cancer, head and neck squamous cell carcinoma, cutaneous melanoma, ocular retinoblastoma, thyroid carcinoma, ovarian adenocarcinoma, and malignant pleural mesothelioma (Li et al. 2021).

Reduction of Pro-Inflammatory Cytokine (IL-6, TNF-α) Release

Numerous investigations have examined the protective properties of quercetin in cardiomyocytes stimulated with TNF-α and have elucidated its underlying mechanisms by utilizing the GEO database to examine variations in gene expression profiles of TNF-α and signal transducer and STAT1. In this study, H9c2 cells were exposed to TNF-α to establish an in vitro model of myocarditis. Cellular viability and apoptosis were quantified using the Cell Counting Kit-8 assay and flow cytometry, respectively. ELISA was conducted to measure the concentrations of pro-inflammatory cytokines IL-6 and IL-17A, as well as the anti-inflammatory cytokine IL-10. To downregulate STAT1 expression, cells underwent transfection with si-STAT1, with knockdown efficiency confirmed via RT-qPCR and Western blot analyses. Western blotting was further employed to assess the expression levels of proteins associated with the MAPK signaling pathway. The findings demonstrated that TNF-α expression was significantly elevated in myocarditis patients, and treatment with TNF-α at a concentration of 20 μg/mL diminished the viability of H9c2 cells. Pretreatment with quercetin partially mitigated the TNF-α-induced reduction in cell viability, the elevation in the incidence of apoptotic cell death, and the secretion of inflammatory cytokines (IL-6, IL-17A, and IL-10). Moreover, TNF-α stimulation upregulated STAT1 expression, which was attenuated by quercetin administration. Importantly, the silencing of STAT1 augmented the protective efficacy of quercetin against TNF-α-induced damage in H9c2 cells. Additionally, quercetin suppressed the activation of the MAPK signaling pathway induced by TNF-α, with STAT1 deficiency further enhancing this inhibitory effect. Collectively, these findings suggest that quercetin confers cytoprotective effects against TNF-α-induced damage in H9c2 cardiomyocytes, potentially through modulation of STAT1 and MAPK signaling pathways (Li et al. 2021).

In a separate investigation, H9C2 cells were randomly allocated into six experimental groups. Cell proliferation was evaluated using the CCK-8 assay, while apoptosis, mitochondrial membrane potential, and ROS levels were quantified via flow cytometry. ELISA and biochemical kits were utilized to quantify the expression levels of eNOS, MDA, and SOD. Western blot analysis was conducted to assess the protein expression of phosphorylated dynamin-related protein 1 (p-DRP1, Ser637), MFN2, p-NF-κB, IκB, and p-IκB. RT-PCR was performed to determine transcriptional levels of IL-10, TNF-α, and IL-1β. The ultrastructural characteristics of mitochondria in H9C2 cells were analyzed through electron microscopy. The findings indicated that, relative to the control group, the model group exhibited markedly increased levels of MDA, p-NF-κB, p-IκB, IL-6, IL-1β, TNF-α, and apoptosis rate. Conversely, the model group showed significantly decreased cell proliferation rates and reduced levels of IL-10, SOD, and ATP ($P < 0.05$). Furthermore, the expression of MDA was markedly reduced in the PVT1 overexpression (OV), quercetin, OV + quercetin, and NAC groups compared to the model group, while SOD and ATP levels were elevated. Electron microscopy analysis demonstrated that either overexpression of PVT1 or therapeutic intervention with quercetin effectively suppressed inflammation-triggered mitochondrial fission and promoted mitochondrial fusion. These results indicate that quercetin enhances the proliferation of H9C2 cells while concurrently attenuating inflammation, oxidative stress, and apoptosis, thereby mitigating structural and functional deficits of mitochondria. Notably, these protective effects are partially mediated through the upregulation of PVT1 expression (Yang et al. 2021).

Intestinal Barrier Repair Effect

Experimental investigations demonstrate quercetin's therapeutic efficacy in mitigating pancreatic and intestinal injuries associated with acute necrotizing pancreatitis (ANP). In ANP-induced rat models, quercetin administration significantly attenuated histopathological damage in both pancreatic and intestinal tissues, evidenced by 42% and 38% reductions in respective pathological scores compared to untreated ANP controls ($P < 0.05$). The compound enhanced intestinal barrier integrity through multiple mechanisms: plasma diamine oxidase (DAO) activity decreased by 57%, D-lactate levels by 49%, and endotoxin concentrations by 63%. This was associated with a 2.1- to 2.4-fold increase in the expression levels of tight junction proteins, including ZO-1 and occludin. Quercetin effectively suppressed inflammatory cascades, reducing intestinal pro-inflammatory cytokines to near-normal levels (IL-1β ↓68%, TNF-α ↓61%, IL-17A ↓59%), while modulating critical signaling pathways. Mechanistically, it inhibited activation of the TLR4/MyD88/p38 MAPK axis, resulting in 54–72% reductions in both expression and phosphorylation levels of pathway components ($P < 0.05$). Concurrently, markers of endoplasmic reticulum stress (ERS) were significantly downregulated—Bip ↓65%, p-IRE1α ↓58%, sXBP1 ↓61%, and ATF6 ↓53% in treated cohorts ($P < 0.05$). These multimodal actions position quercetin as a promising therapeutic candidate for ANP management, targeting both inflammatory signaling (via TLR4/MyD88/p38 MAPK suppression) and cellular stress responses (through ERS mitigation). The demonstrated capacity to preserve pancreatic architecture, restore intestinal barrier function, and modulate stress-adaptive mechanisms underscores its potential for clinical translation in acute pancreatitis treatment. Further pharmacological optimization and clinical trials involving human participants are necessary to confirm the validity of these preclinical results.

A study examining the impact of quercetin on mice with T2DM, with a focus on its potential to enhance insulin resistance and restore intestinal barrier function, yielded several notable results. Regarding body weight and blood glucose levels, from the eighth to the tenth week of intervention, the body weight of mice in the low-dose quercetin group (QR.L) was significantly reduced in comparison to that of the model group, while FBG levels in the high-dose quercetin group (QR.H) were substantially diminished. Regarding inflammation and the repair of the intestinal barrier, treatment with quercetin led to a substantial decrease in the concentrations of MCP-1, D-LA, and LPS, suggesting a mitigation of inflammatory responses and enhancement of intestinal barrier integrity. Furthermore, quercetin administration markedly reduced the proportional presence of the Aspergillus phylum while increasing gut microbiota diversity, indicating that quercetin has the capacity to modulate the constitution of the intestinal microbiota community. Metabolomic profiling demonstrated that quercetin treatment significantly elevated concentrations of L-Dopa and S-adenosylmethionine (SAM), whereas levels of 3-methylhistidine (3-MET) and L-glutamic acid were significantly diminished. These results indicate that quercetin exerts potent antidiabetic effects by regulating the constitution and functionality of the gut microbiota, improving insulin resistance, and restoration of the intestinal barrier integrity (Yuan et al. 2024).

2.2.3 Celastrol

Celastrol, alternatively referred to as tripterine or tripterin, is a triterpenoid compound. Its molecular structure is defined by the presence of an oxo group at the second position, a hydroxyl group at the third position, and methyl groups located at the ninth and thirteenth positions. This compound is naturally occurring in the root of *Rehmannia*, a plant traditionally utilized in medicinal practices. Celastrol has been identified as a potent agent exhibiting both anti-inflammatory and anti-obesity properties (Zhao et al. 2024).

Celastrol was originally known as an antibiotic demonstrating activity against various Gram-positive bacterial strains. Beginning in the 1980s, a substantial body of research has demonstrated that celastrol possesses anticancer activities, resulting in heightened investigation into its fundamental mechanisms of action. Evidence indicates that celastrol modulates tumor cell proliferation and migration and promotes programmed cell death by regulating various cellular signaling pathways, including NF-κB/COX-2, as well as by inhibiting oncogenic proteins such as Hsp90 (Hieronymus et al. 2006; Sethi et al. 2007). Moreover, a growing body of research suggests it may exhibit potential therapeutic efficacy for a diverse range of other human diseases, encompassing inflammation-associated conditions, autoimmune disorders, and protein misfolding disorders (Nanjundaiah et al. 2012). The anti-inflammatory effects of celastrol are consistent with its traditional application in ethnopharmacology for managing RA. The characterization of celastrol's biosynthetic pathway has facilitated the synthesis of this important compound from simple sugars via yeast fermentation. Zhao and colleagues accomplished this by integrating the genes responsible for celastrol biosynthesis, in conjunction with the TwCPR1, within the genetic material of a yeast strain that had been optimized for terpenoid production (Zhao et al. 2023). The engineered strain demonstrates the ability to synthesize calcium acid, which is subsequently released into the culture medium and undergoes auto-oxidation to form celastrol. Research indicates that encapsulating celastrol within albumin nanoparticles markedly enhances its bioavailability while concurrently diminishing systemic toxicity. This delivery approach is especially beneficial in the therapeutic management of inflammatory metabolic syndrome and renal inflammation. Moreover, complexes of celastrol macromolecules conjugated with tissue-specific targeting ligands—such as cancer cell surface marker proteins or aptamers recognizing neutrophil membrane proteins—have been shown to facilitate the targeted delivery of celastrol to colorectal cancer cells and inflamed pancreatic tissues, respectively (Zhou et al. 2019). In light of these developments, it is evident that celastrol is nearing the realization of its potential as a potent and multifaceted anti-inflammatory compound (Zhao et al. 2024).

Regulate the Function of Dendritic Cells

Both tretinoin and dexamethasone (Dex) were found to suppress the maturation process of immature monocyte-derived dendritic cells (MoDCs) via downregulating the expression of surface markers CD1a, CD40, CD86, and HLA-DR, simultaneously enhancing the expression of CD14. These agents also diminished the capacity of MoDCs to induce lymphocyte proliferation in allogeneic mixed lymphocyte cultures. Moreover, both compounds impeded MoDC maturation by completely abrogating the induction of CD83 expression and failing to upregulate the expression levels of CD40, CD80, CD86, and HLA-DR. At elevated concentrations, specifically 20 ng/mL for tretinoin and 10^{-6} M for Dex, apoptosis was induced in MoDCs, as demonstrated by APO2.7 expression and DNA fragmentation identified via the TUNEL assay. Importantly, tretinoin was observed to augment the phagocytic activity of MoDCs, a property not shared by Dex.

Therefore, the inhibition of DC differentiation by tretinoin, its impact on immature DCs, and the suppression of DC maturation collectively may account for certain immunosuppressive effects observed with tretinoin. This study indicates that dendritic cells represent the principal targets of tretinoin's immunosuppressive mechanisms (Zhu et al. 2005).

Targets LRP1 to Inhibit Fibroblast-Macrophage Crosstalk

Recent research conducted by Zhu et al. has elucidated fundamental pathological mechanisms underlying psoriasis, a chronic inflammatory disorder characterized by autoimmune processes and affecting approximately 125 million individuals worldwide. This study particularly emphasizes the role of fibroblast-macrophage interactions mediated by the chemokine CCL2. Through an interdisciplinary approach, the authors identified the natural triterpenoid celastrol as a promising therapeutic agent via systematic screening of 1896 phytochemicals. Celastrol was shown to effectively disrupt pro-inflammatory intercellular signaling within the psoriatic skin microenvironment. Mechanistic investigations revealed that dermal fibroblasts within psoriatic lesions contribute to disease progression by recruiting macrophages in a CCL2-dependent manner, thereby exacerbating inflammatory cascades. Single-cell multi-omics analyses of patient-derived samples further characterized enhanced fibroblast-macrophage interactome networks, highlighting fibroblasts as central regulators of psoriatic pathogenesis. Preclinical validation demonstrated that celastrol administration produced dose-dependent therapeutic benefits in both murine and nonhuman primate models (Zhu et al. 2025).

Acts on Signaling Pathways Such as NF-κB, STAT, MAPK, TLR, PI3K-AKT-mTOR

Nanjundaiah and colleagues demonstrated that celastrol modulates bone-immune crosstalk, thereby preventing bone degradation in autoimmune arthritis. The study further demonstrated that celastrol suppresses osteoclastogenic factors involved in bone remodeling, including IGF-1, OPN, M-CSF, and RANKL. Additionally, celastrol inhibits matrix-degrading enzymes such as MMP-9, as well as proinflammatory cytokines, notably IL-18, IL-6, and IL-1 (Meng et al. 2020). Celastrol inhibits MMP-9 production by suppressing TLR4 signaling. Specifically, celastrol inhibits IL-17A and LPS-induced cellular invasion and migration by suppressing the expression mediated by MMP-9 through the TLR4/NF-κB signaling pathway. Furthermore, celastrol mitigates bone erosion in CIA mouse models by impeding osteoclast differentiation and activity (Gan et al. 2015). Astry et al. provided evidence demonstrating that celastrol suppressed arthritis in AIA rats by regulating the equilibrium between regulatory and pathogenic T lymphocytes within the inflamed synovial tissue (Astry et al. 2015). Cascão et al. provided evidence demonstrating that celastrol markedly reduced the total population of synoviocytes as well as specific subsets of CD68-positive macrophages, inhibited the progression of joint destruction, and mitigated the degradation of cartilage and the resorption of bone (Cascao et al. 2017; Cascao et al. 2015). Fang and colleagues reported that treatment with celastrol markedly reduced the transcriptional activity of several chemokine genes, their corresponding receptors, and associated molecules—including CCR2 and CXCR4—in RA-FLS (Fang et al. 2017). Wong and colleagues demonstrated that celastrol activates calcium signaling pathways, resulting in a decreased cell population in RASF/RAFLS. Furthermore, celastrol was shown to initiate autophagic cell death within these cells and mitigate arthritis symptoms in AIA rat models via mechanisms involving calcium-dependent binding proteins (Wong et al. 2019).

2.2.4 Resveratrol

Resveratrol, a non-flavonoid polyphenolic compound, was first identified and its importance acknowledged upon its isolation from *Veratrum grandiflorum*, commonly referred to as the white hellebore species.

In the context of the worldwide rise in chronic diseases such as cancer, cardiovascular conditions, and diabetes, there has been a growing academic interest in exploring alternative therapeutic strategies. Resveratrol, a bioactive compound recognized for its anti-angiogenic, immunomodulatory, and neuroprotective properties, has demonstrated significant promise in preclinical research for the prevention of chronic diseases and the promotion of longevity. While the practical application of caloric restriction remains challenging, resveratrol has been proposed as a viable substitute. Found naturally in foods including red grapes, berries, peanuts, and dark chocolate, resveratrol modulates key biological processes including apoptosis and inflammation. It produces its effects through the regulation of multiple signaling pathways, notably NF-κB and PI3K/Akt, thereby positioning it as a highly qualified candidate for the management of cardiovascular disease, diabetes, and cancer. Clinical studies have investigated the safety profile of resveratrol, indicating that daily dosages of up to 5 grams are generally well tolerated. Nevertheless, its effectiveness is influenced by factors such as bioavailability and individual variability (Meng et al. 2020).

Regulation of Th17/Treg Balance Through the SIRT1 Pathway

SIRT1 (Sirtuin 1) is an NAD^+-dependent deacetylase that plays a crucial role in maintaining immune homeostasis through epigenetic modifications and metabolic regulation. Research has demonstrated that SIRT1 modulates the equilibrium between Th17 cells and Treg cells through various mechanisms. First, SIRT1 inhibits Th17 differentiation by deacetylating the transcription factor RORγt, thereby suppressing its activity and reducing the differentiation of proinflammatory Th17 cells. Second, SIRT1 enhances Treg function by promoting the stability of Foxp3, which strengthens the immunosuppressive capacity of Treg cells. Furthermore, SIRT1 modulates cellular metabolic processes, including fatty acid oxidation and glycolysis, thereby affecting the differentiation capacity of Th17 and Treg cells. Dysregulation of this balance is strongly linked to autoimmune disorders, comprising multiple sclerosis and rheumatoid arthritis, as well as chronic inflammation, suggesting that SIRT1 may represent a potential therapeutic target.

Resveratrol, recognized as a prominent AhR antagonist, has been thoroughly examined for its potential applications in the management of cardiovascular diseases, metabolic disorders, aging processes, inflammatory responses, and cancer. Furthermore, preliminary research has suggested that resveratrol may reduce the severity of autoimmune disorders (Oliveira et al. 2017), conditions characterized by enhanced differentiation of Th17 cells and impaired Treg functionality. In a current investigation, Yao and colleagues exhibited that the application of resveratrol led to a decrease in terms of relative abundance of Th17 cells linked to an expansion of regulatory T cell populations within a murine model of ulcerative colitis (Yao et al. 2015). Consequently, it can be inferred that employing resveratrol to modulate the Th17/Treg cell imbalance in the therapeutic management of ITP constitutes a compelling and potentially effective therapeutic strategy.

Recent studies conducted by Guo and colleagues demonstrate that resveratrol can reestablish the equilibrium between Th17 cells and Tregs in ITP through the modulation of the aryl hydrocarbon receptor (AhR) signaling pathway. These results highlight the importance of complex, dual function of AhR signaling in the development and progression of ITP. Mechanistically, environmental and endogenous AhR agonists activate T cell-mediated pathways, leading to pathological Th17 hyperactivation, as evidenced by a 2.3-fold increase in CD4 + IL-17A+ cells in ITP patients, while simultaneously impairing immune tolerance mechanisms. This dysregulation promotes autoreactive B cell differentiation, demonstrated by a 58% increase in antiplatelet antibody titers—a hallmark of ITP progression. These findings suggest that AhR modulation represents a novel therapeutic strategy for ITP, with resveratrol serving both as a mechanistic probe and a potential therapeutic agent. The dual role of AhR signaling—as a disease driver through environmental agonist activation and as a therapeutic target via pharmacological inhibition—underscores its central importance in autoimmune hematology research (Guo et al. 2019).

2.2.5 Berberine

Berberine, commonly referred to as the rhizome of *Berberis vulgaris*, is a naturally occurring quaternary isoquinoline alkaloid. This compound is classified within the category of organic substances referred to as protoberberine alkaloids and their respective derivatives. These compounds are distinguished by a structural framework centered on the protoberberine moiety, comprising a 5,6-dihydrodiphenyl segment fused to a quinoline nucleus, thereby constituting the 5,6-dihydrodibenzo[a,g]quinolizine core structure.

Berberine has been recognized as a significant pharmacophore, serving a crucial function in the identification and development of new therapeutic agents targeting heterochromatic diseases. Despite its considerable therapeutic promise, the clinical utilization of this alkaloid is substantially limited by its unfavorable pharmacokinetic characteristics. To address these challenges, extensive structural modifications of the berberine framework have been pursued to improve its therapeutic effectiveness. Collaborative research efforts have led to notable progress in the clinical translation of berberine, with these structural modifications facilitating novel opportunities for therapeutic applications.

Regulation of Macrophage Polarization Through the AMPK-mTOR Axis

The mTOR and AMPK are critical regulators of cellular survival and metabolic processes, responding to a variety of stimuli, for example, fluctuations in amino acid levels, alterations in cellular energy status, changes in oxygen availability, neurotrophic factors, and exposure to xenobiotic compounds. These signaling pathways orchestrate complex, multilayered mechanisms to maintain cellular homeostasis. Accumulating evidence suggests that dysregulation of mTOR and AMPK pathways is linked to neuronal damage, degeneration, and neurotoxic effects. Nevertheless, the precise molecular mechanisms that underlie these associations remain to be thoroughly elucidated. Although earlier research has predominantly emphasized their opposing roles in the regulation of autophagy, recent studies increasingly implicate modifications in protein synthesis, metabolic reprogramming, and mitochondrial functional adaptations as key contributors to the neuroprotective functions mediated by mTOR and AMPK signaling. Elucidating the functional interplay between these two central metabolic regulators is critically important for developing therapeutic strategies to counteract metabolic dysregulation and enhance cell survival in cerebral injuries and neurodegenerative disorders (Garza-Lombo et al. 2018).

This research examined the impact of berberine on the regulation of apoptosis induced by elevated glucose concentrations, as well as its influence on AMPK activation, mTOR signaling pathways, and the regulatory mechanisms governing autophagy in podocytes. The experimental findings revealed that berberine substantially attenuated the reduction in cell viability, the decreased expression of nephrin and podocin, and the elevation in rates of apoptosis caused by high glucose conditions in murine podocytes. The compound markedly enhanced AMPK phosphorylation while counteracting mTOR hyperactivation and apoptosis induced by high glucose exposure or cotreatment with the AMPK inhibitor compound C. Notably, berberine preserved its antiapoptotic efficacy even in AMPK-silenced podocytes under hyperglycemic conditions. Mechanistic analyses revealed that berberine upregulated multiple autophagic markers, including ULK1 phosphorylation at S317 and S555 residues, Beclin-1 expression, the LC3II/LC3I ratio, and autophagosome formation, while suppressing ULK1 S757 phosphorylation in high glucose-treated podocytes. Furthermore, berberine reversed compound C-induced autophagy suppression. Pharmacological suppression of autophagy through the application of 3-methyladenine or bafilomycin A1 markedly diminished the protective effects of berberine against podocyte apoptosis. These findings collectively indicate that berberine mitigates hyperglycemia-induced podocyte injury through AMPK-dependent activation of autophagic pathways. This study provides novel mechanistic insights into berberine's renoprotective potential in diabetic nephropathy, highlighting its therapeutic relevance for developing interventions against glucose-mediated podocytopathy (Jin et al. 2017).

2.3 Challenges and Security Issues

Although the efficacy of phytochemicals has been partially substantiated by experimental research, clinical trials often face challenges such as variability in bioavailability, inconsistencies in dosing protocols, and heterogeneity among study populations, all of which may impact the results. For instance, the limited bioavailability of curcumin restricts its therapeutic potential in certain demographic groups (Khosravi and Seifert 2024). Formulations demonstrate significant heterogeneity, including whole foods and extracts, in addition to participant lifestyle factors such as dietary patterns, physical activity levels, and concurrent medication use, all of which can markedly influence study outcomes. Moreover, the effectiveness of phytochemicals may differ depending on the characteristics of the study population and the experimental design. Numerous studies have reported an absence of significant effects, particularly in trials with small sample sizes or brief intervention periods (Rudzinska et al. 2023). Resveratrol has yielded inconsistent and inconclusive results, with certain studies failing to demonstrate significant improvements in metabolic health or cardiovascular function, thereby raising doubts regarding its clinical effectiveness (Godos et al. 2024). The constraints noted within the experimental framework, medication administration schedules, and the variability noted in the outcome measures emphasize the necessity for standardized methodologies to improve the comprehension and utilization of phytochemicals (Guo et al. 2024). Table 1 offers an extensive summary of recent investigations in epidemiology and clinical science into phytochemicals, emphasizing their associated health benefits and therapeutic applications (Hossain et al. 2025).

3 Phytochemicals in Metabolic Diseases

3.1 Overview of Diabetes, Hypertension, Hyperlipidemia, and Atherosclerosis

Metabolic diseases constitute a category of pathological conditions arising from dysregulated metabolic pathways, predominantly characterized by impairments in glucose and lipid metabolism alongside vascular dysfunction. These disorders frequently present concomitantly, encompassing diabetes mellitus, hypertension, hyperlipidemia, and related comorbidities, which collectively play a significant role in the onset and progression of atherosclerotic cardiovascular disease (ASCVD).

Diabetes mellitus is a multifaceted metabolic disorder characterized by a complex etiology involving genetic, lifestyle, and environmental factors. The development of diabetes primarily results from the interplay between genetic susceptibility and environmental exposures, which culminates in disrupted glucose metabolism and impaired regulation of blood glucose levels. Simultaneously, hypertension-related cardiovascular disease (CVD) remains a major global public health concern,

Table 1 Epidemiological and clinical findings on phytochemicals (Hossain et al. 2025)

Phytochemical	Study details	Findings	Disease risk reduction	Relevance	Reference
Curcumin	5-week animal study with OLETF rats (T2DM model)	Improved glucose homeostasis, lipid profile, cognitive function, and reduced inflammation and ER stress with exercise + curcumin	Potential to mitigate diabetes-related cognitive dysfunction	Suggests combined diet and exercise benefits in T2DM	Cho et al. (2020)
Resveratrol	Phase 2 RCT with 100 COVID-19 outpatients in Ohio	Lower rates of hospitalization, ER visits, and pneumonia vs. placebo	Potential reduction in severe COVID-19 complications	Highlights resveratrol's antiviral and anti-inflammatory potential in COVID-19 treatment	McCreary et al. (2022)
Allicin	4-week study on ethanol-fed mice	Reduced gut permeability, altered microbiota, and suppressed hepatic inflammation via CD14-TLR4 pathway	Potential to mitigate alcohol-induced liver inflammation	Highlights gut-liver axis modulation by allicin	Panyod et al. (2020)
Anthocyanins	24-week RCT with 206 older adults (MCI or cardiometabolic disorders)	No significant group difference in episodic memory, but improved memory slope in weeks 8–24	Potential to slow cognitive decline	Suggests anthocyanins may aid in dementia prevention	Aarsland et al. (2022)
Lycopene	Review of preclinical prostate cancer models	Demonstrated anti-cancer activity in xenograft, chemically induced, and transgenic mouse models; outcomes depend on dose and timing	Potential to reduce prostate cancer risk	Highlights role of lycopene and tomatoes in prostate cancer prevention	Moran et al. (2022)

(continued)

Table 1 (continued)

Phytochemical	Study details	Findings	Disease risk reduction	Relevance	Reference
EGCG	2-month RCT with 50 T2DM patients	Improved antioxidant capacity, lipid profile, blood pressure, and AIP	Reduced cardiovascular risk and oxidative stress	Highlights EGCG's potential benefits in T2DM management	Bazyar et al. (2020)
Soy Isoflavones	48-month prospective study with 1460 BC survivors	Moderate pre- and post-diagnosis intake reduced all-cause and BC-specific mortality (up to 66% lower risk)	Improved survival outcomes in BC survivors	Suggests soy's safety and benefits in BC prognosis	Ho et al. (2021)
Quercetin	8-week study on streptozotocin induced diabetic rat models	Restored body weight, insulin, glucose, and renal parameters; reduced inflammation and oxidative stress; improved kidney histology	Potential prevention of diabetes-associated kidney dysfunction	Highlights quercetin's reno-protective and antidiabetic effects	Rahmani et al. (2023)
Enterolactone	5-year study with 2105 BC survivors	Improved short-term survival; other phytoestrogens linked to poorer prognosis	Potential BC survival benefit	Highlights enterolactone's short-term effects	Jaskulski et al. (2020)

substantially contributing to morbidity and mortality worldwide. Epidemiological studies have consistently demonstrated a positive correlation between elevated arterial blood pressure and an increased risk of adverse clinical events, such as myocardial infarction, stroke, and progression to end-stage renal disease. Atherosclerosis is recognized as the final pathological manifestation of metabolic disturbances, with its progression influenced by multiple interrelated factors. Clinical investigations have further revealed that the prevalence of lower extremity atherosclerosis is significantly higher in diabetic individuals with concomitant hypertension compared to those with diabetes alone.

Metabolic diseases, which represent the most prevalent and frequently occurring chronic conditions, have attracted significant attention both nationally and internationally due to their associated risk factors, underlying pathophysiological mechanisms, and strategies for effective prevention and management. The treatment of metabolic disorders necessitates the implementation of multifaceted interventions aimed at precisely modulating critical nodes within the disease pathways. Lifestyle modification remains the foundational approach, primarily involving calorie-restricted dietary regimens and consistent physical activity. Pharmacotherapeutic options encompass conventional hypoglycemic and lipid-lowering agents, alongside emerging biological therapies. Of particular interest is the regulatory potential of phytochemicals in metabolic diseases, as their multi-targeted mechanisms present a promising avenue for the management of chronic illnesses such as diabetes (Hsu et al. 2005; Psaty et al. 2001).

3.2 *Diabetes*

Diabetes mellitus, a metabolic condition, is distinguished by persistently increased concentrations of blood glucose and is linked to numerous severe complications, such as diabetic nephropathy, diabetic retinopathy, and diabetic foot ulcers. Diabetic foot represents one of the most serious complications associated with diabetes. The normal wound healing process, which involves inflammation, angiogenesis, and ECM remodeling, becomes disrupted and stagnant in diabetic foot ulcers. Persistent, nonhealing wounds are a characteristic feature of these ulcers. Data from the International Diabetes Federation (IDF) indicate that, as of 2021, the global population of individuals diagnosed with diabetes reached 537 million, with approximately 140 million cases reported in China, representing the highest prevalence worldwide. Although current diabetes management primarily relies on pharmacological treatments, traditional medical systems in various countries recognize the therapeutic value of native plant-based resources for diabetes care. Studies reveal that more than 30% of individuals with diabetes utilize complementary and alternative medicine modalities as part of their treatment strategies.

Controlling blood glucose levels and minimizing fluctuations are fundamental to the treatment of diabetes. At present, Western medicine provides a variety of hypoglycemic agents, encompassing conventional drugs such as metformin, sulfonylureas, glinides, thiazolidinediones, and α-glucosidase inhibitors, alongside more recently developed classes including dipeptidyl peptidase IV inhibitors, sodium-glucose cotransporter 2 inhibitors, and GLP-1 receptor agonists. These newer hypoglycemic drugs have multiple mechanisms of action and can promote weight loss, improve lipid and protein metabolism, reduce uric acid levels, and provide cardiovascular and renal benefits. Furthermore, herbs, natural products, and dietary supplements have exhibited notable hypoglycemic properties. As a result, the pursuit of effective alternatives to traditional hypoglycemic medications, including functional foods and dietary components, has attracted growing interest within the domains of medical and nutritional research.

3.2.1 Resveratrol

Resveratrol, a natural bioactive compound, can regulate blood glucose levels through multiple mechanisms. This substance not only facilitates glucose uptake and utilization by cells, but also increases the production of GLUT4 transporters in insulin-sensitive cells, thereby enhancing glucose metabolism efficiency. Research has shown that resveratrol improves insulin secretion and increases insulin sensitivity through the activation of SIRT1 and AMPK expression. Furthermore, resveratrol contributes to the regulation of mitochondrial homeostasis by maintaining the equilibrium between proapoptotic and protective proteins, thereby delaying premature senescence of islet β cells. It also effectively inhibits the overproduction of ROS by facilitating the synthesis of the antioxidant enzyme SOD1. These actions reduce oxidative damage to islet cells and provide a multifaceted protective mechanism for diabetes treatment.

Extended exposure to high levels of glucose and lipid toxicity results in the accumulation of ROS within islet β cells, thereby inducing oxidative stress. This oxidative stress subsequently compromises the functionality of islet β cells and accelerates the progression of diabetes. Furthermore, oxidative stress plays a pivotal role in the development of complications associated with diabetes mellitus. Therefore, mitigating oxidative stress is essential for the effective management of diabetes and its associated chronic complications (Tangvarasittichai 2015). Studies have confirmed that resveratrol can scavenge free radicals, particularly hydroxyl radicals. Resveratrol exhibits stronger antioxidant capacity than vitamin E and vitamin C. Its mechanism of action involves inhibiting the formation of glutathione disulfide, thereby maintaining glutathione in its reduced state to prevent free radical formation (He et al. 2016). RESV can modulate the signaling pathway of HO-1, increase HO-1 expression, and maintain intracellular redox balance. Additionally, resveratrol protects cells from oxidatively modified low-density lipoprotein by inhibiting NADPH oxidase activity (Oshaghi et al. 2017). Elevated concentrations of free fatty acids (FFAs) serve as a direct contributor to oxidative stress in the context of diabetes. The oxidative stress triggered by FFAs is potentially linked to a reduction in the functional activity of the forkhead box transcription factor 1 (FOXO1). Studies have shown that resveratrol can reduce FOXO1 activity by activating SIRT1, thereby mitigating oxidative stress-induced damage caused by FFAs. Resveratrol demonstrates substantial antioxidative properties that mitigate oxidative stress damage caused by elevated glucose or lipid concentrations, thereby contributing critically to the management of diabetes.

Resveratrol has been demonstrated to improve glucose uptake in tissues that are responsive to insulin, including skeletal muscle, adipose tissue, and the liver. Furthermore, it facilitates glycogen synthesis in the liver and reduces insulin resistance. The hypoglycemic properties of RESV are likely mediated by the upregulation of GLUT4 expression in insulin-sensitive cells, as well as the promotion of GLUT4 translocation to the plasma membrane, thereby enhancing cellular glucose uptake. In addition, RESV activates the PI3K and Akt signaling cascade, which contributes to improved insulin signal transduction. Upregulation of SIRT1 expression by RESV increases glucose-stimulated insulin secretion (GSIS) and enhances glucose tolerance. Overall, RESV improves GSIS and insulin sensitivity through activation of SIRT1 (Su et al. 2006).

3.2.2 Momordica Charantia Saponin

Saponins derived from Momordica charantia (MCS) exhibit hypoglycemic effects in diabetic mice through multiple mechanistic pathways. MCS contributes to antidiabetic activity by improving glycemic control, reducing lipid levels, and enhancing antioxidant defenses. Additionally, it enhances the enzymatic activity of hexokinase and promotes glycogen synthesis, promotes the restoration of pancreatic histological structure, and enhances insulin secretion.

The study demonstrated that total saponins extracted from *Momordica charantia* markedly reduced blood glucose concentrations and body weight in rats. Additionally, these compounds elevated the ratio of heart weight to body weight and substantially enhanced cardiac function parameters, including CK and LDH levels. Apoptosis and antiapoptosis mechanisms have long been recognized as critical factors in myocardial injury. Numerous studies have reported significant apoptosis in myocardial cells during the early stages of diabetes, with apoptosis worsening in the middle and late stages. The extent of apoptosis is closely correlated with the severity of cardiomyopathy, and increased apoptosis significantly raises the risk of developing cardiomyopathy. Currently, Bcl-2, Fas, FasL, and p35 are the primary genes identified as regulators of apoptosis and antiapoptosis. Fas and FasL are particularly associated with apoptosis. Fas is a key membrane receptor in the tumor necrosis factor family that mediates apoptotic signal transduction. It primarily interacts with FasL, its natural ligand. Upon binding to FasL, Fas activates the FADD in the cytoplasm, which subsequently triggers the activation of caspase-3, caspase-7, and caspase-8, leading to apoptosis. Total saponins from Momordica charantia significantly reduce the expression of Fas and FasL in myocardial tissue, thereby inhibiting myocardial cell apoptosis and protecting the myocardium (Ebert et al. 2000; Lakhlani et al. 1997; Lou et al. 1992).

Karaviloside XI, a predominant triterpenoid constituent of MCS, has been demonstrated to exhibit hypoglycemic properties by augmenting the phosphorylation of AMPK and facilitating the translocation of GLUT4 in L6 myotube cells and 3 T3-L1 adipocyte cells. MCS regulates glucose metabolism via various molecular targets, including the liver and the small intestine. It governs multiple aspects of glucose metabolism, encompassing glucose absorption, consumption, and the suppression of glucose production. The underlying mechanisms responsible for these effects include the activation of AMPK, the enhancement of GLUT4 translocation, and the suppression of α-glucosidase enzymatic activity (Deng et al. 2023).

3.3 *Hypertension and Cardiovascular Disease*

Hypertension arises from a multitude of factors and pathological conditions and constitutes a primary contributor to damage in critical organs such as the heart, brain, and kidneys, as well as to cardiovascular disease. In recent years, the progression of the national economy, increased life expectancy, enhanced living standards, accelerated lifestyle pace, and dietary shifts toward high salt, fat, and calorie consumption have become prevalent. These changes, combined with occupational and psychological stressors and physical inactivity, have led to a progressive increase in the prevalence of hypertension, notably affecting younger demographics. Hypertension and its associated complications, including coronary heart disease and stroke, are strongly associated with elevated rates of morbidity and mortality. Traditional risk factors for hypertension are classified into non-modifiable and modifiable categories. Extensive research has established significant associations between hypertension and conditions such as dyslipidemia, diabetes mellitus, insulin resistance, and elevated C-reactive protein levels.

Cardiovascular disease, also known as circulatory system disease, refers to abnormalities in the organs and tissues responsible for transporting blood throughout the human body. The principal anatomical locations impacted by these conditions are the heart and the vascular system. This encompasses coronary artery disease, which involves vascular impairment affecting the myocardial blood supply; cerebrovascular disease, characterized by vascular dysfunction compromising cerebral blood flow; and peripheral arterial disease, which pertains to vascular abnormalities reducing blood supply to the extremities; rheumatic heart disease, characterized by injury to the myocardial tissue and cardiac valves, arises as a consequence of rheumatic fever subsequent to streptococcal infection. Congenital heart disease encompasses birth defects stemming from structural malformations that disrupt normal cardiac development and function. Additionally, deep vein thrombosis and pulmonary embolism involve the formation of blood clots within the veins of the lower extremities, which may detach and migrate to the heart and pulmonary vasculature. Risk factors associated with cardiovascular disease can be categorized into modifiable and non-modifiable groups. Modifiable risk factors encompass hypertension, tobacco use, hyperlipidemia, diabetes mellitus, unhealthy dietary patterns, obesity, physical inactivity, and psychological stress. In contrast, non-modifiable risk factors include biological sex, chronological age, ethnicity, and genetic predisposition. Most modifiable risk factors are associated with lifestyle behaviors and patterns of conduct. For instance, hypertension, identified as the principal determinant of risk for cardiovascular and cerebrovascular diseases, is affected by variables including tobacco use and obesity, high sodium consumption, sedentary behavior, and dietary imbalances. Consequently, the adoption of healthier lifestyle practices and behavioral modifications has the potential to substantially decrease the prevalence of cardiovascular and cerebrovascular diseases (Assmann et al. 1999; Grundy et al. 1999).

Research indicates that cardiovascular and cerebrovascular diseases have emerged as the predominant causes of mortality in China, with hypertension recognized as the primary risk factor. Effective prevention and management of hypertension are essential strategies for reducing the incidence of cardiovascular diseases. Phytochemicals have attracted increasing interest in the context of hypertension and cardiovascular disease treatment due to their multicomponent synergistic effects and advantageous safety profiles (Zhou 2002).

3.3.1 Allicin

Garlic (*Allium sativum* L.) is a species within the genus Allium, which is classified under the family Liliaceae. Due to its richness in biologically active compounds and nutrients, garlic has been used for disease prevention for over five thousand years. A considerable volume of research, carried out at both national and international levels, has demonstrated that garlic exhibits notable cardiovascular benefits and holds significant promise in the management of cardiovascular disease.

The pathogenesis of cardiovascular disease is complex and involves multiple interacting factors. Dysfunction of endothelial cells is strongly associated with coronary heart disease, hyperlipidemia, and the initial stages of atherosclerosis. Studies have shown that alliin exhibits significant antioxidant properties, substantially decreasing monocyte adhesion to endothelial cells and mitigating the TNF-α-induced upregulation of VCAM-1 at both the mRNA and protein expression levels. Furthermore, alliin inhibits the generation of superoxide anions and the upregulation of the NADH oxidase subunit NOX4. It also inhibits the initiation of signaling pathways involving JNK, ERK1/2, and IκBα, while inhibiting the dissipation of mitochondrial membrane potential. These findings suggest that alliin effectively alleviates TNF-α-mediated inflammatory damage and may play a protective role in cardiovascular disease. Other studies have reported that alliinase, alliin, and their combination can significantly scavenge ·O2 and ·OH radicals at certain concentrations and inhibit lipid peroxidation. The scavenging ability of the combination is stronger, suggesting that allicin, produced by the reaction of alliinase and alliin, has a potent free radical scavenging effect and serves as an effective antioxidant in vitro. Nrf2 functions as a nuclear transcription factor which is fundamental to the regulation of oxidative stress within cells. (Mann et al. 2007). Experiments conducted in vivo validated that allicin has been demonstrated to significantly enhance cardiovascular function, as well as reduce cardiomyocyte hypertrophy and fibrosis in rats, by augmenting the Nrf2-mediated antioxidant signaling cascade (Li et al. 2012). Components of garlic extract, such as allicin and alliin, can inhibit norepinephrine-induced hypertrophy and apoptosis in rat cardiomyocytes through their antioxidative properties. The fundamental mechanism is likely associated with the generation of NO and H_2S. In summary, the bioactive constituents of garlic demonstrate significant antioxidant properties and free radical scavenging capabilities, which may effectively retard the initiation and advancement of cardiovascular diseases (Louis et al. 2012).

3.3.2 Anthocyanin

Anthocyanin represents a principal pigment responsible for the coloration observed in petals and fruits. This compound is localized within the cell sap of plant tissues and functions as a natural, edible pigment. Anthocyanins are extensively distributed across a variety of fruits and vegetables, including purple sweet potatoes, blueberries, grapes, and black raspberries. Empirical research has revealed that anthocyanins exhibit multiple physiological activities, encompassing antioxidant, anticarcinogenic, hepatoprotective, and vision-enhancing properties (Tsuda et al. 2003).

Anthocyanins exhibit a strong affinity for collagen, enabling them to form a protective antioxidant layer that safeguards cells and tissues against oxidative damage induced by free radicals. Additionally, these compounds contribute to vascular health by enhancing vascular resistance, decreasing capillary fragility, preserving vascular permeability, and improving the functional integrity of capillaries, veins, and arteries. Such effects support the circulatory system and contribute to a reduced risk of cardiovascular diseases. Moreover, anthocyanins have been demonstrated to alleviate conditions such as varicose veins and edema, protect intracellular DNA from damage—thereby potentially diminishing the risk of various cancers—and lower LDL cholesterol levels, which aid in the prevention of atherosclerosis progression.

Recent studies have demonstrated that the vasomotor tone of blood vessels is modulated by vasodilatory agents secreted by vascular endothelial cells, with nitric oxide identified as a principal vasodilator. Investigations into anthocyanins have revealed their potential role in the prevention of cardiovascular diseases, primarily through the enhancement of nitric oxide synthase enzymatic activity. This upregulation leads to elevated nitric oxide concentrations within endothelial cells, promoting vasodilation and thereby facilitating relaxation of the cardiovascular system. Furthermore, anthocyanins exhibit inhibitory effects on vascular endothelial cell collagenase, thereby contributing to the preservation of vascular wall integrity. They also markedly suppress platelet aggregation, exhibiting a safety profile that surpasses that of aspirin. In addition, anthocyanins act as direct scavengers of free radicals and hydroxyl radicals, mitigating oxidative stress during myocardial infarction treatment. Experimental evidence indicates that anthocyanins derived from cranberries can inhibit low-density lipoprotein oxidation, reduce platelet aggregation and adhesion, and diminish foam cell formation by suppressing smooth muscle cell proliferation and lipid phagocytosis. Collectively, these biological activities play a significant role in the prevention of atherosclerosis. Moreover, anthocyanins contribute to atherosclerosis risk reduction by inhibiting endothelial cell proliferation (Inaguma et al. 2011; Renaud and de Lorgeril 1992).

3.3.3 Tanshinone IIA

Salvia miltiorrhiza exhibits pharmacological properties including coronary artery dilation, prevention of myocardial ischemia and infarction, enhancement of microcirculatory function, and reduction of myocardial oxygen demand. Consequently, it is extensively utilized in the management of diverse cardiovascular disorders. The main components of *Salvia miltiorrhiza* include fat-soluble diterpenoids and water-soluble phenolic acids found primarily in the root, as well as flavonoids, triterpenoids, sterols, and other compounds.

Left ventricular hypertrophy frequently occurs as a complication associated with hypertension. Angiotensin II plays a crucial role in stimulating myocardial cell hypertrophy induced by pathological factors such as pressure overload. Research has shown that tanshinone IIA can suppress angiotensin II-mediated cardiac hypertrophy. This effect is predominantly accomplished through the inhibition of angiotensin II interaction with G protein-coupled receptors, which subsequently prevents the activation of PLC and PKC. This action reduces intracellular calcium ion (Ca^{2+}) levels in myocardial cells and disrupts the transmission of hypertrophic signals to the nucleus. Ang II significantly enhances the expression of ANP and β-actin in myocardial cells. Salvianic acid A can inhibit the Ang II-induced upregulation of ANP and β-actin gene expression, thereby reducing protein accumulation in myocardial cells—particularly the accumulation of abnormal proteins—and preventing myocardial hypertrophy. This mechanism is attributed to Salvianic acid A's role as a calcium antagonist, which inhibits the rise in intracellular calcium ion concentration in myocardial cells.

Free radicals exhibit high reactivity and can interact with diverse cellular constituents, including membrane phospholipids, proteins, and nucleic acids, resulting in structural damage and metabolic impairments within cells. *Salvia miltiorrhiza* demonstrates the capacity to neutralize free radicals. Its bioactive compounds, such as tanshinone, danshensu, salvianolic acids, protocatechuic aldehyde, caffeic acid, and rosmarinic acid, possess potent antioxidant activities. Empirical research indicates that tanshinone IIA can suppress the activation of NADH/NADPH oxidase located on the cell membrane, augment SOD activity, scavenge oxygen-derived free radicals, inhibit lipid peroxidation, and thereby provide protective benefits to vascular endothelial cells.

Intracellular calcium overload is recognized as a critical factor in the pathophysiology of myocardial ischemia-reperfusion injury. Research indicates that cellular damage induced by various stimuli disrupts the calcium homeostasis between mitochondria and the sarcoplasmic reticulum, resulting in a marked elevation of intracellular Ca^{2+} levels. This imbalance in calcium homeostasis is a critical pathological feature of this type of injury. The water-soluble components of *Salvia miltiorrhiza* have demonstrated potential protective effects in this process. Since myocardial reperfusion injury is directly related to the disruption of intracellular and extracellular calcium distribution caused by calcium overload, the calcium antagonistic properties of Danshensu are regarded as one of the core mechanisms underlying its cardioprotective effects (Fu et al. 2007; Jang et al. 2006).

The ability of Salvianic acid A to inhibit nitrite is significantly stronger than that of cysteine and ascorbic acid. Peroxynitrite is a key mediator in diseases such as myocardial injury and atherosclerosis. Cysteine and ascorbic acid are two primary antioxidants in the body. Therefore, the presence of Salvianic acid A effectively protects the body from nitrite-induced damage, indicating that its inhibition of peroxynitrite is a crucial molecular mechanism underlying its pharmacological effects, including myocardial protection.

Salvia miltiorrhiza can improve blood viscosity, concentration, aggregation, and stagnation in experimental animals through multiple targets. It protects the function of vascular endothelial cells, thereby enhancing blood circulation, which is beneficial for treating various cardiovascular diseases. With the ongoing progression of technological methodologies and continual enhancements in research, it is imperative to conduct more in-depth investigations into the pharmacological mechanisms of *Salvia miltiorrhiza*, a TCM herb employed to enhance blood circulation and alleviate blood stasis, in order to identify novel therapeutic targets and effects.

3.4 Disorders of Lipid Metabolism and Atherosclerosis

Abnormal lipid metabolism refers to the atypical processes involved in the synthesis, degradation, digestion, absorption, and transport of lipids within the body, resulting in either elevated or reduced lipid levels across various tissues, which in turn affect physiological functions. This condition encompasses both physiological variations and pathological states. The primary lipids circulating in the bloodstream include cholesterol, triacylglycerols (TAG), phospholipids (PL), and free fatty acids. Clinically, dyslipidemia is categorized into two main types: primary and secondary. Primary dyslipidemia is typically linked to genetic and hereditary factors, whereas secondary dyslipidemia arises from metabolic disorders or is influenced by factors such as age, diet, tobacco use, and alcohol consumption. The majority of lipid-lowering agents employed in clinical settings are prescription drugs that necessitate medical oversight due to the potential for adverse effects. For instance, statins, a widely used class of lipid-lowering medications, are associated with side effects including hepatic dysfunction, myalgia, and gastrointestinal disturbances. In traditional medicine, commonly utilized lipid-lowering substances include red yeast rice, hawthorn, ginkgo leaves, and turmeric, many of which are believed to enhance blood circulation, strengthen the spleen, and alleviate digestive stagnation. Empirical studies have substantiated the efficacy of TCM in modulating blood lipid levels, indicating its potential as an effective approach to lipid regulation.

Atherosclerosis (AS) is a vascular disorder distinguished by the gradual buildup of lipids and inflammatory cells within the structural confines of medium and large arterial vessels, resulting in significant incidence of disease and death rates worldwide. It is a critical pathological basis for common cardiovascular and cerebrovascular diseases, including myocardial infarction, stroke, and disabling peripheral arterial diseases. To date, the pathogenesis of AS is not fully understood. Multiple theories exist, involving various risk factors, which has resulted in a lack of effective preventive and therapeutic drugs in clinical practice. Extensive basic and clinical research has delineated multiple risk factors associated with AS, encompassing hyperlipidemia, hyperglycemia (diabetes mellitus), hypercysteinemia, obesity, activation of the RAAS, tobacco use, hypercoagulability (e.g., elevated tissue factor and thrombin levels), disturbances in trace element metabolism (including iron, copper, zinc, selenium, chromium, manganese, and germanium), and imbalances in endogenous bioactive substances (such as 5-hydroxytryptamine, nitric oxide, and endothelin-1), as well as chronic stress and other factors. Various theoretical frameworks have been suggested for the purpose of elucidating the pathogenesis of AS, including the lipid infiltration theory, VSMC proliferation theory, oxidative stress theory, calcium overload theory, shear stress theory, and inflammation theory. Notably, the inflammatory hypothesis of AS represents a relatively recent conceptual advancement that has attracted considerable scientific interest. Extensive research has been conducted, yielding substantial findings and leading to a general consensus (Croca et al. 2021; Mozaffarian et al. 2016; Yu et al. 2019).

Atherosclerosis develops through two distinct stages. The initial stage is characterized by hyperlipidemia (dyslipidemia), which corresponds to the early and intermediate phases of the disease. The subsequent stage involves the middle to late phases, marked by the formation of atherosclerotic plaques. Dietary preferences favoring high-fat intake and unhealthy eating patterns disrupt the homeostasis and composition of the gastrointestinal microbiota. This disruption impairs the digestion and absorption of excess lipids, leading to disorders in lipid metabolism. Such metabolic disturbances alter the body's basal metabolic equilibrium, eliciting stress responses and initiating oxidative stress. These processes manifest as abnormalities in blood lipid profiles and the relative proportions of various biochemical substances, thereby contributing to the onset and progression of hyperlipidemia. Notably, hyperlipidemia, coupled with increased blood viscosity in microvascular and small blood vessels, constitutes the initial stage of atherosclerosis (Ross 1993).

Hyperlipidemia (dyslipidemia) indicates the commencement of oxidative stress injury. The persistent accumulation of oxidative stress plays a role in the advancement of atherosclerosis and its complications during the intermediate and advanced phases. Dyslipidemia causes microcirculatory disorders, disrupting material exchange in the microcirculation and resulting in basal metabolic dysfunction of cells. This dysfunction induces dormancy, decay, and inflammatory damage in vascular wall cells, impairing their function. Consequently, lipid particles, proteoglycans, and other substances accumulate in the intima of the vascular walls of medium and large arteries, promoting the formation and progression of atherosclerotic plaques. This process impacts multiple tissues and organs, resulting in a range of complications and facilitating the advancement of chronic metabolic disorders. Dyslipidemia is integral to the initiation and advancement of atherosclerosis. Consequently, the proactive management of blood lipid concentrations, along with other risk factors associated with atherosclerosis, is imperative for the prevention and mitigation of the onset and progression of this condition (Ness et al. 2000).

3.4.1 Curcumin

Curcumin, a bioactive substance naturally, is extracted from the dried rhizomes of the turmeric plant, turmeric root, and zedoary. It demonstrates a wide array of pharmacological properties characterized by low toxicity and favorable tolerability, highlighting its potential for both economic and therapeutic applications. Contemporary biomedical research has revealed that the pathogenesis of numerous human diseases is closely associated with the production of free radicals and the subsequent activation of inflammatory pathways. The extensive pharmacological effects of curcumin are largely attributed to its potent antioxidant and anti-inflammatory activities. Over the past several decades, curcumin has been extensively utilized in the management of inflammation-related disorders, such as cancer, atherosclerosis, diabetes mellitus, and RA. Recent studies have further clarified the antiatherosclerotic mechanisms of curcumin, emphasizing its ability to exert anti-inflammatory effects, inhibit platelet aggregation, enhance anticoagulant activity, provide antioxidative protection, scavenge reactive oxygen species, suppress smooth muscle cell proliferation, and lower lipid levels. It is now recognized that curcumin mediates its multifaceted and pleiotropic anti-atherosclerotic effects through a complex network of cellular and molecular pathways.

The inflammatory response is involved throughout the entire process of atherosclerosis, from its initiation and progression to the formation and eventual rupture of arterial plaques (Peeters and Chizzolini 2011). Curcumin exhibits potent anti-inflammatory effects on acute, subacute, and chronic inflammatory responses. It can modulate molecular targets associated with inflammation and inhibit the expression of inflammatory mediators. Research has shown that curcumin modulates the activity of multiple transcription factors, cytokines, adhesion molecules, and protein kinases that play critical roles in inflammatory pathways (Aggarwal and Harikumar 2009). Curcumin can effectively inhibit the production of TNF-α cytokines in smooth muscle cells and macrophages by suppressing the breakdown of IκB and the subsequent nuclear translocation of NF-κB. This inhibition of the NF-κB signaling pathway subsequently reduces the expression of COX-2 and iNOS (Gonzales and Orlando 2008). The latter two enzymes serve as essential regulators of the inflammatory response and are intimately linked to the pathological mechanisms involved in human tumors and inflammatory disorders. Additionally, curcumin may prevent angiogenesis by inhibiting COX activation and inhibition of MAPK signaling pathways, thereby decreasing the prevalence of chronic inflammatory disorders, for example, cancer and atherosclerosis, that are driven by angiogenesis (Binion et al. 2008).

In the circulatory system, blood lipids are not present in a free state; rather, they associate with proteins to form lipoprotein complexes, such as chylomicrons, very low-density lipoproteins (VLDL), LDL, and HDL. Hyperlipidemia results from excessive production or impaired clearance of VLDL and the subsequent conversion of VLDL to LDL. Conditions such as obesity, diabetes, alcohol overdose, nephrotic syndrome, and genetic defects can lead to excessive hepatic production of VLDL, abnormal increases in LDL and TC, and impaired LDL clearance, which are often related to structural defects in apolipoprotein B (ApoB). Research has demonstrated that curcumin supplementation markedly decreases concentrations of FFA, TG, TC, and LDL-C. Concurrently, it elevates HDL-C levels, the HDL-C to TC ratio, and the ApoA-1/ApoB ratio. Furthermore, curcumin enhances the expression of apolipoprotein A and paraoxonase in plasma, while also diminishing lipid peroxide accumulation in hepatic tissue (Jang et al. 2008). Numerous investigations employing animal models have established that curcumin significantly reduces cholesterol concentrations in blood lipids, potentially through the reduction of bile acid synthesis in the liver. An increased rate of bile acid uptake and metabolic abnormalities can lead to elevated cholesterol and lipid absorption, thereby accelerating the development of hyperlipidemia. CYP7A1 (7α-hydroxylase) acts as the rate-determining enzyme in the biosynthetic pathway of bile acids and is essential for the regulation of bile acid production. Curcumin can lower blood cholesterol concentrations and reduce the incidence of hyperlipidemia by downregulating the expression of the CYP7A1 gene (Katz et al. 2009; Manjunatha and Srinivasan 2007).

3.4.2 Phenolic Compounds

Tea has historically been a traditional beverage within Chinese culture and continues to rank among the most widely consumed drinks globally. Tea polyphenols, identified as the primary bioactive compounds in tea, demonstrate considerable therapeutic potential in the treatment and prevention of cardiovascular diseases. These compounds represent a class of polyhydroxy phenolic substances found in tea, encompassing more than thirty distinct phenolic constituents. Generally, the mass fraction of tea polyphenols in dried tea leaves ranges from approximately 12% to 25%, including various subclasses such as flavanols, flavonols, flavonoids, anthocyanins, phenolic acids, and other related compounds. Among these, flavanols are the predominant components, primarily catechins. Catechins are flavanol derivatives characterized by the α-phenylbenzodihydropyran structure and constitute about 70% to 80% of many tea polyphenols by mass. Catechins can be categorized into four separate categories grounded in their chemical structures: EC, EGC, ECG, and EGCG. Tea polyphenols, which are found in elevated concentrations in tea, constitute the primary bioactive compounds and have been demonstrated to confer substantial cardioprotective effects. Recent research has further elucidated that the tea polyphenols effectively mitigate and manage medical conditions, for example, atherosclerosis, thrombosis, myocarditis, coronary heart disease, arrhythmia, and myocardial ischemia/reperfusion (I/R) injury. As a natural polyphenol complex, tea polyphenols are easily obtainable and exhibit broad and pronounced biological effects. Consequently, research and development efforts focusing on tea polyphenols as functional food components and medicinal agents have garnered increasing attention (Nakachi et al. 2000; Stangl et al. 2007; Tipoe et al. 2007).

Hyperlipidemia constitutes a significant contributing factor for cardiovascular disorder. Increased concentrations of LDL-C combined with decreased levels of HDL-C in the circulatory system are associated with damage to endothelial cells, heightened vascular permeability, and the accelerated accumulation of LDL-C beneath the endothelial layer. Recent research has indicated that tea polyphenols can effectively lower serum TC, TG, and LDL-C concentrations in individuals with hyperlipidemia, while concurrently elevating HDL-C levels. These effects collectively contribute to the restoration and preservation of vascular endothelial function. Catechins, a major component of tea polyphenols, possess antioxidant properties that scavenge free radicals, inhibit cholesterol oxidation and the formation of rancid substances, and reduce lipid deposition in the blood vessel walls. Additionally, tea polyphenols inhibit the oxidation of unsaturated fatty acids in food, lower serum total cholesterol, and help maintain lipid homeostasis within the arterial wall. Research investigating the impact of tea polyphenols derived from green tea extract on blood lipid profiles has demonstrated decreases in TG, TC, and LDL-C in peripheral blood, accompanied by an elevation in HDL-C levels. The lipid-lowering activity of tea polyphenols was found to be stronger than that of inositol nicotinate, indicating their superior efficacy in inhibiting hyperlipidemia. Furthermore, research suggests that tea polyphenols inhibit the intestinal absorption of both endogenous and exogenous cholesterol and accelerate cholesterol metabolism (Tenore et al. 2015).

The occurrence and progression of AS are closely associated with plasma lipid levels. The accumulation of LDL is associated with an elevated risk of atherosclerosis, while HDL contributes to the reduction of lipid concentrations and thereby attenuates the progression of atherosclerosis. Additionally, apolipoproteins serve a fundamental function in the transport and metabolism of blood lipids, and their dysfunction may result in disruptions of lipid transport and metabolic dysfunctions. Oxidative modification of LDL can cause vascular endothelial injury, and cholesterol deposition in the vascular wall ultimately induces atherosclerosis. A substantial body of research has demonstrated that tea polyphenols exhibit a substantial protective effect against atherosclerosis (Khan and Mukhtar 2013; Santulli 2015). It has been found that tea polyphenols can reduce the activity of phospholipase A2 and cyclooxygenase, while increasing the activity of superoxide dismutase in red blood cells. Additionally, they can decrease platelet aggregation and hemagglutination tendency. Tea polyphenols exhibit anti-atherosclerotic effects by stabilizing the body's redox balance and inhibiting the oxidation of LDL. Recent studies have elucidated that chronic inflammatory responses, mediated by endothelial dysfunction, play a pivotal role in the pathophysiological mechanisms underlying atherosclerosis. The overproduction of inflammatory mediators disrupts the normal physiological functions of endothelial cells, thereby promoting the advancement of atherosclerosis through endothelial injury. Furthermore, tea polyphenols have demonstrated anti-inflammatory properties. In an in vitro inflammatory model employing uric acid to stimulate human umbilical vein endothelial cells, pretreatment with the tea polyphenol EGCG markedly inhibited the release of inflammatory mediators, including IL-6 and TNF-α, through the regulation of the Notch signaling pathway. This attenuation of inflammatory factor release serves to mitigate endothelial cell damage and may exert a considerable influence on the management of cardiovascular diseases (Byun et al. 2014; Ramesh et al. 2010; Widmer et al. 2013).

3.4.3 Piceatannol

Piceatannol is a naturally occurring polyphenolic compound widely distributed across various plant species, such as grapes and sugarcane. Chemically, it exhibits high reactivity and is susceptible to oxidation. The compound exists in both cis and trans isomeric forms, which can interconvert under physiological conditions; however, the naturally occurring isomer is relatively uncommon. Structurally, piceatannol comprises two aromatic rings and several phenolic hydroxyl groups. This distinctive molecular configuration confers notable antioxidant properties. Specifically, the conjugated double bonds in conjunction with the hydroxyl groups constitute the active site, where the position and number of phenolic hydroxyl groups critically influence the compound's free radical scavenging ability and its related biological functions.

The cardioprotective and vasoprotective properties of piceatannol have been demonstrated through a reduction in the severity of myocardial infarction in ischemia-reperfusion (I/R) animal models, a decreased incidence and duration of ventricular tachycardia and ventricular fibrillation, lowered mortality rates, and pronounced vasodilation. The molecular processes that underlie these effects are intricate and multifactorial. Notably, piceatannol inhibits the activation of NF-κB and downregulates the expression of E-selectin, an NF-κB-dependent gene, thereby diminishing monocyte adhesion to endothelial cells. Additionally, piceatannol activates AMPK, which prevents intracellular lipid accumulation and inhibits the development of atherosclerotic plaques. Moreover, piceatannol attenuates the pathological proliferation of injured arterial intimal and vascular smooth muscle cells by regulating cellular concentrations of p53 and p21, inhibiting ROS-mediated activation of SRC kinase, suppressing MAPK activity, and decreasing endothelin (ET) synthesis, thereby contributing to the amelioration of atherosclerosis. In addition, piceatannol enhances the expression of eNOS mRNA, facilitating NO release from the vascular endothelium through the NO-GC-cGMP signaling pathway, which leads to extensive vasodilatory effects. It also protects vascular endothelium and smooth muscle cells by scavenging oxygen free radicals, inhibiting COX, and regulating lipid metabolism (Zang et al. 2006).

4 Phytochemicals on Antitumour Activities

4.1 Mechanism of Tumorigenesis

Tumorigenesis is characterized as the process through which normal cells are transformed into malignant cells via a multistep progression. The initial phase generally involves oncogenic mutations arising within a normal cell, which provide a selective growth advantage for clonal expansion. This advantage promotes the proliferation of the mutant clone and the progressive accumulation of additional genetic and epigenetic alterations. Together, these modifications lead to the formation of an irreversible, highly heterogeneous, and invasive neoplastic lesion (Zhang et al. 2024). A fundamental aspect of tumorigenesis is the gradual accumulation of genetic alterations that compromise normal cellular functions, leading to uncontrolled cell proliferation and increased survival. These genetic changes may arise from various sources, such as exposure to carcinogens, replication errors during DNA synthesis, or inherited genetic predispositions. The sequential acquisition of mutations in pivotal genes that regulate the cell cycle, apoptosis, and DNA repair mechanisms contributes to the neoplastic transformation of cells. Tumorigenesis represents a multifaceted process involving both genetic mutations and epigenetic modifications, which collectively facilitate the transition of normal cells into malignant phenotypes. Of particular importance are mutations in tumor suppressor genes and oncogenes, which disrupt essential cellular pathways responsible for growth regulation, programmed cell death, and genomic integrity maintenance (Kim 2015). These mutations can arise from various sources, including environmental carcinogens, replication errors, and inherited predispositions.

Epigenetic modifications, including DNA methylation, histone modifications, and the dysregulation of microRNAs, play a significant role in tumorigenesis by modulating gene expression without altering the underlying DNA sequence. In particular, aberrant DNA methylation patterns may result in the transcriptional silencing of tumor suppressor genes, while histone modifications can affect chromatin structure, thereby influencing the accessibility of genes for transcriptional regulation (Kanwal and Gupta 2012). These epigenetic changes can cooperate with genetic mutations to promote malignant transformation.

Furthermore, the tumor microenvironment constitutes a critical element in the progression of tumorigenesis. The accumulation of genetic and epigenetic alterations within neoplastic cells can modulate the adjacent stromal cells, thereby creating a supportive microenvironment that promotes tumor development and the metastasis of cancer cells (Takeshima and Ushijima 2019).

In healthy tissues, somatic mutations can occasionally occur and are typically suppressed by tumor-suppressive mechanisms. However, some mutations may confer a growth advantage, leading to the formation of mutant clones. These clones can persist without disrupting tissue homeostasis until they encounter additional stimuli. Upon occurrence of this event, cellular proliferation becomes dysregulated, triggering malignant transformation that advances from early precancerous lesions in cases of advanced malignant neoplasms. Throughout this development, the transformed cells progressively accumulate additional genetic mutations and epigenetic modifications, thereby developing progressively more aggressive phenotypic characteristics, including immune evasion, disruption of tissue architecture, and invasive capabilities. Concurrently, the tumor microenvironment undergoes a transition from a tumor-suppressive to a tumor-promoting milieu. This shift is characterized by impaired immunosurveillance, the development of tumor-facilitating inflammation, the progressive differentiation of fibroblasts into CAFs, increased stiffness of the ECM, and the expansion of MDSCs, collectively fostering tumor progression (Zhang et al. 2024).

Cancer continues to be a predominant contributor to global morbidity and mortality. Based on data from GLOBOCAN 2020, globally, approximately 18.1 million new cases of cancer were diagnosed and 9.6 million fatalities were attributed to cancer. The incidence of cancer exhibits considerable regional variation, with elevated rates predominantly reported in economically advanced nations. Conversely, countries with low to middle income levels are witnessing a rising cancer burden, largely driven by shifts in lifestyle factors and demographic aging (Bray et al. 2024). Therefore, it is both valuable and forward-thinking for human society to conduct more in-depth research on cancer.

4.2 *Multi-Target Intervention of Phytochemicals*

Phytochemicals, which are naturally occurring compounds widely found in plants, have garnered significant attention due to their ability to modulate multiple signaling pathways involved in the onset and development of cancer. These bioactive substances influence a range of cellular processes, including the induction of apoptosis, regulation of cell cycle progression, inhibition of angiogenesis, and suppression of metastasis. By targeting diverse molecular mechanisms, phytochemicals present a multifaceted approach to cancer therapy, with the potential to enhance treatment efficacy while reducing the incidence of adverse side effects.

For example, specific phytochemicals have been demonstrated to regulate critical signaling pathways, for example, PI3K/Akt/mTOR and JAK/STAT, which are essential for regulating the proliferation of cancer cells, survival, and metastasis. The capacity of these compounds to concurrently modulate multiple pathways highlights their promising therapeutic potential in oncological interventions. Moreover, combinations of phytochemicals have demonstrated enhanced anticancer effects by facilitating apoptosis, suppressing cellular proliferation and invasion, enhancing the susceptibility of cancer cells to adjunctive therapies, and augmenting the immune response. This synergistic action emphasizes the prospective effectiveness of phytochemicals as adjunctive agents in oncological treatment. Phytochemicals also show potential in targeting CSCs, which are often resistant to conventional therapies and are responsible for tumor recurrence and metastasis. Several phytochemicals have been demonstrated to influence signaling pathways implicated in CSCs, including the Notch and Hedgehog pathways, resulting in the suppression of CSC proliferation and the promotion of their differentiation. This strategy possesses the potential to contribute to the advancement of more effective and long-lasting cancer treatments. For instance, the concurrent administration of green tea and curcumin has demonstrated a substantial chemopreventive impact in the context of oral carcinogenesis by synergistically triggering programmed cell death and inducing cell cycle arrest at defined phases (Saleh et al. 2023).

4.3 Key Representative Phytochemicals and Pathways of Action

4.3.1 Paclitaxel

Paclitaxel interacts with the β-tubulin subunit of microtubules, facilitating the polymerization of tubulin into stable microtubule structures and concurrently preventing their depolymerization. This stabilization leads to the development of nonfunctional microtubule assemblies that disrupt mitotic spindle assembly. Consequently, cells experience an extended mitotic arrest during the G2/M phase, resulting in the initiation of the spindle assembly checkpoint and subsequently inducing either apoptosis or reentry into the cell cycle without completing division.

Beyond stabilizing microtubules, paclitaxel induces apoptosis by activating the TAK1–JNK signaling pathway. Treatment with paclitaxel increases the levels of TAK1 and its binding partner TAB1 in cells, leading to the phosphorylation and activation of JNK. Activated JNK subsequently phosphorylates and suppresses the antiapoptotic protein Bcl-xL, thereby enhancing the release of proapoptotic factors and promoting the induction of cell death (Di et al. 2020). Paclitaxel disrupts microtubule dynamics, which can induce mitotic catastrophe, a form of cellular demise that transpires during the process of mitosis. This phenomenon is characterized by the activation of the spindle assembly checkpoint, leading to the advancement of cell cycle arrest and, in cases of irreparable damage, subsequent initiation of apoptosis. Mitotic catastrophe serves as a mechanism to inhibit cellular proliferation with genomic instability. Thus, paclitaxel is a potent cancer treatment that interferes with microtubule dynamics, resulting in the cessation of cell cycle progression and the initiation of programmed cell death. The activation of the TAK1-JNK signaling pathway facilitates the promotion of cellular apoptosis while inducing mitotic catastrophe in cells with genomic instability. Furthermore, paclitaxel's mechanisms of action extend beyond microtubule stabilization and apoptosis induction. The drug has been demonstrated to activate several signaling pathways that underlie its antitumor effects. Specifically, paclitaxel induces the production of ROS, which subsequently induces the activation of various stress-responsive protein kinases, for example, JNK and p38 MAPK (Selimovic et al. 2008). These kinases play crucial roles in mediating cell death and modulating the tumor microenvironment. Additionally, paclitaxel's interaction with the microtubule network can influence the function of other cellular structures and processes, such as the endoplasmic reticulum and mitochondria, thereby enhancing its cytotoxic effects. Understanding these multifaceted actions of paclitaxel is essential for optimizing its use in cancer therapy and developing strategies to overcome resistance mechanisms. Despite its effectiveness, additional research is required to effectively address the existing challenges and to optimize its clinical application.

4.3.2 Epigallocatechin Gallate (EGCG)

Epigallocatechin gallate (EGCG) has attracted considerable attention due to its potential anticancer effects. A key mechanism underlying EGCG's biological activity involves the modulation of the PI3K/AKT/mTOR signaling pathway, which plays an essential role in regulating cellular growth and metabolic processes. Aberrations in the regulation of this pathway are frequently observed in various forms of cancer, contributing to unchecked cellular proliferation and evasion of programmed cell death. Consequently, EGCG's ability to inhibit the PI3K/AKT/mTOR axis positions it as a promising agent for both cancer prevention and therapeutic intervention.

The PI3K/AKT/mTOR signaling pathway constitutes a sophisticated cascade integral to the regulation of key cellular functions, including proliferation, survival, metabolic activity, and angiogenesis. The initiation of this pathway occurs upon the interaction of growth factors with RTKs, triggering the activation of PI3K. Activated PI3K catalyzes the phosphorylation of PIP2, producing PIP3, which facilitates the translocation of AKT to the plasma membrane. At this location, AKT experiences phosphorylation and subsequent activation facilitated by PDK1 and the mTORC2. Once activated, AKT phosphorylates a range of downstream substrates that govern cellular survival, growth, and metabolic processes (Ghafouri-Fard et al. 2021). The mTOR, found within two distinct complexes designated as mTORC1 and mTORC2, serves a critical function in regulating these processes through the regulation of protein synthesis and cell cycle progression.

Research has demonstrated that administration of EGCG enhances the expression of PTEN across multiple cancer cell lines, such as those derived from pancreatic, ovarian, and bladder malignancies. PTEN functions as a tumor suppressor gene by means of negative regulation of the PI3K/AKT signaling cascade through the dephosphorylation of PIP3 to PIP2, thereby suppressing the activation of AKT. This upregulation results in a reduction in the levels of PIP3 and reduced AKT activation, resulting in diminished cell proliferation and enhanced apoptosis (Hopkins et al. 2014).

EGCG decreases the phosphorylation of AKT at critical residues, such as Ser473 (Qin et al. 2020). This inhibition reduces AKT's capacity to phosphorylate downstream substrates participating in cellular survival and proliferation processes. For example, EGCG treatment decreases the extent of phosphorylation of mTOR and its downstream effector molecules, including 4E-BP1, resulting in decreased protein synthesis and suppression of cell cycle progression. Furthermore, EGCG has been shown to inhibit mTOR activity by decreasing its phosphorylation and disrupting its interaction with upstream activators. This downregulation leads to reduced translation of proteins essential for cell proliferation and survival, thereby exerting anticancer effects.

EGCG constitutes a prospective strategy for oncological treatment that involves the regulation of the PI3K/AKT/mTOR signaling pathway. By inhibiting critical elements of this pathway, such as AKT and mTOR, EGCG holds potential as a complementary agent alongside standard oncological therapy. Nonetheless, addressing challenges pertaining to its bioavailability, standardization, and clinical validation remains imperative for its effective incorporation into clinical protocols. Ongoing research and development efforts are crucial for optimizing the therapeutic efficacy of EGCG in cancer treatment.

4.3.3 Lycopene

Lycopene, a carotenoid primarily present in tomatoes, has garnered significant attention owing to its potential anticancer properties. Its mechanisms of action incorporate the regulation of IGF-1 signaling pathways, modulation of cyclin expression, and suppression of cellular proliferation signals, thereby emphasizing its prospective applications in oncological prevention and therapeutic interventions.

The IGF-1 signaling pathway is integral to cellular processes, for example, growth, differentiation, and survival. Aberrations in this pathway are frequently involved in the progression of diverse malignancies. Lycopene has been demonstrated to modulate IGF-1 signaling by suppressing the activation of the IGF-1 receptor. Specifically, lycopene attenuates the mitogenic effects of IGF-1 in mammary carcinoma cells by decreasing the tyrosine phosphorylation levels of IRS-1 and decreasing the binding affinity of the AP-1 transcription factor complex. These inhibitory actions are correlated with an upregulation of membrane-associated IGF-binding proteins, which serve as negative regulators of IGF-1 receptor activation (Karas et al. 2000).

Cyclins are regulatory proteins that control cell cycle progression. Alterations in cyclin expression are often associated with uncontrolled cell proliferation in cancer. Lycopene influences cyclins through multiple mechanisms. Initially, lycopene has been demonstrated to reduce the expression of cyclin D1, a protein that promotes the transition from the G1 phase to the S phase of the cell cycle throughout the cell cycle. This reduction in expression leads to the cessation of the cell cycle and a consequent decline in cellular proliferation (Amit Nahum et al. 2006). Second, lycopene treatment leads to the sustained association of the Kip1 with cyclin E-Cdk2 complexes, thereby suppressing their enzymatic activity and triggering cell cycle arrest during the G1 phase (Nahum et al. 2001). In various cancer cell lines, lycopene has been documented to trigger cell cycle arrest at various stages, including G1 and G0/G1, contingent upon the specific cell type and treatment duration (Teodoro et al. 2012).

Lycopene interferes with multiple signaling pathways implicated in the regulation of cellular proliferation. It decreases RAS-dependent activation of NF-κB, a transcription factor that modulates gene expression associated with cell survival and proliferation. This inhibition results in reduced expression of proliferation-related proteins, for example, cyclin D1 and p21, as well as apoptosis-related proteins like Bax and Bcl-2 (Qi et al. 2021). Furthermore, lycopene has been demonstrated to inhibit the MAPK signaling pathway, which is often hyperactivated in cancer cells and serves a crucial function in enabling unregulated cellular proliferation. Through the suppression of this pathway, lycopene reduces the expression of genes associated with cellular proliferation and survival (Han et al. 2019). Subsequently, lycopene inhibits the expression of matrix metalloproteinases (MMPs) and VEGF, key factors implicated in tumor invasion and angiogenesis. Through the suppression of this pathway, lycopene reduces the expression of genes linked to cellular growth and viability.

The diverse mechanisms of lycopene, such as the regulation of IGF-1 signaling pathways, modulation of cyclin expression, and suppression of proliferative signals, emphasize its prospective application as a therapeutic modality in the field of oncology. Although preclinical investigations offer substantial evidence supporting its effectiveness, additional clinical studies are required to determine optimal dosing strategies and to validate its therapeutic efficacy in human subjects.

4.3.4 Curcumin

Curcumin, a polyphenolic compound isolated from *Curcuma longa* L., has garnered significant attention due to its prospective applications in cancer treatment. Recent studies emphasize its capacity to influence the tumor immune microenvironment, notably by modulating exosome-associated microRNAs (miRNAs).

Cancer cells have evolved complex strategies to circumvent the host immune system, a process referred to as tumor immune escape. Among these strategies is the release of exosomes, which are small extracellular vesicles that mediate intercellular communication. These exosomes contain miRNAs, a category of short noncoding RNA molecules that contribute to the modulation of gene expression. Through the transfer of specific miRNAs to immune cells, tumor-derived exosomes can alter immune responses, thereby facilitating tumor progression and the dissemination of malignant cells. The biogenesis of exosomes occurs through the invagination of endosomal membranes, leading to the formation of MVBs (Rincon-Riveros et al. 2021). MVBs have the ability to undergo fusion with the plasma membrane, promoting the secretion of exosomes into the extracellular milieu (Dilsiz 2020). Throughout their biogenesis, exosomes selectively incorporate a range of biomolecules, notably miRNAs. The sorting of these miRNAs into exosomes is mediated by mechanisms that involve RNA-binding proteins as well as the ESCRT machinery. This selective packaging guarantees that exosomes contain particular miRNAs with the capacity to influence the behavior of recipient cells. Exosomal miRNAs modulate immune responses by means of multiple mechanisms, including the suppression of CTL activity, the induction of Treg expansion, the inhibition of DC maturation, and the facilitation of tumor-associated macrophage (TAM) polarization. Tumor cells employ this strategy to evade immune surveillance by secreting exosomes containing miRNAs that transfer to immune cells, thereby altering their function and facilitating immune escape. For example, exosomal miRNAs have the capacity to inhibit the functions of CTLs and NK cells, promote the differentiation of macrophages into an immunosuppressive M2 phenotype, and impede the maturation of DCs. Collectively, these effects facilitate tumor progression.

Curcumin has been shown to influence the biogenesis and content of tumor-derived exosomes, thereby modulating their effects on immune cells. Specifically, curcumin can alter the expression of certain miRNAs within exosomes. For example, curcumin has been demonstrated to inhibit the expression of miR-146a in exosomes originating from cancer-associated fibroblasts (CAFs), which play a critical role in modulating immune responses. Furthermore, curcumin influences the cytokine composition of CAF-derived exosomes by reducing the concentrations of anti-inflammatory cytokines, including IL-6 and TGF-β, which are frequently implicated in immune suppression within the TME (Mirza et al. 2023). Last but not the least, curcumin can promote the maturation of DCs by modulating the miRNA and cytokine content of exosomes. This maturation process augments the capacity of dendritic cells to display antigens and facilitate the activation of T cells, thereby augmenting antitumor immune responses (Mirza et al. 2023).

The capacity of curcumin to regulate exosome-mediated miRNAs signaling highlights its prospective value as a treatment approach within the domain of cancer immunotherapy. Through the modulation of the tumor microenvironment's immune landscape, curcumin may improve the effectiveness of current treatment modalities and support the advancement of innovative therapeutic approaches. Continued investigation is required to comprehensively understand the mechanisms by which curcumin influences exosome-mediated communication and to facilitate the application of these insights within clinical practice.

4.4 The Role of Phytochemicals in Adjuvant Chemotherapy

Phytochemicals have garnered considerable interest due to their potential to enhance the effectiveness of standard cancer therapies, particularly chemotherapy. These compounds may act as adjuvants, providing synergistic effects that improve therapeutic outcomes while potentially reducing side effects. A substantial body of preclinical and clinical investigations has established that natural products, particularly in conjunction with chemotherapeutic agents, exhibit anticancer properties by regulating multiple signaling pathways. These pathways are involved in the initiation of apoptosis, suppression of unregulated cellular proliferation, and augmentation of immune system function. Key phytochemicals such as curcumin and quercetin work synergistically with cancer treatments to reduce cell proliferation, induce apoptosis, and arrest the cell cycle (Ayaz et al. 2022). Currently, researchers have conducted numerous clinical studies to evaluate the safety profile and therapeutic efficacy of curcumin in combination with chemotherapy. For instance, a Phase I clinical study evaluated the safety and tolerability of the concomitant administration of curcumin with FOLFOX chemotherapy in patients diagnosed with metastatic colorectal cancer. The findings demonstrated that the combination regimen was safe and well tolerated, exhibiting no significant increase in adverse effects relative to chemotherapy administered alone (Howells et al. 2019). Phytochemicals may also help overcome chemotherapy resistance by modulating signaling pathways involved in drug resistance mechanisms. For instance, curcumin has been extensively reported to suppress the expression of P-glycoprotein, a protein implicated in multidrug resistance, consequently improving the efficacy of chemotherapeutic drugs (Lopes-Rodrigues et al. 2016). Furthermore, the cytotoxic nature of chemotherapy can cause adverse effects on normal, healthy cells. Phytochemicals demonstrate properties that contribute to antioxidant and anti-inflammatory effects that possess the capacity to safeguard normal cells against oxidative stress and inflammation triggered by chemotherapy. For example, phenethyl isothiocyanate has demonstrated protective effects against chemotherapy-induced toxicity in various studies.

Notable phytochemicals used as adjuvants in chemotherapy include curcumin, resveratrol, quercetin, gingerol, and phenethyl isothiocyanate (PEITC). Curcumin has been extensively investigated for its anticancer properties. It exerts modulatory effects on multiple signaling pathways, comprising NF-κB and PI3K/Akt, which contribute to the potentiation of antineoplastic agents, for example, cisplatin and doxorubicin. Similarly, resveratrol, a polyphenolic substance found in grapes and berries, demonstrates antioxidant and anti-inflammatory properties. It enhances the vulnerability of cancer cells to chemotherapeutic drugs by modulating apoptotic and autophagic mechanisms. Quercetin, a flavonoid present in apples, onions, and tea, has been demonstrated to suppress the activity of drug efflux pumps and increase the cytotoxicity of chemotherapeutic agents. Gingerol, the principal bioactive compound found in ginger, exhibits anti-inflammatory and antioxidant activities. These characteristics contribute to its protective efficacy against toxicity induced by chemotherapy, thereby potentially enhancing the therapeutic efficacy and safety profile of chemotherapeutic treatments. Lastly, PEITC, found in cruciferous vegetables such as watercress, exhibits anticancer properties and enhances the efficacy of chemotherapy agents by modulating multiple signaling pathways.

While the potential benefits of incorporating phytochemicals into cancer therapy are promising, several factors must be considered. The effectiveness of phytochemicals is often limited by their bioavailability, necessitating strategies to enhance absorption and stability to achieve therapeutic concentrations. Additionally, phytochemicals may interact with chemotherapeutic agents, potentially altering their efficacy or toxicity, making it crucial to evaluate these interactions to ensure patient safety. Furthermore, variability in the composition of phytochemical preparations can lead to inconsistent therapeutic outcomes, underscoring the need for standardized formulations to guarantee reliable clinical application.

In conclusion, phytochemicals represent a promising strategy for improving the efficacy and safety of chemotherapy in oncological treatment. The capacity of these compounds to sensitize cancer cells, mitigate resistance, and safeguard normal cells from chemotherapy-induced toxicity underscores their potential as effective adjuvants. Nonetheless, additional clinical investigations are required to determine standardized dosages and formulations, as well as to comprehensively elucidate the interactions between phytochemicals and chemotherapeutic drugs.

4.5 Limitation

While phytochemicals show promise in cancer therapy, several limitations hinder their widespread clinical application. A major obstacle is their limited bioavailability, attributable to low water solubility, rapid metabolic degradation, and inherent instability in physiological conditions. These factors lead to insufficient concentrations at the target site, thereby reducing therapeutic efficacy. Additionally, phytochemicals may interact with conventional chemotherapeutic agents, potentially altering their effectiveness or toxicity. Such interactions require careful evaluation to ensure patient safety. Moreover, variability in the composition of phytochemical preparations can cause inconsistent therapeutic outcomes, highlighting the need for standardized formulations to ensure reliable clinical use. Moreover, the limited availability of extensive clinical data concerning the safety and effectiveness of numerous phytochemicals constrains their integration into conventional oncology practice. To overcome these obstacles, continuous research efforts are required, emphasizing the improvement of bioavailability, standardization, and rigorous clinical validation of therapies derived from phytochemicals.

5 Challenge and Future

5.1 Limitations of Current Research

Although phytochemicals have demonstrated significant potential in the treatment of NCDs, their research and application face several limitations. First, numerous phytochemicals face challenges including limited bioavailability and inadequate chemical stability. For example, polyphenols and flavonoids often exhibit low water solubility, extensive first-pass metabolism, and rapid intestinal degradation, which collectively result in reduced oral bioavailability and limit their in vivo efficacy. Additionally, exposure to factors, for example, light, heat, or pH variations, can degrade their chemical structures; for instance, resveratrol undergoes rapid isomerization when exposed to light, adversely affecting the stability and storage conditions of formulations.

Second, clinical translational evidence remains fragmented, as most studies on phytochemicals are limited to cellular or animal models, with few progressing to phase III trials. Moreover, these studies frequently encounter limitations such as limited sample sizes, brief study periods, and the absence of standardized dosing protocols, resulting in low reproducibility of findings. In terms of mechanistic research, the complexity of multi-target effects complicates the distinction between primary and secondary targets, while the risk of off-target effects increases uncertainty regarding potential side effects. Additionally, individual variability and batch-to-batch differences in raw materials hinder standardized application. Lastly, there exists a considerable deficiency in long-term toxicity data and investigations into drug interactions, resulting in an insufficient characterization of potential safety risks.

Therefore, current research must systematically address these bottlenecks by employing interdisciplinary technologies, such as computational pharmacology and precision delivery, while also fostering global collaboration through data-sharing platforms and policy coordination. This method aims to utilize the potential properties of phytochemicals for management of NCDs and to promote systematic innovation spanning from fundamental research to clinical implementation.

5.2 Breakthrough on Phytochemicals

5.2.1 Nano Delivery System

Although phytochemicals are naturally abundant, their poor water solubility leads to low concentrations in the body and consequently low bioavailability, which limits their efficacy and presents challenges for clinical application (Baldassari et al. 2023). To effectively tackle this issue, scholars have devised various methodologies aimed at improving the bioavailability of phytochemicals. Nanodelivery systems, through the utilization of advanced materials and design principles, have markedly enhanced the stability, bioavailability, and targeted delivery of these compounds. Consequently, these systems have become a pivotal strategy in addressing the limitations inherent in the use of plant-derived substances.

Phytochemicals can be conjugated, encapsulated, or combined with nanomaterials to form complexes—such as nanoparticles and nanocarriers—that enhance their solubility and stability. This method enables precise targeting in drug delivery (Chavda et al. 2023). The nanodelivery system presents several significant benefits, such as enabling precise drug targeting to specific tissues with enhanced specificity and diminished adverse effects. Furthermore, it facilitates sustained drug release, improves target selectivity, and reduces both the required dosage and associated toxicity (Bartosz and Irene 2016; Mehan et al. 2022).

The deep integration of materials science and biomedicine in nanodelivery systems presents a novel approach for phytochemicals to overcome inherent limitations and is expected to transform the therapeutic landscape of NCDs.

5.2.2 Artificial Intelligence Application

Due to the time-consuming and costly nature of pharmacological screening for phytochemicals, the application of artificial intelligence (AI) in designing new drugs derived from medicinal plants has garnered increasing attention and anticipation. Computational methods such as molecular docking, molecular dynamics simulations, and deep learning are essential tools in phytochemical research. Molecular docking elucidates the interactions and biological therapeutic properties of potential phytochemicals by modeling their binding mechanisms with target active sites. Molecular dynamics simulations reveal the dynamic behavior of biomolecules at the atomic level, providing detailed characterizations. Artificial intelligence is fundamentally reshaping the framework of phytochemical research by employing advanced technologies, for example, deep learning, GANs, and NLP. This integration significantly expedites the comprehensive innovation process, spanning from target identification to clinical application. Advanced algorithms, including artificial neural networks and deep neural networks, hold significant potential to reduce the time required for traditional experimental approaches. These remarkable advancements in AI have paved the way for a deeper understanding of the pharmacological effects of phytochemicals in NCDs and have introduced novel concepts for drug design and development.

6 Conclusion

The significance of phytochemicals in NCDs research is evident not only in their substantial scientific value but also in their potential to inspire innovative approaches in clinical practice, public health, and industrial development. First, the traditional drug development model struggles to address the multifactorial pathogenic characteristics of NCDs. In contrast, the synergistic effects of multicomponent phytochemicals provide a robust theoretical foundation for developing multi-target therapies. Second, phytochemicals have the potential to either substitute for or complement existing pharmacological treatments and to improve the efficacy of adjuvant therapies by providing innovative therapeutic approaches, thereby substantially enhancing current treatment protocols. Additionally, the diversity of phytochemicals offers a wealth of candidate molecules for precision medicine. Widely sourced phytochemicals can serve as a cost-effective means of disease prevention and control in resource-limited areas, facilitating low-cost intervention strategies. Furthermore, the global expansion of phytochemical-derived drugs, coupled with the principles of a green economy, has fostered sustainable development. Finally, the investigation of phytochemicals offers molecular-level evidence that underpins the modernization of Traditional Chinese Medicine and Ayurveda, thereby facilitating the progressive development of these traditional medical systems.

Therefore, the study of phytochemicals serves as a vital link between traditional knowledge and modern science, representing a significant breakthrough in addressing the global challenges posed by NCDs. Through mechanistic analysis, technological innovation, and interdisciplinary collaboration, the application of phytochemicals is expected to facilitate a shift from disease treatment to health management, thereby providing scientific support for "Healthy China 2030 and the United Nations Sustainable Development Goals" (SDG 3).

References

Aarsland D, Khalifa K, Bergland AK, Soennesyn H, Oppedal, K, Holteng LBA, Oesterhus R, Nakling A, Jarholm JA, de Lucia C, Fladby T, Brooker H, Dalen I, Ballard C (2022) A Randomised Placebo-Controlled Study of Purified Anthocyanins on Cognition in Individuals at Increased Risk for Dementia. Randomized Controlled Trial 31(2):141–151. https://doi.org/10.1016/j.jagp.2022.10.002

Aggarwal BB, Harikumar KB (2009) Potential therapeutic effects of curcumin, the anti-inflammatory agent, against neurodegenerative, cardiovascular, pulmonary, metabolic, autoimmune and neoplastic diseases. Int J Biochem Cell Biol 41(1):40–59. https://doi.org/10.1016/j.biocel.2008.06.010

Aggarwal BB, Kumar A, Bharti AC (2003) Anticancer potential of curcumin: preclinical and clinical studies. Anticancer Res 23(1A):363–398

Agustín RM, Claudia A, Mariela VC, Elio AS (2018) Pharmacology and toxicology of polyphenols with potential as neurotropic agents in non-communicable diseases. Curr Drug Targets 19(2):97–110. https://doi.org/10.2174/1389450117666161220152336

Ak T, Gulcin I (2008) Antioxidant and radical scavenging properties of curcumin. Chem Biol Interact 174(1):27–37. https://doi.org/10.1016/j.cbi.2008.05.003

Alivernini S, Firestein GS, McInnes IB (2022) The pathogenesis of rheumatoid arthritis. Immunity 55(12):2255–2270. https://doi.org/10.1016/j.immuni.2022.11.009

Alvarez-Rodriguez L, Martinez-Taboada V, Calvo-Alen J, Beares I, Villa I, Lopez-Hoyos M (2019) Altered Th17/Treg ratio in peripheral blood of systemic lupus erythematosus but not primary antiphospholipid syndrome. Front Immunol 10:391. https://doi.org/10.3389/fimmu.2019.00391

Assmann G, Carmena R, Cullen P, Fruchart JC, Jossa F, Lewis B, Paoletti R (1999) Coronary heart disease: reducing the risk: a worldwide view. International Task Force for the Prevention of Coronary Heart Disease. Circulation 100(18):1930–1938. https://doi.org/10.1161/01.cir.100.18.1930

Astry B, Venkatesha SH, Laurence A, Christensen-Quick A, Garzino-Demo A, Frieman MB, Moudgil KD (2015) Celastrol, a Chinese herbal compound, controls autoimmune inflammation by altering the balance of pathogenic and regulatory T cells in the target organ. Clin Immunol 157(2):228–238. https://doi.org/10.1016/j.clim.2015.01.011

Atreya R, Neurath MF (2008) New therapeutic strategies for treatment of inflammatory bowel disease. Mucosal Immunol 1(3):175–182. https://doi.org/10.1038/mi.2008.7

Ayaz M, Nawaz A, Ahmad S, Mosa OF, Hamdoon AAE, Khalifa MA, Murthy HCA (2022) Underlying anticancer mechanisms and synergistic combinations of phytochemicals with cancer chemotherapeutics: potential benefits and risks. J Food Qual 2022:1189034. https://doi.org/10.1155/2022/1189034

Baldassari S, Balboni A, Drava G, Donghia D, Canepa P, Ailuno G, Caviglioli G (2023) Phytochemicals and cancer treatment: cell-derived and biomimetic vesicles as promising carriers. Pharmaceutics 15(5):1445. https://doi.org/10.3390/pharmaceutics15051445

Banfi D, Moro E, Bosi A, Bistoletti M, Cerantola S, Crema F, Baj A (2021) Impact of microbial metabolites on microbiota-gut-brain axis in inflammatory bowel disease. Int J Mol Sci 22(4). https://doi.org/10.3390/ijms22041623

Barnabei L, Laplantine E, Mbongo W, Rieux-Laucat F, Weil R (2021) NF-kappaB: at the borders of autoimmunity and inflammation. Front Immunol 12:716469. https://doi.org/10.3389/fimmu.2021.716469

Bar-Or A, Oliveira EM, Anderson DE, Krieger JI, Duddy M, O'Connor KC, Hafler DA (2001) Immunological memory: contribution of memory B cells expressing costimulatory molecules in the resting state. J Immunol 167(10):5669–5677. https://doi.org/10.4049/jimmunol.167.10.5669

Barry J, Fritz M, Brender JR, Smith PE, Lee DK, Ramamoorthy A (2009) Determining the effects of lipophilic drugs on membrane structure by solid-state NMR spectroscopy: the case of the antioxidant curcumin. J Am Chem Soc 131(12):4490–4498. https://doi.org/10.1021/ja809217u

Bartosz T, Irene T (2016) Polyphenols encapsulation – application of innovation technologies to improve stability of natural products. De Gruyter 1(2):20150005. https://doi.org/10.1515/psr-2015-0005

Bazyar H, Hosseini SA, Saradar S, Mombaini D, Allivand M, Labibzade M, Alipour M (2020) Effects of epigallocatechin-3-gallate of Camellia sinensis leaves on blood pressure, lipid profile, atherogenic index of plasma and some inflammatory and antioxidant markers in type 2 diabetes mellitus patients: a clinical trial. Randomized Controlled Trial 18(2):405–411. https://doi.org/10.1515/jcim-2020-0090

Bayet-Robert M, Kwiatkowski F, Leheurteur M, Gachon F, Planchat E, Abrial C, Chollet P (2010) Phase I dose escalation trial of docetaxel plus curcumin in patients with advanced and metastatic breast cancer. Cancer Biol Ther 9(1):8–14. https://doi.org/10.4161/cbt.9.1.10392

Bharti AC, Aggarwal BB (2002) Chemopreventive agents induce suppression of nuclear factor-kappaB leading to chemosensitization. Ann N Y Acad Sci 973:392–395. https://doi.org/10.1111/j.1749-6632.2002.tb04671.x

Bharti AC, Donato N, Singh S, Aggarwal BB (2003) Curcumin (diferuloylmethane) down-regulates the constitutive activation of nuclear factor-kappa B and IkappaBalpha kinase in human multiple myeloma cells, leading to suppression of proliferation and induction of apoptosis. Blood 101(3):1053–1062. https://doi.org/10.1182/blood-2002-05-1320

Bhattacharya S, Heidler P, Varshney S (2023) Incorporating neglected non-communicable diseases into the national health program—A review. Front Public Health 10:1093170. https://doi.org/10.3389/fpubh.2022.1093170

Binion DG, Otterson MF, Rafiee P (2008) Curcumin inhibits VEGF-mediated angiogenesis in human intestinal microvascular endothelial cells through COX-2 and MAPK inhibition. Gut 57(11):1509–1517. https://doi.org/10.1136/gut.2008.152496

Bray F, Laversanne M, Sung H, Ferlay J, Siegel RL, Soerjomataram I, Jemal A (2024) Global cancer statistics 2022: GLOBOCAN estimates of incidence and mortality worldwide for 36 cancers in 185 countries. CA Cancer J Clin 74(3):229–263. https://doi.org/10.3322/caac.21834

Britton GJ, Contijoch EJ, Mogno I, Vennaro OH, Llewellyn SR, Ng R, Faith JJ (2019) Microbiotas from humans with inflammatory bowel disease alter the balance of gut Th17 and RORgammat(+) regulatory T cells and exacerbate colitis in mice. Immunity 50(1):212–224 e214. https://doi.org/10.1016/j.immuni.2018.12.015

Brown EM, Kenny DJ, Xavier RJ (2019) Gut microbiota regulation of T cells during inflammation and autoimmunity. Annu Rev Immunol 37:599–624. https://doi.org/10.1146/annurev-immunol-042718-041841

Budreviciute A, Damiati S, Sabir DK, Onder K, Schuller-Goetzburg P, Plakys G, Kodzius R (2020) Management and prevention strategies for non-communicable diseases (NCDs) and their risk factors. Front Public Health 8:574111. https://doi.org/10.3389/fpubh.2020.574111

Buhrmann C, Shayan P, Banik K, Kunnumakkara AB, Kubatka P, Koklesova L, Shakibaei M (2020) Targeting NF-kappaB signaling by Calebin A, a compound of turmeric, in multicellular tumor microenvironment: potential role of apoptosis induction in CRC cells. Biomedicine 8(8). https://doi.org/10.3390/biomedicines8080236

Byun EB, Mi S, Kim JH, Song DS, Lee BS, Park JN, Byun EH (2014) Epigallocatechin-3-gallate-mediated Tollip induction through the 67-kDa laminin receptor negatively regulating TLR4 signaling in endothelial cells. Immunobiology 219(11):866–872. https://doi.org/10.1016/j.imbio.2014.07.010

Carlos Kusano Bucalen F, Sandro P, José Carlos Costa Baptista S, Elizabeth Aparecida Ferraz da Silva T (2016) An apple plus a Brazil nut a day keeps the doctors away: antioxidant capacity of foods and their health benefits. Curr Pharm Des 22(2):189–195. https://doi.org/10.2174/1381612822666151117122715

Cascao R, Vidal B, Lopes IP, Paisana E, Rino J, Moita LF, Fonseca JE (2015) Decrease of CD68 synovial macrophages in celastrol treated arthritic rats. PLoS One 10(12):e0142448. https://doi.org/10.1371/journal.pone.0142448

Cascao R, Vidal B, Jalmari Finnila MA, Lopes IP, Teixeira RL, Saarakkala S, Fonseca JE (2017) Effect of celastrol on bone structure and mechanics in arthritic rats. RMD Open 3(2):e000438. https://doi.org/10.1136/rmdopen-2017-000438

Cervera R, Khamashta MA, Font J, Sebastiani GD, Gil A, Lavilla P, European Working Party on Systemic Lupus, E (2003) Morbidity and mortality in systemic lupus erythematosus during a 10-year period: a comparison of early and late manifestations in a cohort of 1,000 patients. Medicine (Baltimore) 82(5):299–308. https://doi.org/10.1097/01.md.0000091181.93122.55

Chavda VP, Nalla LV, Balar P, Bezbaruah R, Apostolopoulos V, Singla RK, Uversky VN (2023) Advanced phytochemical-based nanocarrier systems for the treatment of breast cancer. Cancer 15(4):1023. https://doi.org/10.3390/cancers15041023

Chen M, Chen X, Wan Q (2018) Altered frequency of Th17 and Treg cells in new-onset systemic lupus erythematosus patients. Eur J Clin Invest 48(11):e13012. https://doi.org/10.1111/eci.13012

Chervy M, Barnich N, Denizot J (2020) Adherent-Invasive E. coli: update on the lifestyle of a troublemaker in Crohn's disease. Int J Mol Sci 21(10). https://doi.org/10.3390/ijms21103734

Cho, JA, Park SH, Cho J, Kim J.-O, Yoon, JH, & Park, E. (2020) Exercise and Curcumin in Combination Improves Cognitive Function and Attenuates ER Stress in Diabetic Rats. Nutrients 12(5):1309. https://doi.org/10.3390/nu12051309

Choi SR, Howell OW, Carassiti D, Magliozzi R, Gveric D, Muraro PA, Reynolds R (2012) Meningeal inflammation plays a role in the pathology of primary progressive multiple sclerosis. Brain 135(Pt 10):2925–2937. https://doi.org/10.1093/brain/aws189

Choudhari AS, Mandave PC, Deshpande M, Ranjekar P, Prakash O (2020) Phytochemicals in cancer treatment: from preclinical studies to clinical practice. Front Pharmacol 10:1614. https://doi.org/10.3389/fphar.2019.01614

Chow S-E, Hshu Y-C, Wang J-S, Chen J-K (2007) Resveratrol attenuates oxLDL-stimulated NADPH oxidase activity and protects endothelial cells from oxidative functional damages. J Appl Physiol 102(4):1520–1527. https://doi.org/10.1152/japplphysiol.00881.2006

Chu AJ (2022) Quarter-century explorations of bioactive polyphenols: diverse health benefits. Front Biosci-Landmark 27(4):134. https://doi.org/10.31083/j.fbl2704134

Cluxton D, Petrasca A, Moran B, Fletcher JM (2019) Differential regulation of human Treg and Th17 cells by fatty acid synthesis and glycolysis. Front Immunol 10:115. https://doi.org/10.3389/fimmu.2019.00115

Costello SP, Hughes PA, Waters O, Bryant RV, Vincent AD, Blatchford P, Andrews JM (2019) Effect of fecal microbiota transplantation on 8-week remission in patients with ulcerative colitis: a randomized clinical trial. JAMA 321(2):156–164. https://doi.org/10.1001/jama.2018.20046

Croca SC, Griffin M, Farinha F, Isenberg DA, Nicolaides A, Rahman A (2021) Total plaque area and plaque echogenicity are novel measures of subclinical atherosclerosis in patients with systemic lupus erythematosus. Rheumatology (Oxford) 60(9):4185–4198. https://doi.org/10.1093/rheumatology/keaa905

Crowl JT, Gray EE, Pestal K, Volkman HE, Stetson DB (2017) Intracellular nucleic acid detection in autoimmunity. Annu Rev Immunol 35:313–336. https://doi.org/10.1146/annurev-immunol-051116-052331

Dalile B, Van Oudenhove L, Vervliet B, Verbeke K (2019) The role of short-chain fatty acids in microbiota-gut-brain communication. Nat Rev Gastroenterol Hepatol 16(8):461–478. https://doi.org/10.1038/s41575-019-0157-3

Davidson A, Diamond B (2001) Autoimmune diseases. N Engl J Med 345(5):340–350. https://doi.org/10.1056/NEJM200108023450506

de Bock M, Derraik JGB, Brennan CM, Biggs JB, Morgan PE, Hodgkinson SC, Cutfield WS (2013) Olive (Olea europaea L.) leaf polyphenols improve insulin sensitivity in middle-aged overweight men: a randomized, placebo-controlled, crossover trial. PLoS One 8(3):e57622. https://doi.org/10.1371/journal.pone.0057622

Deng Y, Zhang Y, Liu G, Zhou P, Li P, Zhao Z, Zhang R, Tang X, Wang Z, Wei Z, Zhang M (2023) Saponins from Momordica charantia exert hypoglycemic effect in diabetic mice by multiple pathways. Food Sci Nutr 11(12):7626–7637. https://doi.org/10.1002/fsn3.3682

Dhillon N, Aggarwal BB, Newman RA, Wolff RA, Kunnumakkara AB, Abbruzzese JL, Kurzrock R (2008) Phase II trial of curcumin in patients with advanced pancreatic cancer. Clin Cancer Res 14(14):4491–4499. https://doi.org/10.1158/1078-0432.CCR-08-0024

Di Y-W, Li Z-s, Xiong S-m, Huang G, Luo Y-f, Huo T-y, Zheng Y-w (2020) Paclitaxel induces apoptosis through the TAK1-JNK activation pathway. FEBS Open Bio 10(8):1655–1667. https://doi.org/10.1002/2211-5463.12917

Dilsiz N (2020) Role of exosomes and exosomal microRNAs in cancer. Future Sci OA 6(4). https://doi.org/10.2144/fsoa-2019-0116

Doria A, Arienti S, Rampudda M, Canova M, Tonon M, Sarzi-Puttini P (2008) Preventive strategies in systemic lupus erythematosus. Autoimmun Rev 7(3):192–197. https://doi.org/10.1016/j.autrev.2007.11.004

Ebert TJ, Hall JE, Barney JA, Uhrich TD, Colinco MD (2000) The effects of increasing plasma concentrations of dexmedetomidine in humans. Anesthesiology 93(2):382–394. https://doi.org/10.1097/00000542-200008000-00016

Ebner K, Bandion A, Binder BR, de Martin R, Schmid JA (2003) GMCSF activates NF-kappaB via direct interaction of the GMCSF receptor with IkappaB kinase beta. Blood 102(1):192–199. https://doi.org/10.1182/blood-2002-12-3753

Fan G, Li F, Wang P, Jin X, Liu R (2022) Natural-product-mediated autophagy in the treatment of various liver diseases. Int J Mol Sci 23(23). https://doi.org/10.3390/ijms232315109

Fang Z, He D, Yu B, Liu F, Zuo J, Li Y, Wang Q (2017) High-throughput study of the effects of celastrol on activated fibroblast-like synoviocytes from patients with rheumatoid arthritis. Genes (Basel) 8(9). https://doi.org/10.3390/genes8090221

Frank DN, St Amand AL, Feldman RA, Boedeker EC, Harpaz N, Pace NR (2007) Molecular-phylogenetic characterization of microbial community imbalances in human inflammatory bowel diseases. Proc Natl Acad Sci USA 104(34):13780–13785. https://doi.org/10.1073/pnas.0706625104

Fu J, Huang H, Liu J, Pi R, Chen J, Liu P (2007) Tanshinone IIA protects cardiac myocytes against oxidative stress-triggered damage and apoptosis. Eur J Pharmacol 568(1–3):213–221. https://doi.org/10.1016/j.ejphar.2007.04.031

Gan K, Xu L, Feng X, Zhang Q, Wang F, Zhang M, Tan W (2015) Celastrol attenuates bone erosion in collagen-induced arthritis mice and inhibits osteoclast differentiation and function in RANKL-induced RAW264.7. Int Immunopharmacol 24(2):239–246. https://doi.org/10.1016/j.intimp.2014.12.012

Garza-Lombo C, Schroder A, Reyes-Reyes EM, Franco R (2018) mTOR/AMPK signaling in the brain: cell metabolism, proteostasis and survival. Curr Opin Toxicol 8:102–110. https://doi.org/10.1016/j.cotox.2018.05.002

Gerondakis S, Grossmann M, Nakamura Y, Pohl T, Grumont R (1999) Genetic approaches in mice to understand Rel/NF-kappaB and IkappaB function: transgenics and knockouts. Oncogene 18(49):6888–6895. https://doi.org/10.1038/sj.onc.1203236

Ghafouri-Fard S, Abak A, Anamag FT, Shoorei H, Majidpoor J, Taheri M (2021) The emerging role of non-coding RNAs in the regulation of PI3K/AKT pathway in the carcinogenesis process. Biomed Pharmacother 137. https://doi.org/10.1016/j.biopha.2021.111279

Gharibi T, Majidi J, Kazemi T, Dehghanzadeh R, Motallebnezhad M, Babaloo Z (2016) Biological effects of IL-21 on different immune cells and its role in autoimmune diseases. Immunobiology 221(2):357–367. https://doi.org/10.1016/j.imbio.2015.09.021

Godos J, Romano GL, Gozzo L, Laudani S, Paladino N, Dominguez Azpiroz I, Grosso G (2024) Resveratrol and vascular health: evidence from clinical studies and mechanisms of actions related to its metabolites produced by gut microbiota. Front Pharmacol 15:1368949. https://doi.org/10.3389/fphar.2024.1368949

Gong T, Liu L, Jiang W, Zhou R (2020) DAMP-sensing receptors in sterile inflammation and inflammatory diseases. Nat Rev Immunol 20(2):95–112. https://doi.org/10.1038/s41577-019-0215-7

Gonzales AM, Orlando RA (2008) Curcumin and resveratrol inhibit nuclear factor-kappaB-mediated cytokine expression in adipocytes. Nutr Metab (Lond) 5:17. https://doi.org/10.1186/1743-7075-5-17

Govindarajan VS (1980) Turmeric--chemistry, technology, and quality. Crit Rev Food Sci Nutr 12(3):199–301. https://doi.org/10.1080/10408398009527278

Greco CM, Rudy TE, Manzi S (2003) Adaptation to chronic pain in systemic lupus erythematosus: applicability of the multidimensional pain inventory. Pain Med 4(1):39–50. https://doi.org/10.1046/j.1526-4637.2003.03001.x

Greth W, Robbie GJ, Brohawn P, Hultquist M, Yao B (2017) Targeting the interferon pathway with sifalimumab for the treatment of systemic lupus erythematosus. Immunotherapy 9(1):57–70. https://doi.org/10.2217/imt-2016-0090

Grundy SM, Pasternak R, Greenland P, Smith S Jr, Fuster V (1999) AHA/ACC scientific statement: assessment of cardiovascular risk by use of multiple-risk-factor assessment equations: a statement for healthcare professionals from the American Heart Association and the American College of Cardiology. J Am Coll Cardiol 34(4):1348–1359. https://doi.org/10.1016/s0735-1097(99)00387-3

Guo Q, Wang Y, Xu D, Nossent J, Pavlos NJ, Xu J (2018) Rheumatoid arthritis: pathological mechanisms and modern pharmacologic therapies. Bone Res 6:15. https://doi.org/10.1038/s41413-018-0016-9

Guo NH, Fu X, Zi FM, Song Y, Wang S, Cheng J (2019) The potential therapeutic benefit of resveratrol on Th17/Treg imbalance in immune thrombocytopenic purpura. Int Immunopharmacol 73:181–192. https://doi.org/10.1016/j.intimp.2019.04.061

Guo J, Li Z, Yao Y, Fang L, Yu M, Wang Z (2024) Curcumin in the treatment of inflammation and oxidative stress responses in traumatic brain injury: a systematic review and meta-analysis. Front Neurol 15:1380353. https://doi.org/10.3389/fneur.2024.1380353

Hahn BH (2003) Systemic lupus erythematosus and accelerated atherosclerosis. N Engl J Med 349(25):2379–2380. https://doi.org/10.1056/NEJMp038168

Han H, Lim JW, Kim H (2019) Lycopene inhibits activation of epidermal growth factor receptor and expression of cyclooxygenase-2 in gastric cancer cells. Nutrients 11(9). https://doi.org/10.3390/nu11092113

Hauser SL, Bhan AK, Gilles F, Kemp M, Kerr C, Weiner HL (1986) Immunohistochemical analysis of the cellular infiltrate in multiple sclerosis lesions. Ann Neurol 19(6):578–587. https://doi.org/10.1002/ana.410190610

Hauser SL, Chan JR, Oksenberg JR (2013) Multiple sclerosis: prospects and promise. Ann Neurol 74(3):317–327. https://doi.org/10.1002/ana.24009

Hayden MS, Ghosh S (2011) NF-kappaB in immunobiology. Cell Res 21(2):223–244. https://doi.org/10.1038/cr.2011.13

He T, Xiong J, Nie L, Yu Y, Guan X, Xu X, Zhao J (2016) Resveratrol inhibits renal interstitial fibrosis in diabetic nephropathy by regulating AMPK/NOX4/ROS pathway. J Mol Med 94(12):1359–1371. https://doi.org/10.1007/s00109-016-1451-y

Hewlings SJ, Kalman DS (2017) Curcumin: a review of its effects on human health. Foods 6(10). https://doi.org/10.3390/foods6100092

Hieronymus H, Lamb J, Ross KN, Peng XP, Clement C, Rodina A, Golub TR (2006) Gene expression signature-based chemical genomic prediction identifies a novel class of HSP90 pathway modulators. Cancer Cell 10(4):321–330. https://doi.org/10.1016/j.ccr.2006.09.005

Ho SC, Yeo W, Goggins W, Kwok C, Cheng A, Chong M, Lee R, Cheung KL (2021) Pre-diagnosis and early post-diagnosis dietary soy isoflavone intake and survival outcomes: a prospective cohort study of early stage breast cancer survivors. Cancer Treat Res Commun 27:100350. https://doi.org/10.1016/j.ctarc.2021.100350

Hopkins BD, Hodakoski C, Barrows D, Mense SM, Parsons RE (2014) PTEN function: the long and the short of it. Trends Biochem Sci 39(4):183–190. https://doi.org/10.1016/j.tibs.2014.02.006
Hossain MS, Wazed MA, Asha S, Amin MR, Shimul IM (2025) Dietary phytochemicals in health and disease: mechanisms, clinical evidence, and applications-A comprehensive review. Food Sci Nutr 13(3):e70101. https://doi.org/10.1002/fsn3.70101
Howells LM, Iwuji COO, Irving GRB, Barber S, Walter H, Sidat Z, Brown K (2019) Curcumin combined with FOLFOX chemotherapy is safe and tolerable in patients with metastatic colorectal cancer in a randomized phase IIa trial. J Nutr 149(7):1133–1139. https://doi.org/10.1093/jn/nxz029
Hsu C-Y, McCulloch CE, Darbinian J, Go A S, Iribarren C (2005) Elevated blood pressure and risk of end-stage renal disease in subjects without baseline kidney disease. Comp Stud 165(8):923–928. https://doi.org/10.1001/archinte.165.8.923
Hu Y, Chen B, Yang F, Su Y, Yang D, Yao Y, Xu T (2022) Emerging role of the cGAS-STING signaling pathway in autoimmune diseases: biologic function, mechanisms and clinical prospection. Autoimmun Rev 21(9):103155. https://doi.org/10.1016/j.autrev.2022.103155
Huang WJ, Chen WW, Zhang X (2017) Multiple sclerosis: pathology, diagnosis and treatments. Exp Ther Med 13(6):3163–3166. https://doi.org/10.3892/etm.2017.4410
Inaguma T, Han J, Isoda H (2011) Improvement of insulin resistance by Cyanidin 3-glucoside, anthocyanin from black beans through the up-regulation of GLUT4 gene expression. BMC Proc 5 Suppl 8(Suppl 8):P21. https://doi.org/10.1186/1753-6561-5-s8-p21
Ishikawa Y, Ikari K, Hashimoto M, Ohmura K, Tanaka M, Ito H, Terao C (2019) Shared epitope defines distinct associations of cigarette smoking with levels of anticitrullinated protein antibody and rheumatoid factor. Ann Rheum Dis 78(11):1480–1487. https://doi.org/10.1136/annrheumdis-2019-215463
Iwata S, Tanaka Y (2015) The importance of B cell-T cell interaction in autoimmune diseases. Nihon Rinsho Meneki Gakkai Kaishi 38(5):398–402. https://doi.org/10.2177/jsci.38.398
Jang SI, Kim HJ, Kim YJ, Jeong SI, You YO (2006) Tanshinone IIA inhibits LPS-induced NF-κB activation in RAW 264.7 cells: possible involvement of the NIK-IKK, ERK1/2, p38 and JNK pathways. Eur J Pharmacol 542(1–3):1–7. https://doi.org/10.1016/j.ejphar.2006.04.044
Jang EM, Choi MS, Jung UJ, Kim MJ, Kim HJ, Jeon SM, Lee MK (2008) Beneficial effects of curcumin on hyperlipidemia and insulin resistance in high-fat-fed hamsters. Metabolism 57(11):1576–1583. https://doi.org/10.1016/j.metabol.2008.06.014
Jaskulski S, Jung AY, Huebner M, Poschet G, Hell R, Hüsing A, Gonzalez-Maldonado S, Behrens S, Obi N, Becher H, Chang-Claude J (2020) Prognostic associations of circulating phytoestrogens and biomarker changes in long-term survivors of postmenopausal breast cancer. Nutr Cancer 72(7):1155–1169. https://doi.org/10.1080/01635581.2019.1672762
Jin Y, Liu S, Ma Q, Xiao D, Chen L (2017) Berberine enhances the AMPK activation and autophagy and mitigates high glucose-induced apoptosis of mouse podocytes. Eur J Pharmacol 794:106–114. https://doi.org/10.1016/j.ejphar.2016.11.037
Kadakol A, Sharma N, Kulkarni YA, Gaikwad AB (2016) Esculetin: A phytochemical endeavor fortifying effect against non-communicable diseases. Biomed Pharmacother 84:1442–1448. https://doi.org/10.1016/j.biopha.2016.10.072
Kalim KW, Yang JQ, Li Y, Meng Y, Zheng Y, Guo F (2018) Reciprocal regulation of glycolysis-driven Th17 pathogenicity and regulatory T cell stability by Cdc42. J Immunol 200(7):2313–2326. https://doi.org/10.4049/jimmunol.1601765
Kanwal R, Gupta S (2012) Epigenetic modifications in cancer. Clin Genet 81(4):303–311. https://doi.org/10.1111/j.1399-0004.2011.01809.x
Karar J, Maity A (2011) PI3K/AKT/mTOR pathway in angiogenesis. Front Mol Neurosci 4:51. https://doi.org/10.3389/fnmol.2011.00051
Karas M, Amir H, Fishman D, Danilenko M, Segal S, Nahum A, Sharoni Y (2000) Lycopene interferes with cell cycle progression and insulin-like growth factor I signaling in mammary cancer cells. Nutr Cancer 36(1):101–111. https://doi.org/10.1207/s15327914nc3601_14

Katz PS, Trask AJ, Lucchesi PA (2009) Curcuminoids: spicing up sympathovagal tone. Nutrition 25(7–8):879–880. https://doi.org/10.1016/j.nut.2009.03.007

Kaur H, He B, Zhang C, Rodriguez E, Hage DS, Moreau R (2018) Piperine potentiates curcumin-mediated repression of mTORC1 signaling in human intestinal epithelial cells: implications for the inhibition of protein synthesis and TNFalpha signaling. J Nutr Biochem 57:276–286. https://doi.org/10.1016/j.jnutbio.2018.04.010

Khan N, Mukhtar H (2013) Tea and health: studies in humans. Curr Pharm Des 19(34):6141–6147. https://doi.org/10.2174/1381612811319340008

Khosravi MA, Seifert R (2024) Clinical trials on curcumin in relation to its bioavailability and effect on malignant diseases: critical analysis. Naunyn Schmiedeberg's Arch Pharmacol 397(5):3477–3491. https://doi.org/10.1007/s00210-023-02825-7

Kim S (2015) New and emerging factors in tumorigenesis: an overview. Cancer Manag Res 7:225–239. https://doi.org/10.2147/cmar.S47797

Kinnunen T, Chamberlain N, Morbach H, Cantaert T, Lynch M, Preston-Hurlburt P, Meffre E (2013) Specific peripheral B cell tolerance defects in patients with multiple sclerosis. J Clin Invest 123(6):2737–2741. https://doi.org/10.1172/JCI68775

Klareskog L, Stolt P, Lundberg K, Kallberg H, Bengtsson C, Grunewald J, Alfredsson L (2006) A new model for an etiology of rheumatoid arthritis: smoking may trigger HLA-DR (shared epitope)-restricted immune reactions to autoantigens modified by citrullination. Arthritis Rheum 54(1):38–46. https://doi.org/10.1002/art.21575

Koh Y-C, Ho C-T, Pan M-H (2020) Recent advances in cancer chemoprevention with phytochemicals. J Food Drug Anal 28(1):14–37. https://doi.org/10.1016/j.jfda.2019.11.001

Kono M, Yoshida N, Maeda K, Skinner NE, Pan W, Kyttaris VC, Tsokos GC (2018) Pyruvate dehydrogenase phosphatase catalytic subunit 2 limits Th17 differentiation. Proc Natl Acad Sci USA 115(37):9288–9293. https://doi.org/10.1073/pnas.1805717115

La Cava A (2018) Tregs in SLE: an update. Curr Rheumatol Rep 20(2):6. https://doi.org/10.1007/s11926-018-0714-8

Lakhlani PP, MacMillan LB, Guo TZ, McCool BA, Lovinger DM, Maze M, Limbird LE (1997) Substitution of a mutant alpha2a-adrenergic receptor via "hit and run" gene targeting reveals the role of this subtype in sedative, analgesic, and anesthetic-sparing responses in vivo. Proc Natl Acad Sci USA 94(18):9950–9955. https://doi.org/10.1073/pnas.94.18.9950

Leppkes M, Neurath MF (2020) Cytokines in inflammatory bowel diseases - update 2020. Pharmacol Res 158:104835. https://doi.org/10.1016/j.phrs.2020.104835

Li XH, Li CY, Xiang ZG, Hu JJ, Lu JM, Tian RB, Jia W (2012) Allicin ameliorates cardiac hypertrophy and fibrosis through enhancing of Nrf2 antioxidant signaling pathways. Cardiovasc Drugs Ther 26(6):457–465. https://doi.org/10.1007/s10557-012-6415-z

Li R, Rezk A, Miyazaki Y, Hilgenberg E, Touil H, Shen P et al (2015) Proinflammatory GM-CSF-producing B cells in multiple sclerosis and B cell depletion therapy. Sci Transl Med 7(310):310ra166. https://doi.org/10.1126/scitranslmed.aab4176

Li F, Xiong F, Xu ZL, Zhang DG, Yao J, Wang LS (2020) Polyglycolic acid sheets decrease post-endoscopic submucosal dissection bleeding in early gastric cancer: A systematic review and meta-analysis. J Dig Dis 21(8):437–444. https://doi.org/10.1111/1751-2980.12908

Li F, Liu J, Tang S, Yan J, Chen H, Li D, Yan X (2021) Quercetin regulates inflammation, oxidative stress, apoptosis, and mitochondrial structure and function in H9C2 cells by promoting PVT1 expression. Acta Histochem 123(8):151819. https://doi.org/10.1016/j.acthis.2021.151819

Lin J, Della-Fera MA, Baile CA (2005) Green tea polyphenol epigallocatechin gallate inhibits adipogenesis and induces apoptosis in 3T3-L1 adipocytes. Obes Res 13(6):982–990. https://doi.org/10.1038/oby.2005.115

Liochev SI (2013) Reactive oxygen species and the free radical theory of aging. Free Radic Biol Med 60:1–4. https://doi.org/10.1016/j.freeradbiomed.2013.02.011

Liu RH (2004) Potential synergy of phytochemicals in cancer prevention: mechanism of action. J Nutr 134(12):3479S–3485S. https://doi.org/10.1093/jn/134.12.3479S

Liu S, Zhao W, Lan P, Mou X (2021) The microbiome in inflammatory bowel diseases: from pathogenesis to therapy. Protein Cell 12(5):331–345. https://doi.org/10.1007/s13238-020-00745-3

Lloyd-Price J, Arze C, Ananthakrishnan AN, Schirmer M, Avila-Pacheco J, Poon TW, Huttenhower C (2019) Multi-omics of the gut microbial ecosystem in inflammatory bowel diseases. Nature 569(7758):655–662. https://doi.org/10.1038/s41586-019-1237-9

Lopes-Rodrigues V, Sousa E, Vasconcelos MH (2016) Curcumin as a modulator of P-glycoprotein in cancer: challenges and perspectives. Pharmaceuticals (Basel, Switzerland) 9(4). https://doi.org/10.3390/ph9040071

López-Alarcón C, Denicola A (2013) Evaluating the antioxidant capacity of natural products: a review on chemical and cellular-based assays. Anal Chim Acta 763:1–10. https://doi.org/10.1016/j.aca.2012.11.051

Lou YP, Franco-Cereceda A, Lundberg JM (1992) Variable alpha 2-adrenoceptor-mediated inhibition of bronchoconstriction and peptide release upon activation of pulmonary afferents. Eur J Pharmacol 210(2):173–181. https://doi.org/10.1016/0014-2999(92)90668-t

Louis XL, Murphy R, Thandapilly SJ, Yu L, Netticadan T (2012) Garlic extracts prevent oxidative stress, hypertrophy and apoptosis in cardiomyocytes: a role for nitric oxide and hydrogen sulfide. BMC Complement Altern Med 12:140. https://doi.org/10.1186/1472-6882-12-140

Magliozzi R, Howell O, Vora A, Serafini B, Nicholas R, Puopolo M, Aloisi F (2007) Meningeal B-cell follicles in secondary progressive multiple sclerosis associate with early onset of disease and severe cortical pathology. Brain 130(Pt 4):1089–1104. https://doi.org/10.1093/brain/awm038

Mahammedi H, Planchat E, Pouget M, Durando X, Cure H, Guy L, Eymard JC (2016) The new combination docetaxel, prednisone and curcumin in patients with castration-resistant prostate cancer: a pilot phase II study. Oncology 90(2):69–78. https://doi.org/10.1159/000441148

Malmstrom V, Catrina AI, Klareskog L (2017) The immunopathogenesis of seropositive rheumatoid arthritis: from triggering to targeting. Nat Rev Immunol 17(1):60–75. https://doi.org/10.1038/nri.2016.124

Manichanh C, Rigottier-Gois L, Bonnaud E, Gloux K, Pelletier E, Frangeul L, Dore J (2006) Reduced diversity of faecal microbiota in Crohn's disease revealed by a metagenomic approach. Gut 55(2):205–211. https://doi.org/10.1136/gut.2005.073817

Manjunatha H, Srinivasan K (2007) Hypolipidemic and antioxidant effects of curcumin and capsaicin in high-fat-fed rats. Can J Physiol Pharmacol 85(6):588–596. https://doi.org/10.1139/y07-044

Mann GE, Niehueser-Saran J, Watson A, Gao L, Ishii T, de Winter P, Siow RC (2007) Nrf2/ARE regulated antioxidant gene expression in endothelial and smooth muscle cells in oxidative stress: implications for atherosclerosis and preeclampsia. Sheng Li Xue Bao 59(2):117–127

Marchiani A, Rozzo C, Fadda A, Delogu G, Ruzza P (2014) Curcumin and curcumin-like molecules: from spice to drugs. Curr Med Chem 21(2):204–222. https://doi.org/10.2174/092986732102131206115810

McCreary MR, Schnell PM, & Rhoda DA (2022) Randomized double-blind placebo-controlled proof-of-concept trial of resveratrol for outpatient treatment of mild coronavirus disease (COVID-19). Randomized Controlled Trial 12(1):10978. https://doi.org/10.1038/s41598-022-13920-9

Mas-Orea X, Sebert M, Benamar M, Petitfils C, Blanpied C, Saoudi A, Dietrich G (2021) Peripheral opioid receptor blockade enhances epithelial damage in piroxicam-accelerated colitis in IL-10-deficient mice. Int J Mol Sci 22(14). https://doi.org/10.3390/ijms22147387

Mehan S, Arora N, Bhalla S, Khan A, U Rehman M, Alghamdi BS, Ashraf GM (2022) Involvement of phytochemical-encapsulated nanoparticles' interaction with cellular signalling in the amelioration of benign and malignant brain tumours. Molecules 27(11):3561. https://doi.org/10.3390/molecules27113561

Meng X, Zhou J, Zhao CN, Gan RY, Li HB (2020) Health benefits and molecular mechanisms of resveratrol: a narrative review. Foods 9(3). https://doi.org/10.3390/foods9030340

Miljkovic D, Spasojevic I (2013) Multiple sclerosis: molecular mechanisms and therapeutic opportunities. Antioxid Redox Signal 19(18):2286–2334. https://doi.org/10.1089/ars.2012.5068

Mirza S, Penny C, Jain NK, Rawal RM (2023) Curcumin mediated dendritic cell maturation by modulating cancer associated fibroblasts-derived exosomal miRNA-146a. J Cancer Res Ther 19:S649–S657. https://doi.org/10.4103/jcrt.jcrt_1286_22

Mogensen TH (2009) Pathogen recognition and inflammatory signaling in innate immune defenses. Clin Microbiol Rev 22(2):240–273, Table of Contents. https://doi.org/10.1128/CMR.00046-08

Moran NE, Thomas-Ahner JM, Wan L, Zuniga KE, Erdman JW, Clinton SK (2022) Tomatoes, lycopene, and prostate cancer: what have we learned from experimental models? J Nutr 152(6):1381–1403. https://doi.org/10.1093/jn/nxac066

Mozaffarian D, Benjamin EJ, Go AS, Arnett DK, Blaha MJ, Cushman M, Turner MB (2016) Heart disease and stroke statistics-2016 update: a report from the American Heart Association. Circulation 133(4):e38–e360. https://doi.org/10.1161/cir.0000000000000350

Mukhopadhyay A, Bueso-Ramos C, Chatterjee D, Pantazis P, Aggarwal BB (2001) Curcumin downregulates cell survival mechanisms in human prostate cancer cell lines. Oncogene 20(52):7597–7609. https://doi.org/10.1038/sj.onc.1204997

Nahum A, Hirsch K, Danilenko M, Watts CKW, Prall OWJ, Levy J, Sharoni Y (2001) Lycopene inhibition of cell cycle progression in breast and endometrial cancer cells is associated with reduction in cyclin D levels and retention of p27 (Kip1) in the cyclin E-cdk2 complexes. Oncogene 20(26):3428–3436. https://doi.org/10.1038/sj.onc.1204452

Nahum A, Zeller L, Danilenko M, Prall OWJ, Watts CKW, Sutherland RL, Sharoni Y (2006) Lycopene inhibition of IGF-induced cancer cell growth depends on the level of cyclin D1. Eur J Nutr 45(5):275–282. https://doi.org/10.1007/s00394-006-0595-x

Nakachi K, Matsuyama S, Miyake S, Suganuma M, Imai K (2000) Preventive effects of drinking green tea on cancer and cardiovascular disease: epidemiological evidence for multiple targeting prevention. Biofactors 13(1–4):49–54. https://doi.org/10.1002/biof.5520130109

Nanjundaiah SM, Venkatesha SH, Yu H, Tong L, Stains JP, Moudgil KD (2012) Celastrus and its bioactive celastrol protect against bone damage in autoimmune arthritis by modulating osteoimmune cross-talk. J Biol Chem 287(26):22216–22226. https://doi.org/10.1074/jbc.M112.356816

Ness J, Aronow WS, Ahn C (2000) Risk factors for coronary artery disease in old persons in an academic hospital-based geriatrics practice. Coron Artery Dis 11(5):437–439. https://doi.org/10.1097/00019501-200007000-00009

Ohl K, Tenbrock K (2015) Regulatory T cells in systemic lupus erythematosus. Eur J Immunol 45(2):344–355. https://doi.org/10.1002/eji.201344280

Oliveira ALB, Monteiro VVS, Navegantes-Lima KC, Reis JF, Gomes RS, Rodrigues DVS, Monteiro MC (2017) Resveratrol role in autoimmune disease-a mini-review. Nutrients 9(12). https://doi.org/10.3390/nu9121306

Oshaghi EA, Goodarzi MT, Higgins V, Adeli K (2017) Role of resveratrol in the management of insulin resistance and related conditions: mechanism of action. Crit Rev Clin Lab Sci 54(4):267–293. https://doi.org/10.1080/10408363.2017.1343274

Panyod S, Wu W-K, Lu K-H, Liu C-T, Chu Y-L, Ho C-T, Hsiao W-L. W, Lai Y-S, Chen W-C, Lin Y-E, Lin S-H, Wu M-S, Sheen L-Y (2020) Allicin modifies the composition and function of the gut microbiota in alcoholic hepatic steatosis mice. J Agric Food Chem 68(10):3088–3098. https://doi.org/10.1021/acs.jafc.9b07555

Paramsothy S, Kamm MA, Kaakoush NO, Walsh AJ, van den Bogaerde J, Samuel D, Borody TJ (2017) Multidonor intensive faecal microbiota transplantation for active ulcerative colitis: a randomised placebo-controlled trial. Lancet 389(10075):1218–1228. https://doi.org/10.1016/S0140-6736(17)30182-4

Parent K, Mitchell P (1978) Cell wall-defective variants of pseudomonas-like (group Va) bacteria in Crohn's disease. Gastroenterology 75(3):368–372

Patel SS, Acharya A, Ray RS, Agrawal R, Raghuwanshi R, Jain P (2020) Cellular and molecular mechanisms of curcumin in prevention and treatment of disease. Crit Rev Food Sci Nutr 60(6):887–939. https://doi.org/10.1080/10408398.2018.1552244

Peeters MA, Chizzolini C (2011) Cardiovascular risk in autoimmune and inflammatory disorders. Rev Med Suisse 7(291):867–871

Perry MC, Demeule M, Regina A, Moumdjian R, Beliveau R (2010) Curcumin inhibits tumor growth and angiogenesis in glioblastoma xenografts. Mol Nutr Food Res 54(8):1192–1201. https://doi.org/10.1002/mnfr.200900277

Petri M (2007) Monitoring systemic lupus erythematosus in standard clinical care. Best Pract Res Clin Rheumatol 21(4):687–697. https://doi.org/10.1016/j.berh.2007.01.003

Pichersky E, Gang DR (2000) Genetics and biochemistry of secondary metabolites in plants: an evolutionary perspective. Trends Plant Sci 5(10):439–445. https://doi.org/10.1016/S1360-1385(00)01741-6

Pisetsky DS (2023) Pathogenesis of autoimmune disease. Nat Rev Nephrol 19(8):509–524. https://doi.org/10.1038/s41581-023-00720-1

Poljsak B, Šuput D, Milisav I (2013) Achieving the balance between ROS and antioxidants: when to use the synthetic antioxidants. Oxidative Med Cell Longev 2013(1):956792. https://doi.org/10.1155/2013/956792

Pooja R, Kaid Johar SR (2019) Metabolism and pharmacokinetics of phytochemicals in the human body. Curr Drug Metab 20(14):1085–1102. https://doi.org/10.2174/1389200221666200103090757

Postal M, Vivaldo JF, Fernandez-Ruiz R, Paredes JL, Appenzeller S, Niewold TB (2020) Type I interferon in the pathogenesis of systemic lupus erythematosus. Curr Opin Immunol 67:87–94. https://doi.org/10.1016/j.coi.2020.10.014

Powrie F, Leach MW, Mauze S, Menon S, Caddle LB, Coffman RL (1994) Inhibition of Th1 responses prevents inflammatory bowel disease in scid mice reconstituted with CD45RBhi CD4+ T cells. Immunity 1(7):553–562. https://doi.org/10.1016/1074-7613(94)90045-0

Qi WJ, Sheng WS, Peng C, Ma X, Yao TZ (2021) Investigating into anti-cancer potential of lycopene: molecular targets. Biomed Pharmacother 138:111546. https://doi.org/10.1016/j.biopha.2021.111546

Qin J, Fu M, Wang J, Huang F, Liu H, Huangfu M, Chen X (2020) PTEN/AKT/mTOR signaling mediates anticancer effects of epigallocatechin-3-gallate in ovarian cancer. Oncol Rep 43(6):1885–1896. https://doi.org/10.3892/or.2020.7571

Rahmani AH, Alsahli MA, Khan AA, Almatroodi SA (2023) Quercetin, a Plant Flavonol Attenuates Diabetic Complications, Renal Tissue Damage, Renal Oxidative Stress and Inflammation in Streptozotocin-Induced Diabetic Rats. Metabolites 13(1):130. https://doi.org/10.3390/metabo13010130

Ramaswamy M, Tummala R, Streicher K, Nogueira da Costa A, Brohawn PZ (2021) The pathogenesis, molecular mechanisms, and therapeutic potential of the interferon pathway in systemic lupus erythematosus and other autoimmune diseases. Int J Mol Sci 22(20). https://doi.org/10.3390/ijms222011286

Ramesh E, Geraldine P, Thomas PA (2010) Regulatory effect of epigallocatechin gallate on the expression of C-reactive protein and other inflammatory markers in an experimental model of atherosclerosis. Chem Biol Interact 183(1):125–132. https://doi.org/10.1016/j.cbi.2009.09.013

Renaud S, de Lorgeril M (1992) Wine, alcohol, platelets, and the French paradox for coronary heart disease. Lancet 339(8808):1523–1526. https://doi.org/10.1016/0140-6736(92)91277-f

Rincon-Riveros A, Lopez L, Villegas EV, Antonia Rodriguez J (2021) Regulation of antitumor immune responses by exosomes derived from tumor and immune cells. Cancer 13(4). https://doi.org/10.3390/cancers13040847

Roda G, Jharap B, Neeraj N, Colombel JF (2016) Loss of response to anti-TNFs: definition, epidemiology, and management. Clin Transl Gastroenterol 7(1):e135. https://doi.org/10.1038/ctg.2015.63

Ronnblom L, Leonard D (2019) Interferon pathway in SLE: one key to unlocking the mystery of the disease. Lupus Sci Med 6(1):e000270. https://doi.org/10.1136/lupus-2018-000270

Ross R (1993) The pathogenesis of atherosclerosis: a perspective for the 1990s. Nature 362(6423):801–809. https://doi.org/10.1038/362801a0

Rossen NG, Fuentes S, van der Spek MJ, Tijssen JG, Hartman JH, Duflou A, Ponsioen CY (2015) Findings from a randomized controlled trial of fecal transplantation for patients with ulcerative colitis. Gastroenterology 149(1):110–118 e114. https://doi.org/10.1053/j.gastro.2015.03.045

Rudzinska A, Juchaniuk P, Oberda J, Wisniewska J, Wojdan W, Szklener K, Mandziuk S (2023) Phytochemicals in cancer treatment and cancer prevention-review on epidemiological data and clinical trials. Nutrients 15(8). https://doi.org/10.3390/nu15081896

Saha P, Golonka RM, Abokor AA, Yeoh BS, Vijay-Kumar M (2021) IL-10 receptor neutralization-induced colitis in mice: a comprehensive guide. Curr Protoc 1(8):e227. https://doi.org/10.1002/cpz1.227

Saleh MM, Darwish ZE, El Nouaem MI, Fayed NA, Mourad GM, Ramadan OR (2023) The potential preventive effect of dietary phytochemicals in vivo. BDJ Open 9(1). https://doi.org/10.1038/s41405-023-00157-5

Santulli G (2015) MicroRNAs distinctively regulate vascular smooth muscle and endothelial cells: functional implications in angiogenesis, atherosclerosis, and in-stent restenosis. Adv Exp Med Biol 887:53–77. https://doi.org/10.1007/978-3-319-22380-3_4

Saraiva M, O'Garra A (2010) The regulation of IL-10 production by immune cells. Nat Rev Immunol 10(3):170–181. https://doi.org/10.1038/nri2711

Schiering C, Krausgruber T, Chomka A, Frohlich A, Adelmann K, Wohlfert EA, Powrie F (2014) The alarmin IL-33 promotes regulatory T-cell function in the intestine. Nature 513(7519):564–568. https://doi.org/10.1038/nature13577

Schlee M, Hartmann G (2016) Discriminating self from non-self in nucleic acid sensing. Nat Rev Immunol 16(9):566–580. https://doi.org/10.1038/nri.2016.78

Selimovic D, Hassan M, Haikel Y, Hengge UR (2008) Taxol-induced mitochondrial stress in melanoma cells is mediated by activation of c-Jun N-terminal kinase (JNK) and p38 pathways via uncoupling protein. Cell Signal 20(2):311–322. https://doi.org/10.1016/j.cellsig.2007.10.015

Serafini B, Rosicarelli B, Magliozzi R, Stigliano E, Aloisi F (2004) Detection of ectopic B-cell follicles with germinal centers in the meninges of patients with secondary progressive multiple sclerosis. Brain Pathol 14(2):164–174. https://doi.org/10.1111/j.1750-3639.2004.tb00049.x

Sergott RC, Bennett JL, Rieckmann P, Montalban X, Mikol D, Freudensprung U, Group, A. T (2015) ATON: results from a phase II randomized trial of the B-cell-targeting agent atacicept in patients with optic neuritis. J Neurol Sci 351(1–2):174–178. https://doi.org/10.1016/j.jns.2015.02.019

Sethi G, Ahn KS, Pandey MK, Aggarwal BB (2007) Celastrol, a novel triterpene, potentiates TNF-induced apoptosis and suppresses invasion of tumor cells by inhibiting NF-kappaB-regulated gene products and TAK1-mediated NF-kappaB activation. Blood 109(7):2727–2735. https://doi.org/10.1182/blood-2006-10-050807

Shakeel L, Shaukat A, Khaliq N, Kashif A, Mujeeb A, Adnan Z, Akilimali A (2025) Rheumatoid arthritis: a comprehensive overview of genetic markers, emerging therapies, and personalized medicine. Ann Med Surg (Lond) 87(2):696–710. https://doi.org/10.1097/MS9.0000000000002890

Shakibaei M, John T, Schulze-Tanzil G, Lehmann I, Mobasheri A (2007) Suppression of NF-kappaB activation by curcumin leads to inhibition of expression of cyclo-oxygenase-2 and matrix metalloproteinase-9 in human articular chondrocytes: implications for the treatment of osteoarthritis. Biochem Pharmacol 73(9):1434–1445. https://doi.org/10.1016/j.bcp.2007.01.005

Shakibaei M, Mobasheri A, Lueders C, Busch F, Shayan P, Goel A (2013) Curcumin enhances the effect of chemotherapy against colorectal cancer cells by inhibition of NF-kappaB and Src protein kinase signaling pathways. PLoS One 8(2):e57218. https://doi.org/10.1371/journal.pone.0057218

Shakibaei M, Buhrmann C, Kraehe P, Shayan P, Lueders C, Goel A (2014) Curcumin chemosensitizes 5-fluorouracil resistant MMR-deficient human colon cancer cells in high density cultures. PLoS One 9(1):e85397. https://doi.org/10.1371/journal.pone.0085397

Shakibaei M, Kraehe P, Popper B, Shayan P, Goel A, Buhrmann C (2015) Curcumin potentiates antitumor activity of 5-fluorouracil in a 3D alginate tumor microenvironment of colorectal cancer. BMC Cancer 15:250. https://doi.org/10.1186/s12885-015-1291-0

Shin S-A, Moon SY, Kim W-Y, Paek S-M, Park HH, Lee CS (2018) Structure-based classification and anti-cancer effects of plant metabolites. Int J Mol Sci 19(9):2651. https://doi.org/10.3390/ijms19092651

Skopelja-Gardner S, An J, Tai J, Tanaka L, Sun X, Hermanson P, Elkon KB (2020) The early local and systemic Type I interferon responses to ultraviolet B light exposure are cGAS dependent. Sci Rep 10(1):7908. https://doi.org/10.1038/s41598-020-64865-w

Song Y, Li J, Wu Y (2024) Evolving understanding of autoimmune mechanisms and new therapeutic strategies of autoimmune disorders. Signal Transduct Target Ther 9(1):263. https://doi.org/10.1038/s41392-024-01952-8

Srimal RC, Dhawan BN (1973) Pharmacology of diferuloyl methane (curcumin), a non-steroidal anti-inflammatory agent. J Pharm Pharmacol 25(6):447–452. https://doi.org/10.1111/j.2042-7158.1973.tb09131.x

Stangl V, Dreger H, Stangl K, Lorenz M (2007) Molecular targets of tea polyphenols in the cardiovascular system. Cardiovasc Res 73(2):348–358. https://doi.org/10.1016/j.cardiores.2006.08.022

Su HC, Hung LM, Chen JK (2006) Resveratrol, a red wine antioxidant, possesses an insulin-like effect in streptozotocin-induced diabetic rats. Am J Physiol Endocrinol Metab 290(6):E1339–E1346. https://doi.org/10.1152/ajpendo.00487.2005

Takeshima H, Ushijima T (2019) Accumulation of genetic and epigenetic alterations in normal cells and cancer risk. NPJ Precis Oncol 3:7. https://doi.org/10.1038/s41698-019-0079-0

Takeuchi O, Akira S (2010) Pattern recognition receptors and inflammation. Cell 140(6):805–820. https://doi.org/10.1016/j.cell.2010.01.022

Talaat RM, Mohamed SF, Bassyouni IH, Raouf AA (2015) Th1/Th2/Th17/Treg cytokine imbalance in systemic lupus erythematosus (SLE) patients: correlation with disease activity. Cytokine 72(2):146–153. https://doi.org/10.1016/j.cyto.2014.12.027

Tangvarasittichai S (2015) Oxidative stress, insulin resistance, dyslipidemia and type 2 diabetes mellitus. World J Diabetes 6(3):456–480. https://doi.org/10.4239/wjd.v6.i3.456

Taniguchi K, Karin M (2018) NF-kappaB, inflammation, immunity and cancer: coming of age. Nat Rev Immunol 18(5):309–324. https://doi.org/10.1038/nri.2017.142

Teng MW, Bowman EP, McElwee JJ, Smyth MJ, Casanova JL, Cooper AM, Cua DJ (2015) IL-12 and IL-23 cytokines: from discovery to targeted therapies for immune-mediated inflammatory diseases. Nat Med 21(7):719–729. https://doi.org/10.1038/nm.3895

Tenore GC, Campiglia P, Giannetti D, Novellino E (2015) Simulated gastrointestinal digestion, intestinal permeation and plasma protein interaction of white, green, and black tea polyphenols. Food Chem 169:320–326. https://doi.org/10.1016/j.foodchem.2014.08.006

Teodoro AJ, Oliveira FL, Martins NB, Maia G d A, Martucci RB, Borojevic R (2012) Effect of lycopene on cell viability and cell cycle progression in human cancer cell lines. Cancer Cell Int 12:36. https://doi.org/10.1186/1475-2867-12-36

Tipoe GL, Leung TM, Hung MW, Fung ML (2007) Green tea polyphenols as an anti-oxidant and anti-inflammatory agent for cardiovascular protection. Cardiovasc Hematol Disord Drug Targets 7(2):135–144. https://doi.org/10.2174/187152907780830905

Trinchieri G (2003) Interleukin-12 and the regulation of innate resistance and adaptive immunity. Nat Rev Immunol 3(2):133–146. https://doi.org/10.1038/nri1001

Tsuda T, Horio F, Uchida K, Aoki H, Osawa T (2003) Dietary cyanidin 3-O-beta-D-glucoside--rich purple corn color prevents obesity and ameliorates hyperglycemia in mice. J Nutr 133(7):2125–2130. https://doi.org/10.1093/jn/133.7.2125

Vanpouille-Box C, Hoffmann JA, Galluzzi L (2019) Pharmacological modulation of nucleic acid sensors - therapeutic potential and persisting obstacles. Nat Rev Drug Discov 18(11):845–867. https://doi.org/10.1038/s41573-019-0043-2

Wang GE, Li YF, Wu YP, Tsoi B, Zhang SJ, Cao LF, He RR (2014) Phloridzin improves lipoprotein lipase activity in stress-loaded mice via AMPK phosphorylation. Int J Food Sci Nutr 65(7):874–880. https://doi.org/10.3109/09637486.2014.925429

Wang J, Zhao X, Wan YY (2023) Intricacies of TGF-beta signaling in Treg and Th17 cell biology. Cell Mol Immunol 20(9):1002–1022. https://doi.org/10.1038/s41423-023-01036-7

Wei H, Li B, Sun A, Guo F (2019) Interleukin-10 family cytokines immunobiology and structure. Adv Exp Med Biol 1172:79–96. https://doi.org/10.1007/978-981-13-9367-9_4

Weyand CM, Hicok KC, Conn DL, Goronzy JJ (1992) The influence of HLA-DRB1 genes on disease severity in rheumatoid arthritis. Ann Intern Med 117(10):801–806. https://doi.org/10.7326/0003-4819-117-10-801

Widmer RJ, Freund MA, Flammer AJ, Sexton J, Lennon R, Romani A, Lerman A (2013) Beneficial effects of polyphenol-rich olive oil in patients with early atherosclerosis. Eur J Nutr 52(3):1223–1231. https://doi.org/10.1007/s00394-012-0433-2

Wolf C, Lim EL, Mokhtari M, Kind B, Odainic A, Lara-Villacanas E, Lee-Kirsch MA (2024) UNC93B1 variants underlie TLR7-dependent autoimmunity. Sci Immunol 9(92):eadi9769. https://doi.org/10.1126/sciimmunol.adi9769

Wong VKW, Qiu C, Xu SW, Law BYK, Zeng W, Wang H, Liu L (2019) Ca(2+) signalling plays a role in celastrol-mediated suppression of synovial fibroblasts of rheumatoid arthritis patients and experimental arthritis in rats. Br J Pharmacol 176(16):2922–2944. https://doi.org/10.1111/bph.14718

Xiao QP, Zhong YB, Kang ZP, Huang JQ, Fang WY, Wei SY, Liu DY (2022) Curcumin regulates the homeostasis of Th17/Treg and improves the composition of gut microbiota in type 2 diabetic mice with colitis. Phytother Res 36(4):1708–1723. https://doi.org/10.1002/ptr.7404

Xu H, Zhang X, Wang X, Li B, Yu H, Quan Y, Cao X (2024) Cellular spermine targets JAK signaling to restrain cytokine-mediated autoimmunity. Immunity 57(8):1796–1811 e1798. https://doi.org/10.1016/j.immuni.2024.05.025

Yang B, Zheng CY, Zhang R, Zhao C, Li S, An Y (2021) Quercetin efficiently alleviates TNF-alpha-stimulated injury by signal transducer and activator of transcription 1 and mitogen-activated protein kinase pathway in H9c2 cells: a protective role of quercetin in myocarditis. J Cardiovasc Pharmacol 77(5):570–577. https://doi.org/10.1097/FJC.0000000000001000

Yao J, Wei C, Wang JY, Zhang R, Li YX, Wang LS (2015) Effect of resveratrol on Treg/Th17 signaling and ulcerative colitis treatment in mice. World J Gastroenterol 21(21):6572–6581. https://doi.org/10.3748/wjg.v21.i21.6572

Yu XH, Zhang DW, Zheng XL, Tang CK (2019) Cholesterol transport system: an integrated cholesterol transport model involved in atherosclerosis. Prog Lipid Res 73:65–91. https://doi.org/10.1016/j.plipres.2018.12.002

Yuan M, Sun T, Zhang Y, Guo C, Wang F, Yao Z, Yu L (2024) Quercetin alleviates insulin resistance and repairs intestinal barrier in db/db mice by modulating gut microbiota. Nutrients 16(12). https://doi.org/10.3390/nu16121870

Zang M, Xu S, Maitland-Toolan KA, Zuccollo A, Hou X, Jiang B, Cohen RA (2006) Polyphenols stimulate AMP-activated protein kinase, lower lipids, and inhibit accelerated atherosclerosis in diabetic LDL receptor-deficient mice. Diabetes 55(8):2180–2191. https://doi.org/10.2337/db05-1188

Zhang R, Miao J, Zhu P (2021) Regulatory T cell heterogeneity and therapy in autoimmune diseases. Autoimmun Rev 20(5):102715. https://doi.org/10.1016/j.autrev.2020.102715

Zhang S, Xiao X, Yi Y, Wang X, Zhu L, Shen Y et al (2024) Tumor initiation and early tumorigenesis:molecular mechanisms and interventional targets. Signal Transduct Target Ther 9(7):2900–2935. https://doi.org/10.1038/s41392-024-01848-7

Zhao Y, Hansen NL, Duan YT, Prasad M, Motawia MS, Moller BL, Kampranis SC (2023) Biosynthesis and biotechnological production of the anti-obesity agent celastrol. Nat Chem 15(9):1236–1246. https://doi.org/10.1038/s41557-023-01245-7

Zhao Y, Miettinen K, Kampranis SC (2024) Celastrol: A century-long journey from the isolation to the biotechnological production and the development of an antiobesity drug. Curr Opin Plant Biol 81:102615. https://doi.org/10.1016/j.pbi.2024.102615

Zhou B (2002) Predictive values of body mass index and waist circumference to risk factors of related diseases in Chinese adult population. Zhonghua Liu Xing Bing Xue Za Zhi 23(1):5–10

Zhou X, Cao X, Tu H, Zhang ZR, Deng L (2019) Inflammation-targeted delivery of celastrol via neutrophil membrane-coated nanoparticles in the management of acute pancreatitis. Mol Pharm 16(3):1397–1405. https://doi.org/10.1021/acs.molpharmaceut.8b01342

Zhu KJ, Shen QY, Cheng H, Mao XH, Lao LM, Hao GL (2005) Triptolide affects the differentiation, maturation and function of human dendritic cells. Int Immunopharmacol 5(9):1415–1426. https://doi.org/10.1016/j.intimp.2005.03.020

Zhu Y, Huang Y, Ming B, Wu X, Chen Y, Dong L (2019) Regulatory T-cell levels in systemic lupus erythematosus patients: a meta-analysis. Lupus 28(4):445–454. https://doi.org/10.1177/0961203319828530

Zhu Y, Zhao L, Yan W, Ma H, Zhao W, Qu J, Ouyang Z (2025) Celastrol directly targets LRP1 to inhibit fibroblast-macrophage crosstalk and ameliorates psoriasis progression. Acta Pharm Sin B 15(2):876–891. https://doi.org/10.1016/j.apsb.2024.12.041

Phytochemicals Potentially Applied for Dermatological Diseases

Sandipan Dash, Arghya Kusum Dhar, and Subhadas Chatterjee

Abstract Dermatological disorders impose a significant global burden, driving the need for novel, cost-effective therapeutic strategies that transcend the limitations of conventional treatments. This chapter highlights the potential of phytochemicals, including flavonoids, phenolic acids, terpenoids, alkaloids, tannins, and saponins, in managing diverse dermatological disorders such as eczema, acne, hyperpigmentation, photoageing, and even skin cancers. These naturally derived compounds exert multifaceted effects by neutralising oxidative stress, modulating inflammatory pathways, inhibiting critical enzymes like tyrosinase and matrix metalloproteinases, and promoting collagen synthesis and wound healing, thereby enhancing skin barrier integrity and repair. Collectively, the convergence of traditional herbal wisdom with modern scientific methodologies foresees a transformative era in personalised dermatological care, where phytochemical-based formulations offer sustainable and effective alternatives for skin protection and rejuvenation.

Keywords Phytochemicals · Dermatological disorders · Anti-ageing · Skin protector · Derma-therapy

---

S. Dash
University Institute of Pharma Sciences, Chandigarh University, Mohali, Punjab, India

A. K. Dhar (✉)
School of Pharmacy, The Neotia University, Sarisha, West Bengal, India

S. Chatterjee
School of Pharmacy, The Neotia University, Sarisha, West Bengal, India

Bengal School of Technology, Sugandha, Chuchura, Hooghly, West Bengal, India

S. Kumar Tripathi et al. (eds.), *Phytoceuticals for Sustainable Medication*, Interdisciplinary Biotechnological Advances,
https://doi.org/10.1007/978-981-95-7588-6_9

1 Introduction

Dermatological conditions constitute a prominent worldwide health concern; they are the fourth prevalent cause of human illness, impacting nearly one-third of the global population. Employing measures such as disability-adjusted life years to quantify both early death and impairment (Hay et al. 2014; Karimkhani et al. 2017), the impact of these ailments is remarkable: atopic dermatitis by itself is positioned 15th among all non-lethal diseases, reaching its highest levels in early childhood and recurring in middle-aged and elderly persons; acne, occurring increasingly in adolescents and females, and psoriasis, with its distinct bimodal occurrence peaking between 30–39 and 60–69 years (Iskandar et al. 2021; Gonçalo et al. 2021), further exemplify these patterns. Furthermore, chronic urticaria incurs an annual expense approaching 15,550 purchasing power parity dollars, accompanied by more than 30% of sufferers reporting substantial psychological health problems like anxiety and depression (Cox et al. 2021; Loney et al. 2021). These quantitative observations, combined with proof of the financial demands from occupational skin cancers and overlooked tropical skin afflictions, emphasise the critical requirement for novel, economical treatments such as phytochemicals to alleviate the substantial burden of skin diseases (Engelman et al. 2020; Murdoch 2021; Flohr and Hay 2021).

As the body's largest organ, the human integument plays a crucial role in protecting against pathogenic microorganisms and excessive transepidermal water loss. This protective function is ensured by the skin's anatomical structure, which comprises three main layers: the epidermis, dermis, and hypodermis (Tomczyk and Latté 2009). The outermost layer of the epidermis, known as the stratum corneum, consists of multiple layers of corneocytes encased in a lipid bilayer, forming a "brick and mortar" arrangement where keratin-rich corneocytes serve as the "bricks" and intercellular lipids act as the "mortar." While this layer serves as a barrier against pathogens, it also hinders the absorption of cosmeceutical active compounds into the underlying skin tissues (Alencastre et al. 2006; Scalia et al. 2015). However, continuous exposure to external chemical agents and environmental factors can lead to various complex dermatological conditions, such as eczematous disorders (including Atopic Dermatitis), dyschromia/pigmentation disorders, impaired wound healing, photocarcinogenesis, fibrotic dermal pathologies (e.g., Scleroderma), photoinduced ageing, and Acne Vulgaris.

Recent advances in phytochemical research have illuminated the remarkable potential of plant-derived compounds in managing dermatological diseases. A wide spectrum of botanicals from *Viola tricolor* and *Veronica officinalis* to *Achillea millefolium*, *Allium cepa*, *Withania somnifera*, and many others have been found to harbour an impressive variety of bioactive constituents. Flavonoids, phenolic acids, terpenoids, alkaloids, tannins, saponins, and other secondary metabolites have been identified as key players in neutralising oxidative stress, modulating inflammatory pathways, and enhancing skin repair mechanisms (Melnyk et al. 2022). These natural compounds not only combat the damaging effects of ultraviolet radiation, pathogen-induced inflammation, and free radical activity, but also support the maintenance and restoration of the skin barrier through intricate actions such as enzyme inhibition (e.g., tyrosinase, collagenase, elastase) and the regulation of cell growth and apoptosis. The dermatological benefits of these phytochemicals have been validated through a myriad of studies employing both traditional extraction methods and innovative technologies such as ultrasound-assisted and superheated water extraction (Gwiazdowska et al. 2022). For instance, advanced analyses demonstrate that compounds derived from plants like *Pentanema verbascifolium*, *Cuphea hookeriana*, and *Coffea arabica L.*, when integrated into novel formulations, can significantly reduce signs of photoageing, improve wound healing, and even counter hyperpigmentation. Moreover, the implementation of advanced delivery systems, such as liposomes, nanoemulsions, and solid lipid nanoparticles, has improved the bioavailability and targeted effectiveness of these compounds. This advancement not only strengthens their role as cosmeceutical ingredients, but also highlights their potential as therapeutic agents for various skin disorders. The fusion of traditional medicinal knowledge with modern scientific research marks a promising new frontier in dermatology. By integrating empirical evidence from in vitro studies, in vivo models, and emerging clinical evaluations, the current landscape supports the use of phytochemicals as versatile, naturally derived agents that may provide safer and more cost-effective alternatives to conventional treatments (Młynarczyk et al. 2018). This chapter delved into the diverse applications of these phytochemicals in skin protection and regeneration.

2 Structure of Skin

The skin is a dynamic, multilayered organ consisting of three primary layers (Fig. 1) that work in harmony to protect the body, regulate temperature, and facilitate sensory perception (Brito et al. 2024; Meindl et al. 2024). At the surface, the epidermis is primarily made up of keratinocytes, which transform into a hardened, keratin-filled barrier. Meanwhile, melanocytes provide pigmentation to shield against harmful UV rays, and Langerhans and Merkel cells contribute to immune defence and tactile sensing (Lee et al. 2024). Just below, the dermis is a robust matrix of connective tissue, rich in collagen and elastin fibres produced by fibroblasts, which grant the skin both strength and elasticity. This layer houses hair follicles, accompanied by sebaceous glands that lubricate and protect, as well as sweat glands crucial for cooling, along with an intricate network of blood vessels and sensory nerve endings that continuously supply nutrients and alert the body to environmental changes (Prausnitz 2004). Finally, the innermost hypodermis, or subcutaneous tissue, is primarily composed of adipose tissue, which not only cushions underlying muscles and bones but also provides insulation and serves as an energy reserve, anchoring the skin to deeper structures and allowing for flexible movement (Hymes 1984).

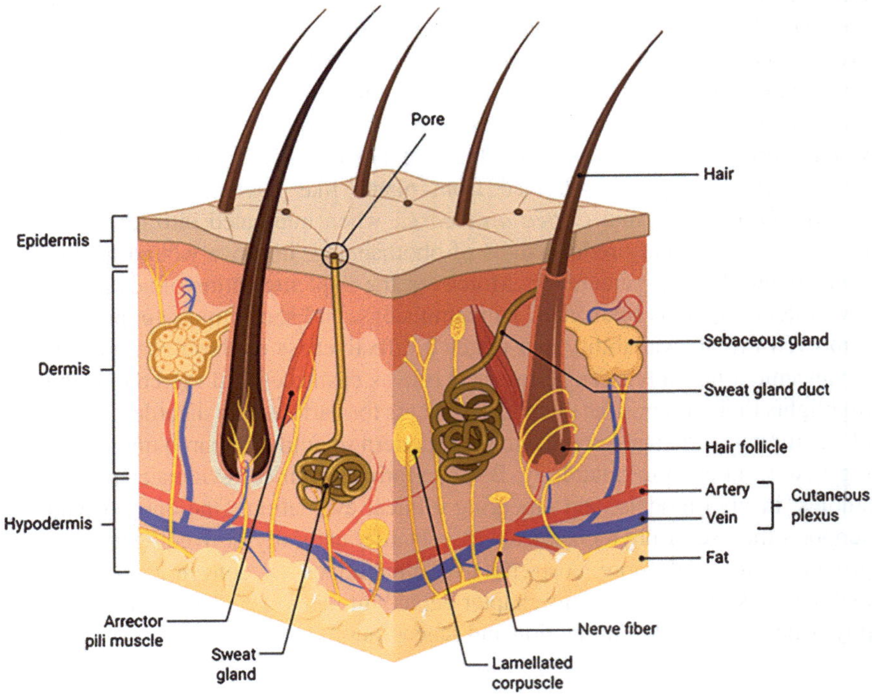

Fig. 1 Structure of skin

3 Normal Skin Function and Factors Affecting the Function

The figure below illustrates the skin's multifaceted role as a dynamic and complex organ, highlighting its functions as a protective barrier, an active participant in wound healing, and a vigilant immune defence system. It also details the various factors (Fig. 2) that can disrupt these functions (Patel and Hussain 2021; Guo et al. 2021; Mistry et al. 2023). The outermost layer, known as the stratum corneum, acts as a physical barricade, preventing the entry of pathogens, harmful chemicals, and excessive moisture loss. This layer is reinforced by chemical defences such as antimicrobial peptides and immune cells like Langerhans cells, which help detect and neutralise potential threats (Agaimy et al. 2018; Goodlad et al. 2023). Simultaneously, when injury occurs, the skin initiates a meticulously coordinated healing process. This begins with an inflammatory phase where cells release histamines and cytokines to trigger a cascade of immune activities, progresses into a proliferation phase marked by the actions of neutrophils and macrophages that clear debris and foster new cell and blood vessel formation, and culminates in a remodeling phase that reinforces tissue strength (Claudel et al. 2018; Bakry et al. 2021; Carrilho and Lunet 2023). However, this robust defence mechanism can be compromised by several factors: microbial infections that breach an already weakened barrier; genetic

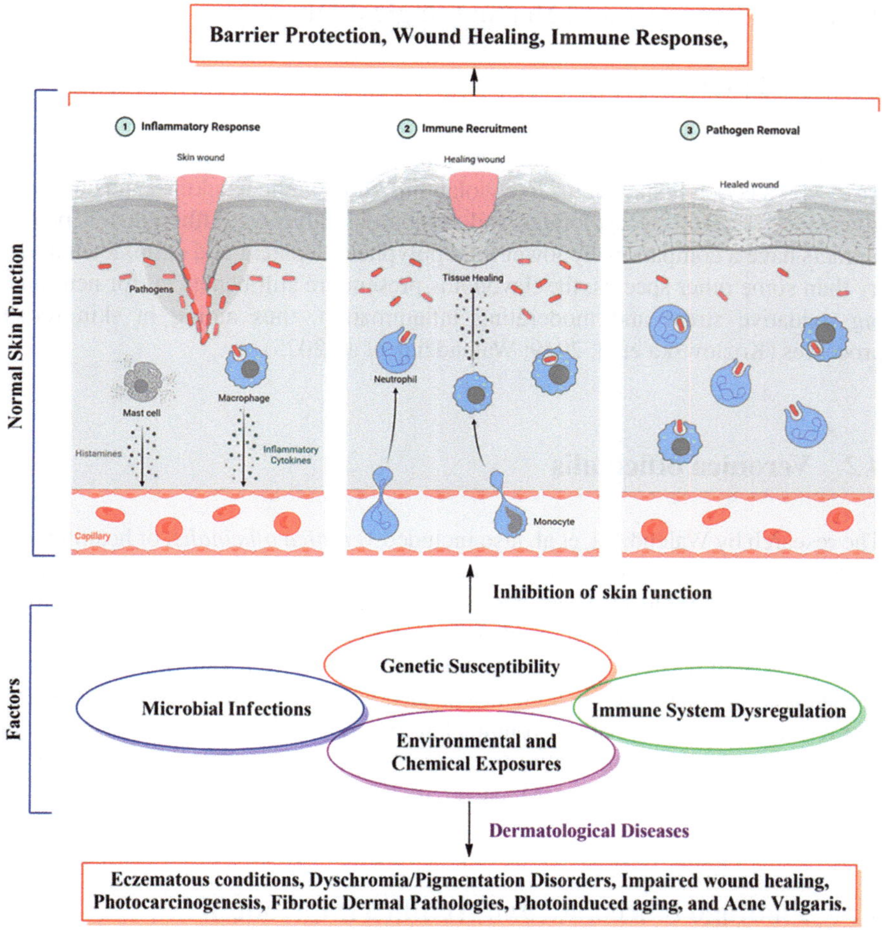

Fig. 2 Normal function of skin and functions affecting the normal functions of the skin, which lead to dermatological problems

predispositions, such as those seen in individuals prone to eczema or psoriasis, which affect the skin's ability to repair itself; environmental and chemical exposures, including ultraviolet radiation, pollutants, and harsh chemicals that gradually degrade structural proteins and accelerate ageing; and immune system dysregulation, which may lead to overactive inflammatory responses, contributing to conditions like acne or autoimmune disorders. Ultimately, disturbances in these normal functions can lead to a spectrum of issues ranging from delayed wound healing and increased infection risk to chronic skin conditions and premature ageing, underscoring the delicate balance and intricate interplay of factors that sustain skin health (Fujii et al. 2019).

4 Phytochemicals and Dermatological Diseases

4.1 Viola tricolor

Walendziak et al. investigated *Viola tricolor*, also known as wild pansy or heartsease, which is rich in flavonoids like violanthin, rutin, anthocyanidins, and quercetin glycosides, as well as cyclotides and bisabolol (Table 1). Although the plant's extracts have a comparatively lower total polyphenol content and antioxidant activity than some other species, the flavonoids present are still beneficial for neutralising oxidative stress and moderating inflammation, thus aiding in skin repair processes (Kozlowska et al. 2019; Walendziak et al. 2025).

4.2 Veronica officinalis

The research by Walendziak et al. also included *Veronica officinalis*, or heath speedwell, which contains quercitrin, p-coumaric acid, ferulic acid, luteolin, hispidulin, and β-sitosterol (Table 1). These compounds enhance the skin's regenerative abilities by strengthening antioxidant defences and reducing inflammation while preserving the skin barrier's integrity. In Glechoma hederacea, known as ground ivy, the main components are phenolic acids, such as chlorogenic, rosmarinic, caffeic, and ferulic acids, along with flavonoids like rutin and genistin (Fig. 3). These substances work together to neutralise free radicals and alleviate inflammation, contributing to a stronger skin barrier (Mocan et al. 2015).

4.3 Plantago lanceolata *and* Achillea millefolium

Walendziak et al. examined *Plantago lanceolata*, or ribwort plantain, which contains a complex mix of polyphenols, tannins, flavonoids, alkaloids, terpenoids, and iridoid glycosides (Table 1) (including p-hydroxybenzoic, vanillic, gallic, and chlorogenic acids, as well as derivatives of apigenin and luteolin). This diverse range of constituents is linked to antimicrobial and anti-inflammatory benefits that soothe irritated skin and promote barrier restoration. *Achillea millefolium*, commonly known as yarrow, is notable for its high levels of specific flavonoids (notably luteolin O-acetylhexoside and apigenin O-acetylhexoside), organic acids such as malic, oxalic, and quinic acids, and tocopherols. Its strong anti-inflammatory and wound-healing properties make it effective in reducing skin irritation and speeding up the healing of minor abrasions, while its antioxidant features further support skin detoxification (Zillich et al. 2015).

Table 1 Summary of phytoconstituents potentially applied for the treatment of different classes of dermatological diseases

Class of disorders	Plant source	Key phytoconstituents	Target skin disorder	Mechanism
Inflammatory and barrier disorders	*Allium cepa*	Quercetin, organosulfur	Psoriasis, atopic dermatitis, acne	Alleviates oxidative stress; antimicrobial; anti-inflammatory
	Paeonia suffruticosa, Mentha haplocalyx, Portulaca oleracea L., Azadirachta indica	Flavonoids, polyphenols, terpenoids, essential oils	Eczema, atopic dermatitis	Reduce inflammation; improve barrier function
	Plantago lanceolata	Polyphenols, tannins, flavonoids, iridoids	Eczema	Antimicrobial; anti-inflammatory; promotes barrier restoration
	Achillea millefolium	Luteolin O-acetylhexoside, organic acids, tocopherols	Inflammatory skin conditions	Anti-inflammatory; wound healing
	Veronica officinalis	Quercitrin, p-Coumaric acid, ferulic acid, luteolin	Barrier disorders	Enhance skin regeneration; antioxidant; preserve barrier integrity
	Sambucus nigra	Rutin, quercetin, caffeoylquinic acid	UV damage, barrier dysfunction	UV protection; maintain hydration and barrier performance
	Thymus vulgaris, Ocimum basilicum, Salvia Rosmarinus	Ursolic acid (UA)	Inflammatory skin conditions, skin cancer	Anti-inflammatory; anti-proliferative; induces apoptosis
	Tilia tomentosa	Polyphenols, phytohormones, saponins	Skin hydration loss	Improve hydration; chemo-protective

(continued)

Table 1 (continued)

Class of disorders	Plant source	Key phytoconstituents	Target skin disorder	Mechanism
Hyperpigmentation	*Pentanema verbascifolium*	Chlorogenic acid, apigenin, kaempferol, luteolin	Hyperpigmentation	Tyrosinase inhibition (IC_{50} ~1.16 mg/mL)
	Nelumbo nucifera	Kaempferol-3-O-robinobioside (Kae-3-Rob)	Hyperpigmentation	Inhibits tyrosinase (~70%)
	Cuphea hookeriana	Myricitrin, tellimoside, galloylglucoses	Hyperpigmentation, photoageing	Tyrosinase inhibition (~70.5%); reduces UVB-induced melanin
	Aloe barbadensis	Aloesin	Hyperpigmentation	Competitive tyrosinase inhibitor; reduces melanin
	Arctostaphylos uva-ursi	Arbutin	Hyperpigmentation	Competitive tyrosinase inhibition
	Glycyrrhiza glabra	Glabridin, liquiritin	Hyperpigmentation, melasma	Inhibits tyrosinase; anti-inflammatory; clinically effective for melasma
	Ximenia americana var. caffra	Rutin, isoquercetin, avicularin, tannins	Hyperpigmentation, ageing	Tyrosinase inhibition; antioxidant; inhibits collagenase/elastase

Photoageing and UV damage	*Capsicum annuum*	Capsaicin	Photoageing	Reverses UV-induced collagen decline; inhibits MMPs
	Camellia sinensis	Epigallocatechin Gallate	Photoageing, Photocarcinogenesis	Activates Nrf2; combats ROS/DNA damage; inhibits MMPs
	Prunus dulcis	α-Tocopherol, quercetin, catechin	UV damage	Antioxidant; UV absorption; reduces photodamage
	Diospyros kaki	Phenolic acids, flavonoids, carotenoids	Wrinkles, hyperpigmentation	Neutralises ROS; inhibits collagenase/elastase/tyrosinase
	Glycine max	Genistein, daidzein, lunasin, anthocyanins	Photoageing, skin cancer	Inhibits MMP-1; enhances collagen I/III; antioxidant
	Polygonum cuspidatum	Resveratrol	Photoageing, skin cancer	Counters UV-induced DNA damage; modulates NF-κB/MAPK pathways
Acne and infections	*Garcinia mangostana*	α-Mangostin	Acne	Reduces sebum; inhibits C. acnes; anti-inflammatory
	Hypoxis hemerocallidea	α-Myrcene, n-Hexadecanoic acid	Skin infections	Antimicrobial (MIC <1 mg/mL)
	Thymus satureioides	Phenolic acids, flavonoids	Pseudomonas aeruginosa infections	Antimicrobial (MIC 50 mg/mL); reduces biofilm

(continued)

Table 1 (continued)

Class of disorders	Plant source	Key phytoconstituents	Target skin disorder	Mechanism
Wound healing	*Coffea arabica*	Chlorogenic acid	Wound repair	Promotes wound contraction (78.20% in vivo)
	Withania somnifera	Withaferin A	Scleroderma, wound healing	Antifibrotic (interferes with TGF-β/Smad); influences melanogenesis
	Labisia pumila	Quercetin, kaempferol, saponins	Tissue repair	Promotes collagen synthesis in fibroblasts
Skin cancer	*Honey*	Caffeic Acid Phenethyl Ester (CAPE)	Skin cancer	Anticarcinogenic; suppresses angiogenesis
	Curcuma longa	Curcumin	Skin cancer	Targets NF-κB/COX-2; reduces inflammation/ oxidative stress

MMPs Matrix Metalloproteinases, *ROS* Reactive Oxygen Species, *MIC* Minimum Inhibitory Concentration, *NF-κB/MAPK* Signalling pathways involved in inflammation and cancer, *TGF-β* Transforming Growth Factor beta (fibrosis regulator)

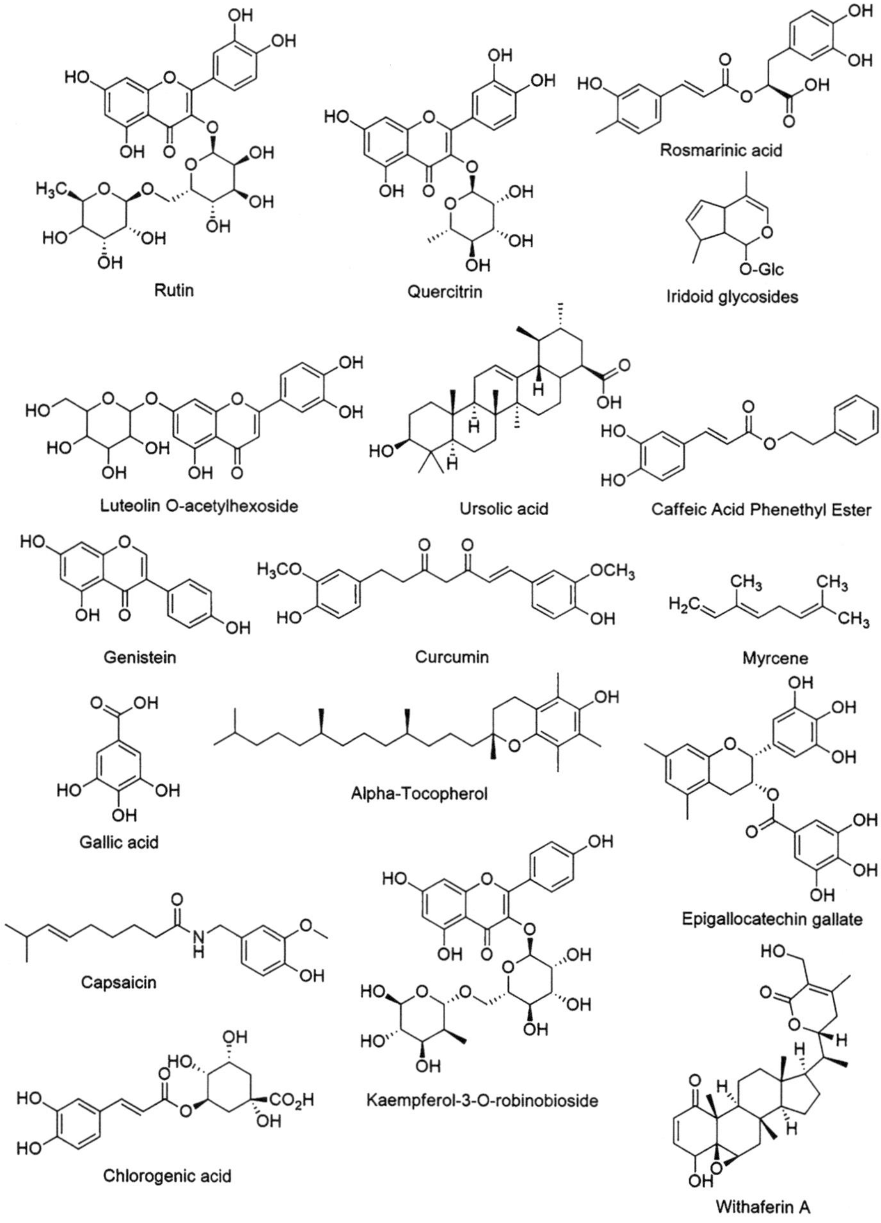

Fig. 3 Phytoconstituents having applications in the treatment of dermatological diseases

4.4 Sambucus nigra

Walendziak et al. extracted and studied *Sambucus nigra*, or elderberry, which is recognised for its strong antioxidant potential, largely due to high concentrations of flavonoids, such as rutin, quercetin, and kaempferol, and phenolic acids, such as caffeoylquinic acid (Table 1). This robust antioxidant capacity is crucial for protecting the skin from UV-induced damage and maintaining optimal hydration and barrier performance. Tilia cordata, rich in vanillic acid, rutoside, and (±)-epicatechin, enhances skin hydration and provides additional anti-inflammatory benefits. Lastly, Potentilla erecta, known as tormentil or septfoil, is abundant in tannins, ellagitannins, various phenolic acids, flavonoids, and triterpene saponins. Its compounds demonstrate significant antimicrobial and anti-inflammatory properties, reducing redness and enhancing skin tightness by supporting overall barrier function (Boroduske et al. 2021).

4.5 Thymus vulgaris, Ocimum basilicum, Salvia Rosmarinus

Iqbal et al. highlighted several herbs, including thyme (*Thymus vulgaris*), basil (*Ocimum basilicum*), and rosemary (*Salvia Rosmarinus*), as abundant sources of Ursolic Acid (UA). This compound is renowned for its anti-proliferative, antioxidant, and anti-inflammatory effects (Table 1). UA promotes health by inducing apoptosis through caspase activation and influencing critical cell cycle regulators, emphasising its potential in cancer prevention and treatment. Honey, a product of bees, is a recognised source of Caffeic Acid Phenethyl Ester (CAPE), a phytochemical with significant anticarcinogenic properties. It can suppress angiogenic factors, essential for tumour development, by restricting the formation of new blood vessels to cancer cells. Soybeans are known for genistein, an isoflavone with potent antioxidant, anti-inflammatory, and antiproliferative properties. Genistein aids in maintaining cellular balance by disrupting various signalling pathways that control cell growth and apoptosis, thus lowering the risk of unchecked cell proliferation. A variety of vegetables and fruits, such as carrots, celery, olives, and peppers, contain luteolin. This bioactive compound is crucial in hindering cancer progression by modulating several signalling pathways, including the focal adhesion kinase pathway, which is important for cell adhesion and migration. Lastly, the rhizome of *Curcuma longa*, or turmeric, produces curcumin. This powerful phytochemical targets various molecular pathways, such as NF-κB and COX-2, aiding in cancer prevention and treatment by reducing inflammation and oxidative stress (Allen-Mersh 1997; Imanbayev et al. 2018; Iqbal et al. 2019).

4.6 Allium cepa

Gupta et al. explored *Allium cepa* (Onion) and identified flavonoids like Quercetin and Kaempferol, with Quercetin being the most prominent (Table 1). This compound is a strong antioxidant and anti-inflammatory agent. Neutralising free radicals, it alleviates oxidative stress, a key factor in skin ageing, inflammation, and conditions like psoriasis and atopic dermatitis. Quercetin also regulates collagen production, which can enhance scar appearance and diminish hypertrophic scars. Organosulfur compounds, such as Allicin, Diallyl disulfide, and Diallyl trisulfide, are initially responsible for onions' strong aroma. They have significant antimicrobial properties, making them effective against skin pathogens that can cause acne and other infections. Additionally, their anti-inflammatory properties support their use in treating inflammatory skin conditions. Phenolic acids add to the antioxidant capacity, shielding skin cells from UV damage and environmental pollutants. In red onions and even in waste parts like the peel, anthocyanins provide colour and bioactivity by strengthening the skin's antioxidant defences and modulating inflammatory responses (Borlinghaus et al. 2014; Brüll et al. 2015; Gupta et al. 2025).

4.7 Pentanema verbascifolium

Selvi et al. explored *Pentanema verbascifolium*, focusing on the leaves extracted using ultrasound-assisted methanol extraction, which revealed a diverse range of bioactive phytochemicals (Table 1). These included significant total phenolic (94.38 mg GAEs/g extract) and flavonoid contents (67.54 mg REs/g extract), with chlorogenic acid levels reaching 9739 μg/g, along with notable amounts of apigenin, kaempferol, luteolin, and vanillin. These compounds collectively contribute to strong antioxidant and anti-inflammatory properties, making them highly relevant for treating skin disorders. Extensive in vitro tests, including phosphomolybdenum, CUPRAC, FRAP, DPPH, and ABTS assays, showed that the leaf extracts have excellent free radical scavenging and reducing abilities. Enzyme inhibition studies indicated that the extracts, particularly the root extracts, exhibit strong tyrosinase inhibitory activity (IC_{50} around 1.16 mg/mL), which may help regulate melanin production and offer potential as natural treatments for hyperpigmentation. They also have the potential to alleviate oxidative stress and inflammation associated with various skin conditions, although further in vivo and clinical studies are needed to confirm these initial findings and fully utilise their therapeutic potential in managing skin disorders (Sarikurkcu et al. 2019; Sezen Karaoğlan et al. 2023; Selvi 2025).

4.8 Hypoxis hemerocallidea

Mwinga et al. thoroughly examined the dermatological potential of *Hypoxis hemerocallidea* by extracting the plant's bulbs with both 50% methanol and petroleum ether to evaluate their antimicrobial, antioxidant, phytochemical, and cytotoxic properties (Table 1). The antimicrobial tests showed that both extracts effectively inhibited six skin-related pathogens, with particularly strong activity against Shigella flexneri and Trichophyton tonsurans, with minimum inhibitory concentrations (MICs) below 1 mg/mL, while other pathogens had MICs up to 12.5 mg/mL. Antioxidant assessments using the DPPH assay revealed an EC_{50} of 29.8 μg/mL, and a β-carotene-linoleic acid model showed 76.91% inhibition of bleaching, highlighting the extracts' ability to combat oxidative stress. Phytochemical analyses measured 41 mg GAE/g total phenolics and 10 mg CE/g total flavonoids, and GC-MS profiling identified 29 compounds in the methanol extract (with an even broader range in the petroleum ether extract), including bioactives like α-myrcene and n-hexadecanoic acid that likely contribute to the observed biological activities. Additionally, cytotoxicity evaluations using the MTT assay on Vero kidney cells showed LC_{50} values of 210.9 ± 18.4 μg/mL for the petroleum ether extract and 95.5 ± 13.3 μg/mL for the methanol extract, indicating a moderate safety profile that supports further in vivo studies to confirm these promising results for potential cosmetic and dermatological applications (Kaur et al. 2006; Thein et al. 2009; Mwinga et al. 2019).

4.9 Labisia pumila

Chua et al. discussed studies on *Labisia pumila*, also known as Kacip Fatimah, a traditional Malay herb known for its wide variety of bioactive phytochemicals, including flavonoids (quercetin, kaempferol, myricetin, and catechin), phenolic acids, and saponins (Fig. 3 and Table 1). These compounds not only exhibit strong antioxidant and anti-inflammatory properties, but also promote collagen synthesis in dermal fibroblasts, which is crucial for maintaining skin elasticity and reducing signs of photoageing. By neutralizing free radicals generated by UV exposure and environmental stress, these compounds help protect skin cells from oxidative damage and modulate inflammatory pathways, thereby enhancing skin repair and rejuvenation, while the herb's phytoestrogenic effects may further support hormonal balance and cellular proliferation, making *Labisia pumila* a promising natural candidate for innovative dermatological formulations aimed at improving skin texture and resilience (Kour et al. 2010; Chua et al. 2012; Mohd Zain et al. 2021).

4.10 Gentiana lutea *and* Camphora officinarum

According to Gradinaru et al., *Gentiana lutea* and the Camphor tree (*Camphora officinarum*) are rich sources of bioactive bitter compounds, including alkaloids, flavonoids, terpenoids, tannins, steroids, and phenolics (Table 1). These compounds have been thoroughly researched for their antioxidant, anti-inflammatory, antimicrobial, and wound-healing effects on skin disorders. Special focus is placed on bitter phytochemicals that interact with extraoral bitter taste receptors (TAS2Rs) in skin cells, influencing essential processes such as keratinocyte differentiation, collagen production, and calcium signalling. These mechanisms offer a molecular explanation for the benefits observed in skin ageing, inflammatory conditions, wound healing, and even skin cancer. This is supported by comprehensive in vitro studies (using HaCaT cells and primary keratinocytes), histological assessments, and in vivo experiments that combine traditional phytochemical screening with modern analytical methods to confirm efficacy and safety. Additionally, new formulations like nanotechnology-based delivery systems improve the bioavailability of these natural compounds, leading to innovative, cost-effective, and side-effect-free dermatological treatments (Luongo et al. 2022; Grădinaru et al. 2024).

4.11 Diospyros kaki

Kashif et al. highlighted that *Diospyros kaki*, or persimmon, has attracted considerable interest due to its wide array of bioactive phytoconstituents and its promising uses in dermatology and cosmeceuticals (Fig. 1). Traditionally employed in Chinese medicine for skin issues like pimples, eruptions, and eczema, modern studies show that extracts from different parts of the plant contain powerful antioxidant and anti-inflammatory compounds, including phenolic acids (gallic, chlorogenic, and caffeic acids), flavonoids (isoquercitrin, hyperin, and astragalin), carotenoids (beta-carotene, lutein, zeaxanthin, lycopene), tannins, terpenoids, and essential vitamins (A, D, E, and ascorbic acid). These compounds work together to neutralise reactive oxygen species, inhibit enzymes such as tyrosinase, collagenase, and elastase, decrease the release of pro-inflammatory cytokines, and strengthen skin barrier integrity. Collectively, they contribute to skin lightening, wrinkle reduction, photoprotection, and overall skin rejuvenation. This multifaceted effectiveness highlights the potential of persimmons as a natural ingredient in cosmetic products, although further clinical research is needed to determine optimal dosages, delivery systems, and long-term safety for human use (Fölster-Holst and Latussek 2007; Kashif et al. 2017).

4.12 Prunus dulcis

Evans-Johnson et al. explored the phytochemicals in almond (*Prunus dulcis*), particularly vitamin E (α-tocopherol) and a mix of polyphenolic flavonoids like quercetin, catechin, kaempferol, epicatechin, and isorhamnetin (Fig. 3 and Table 1), which have gained significant attention for their diverse roles in protecting and repairing skin from various disorders, especially those caused by UV radiation. These compounds exhibit strong antioxidant activity that reduces oxidative stress and lipid peroxidation, UV absorption that lessens photodamage, and anti-inflammatory effects that help regulate cellular signalling pathways involved in both cell death and repair. In advanced in vitro studies using three-dimensional human skin equivalent (HSE) models, these bioactive ingredients have shown promising outcomes. Pre-treatment with almond phytochemicals, applied either topically or through culture medium, improved UVA-induced morphological changes, maintained normal keratinocyte proliferation, reduced fibroblast apoptosis, and restored proper cellular differentiation, thereby re-establishing a more natural and resilient skin structure. Notably, topical application in these models achieved substantially higher local concentrations of the active agents compared to medium application, translating into more effective photoprotection, which not only suggests superior efficacy in preventing photodamage but also indicates potential benefits in countering chronic inflammatory conditions and premature ageing (Bernerd and Asselineau 1998; Evans-Johnson et al. 2013).

4.13 Camellia sinensis

Chaiprasongsuk and Panich (2022) investigated the bioactive phytochemicals found in *Camellia sinensis*, which present promising natural methods for safeguarding the skin against damage caused by ultraviolet radiation (UVR) by activating the nuclear factor erythroid 2-related factor 2 (Nrf2) pathway (Table 1). Although UVR is crucial for processes like vitamin D production and melanin synthesis, excessive exposure leads to the formation of reactive oxygen species (ROS) that initiate harmful intracellular signalling pathways, such as MAPK/AP-1, NF-κB, and STAT. This results in DNA damage, cell apoptosis, inflammation, and the breakdown of the extracellular matrix through matrix metalloproteinases (MMPs), collectively contributing to photoageing, abnormal pigmentation, and even photocarcinogenesis. However, during oxidative stress, Nrf2 separates from its inhibitor, Keap1, and moves into the nucleus to trigger the expression of antioxidant and cytoprotective enzymes, such as HO-1, NQO-1, and GST, thereby restoring redox balance and reducing inflammation. By boosting these natural defences, phytochemicals not only help prevent photoageing and maintain skin integrity but also influence pathways involved in melanogenesis, making them effective candidates for managing

UVR-related skin disorders and suggesting their potential as complementary agents in dermatological treatments. (Yamamoto et al. 2008; Chaiprasongsuk and Panich 2022).

4.14 Capsicum annuum

Wu et al. examined capsaicin, a key phytochemical from chilli pepper (*Capsicum annuum*), known for its anti-inflammatory, analgesic, and anti-psoriatic properties, as well as its protective effects on the skin (Table 1), particularly against UV-induced photoageing. They demonstrated that capsaicin reverses the UV-induced decline in collagen synthesis and the associated increase in matrix metalloproteinases (MMPs) in both in vivo mouse models and in vitro cultured dermal fibroblasts. The study showed that UV exposure raised reactive oxygen species (ROS) levels, which activated the Erk/c-Jun signalling pathway, leading to increased MMP expression and subsequent collagen degradation. Pre-treatment with capsaicin significantly reduced ROS production, inhibited the phosphorylation of Erk and c-Jun, and restored collagen levels in a dose-dependent manner, with its mechanism of action occurring independently of the TRPV1 receptor typically linked to its irritant effects. This suggests the high potential of capsaicin as a therapeutic agent for anti-photoageing skincare formulations and broader dermatological applications (Rosenbaum et al. 2004; Wu et al. 2022).

4.15 Stizolophus balsamita inflorescences

Nawrot et al. conducted several experiments on *Stizolophus balsamita inflorescences* and discovered that they contain a wide range of bioactive compounds that offer promising benefits for skin disorders and protection (Table 1). These include four main groups: sesquiterpene lactones (specifically germacranolides such as izospiciformin, stizolin, and stizolicin, which feature a 4,5-epoxide group enhancing their anti-inflammatory and antiserotonin activities), flavonoids (comprising quercetin, kaempferol, rhamnetin, taxifolin, and kaempferol 3-O-α-rhamnopyranoside, which deliver potent antioxidant and anti-inflammatory effects, with taxifolin notably demonstrating excellent safety in human fibroblast assays), a natural steroid (ajugasterone C, which may offer advantages as a safer, plant-derived alternative to synthetic steroids), and simple phenolic compounds (including arbutin, known for its skin-lightening properties, and protocatechuic acid methyl ester with additional health-promoting activities). When evaluated in a dermatological context, a 3% topical formulation of the *Stizolophus balsamita* extract significantly reduced transepidermal water loss (TEWL), thereby enhancing the skin's barrier function, while also showing a trend toward improved hydration without any significant cytotoxicity, making these phytoconstituents a compelling basis for developing new cosmetic and therapeutic strategies targeted at inflammatory skin conditions and overall barrier protection (Suedee et al. 2017; Nawrot et al. 2021).

4.16 Nelumbo nucifera

Nutho et al. conducted a study on *Nelumbo nucifera*, also known as the sacred lotus, which has been highly regarded in traditional medicine for its wide array of bioactive flavonoids, especially those in its stamen extract, showing promising potential for skin protection and anti-ageing uses (Table 1). Recent research utilising in silico molecular docking, molecular dynamics simulations, and in vitro enzyme assays has identified that significant compounds like kaempferol-3-O-robinobioside (Kae-3-Rob) effectively inhibit skin ageing enzymes such as collagenase, elastase, and tyrosinase, with inhibition rates of about 58% for collagenase and 70% for tyrosinase, and a moderate impact on elastase. These compounds interact with crucial residues in the enzymes' active sites, disrupting essential metalloprotein interactions and reducing oxidative and inflammatory processes involved in skin ageing, thereby supporting and expanding the traditional use of the lotus for skin health. This comprehensive evaluation not only provides a molecular basis for the empirical use of N. nucifera in skincare, but also opens avenues for developing new natural cosmeceutical products that utilise these powerful phytochemicals for improved skin protection and rejuvenation (Wagle et al. 2018; Nutho and Tungmunnithum 2023).

4.17 Paeonia suffruticosa, Mentha haplocalyx, Portulaca oleracea L., *and* Azadirachta indica

Radhakrishnan et al. *examined Paeonia suffruticosa, Mentha haplocalyx, Portulaca oleracea L., and Azadirachta indica*, whose phytochemicals have emerged as promising alternatives for managing eczema by addressing both the inflammatory response and skin barrier dysfunction characteristic of atopic dermatitis (Table 1). Various bioactive compounds, including flavonoids, polyphenols, terpenoids, and essential oils, exhibit anti-inflammatory, antioxidant, and immunomodulatory effects that reduce key mediators like interleukins, TNF-α, and immunoglobulin E, while simultaneously enhancing essential skin proteins such as filaggrin and loricrin to improve barrier integrity and reduce transepidermal water loss. Biological evaluations through in vitro assays and animal models, along with early-phase clinical studies, have shown improvements in clinical indices like SCORAD and EASI and patient-reported outcomes, indicating that these natural compounds can effectively reduce inflammation and restore skin hydration. Additionally, the development of advanced delivery systems, such as liposomes, ethosomes, and nanoemulsions, has improved the stability, penetration, bioavailability, and targeted release of these phytochemicals, offering the dual benefit of increased efficacy and reduced side effects compared to conventional topical therapies like corticosteroids and calcineurin inhibitors (Lin et al. 2013; Radhakrishnan et al. 2024).

4.18 Withania somnifera

Bungau et al. researched *Withania somnifera*, commonly known as Ashwagandha, a well-known medicinal plant whose therapeutic potential is largely attributed to its main bioactive compound, withaferin A (WFA) (Table 1). This potent withanolide is at the forefront of research exploring dermatological applications, as preclinical studies have demonstrated its multifaceted efficacy in treating various skin disorders. For instance, in skin cancers, WFA shows strong anticancer activity by inhibiting tumour cell proliferation and migration, inducing apoptosis, and modulating crucial metabolic and signalling pathways, including the stabilisation of isocitrate dehydrogenase 1 (IDH1) and repression of acetyl coenzyme A carboxylase-1 (ACC1) and NF-κB activation. Beyond its antitumour properties, withaferin A also shows promising antifibrotic effects in conditions such as scleroderma by interfering with TGF-β/Smad signalling and preventing fibroblast-to-myofibroblast transition, thereby reducing inflammation and skin hardening. Moreover, its potential role in managing pigmentation disorders by influencing melanogenesis further highlights its versatility in skin protection and repair is noteworthy. Together, these biological evaluations underline the significant promise of withaferin A as a natural therapeutic agent capable of bridging traditional Ayurvedic wisdom with modern dermatological treatment strategies (Bale et al. 2018; Bungau et al. 2021).

4.19 Garcinia mangostana, Eucalyptus globulus, Vitis vinifera, Curcuma longa, Camellia sinensis, Syzygium aromaticum, Hibiscus rosa-sinensis, *and* Salix species

Chutoprapat et al. explored the potential of various plant-derived phytochemicals, including *Garcinia mangostana, Eucalyptus globulus, Vitis vinifera, Curcuma longa, Camellia sinensis, Syzygium aromaticum, Hibiscus rosa-sinensis, and Salix species,* to address Acne vulgaris (Table 1). This common skin condition is characterised by excessive sebum production, bacterial growth, and inflammation, prompting interest in botanical solutions that offer multiple benefits with fewer side effects compared to conventional synthetic treatments. Mangosteen *(Garcinia mangostana)* contains xanthones, especially α-mangostin, which have been found to decrease keratinocyte growth and reduce inflammation caused by Cutibacterium acnes. Eucalyptus *(Eucalyptus globulus)* provides essential oils like 1,8-cineole and α-pinene, which help lower sebum levels and prevent bacterial proliferation in experimental settings. Similarly, resveratrol from grapes *(Vitis vinifera)* offers strong antioxidant and antimicrobial effects that help reduce acne lesions, while turmeric *(Curcuma longa)* curcuminoids exhibit notable anti-inflammatory and antimicrobial properties, particularly when advanced carriers enhance their skin retention. Green Tea *(Camellia sinensis)* contains epigallocatechin gallate (EGCG), which reduces inflammatory mediators and fights bacterial survival, and Clove *(Syzygium aromaticum)* provides eugenol, which targets *P. acnes* and improves skin hydration when properly formulated. Additionally, hibiscus *(Hibiscus rosa-sinensis)* and Willow Bark *(Salix species)* extracts offer anthocyanins, flavonoids, and salicin that aid in skin repair and inflammation reduction, with quercetin adding further antioxidant support. These botanicals are often incorporated into advanced topical formulations using delivery systems like solid lipid nanoparticles (SLNs) and nanostructured lipid carriers (NLCs) to address challenges such as instability and limited skin penetration. Their effectiveness has been confirmed through various in vitro antimicrobial tests, ex vivo skin penetration studies, and clinical evaluations, highlighting their potential as complementary agents in acne treatment (Raza et al. 2013; Chutoprapat et al. 2022).

4.20 Cucurbita *spp.* Peel

Gaweł-Beben et al. investigated the use of *Cucurbita* spp. *peel* extracts as multifunctional active ingredients for skincare and dermatology, employing sustainable, green extraction methods like ultrasound-assisted extraction with water, hydroglycolic, and ethanolic solvents to extract valuable bioactive compounds from the peels of Cucurbita maxima and Cucurbita moschata cultivars (Table 1). Detailed phytochemical analyses showed that these extracts are rich in phenolic acids (such as chlorogenic and p-coumaric acids), flavonoids (including apigenin and kaempferol derivatives), essential amino acids (such as L-tyrosine and L-valine, which contribute to the skin's natural moisturizing factor), and fatty acids (notably palmitic, oleic, and linoleic acids), each playing a crucial role in enhancing skin health. The extracts demonstrated high antioxidant potential using ABTS and DPPH assays, exhibited promising in vitro sun protection factor (SPF) values, and showed a nuanced influence on tyrosinase activity, which is important for melanin synthesis. Certain extracts enhanced enzyme activity, suggesting potential applications in skin-lightening and repigmentation therapies. Additionally, safety tests confirmed that these extracts were non-cytotoxic to human keratinocytes at concentrations up to 1000 μg/mL, thereby supporting their safe topical use. Overall, this study highlights the innovative use of pumpkin peel, a typically discarded agricultural by-product, for the development of eco-friendly cosmetic formulations that combine antioxidant, photoprotective, and skin-regenerative properties (Gaweł-Bęben et al. 2022; Sroczyk et al. 2024).

4.21 Cupressus arizonica

Research by Tawfeek et al. on *Cupressus arizonica* leaf extracts revealed significant potential for skincare applications due to their rich phytochemical and biological properties (Table 1). Through a detailed study employing both aqueous and ethanolic extraction techniques, 67 compounds were identified using LC-MS/MS. These included phenolic acids, fatty acids, diterpene acids, proanthocyanidins, and various flavonoid and biflavonoid glycosides, with the aqueous extract showing a higher concentration of polyphenolic content. This diverse phytochemical profile is the basis for its strong antioxidant activity, as evidenced by DPPH and FRAP assays, which are crucial for neutralising reactive oxygen species that contribute to skin ageing. Furthermore, both extracts effectively inhibited key enzymes such as collagenase, elastase, tyrosinase, and hyaluronidase, which are involved in the degradation of the skin's extracellular matrix and the acceleration of ageing processes, with IC50 values nearly matching those of standard inhibitors. Beyond its anti-ageing potential, the extract, especially at sub-inhibitory doses, reduced biofilm formation and decreased the motility of Pseudomonas aeruginosa, a common pathogen linked to skin infections. Overall, these findings indicate that *Cupressus arizonica* leaf extracts could be promising natural agents for developing innovative cosmeceutical and dermatological formulations aimed at protecting, preserving, and rejuvenating ageing skin while reducing bacterial infections (Elgamal et al. 2021; Tawfeek et al. 2023).

4.22 Thymus satureioides Coss.

Thymus satureioides Coss., a perennial aromatic herb native to Morocco's semiarid regions, was studied by Magdi et al. and has been traditionally used to treat various ailments, including skin disorders (Table 1). Modern research has confirmed its medicinal potential through extensive phytochemical and biological evaluations. The aqueous extract of its aerial parts is nutritionally rich, containing high levels of essential minerals like calcium and iron, moderate amounts of magnesium, manganese, and zinc, and a significant amino acid profile with notable levels of asparagine, 4-hydroxyproline, isoleucine, and leucine, the latter contributing to structural proteins such as collagen. Additionally, the extract is enriched with bioactive compounds, as indicated by its high total polyphenol (118.17 mg GAE/g extract) and flavonoid (32.32 mg quercetin extract) contents. LC-MS/MS analysis identified 46 secondary metabolites, including various phenolic acids, chalcones, and flavonoids, which support its strong antioxidant activity, as demonstrated in DPPH and ABTS assays. Its antimicrobial effectiveness is equally notable, as the extract completely inhibits the growth of Pseudomonas aeruginosa at a minimum inhibitory concentration of 50 mg/mL, while sub-inhibitory doses significantly reduce biofilm formation by over 35%, decrease extracellular protein secretion by up to 46%, lower exopolysaccharide production by nearly 69%, and impair bacterial motility. Moreover, in silico assessments predicted that 33 of these 46 compounds have minimal skin sensitisation risk and favourable permeability profiles, highlighting their potential safety in topical applications. Together, these integrated nutritional, antioxidant, and antimicrobial properties support the traditional use of T. satureioides in managing skin disorders and underscore its promising application in developing innovative dermacosmeceutical formulations aimed at enhancing skin hydration, elasticity, and protection against environmental stressors (Matić et al. 2017; Mahdi et al. 2023).

4.23 Cuphea hookeriana

Research by Wu et al. on *Cuphea hookeriana* uncovered that the fine active fraction derived from the plant's ethanolic extract is abundant in synergistic polyphenolic compounds, including myricitrin (Fig. 4), tellimoside, myricetin 3-O-(6″-O-galloyl) β-D-glucopyranoside, myricetin, desmanthin-1, penta-O-galloyl-β-D-glucose, and quercetin 3-O-β-(2″-O-galloylxylopyranoside), which collectively enhance its strong cosmeceutical properties (Table 1). This fraction demonstrated impressive antioxidant capabilities, with an ABTS IC50 of 1.66 μg/mL, comparable to standard

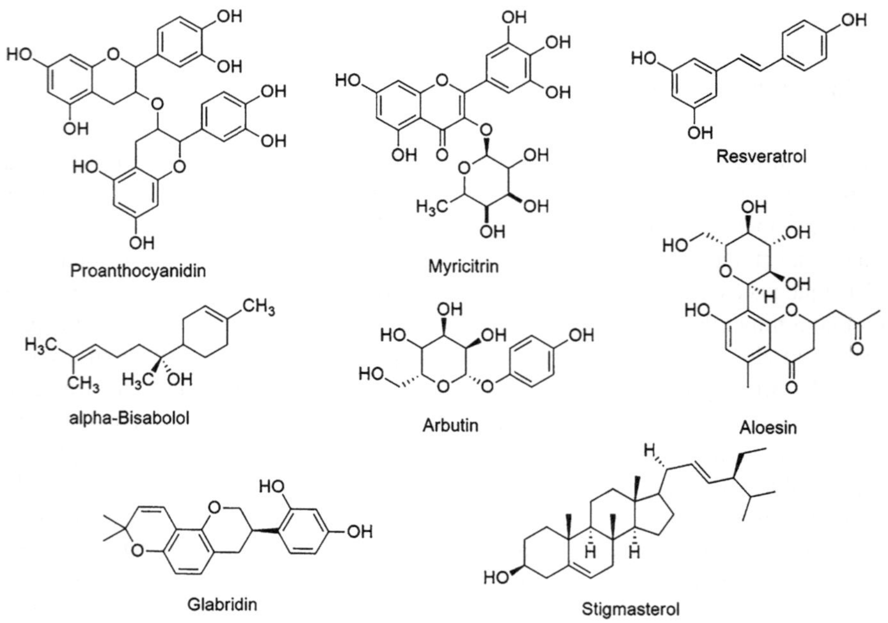

Fig. 4 Phytochemicals having a potential role in the management of dermatological disorders

compounds like α-arbutin. It also showed notable inhibition of key enzymes related to skin issues, reducing tyrosinase activity by about 70.5% and effectively inhibiting matrix metalloproteinase-1 (MMP-1) activity with an IC50 of 55.0 μg/mL, indicating its potential in skin-whitening and anti-ageing products. Additionally, acute toxicity tests in mice confirmed its safety at doses up to 2000 mg/kg. In vivo studies using a UVB-induced skin pigmentation model in guinea pigs further revealed that the fraction not only reduced melanin production more effectively than α-arbutin but also mitigated UV-induced skin thickening and encouraged collagen fibre growth. Overall, these findings suggest that *Cuphea hookeriana* has significant potential as a natural, plant-based ingredient for cosmeceutical applications, addressing skin ageing and hyperpigmentation through a multifaceted mechanism involving antioxidant protection and enzymatic inhibition (Song et al. 2021; Wu et al. 2025).

4.24 Coffea arabica L.

Affonso et al. investigated *Coffea arabica L.*, focusing on the rich phytochemical composition and bioactive potential of aqueous extracts from the residual press cake of coffee beans, highlighting their promising applications in managing and protecting against skin disorders (Table 1). The study thoroughly analysed the extract's contents using methods like the Folin-Ciocalteu assay and RP-HPLC, revealing that the green coffee extract contains a significantly higher concentration of phenolic compounds, particularly chlorogenic acid and related metabolites, compared to its roasted counterpart, a difference largely due to the degradation of these heat-sensitive compounds during roasting. Furthermore, the antioxidant potential of these extracts was confirmed using the DPPH assay, which showed a radical-scavenging capacity nearly equivalent to standard antioxidants like Trolox, emphasising the extracts' ability to reduce oxidative stress. In vitro evaluations using L929 mouse fibroblasts confirmed that the green coffee extract was non-cytotoxic at effective concentrations, while in vivo experiments using a murine excisional wound model demonstrated that hydrogel formulations enriched with green coffee extract achieved remarkable wound contraction (78.20%), outperforming both the roasted coffee extract (53.71%) and the widely used positive control, allantoin (70.83%). This comprehensive phytochemical and biological assessment suggests that the bioactive constituents of *Coffea arabica L.*, particularly from green coffee press cake, hold significant promise for developing sustainable, natural formulations in dermatological applications aimed at enhancing skin repair and protection (Farah et al. 2005; Affonso et al. 2016).

4.25 Althea officinalis

Curnow et al. conducted an evaluation of aqueous extracts from the roots of *Althea officinalis* (marshmallow) and Astragalus membranaceus to assess their potential as natural ingredients in UV-protective skin care products. The study employed a novel method involving superheated water extraction followed by ultrafiltration to isolate bioactive components, aiming to determine if these extracts could mitigate UVA-induced oxidative stress and DNA damage in cultured human fibroblasts (Table 1). The alkaline comet assay indicated that while Astragalus membranaceus extracts occasionally showed inherent genotoxic effects, especially in early ultrafiltrated fractions, *Althea officinalis* extracts consistently reduced DNA damage caused by UVA exposure. Additionally, the method of cultivation influenced efficacy, with hydroponically and glasshouse soil-grown Althea roots offering more sustained protection than commercially sourced, field-grown roots. Although the extracts showed promise against indirect UVA-induced oxidative damage, they did not significantly counteract the direct DNA-damaging effects of UVB radiation, implying that these phytochemicals are mainly effective against oxidative stress rather than direct UV-induced damage (Haywood et al. 2003; Curnow and Owen 2016).

4.26 Achillea millefolium

Strzępek-Gomółka et al. highlighted research on *Achillea millefolium*, or yarrow, which is well-known for its wide range of bioactive compounds and its traditional use in treating skin conditions, now validated by modern phytochemical and biological studies (Table 1). Extracts from *Achillea millefolium* are particularly rich in flavonoids, phenolic acids, terpenes, and guaianolides, which provide strong antioxidant, anti-inflammatory, antimicrobial, and tyrosinase inhibitory properties that help reduce oxidative stress and inflammation while aiding in wound healing and tissue regeneration. Research has shown that these extracts effectively downregulate pro-inflammatory mediators like TNF-α, IL-6, and COX-2 by influencing key signalling pathways (e.g., MAPK and STAT), thereby calming irritated skin and restoring its barrier function. Furthermore, advanced extraction methods such as ultrasound-assisted extraction have been found to increase the yield of these beneficial phytochemicals, enhancing their dermatological advantages and ensuring safety in use, as confirmed by non-irritant results in human patch tests. Overall, the complex phytochemistry and diverse bioactivity of Achillea support its increasing importance in developing innovative cosmeceutical and therapeutic products for effective skin protection and rejuvenation (Spiker and Mowad 2016; Strzępek-Gomółka et al. 2021).

4.27 Ximenia americana var. caffra

The study on *Ximenia americana var. caffra* done by Bakrim et al. elucidates a comprehensive phytochemical profile and a series of promising biological activities relevant to skin protection and anti-ageing (Table 1). Using advanced HPLC-PDA-ESI-MS/MS techniques, the leaf extract was found to contain 23 secondary metabolites, including a variety of quercetin-related flavonoids such as rutin, isoquercetin, and avicularin, as well as several kaempferol derivatives and condensed tannins. These compounds contribute not only to potent in vitro antioxidant effects demonstrated by low IC_{50} values in DPPH and robust FRAP assay results, but also to the inhibition of key enzymes involved in skin ageing processes, namely collagenase, elastase, hyaluronidase, and tyrosinase. Such enzyme inhibition is pivotal in preventing collagen and elastin degradation, preserving skin hydration, and managing hyperpigmentation. Furthermore, the extract showed effective antibacterial activity against Pseudomonas aeruginosa by reducing biofilm formation and interfering with bacterial motility, suggesting a role in the prevention of skin infections. In vivo, evaluations using Caenorhabditis elegans confirmed the extract's capacity to mitigate oxidative stress, as evidenced by increased survival rates upon juglone-induced stress, a dose-dependent reduction in intracellular reactive oxygen species (ROS), decreased expression of the heat shock protein HSP 16.2, and enhanced nuclear localisation of the DAF-16 transcription factor. Together, these findings underscore the potential of *X. americana var. caffra* leaf extract as a natural cosmeceutical agent capable of preventing oxidative stress-induced skin ageing and disorders (Zou et al. 2004; Bakrim et al. 2022).

4.28 Polygonum cuspidatum

Oca et al. mentioned that studies of phytochemicals derived from *Polygonum cuspidatum* plants have emerged as promising agents for skin protection and the prevention of photocarcinogenesis (Table 1). These natural compounds, including resveratrol (Fig. 4) from grapes and peanuts and epigallocatechin-3-gallate (EGCG) from green tea, exhibit potent antioxidant, anti-inflammatory, and antiproliferative properties that counteract UV-induced damage. UV radiation damages the skin by forming cyclobutane pyrimidine dimers (CPDs), generating reactive oxygen species (ROS), and triggering inflammatory cascades that contribute to DNA mutations and skin cancer development. Phytochemicals mitigate these effects by scavenging ROS, modulating critical signalling pathways such as NF-κB, MAPK, and AP-1, and upregulating protective markers like p53 and Nrf2, which promote DNA repair and induce the apoptosis of damaged cells. Additionally, advances in delivery systems such as nanostructured formulations and microemulsions enhance the bioavailability and stability of these compounds, thereby increasing their therapeutic potential as chemopreventive agents against nonmelanoma skin cancers and other UV-induced skin disorders (Altieri 2001; Montes de Oca et al. 2017).

4.29 Aloe barbadensis Miller., Matricaria chamomilla, Arctostaphylos uva-ursi, Glycyrrhiza glabra, *and* Silybum marianum

Aloesin from aloe vera (*Aloe barbadensis Miller.*) acts as a competitive inhibitor of tyrosinase by suppressing the oxidation of l-DOPA, thereby reducing melanin production (Table 1). This study was conducted by Clark et al. Similarly, alpha-bisabolol, the primary component of chamomile (*Matricaria chamomilla*), decreases melanogenesis by lowering intracellular cyclic AMP levels generated in response to melanocyte-stimulating hormone. Arbutin, found in bearberry (*Arctostaphylos uva-ursi*), California buckeye, and related plants, structurally mimics tyrosine to competitively inhibit both tyrosinase and downstream polymerase activities, resulting in marked reductions in melanin synthesis. Meanwhile, ellagic acid, a polyphenolic compound present in green tea, strawberries, grapes, and walnuts, exerts its effect by chelating the copper ions essential for tyrosinase's activity, thereby diminishing UV-induced pigmentation. Licorice (*Glycyrrhiza glabra*) provides further beneficial agents such as glabridin, which not only inhibits tyrosinase but also mitigates inflammation, and liquiritin, which has demonstrated superior efficacy in clinical settings for conditions like melasma when compared to lower concentrations or even to hydroquinone. Although hesperidin from citrus fruits offers potential through its flavonoid structure, conflicting evidence suggests it may either inhibit or induce melanogenesis, underscoring the need for more rigorous trials. Moreover, procyanidin from Pinus pinaster exhibits antioxidant and anti-inflammatory properties that help alleviate pigmentation disorders when used in combination with vitamins, and silymarin from milk thistle (*Silybum marianum*) provides potent photoprotective benefits by reducing UV-induced oxidative stress and suppressing melanogenic enzyme expression. Collectively, these botanically derived cosmeceuticals represent a diverse and compelling therapeutic arsenal for managing hyperpigmentation, paving the way for safer and more effective treatment strategies (Kren and Walterová 2005; Clark and Sivamani 2016).

4.30 Drimia sanguinea, Elephantorrhiza elephantine, Helichrysum paronychioides, *and* Senecio longiflorus

A recent study evaluating four medicinal plants traditionally used to treat skin disorders by Asong et al., including *Drimia sanguinea, Elephantorrhiza elephantine, Helichrysum paronychioides,* and *Senecio longiflorus,* revealed that their phytochemical profiles and biological activities strongly support their folkloric application (Table 1). The research demonstrated that both petroleum ether and 50% methanol extracts from these plants exhibit significant antimicrobial effects against pathogens responsible for skin infections, including bacteria such as Bacillus cereus and Shigella flexneri and fungi like Candida glabrata, Candida Kruse, Trichophyton rubrum, and Trichophyton tonsurans, with several extracts showing noteworthy minimum inhibitory concentrations. In addition, the extracts displayed potent antioxidant activities in DPPH-free radical scavenging and β-carotene-linoleic acid assays, a performance that correlated well with their total phenolic and flavonoid contents, particularly high in *Elephantorrhiza elephantina* and relatively lower in *Senecio longiflorus*. Gas chromatography-mass spectrometry analysis further identified a diverse range of bioactive compounds common to all four plants, such as dotriacontane, benzothiazole, heptacosane, stigmasterol (Fig. 4), and various fatty acids, which likely work synergistically to contribute to their antimicrobial, anti-inflammatory, and protective effects against oxidative stress-related skin damage. However, the study also noted varying degrees of cytotoxicity among the extracts, emphasising that while these botanicals hold significant promise as natural and cost-effective dermatological agents, careful consideration must be given to their safety profiles, particularly for extracts like that of Drimia sanguinea (Loizou et al. 2010; Asong et al. 2019).

4.31 Glycine max

A review by Kim et al. presents soybean (*Glycine max*) phytochemicals as potent agents for enhancing skin health by addressing common dermatological concerns such as ageing, pigmentation, and inflammation (Table 1). It shows that soybean extracts can modulate enzymes like matrix metalloproteinase-1 (MMP-1), especially after fermentation converts glycosides into more bioactive aglycon isoflavones, thereby preserving collagen integrity and reducing wrinkles; meanwhile, soybean peptides like lunasin enhance the synthesis of collagen types I and III and strengthen skin barrier proteins, contributing to a more resilient and moisturised epidermis. Additionally, soy isoflavones such as genistein and daidzein act as phytoestrogens with antioxidant properties that mitigate UV-induced damage, and soybean-derived anthocyanins further protect the skin by scavenging reactive oxygen species and inhibiting melanogenesis, which aids in skin whitening. Collectively, these findings suggest that soybean compounds offer versatile benefits for preventing and treating skin disorders, although further studies on their bioavailability and precise mechanisms are needed to fully optimise their application in cosmetic and dermatological products (Wölfle et al. 2014; Kim et al. 2017).

4.32 Tilia tomentosa

The study on *Tilia tomentosa* (Silver Linden) foliar bud by Peev et al. reveals a multifaceted phytochemical profile and promising dermatological benefits for skin care applications (Table 1). The buds, which exhibit a seasonal variation in water content (33.90% in winter rising to 57.93% in early spring), contain significant levels of bioactive compounds: chlorophyll A (6%), chlorophyll B (4%), carotenoids (1.99 mg/100 g buds), provitamin A (0.77 mg/100 g buds), and total polyphenols (380 mg/100 g buds), along with phyto-hormones such as auxins, cytokinins, and gibberellins identified via TLC, and a notable concentration of hemolytic saponins (5.21%). In vitro assessment using the Lepidium sativum biotest demonstrated potent antiproliferative activity with a 2% extract dilution achieving an 83.33% inhibition rate, while dermatological testing on human volunteers showed that semisolid formulations containing the extract significantly improved skin hydration (with hydration values increasing from approximately 66.5 to over 92) and reduced transepidermal water loss (TEWL dropping from around 14.08 to 11.09 g/hm^2) without causing any irritation. These findings suggest that the balanced composition of the hydro-glycerol-alcoholic extract, enriched with natural antioxidants, phytohormones, and saponins, holds great potential for the development of chemoprotective and anti-ageing topical formulations (Toker et al. 2004; Ieri et al. 2015).

4.33 Haplophyllum myrtifolium Boiss.

Haplophyllum myrtifolium Boiss., an endemic species from Turkey explored by Zengin et al., has been comprehensively characterised for its rich phytochemical composition and promising biological activities, particularly for managing skin disorders and protecting against oxidative damage (Table 1). Detailed extraction studies using solvents of varying polarities (petroleum ether, ethyl acetate, methanol, and water) have revealed a diverse array of bioactive compounds, including significant amounts of total phenolics, flavonoids, condensed tannins, saponins, and flavanols. Notably, the ethyl acetate extract demonstrated the highest phenolic content, which correlates with its robust antioxidant capacity as shown by various assays such as DPPH, ABTS, FRAP, CUPRAC, and metal chelation tests. These antioxidant properties are vital for scavenging free radicals and mitigating oxidative stress in skin cells, while the enzyme inhibitory activities, particularly the potent inhibition of tyrosinase, suggest its potential in regulating melanogenesis and treating hyperpigmentation disorders. Consequently, the multifaceted actions of *Haplophyllum myrtifolium* underscore its potential as a natural candidate for developing dermatological formulations aimed at skin protection and rejuvenation (Limoncu et al. 1997; Wintola and Afolayan 2011; Mendez et al. 2012; Zengin et al. 2014).

5 Future Prospective

The future of phytochemical applications in dermatology is set to flourish as advancements in extraction techniques and innovative delivery systems unlock the full potential of these natural compounds. By integrating traditional medicinal knowledge with emerging scientific insights, upcoming research is expected to refine methods such as ultrasound-assisted extraction, superheated water extraction, and nanotechnology-based formulations to enhance bioavailability, targeting precision, and safety. This progress is likely to transform phytochemicals into versatile, cost-effective therapeutic agents that not only address inflammatory, hyperpigmentary, and photoageing disorders but also extend to managing complex pathologies like skin cancers and chronic barrier dysfunctions. As in vivo and clinical evaluations continue to substantiate their efficacy, the convergence of sustainable sourcing and personalised medicine could revolutionise modern dermatological care, bridging the gap between centuries-old herbal remedies and contemporary therapeutic innovations.

6 Conclusion

The comprehensive exploration of phytochemicals reveals an inspiring horizon for dermatological innovation, where time-honoured herbal remedies meld seamlessly with cutting-edge scientific methodologies. The diverse tableau of bioactive compounds from flavonoids and phenolic acids to terpenoids and alkaloids demonstrates potent antioxidant, anti-inflammatory, and enzyme-inhibitory effects that address a range of skin conditions, including inflammatory disorders, hyperpigmentation, photoageing, and even skin cancers. Enhanced extraction techniques and advanced delivery systems like nanoemulsions and solid lipid nanoparticles further amplify the efficacy and safety of these natural agents, paving the way for cost-effective and sustainable therapeutic options. This convergence not only validates traditional knowledge, but also sets the stage for a new era in personalised dermatological care, where phytochemicals promise to rejuvenate and protect skin with precision and care.

References

Affonso RCL, Voytena APL, Fanan S, Pitz H, Coelho DS, Horstmann AL, Pereira A, Uarrota VG, Hillmann MC, Varela LAC, Ribeiro-do-Valle RM, Maraschin M (2016) Phytochemical composition, antioxidant activity, and the effect of the aqueous extract of coffee (Coffea arabica L.) bean residual press cake on the skin wound healing. Oxid Med Cell Longev 2016:1923754. https://doi.org/10.1155/2016/1923754

Agaimy A, Mueller SK, Harrer T, Bauer S, Thompson LDR (2018) Head and neck Kaposi sarcoma: clinicopathological analysis of 11 cases. Head Neck Pathol 12:511–516. https://doi.org/10.1007/s12105-018-0902-x

Alencastre JB, Vitoria M, Badra L, Garcia FS, De M, Viladot JL, Marchetti JM (2006) A study of the characteristics and in vitro permeation properties of CMC/chitosan microparticles as a skin delivery system for vitamin E. Rev Bras Cienc Farm 42:69–76

Allen-Mersh TG (1997) Cancer: principles and practice of oncology. 5th ed. V. T. Devita Jr, S. Hellman and S. A. Rosenberg (eds). 286 × 220 mm. Pp. 3312. Illustrated. 1996. Philadelphia,

Pennsylvania: Lippincott-Raven. £160. Br J Surg 84:1036. https://doi.org/10.1002/bjs.1800840754

Altieri DC (2001) The molecular basis and potential role of survivin in cancer diagnosis and therapy. Trends Mol Med 7:542–547. https://doi.org/10.1016/s1471-4914(01)02243-2

Asong JA, Amoo SO, McGaw LJ, Nkadimeng SM, Aremu AO, Otang-Mbeng W (2019) Antimicrobial activity, antioxidant potential, cytotoxicity and phytochemical profiling of four plants locally used against skin diseases. Plants (Basel, Switz) 8. https://doi.org/10.3390/plants8090350

Bakrim WB, Nurcahyanti ADR, Dmirieh M, Mahdi I, Elgamal AM, El Raey MA, Wink M, Sobeh M (2022) Phytochemical profiling of the leaf extract of Ximenia americana var. caffra and its antioxidant, antibacterial, and antiaging activities in vitro and in Caenorhabditis elegans: a cosmeceutical and dermatological approach. Oxidative Med Cell Longev 2022:3486257. https://doi.org/10.1155/2022/3486257

Bakry O, Shoeib M, Soliman S, Kamal L (2021) Neutrophil cytosolic factor-1 genotyping in acne vulgaris. Skin Pharmacol Physiol 34:51–56. https://doi.org/10.1159/000513053

Bale S, Pulivendala G, Godugu C (2018) Withaferin A attenuates bleomycin-induced scleroderma by targeting FoxO3a and NF-κβ signaling: connecting fibrosis and inflammation. Biofactors 44:507–517. https://doi.org/10.1002/biof.1446

Bernerd F, Asselineau D (1998) UVA exposure of human skin reconstructed in vitro induces apoptosis of dermal fibroblasts: subsequent connective tissue repair and implications in photoaging. Cell Death Differ 5:792–802. https://doi.org/10.1038/sj.cdd.4400413

Borlinghaus J, Albrecht F, Gruhlke MCH, Nwachukwu ID, Slusarenko AJ (2014) Allicin: chemistry and biological properties. Molecules 19:12591–12618. https://doi.org/10.3390/molecules190812591

Boroduske A, Jekabsons K, Riekstina U, Muceniece R, Rostoks N, Nakurte I (2021) Wild Sambucus nigra L. from north-east edge of the species range: a valuable germplasm with inhibitory capacity against SARS-CoV2 S-protein RBD and hACE2 binding in vitro. Ind Crop Prod 165:113438. https://doi.org/10.1016/j.indcrop.2021.113438

Brito S, Baek M, Bin B-H (2024) Skin structure, physiology, and pathology in topical and transdermal drug delivery. Pharmaceutics 16:1403

Brüll V, Burak C, Stoffel-Wagner B, Wolffram S, Nickenig G, Müller C, Langguth P, Alteheld B, Fimmers R, Naaf S, Zimmermann BF, Stehle P, Egert S (2015) Effects of a quercetin-rich onion skin extract on 24 h ambulatory blood pressure and endothelial function in overweight-to-obese patients with (pre-)hypertension: a randomised double-blinded placebo-controlled cross-over trial. Br J Nutr 114:1263–1277. https://doi.org/10.1017/S0007114515002950

Bungau S, Vesa CM, Abid A, Behl T, Tit DM, Purza AL, Pasca B, Todan LM, Endres L (2021) Withaferin A-A promising phytochemical compound with multiple results in dermatological diseases. Molecules 26. https://doi.org/10.3390/molecules26092407

Carrilho C, Lunet N (2023) Global trends in Kaposi sarcoma incidence and mortality: the need for action to reduce inequalities. Lancet Glob Health 11:e1479. https://doi.org/10.1016/S2214-109X(23)00413-8

Chaiprasongsuk A, Panich U (2022) Role of phytochemicals in skin photoprotection via regulation of Nrf2. Front Pharmacol 13:823881. https://doi.org/10.3389/fphar.2022.823881

Chua LS, Lee SY, Abdullah N, Sarmidi MR (2012) Review on Labisia pumila (Kacip Fatimah): bioactive phytochemicals and skin collagen synthesis promoting herb. Fitoterapia 83:1322–1335. https://doi.org/10.1016/j.fitote.2012.04.002

Chutoprapat R, Kopongpanich P, Chan LW (2022) A mini-review on solid lipid nanoparticles and nanostructured lipid carriers: topical delivery of phytochemicals for the treatment of acne vulgaris. Molecules 27. https://doi.org/10.3390/molecules27113460

Clark AK, Sivamani RK (2016) Phytochemicals in the treatment of hyperpigmentation. Bot Targets Ther 6:89–96. https://doi.org/10.2147/BTAT.S69113

Claudel JP, Auffret N, Leccia MT, Poli F, Dréno B (2018) Acne and nutrition: hypotheses, myths and facts. J Eur Acad Dermatol Venereol 32:1631–1637. https://doi.org/10.1111/jdv.14998

Cox V, Fuller LC, Engelman D, Steer A, Hay RJ (2021) Estimating the global burden of scabies: what else do we need? Br J Dermatol 184:237–242. https://doi.org/10.1111/bjd.19170

Curnow A, Owen SJ (2016) An evaluation of root phytochemicals derived from Althea officinalis (marshmallow) and Astragalus membranaceus as potential natural components of UV protecting dermatological formulations. Oxidative Med Cell Longev 2016:7053897. https://doi.org/10.1155/2016/7053897

Elgamal AM, El Raey MA, Gaara A, Abdelfattah MAO, Sobeh M (2021) Phytochemical profiling and anti-aging activities of Euphorbia retusa extract: in silico and in vitro studies. Arab J Chem 14:103159. https://doi.org/10.1016/j.arabjc.2021.103159

Engelman D, Yoshizumi J, Hay RJ, Osti M, Micali G, Norton S, Walton S, Boralevi F, Bernigaud C, Bowen AC, Chang AY, Chosidow O, Estrada-Chavez G, Feldmeier H, Ishii N, Lacarrubba F, Mahé A, Maurer T, Mahdi MMA, Murdoch ME, Pariser D, Nair PA, Rehmus W, Romani L, Tilakaratne D, Tuicakau M, Walker SL, Wanat KA, Whitfeld MJ, Yotsu RR, Steer AC, Fuller LC (2020) The 2020 international alliance for the control of scabies consensus criteria for the diagnosis of scabies. Br J Dermatol 183:808–820. https://doi.org/10.1111/bjd.18943

Evans-Johnson JA, Garlick JA, Johnson EJ, Wang X-D, Oliver Chen C-Y (2013) A pilot study of the photoprotective effect of almond phytochemicals in a 3D human skin equivalent. J Photochem Photobiol B 126:17–25. https://doi.org/10.1016/j.jphotobiol.2013.07.006

Farah A, de Paulis T, Trugo LC, Martin PR (2005) Effect of roasting on the formation of chlorogenic acid lactones in coffee. J Agric Food Chem 53:1505–1513. https://doi.org/10.1021/jf048701t

Flohr C, Hay R (2021) Putting the burden of skin diseases on the global map. Br J Dermatol 184:189–190. https://doi.org/10.1111/bjd.19704

Fölster-Holst R, Latussek E (2007) Synthetic tannins in dermatology--a therapeutic option in a variety of pediatric dermatoses. Pediatr Dermatol 24:296–301. https://doi.org/10.1111/j.1525-1470.2007.00406.x

Fujii H, Endo Y, Dainichi T, Otsuka A, Fujisawa A, Tanioka M, Miyachi Y, Kabashima K (2019) Predictive factors of response to pulse methylprednisolone therapy in patients with alopecia areata: a follow-up study of 105 Japanese patients. J Dermatol 46:522–525. https://doi.org/10.1111/1346-8138.14871

Gaweł-Bęben K, Czech K, Strzępek-Gomółka M, Czop M, Szczepanik M, Lichtarska A, Kukula-Koch W (2022) Assessment of Cucurbita spp. Peel extracts as potential sources of active substances for skin care and dermatology. Molecules 27. https://doi.org/10.3390/molecules27217618

Gonçalo M et al (2021) The global burden of chronic urticaria for the patient and society. Br J Dermatol 184:e36–e36. https://doi.org/10.1111/bjd.19727

Goodlad JR, Cerroni L, Swerdlow SH (2023) Recent advances in cutaneous lymphoma-implications for current and future classifications. Virchows Arch 482:281–298. https://doi.org/10.1007/s00428-022-03421-5

Grădinaru T-C, Vlad A, Gilca M (2024) Bitter phytochemicals as novel candidates for skin disease treatment. Curr Issues Mol Biol 46:299–326

Guo W, Wang H, Li C (2021) Signal pathways of melanoma and targeted therapy. Signal Transduct Target Ther 6:424. https://doi.org/10.1038/s41392-021-00827-6

Gupta AJ, Kaldate S, Volaguthala S, Mahajan V (2025) Onion nutritional and nutraceutical composition and therapeutic potential of its phytochemicals assessed through preclinical and clinical studies. J Funct Foods 129:106889. https://doi.org/10.1016/j.jff.2025.106889

Gwiazdowska D, Uwineza PA, Frąk S, Juś K, Marchwińska K, Gwiazdowski R, Waśkiewicz A (2022) Antioxidant, antimicrobial and antibiofilm properties of Glechoma hederacea extracts obtained by supercritical fluid extraction, using different extraction conditions. Appl Sci 12:3572

Hay RJ, Johns NE, Williams HC, Bolliger IW, Dellavalle RP, Margolis DJ, Marks R, Naldi L, Weinstock MA, Wulf SK, Michaud C, J.L. Murray C, Naghavi M (2014) The global burden

of skin disease in 2010: an analysis of the prevalence and impact of skin conditions. J Invest Dermatol 134:1527–1534. https://doi.org/10.1038/jid.2013.446
Haywood R, Wardman P, Sanders R, Linge C (2003) Sunscreens inadequately protect against ultraviolet-A-induced free radicals in skin: implications for skin aging and melanoma? J Invest Dermatol 121:862–868. https://doi.org/10.1046/j.1523-1747.2003.12498.x
Hymes AC (1984) Transdermal drug delivery from a solid state hydrophilic reservoir system BT - recent advances in drug delivery systems. In: Anderson JM, Kim SW (eds) Signal transduction and targeted therapy. Springer US, Boston, MA, pp 309–313
Ieri F, Innocenti M, Possieri L, Gallori S, Mulinacci N (2015) Phenolic composition of "bud extracts" of Ribes nigrum L., Rosa canina L. and Tilia tomentosa M. J Pharm Biomed Anal 115:1–9. https://doi.org/10.1016/j.jpba.2015.06.004
Imanbayev K, Makishev A, Zhagiparov M, McLoone P (2018) Non-melanoma skin cancers at sites of previous frostbite: case report and review. Case Rep Dermatol 10:17–23. https://doi.org/10.1159/000486477
Iqbal J, Abbasi BA, Ahmad R, Batool R, Mahmood T, Ali B, Khalil AT, Kanwal S, Afzal Shah S, Alam MM, Bashir S, Badshah H, Munir A (2019) Potential phytochemicals in the fight against skin cancer: current landscape and future perspectives. Biomed Pharmacother 109:1381–1393. https://doi.org/10.1016/j.biopha.2018.10.107
Iskandar IYK, Parisi R, Griffiths CEM, Ashcroft DM, Atlas on behalf of the GP (2021) Systematic review examining changes over time and variation in the incidence and prevalence of psoriasis by age and gender. Br J Dermatol 184:243–258. https://doi.org/10.1111/bjd.19169
Karimkhani C, Dellavalle RP, Coffeng LE, Flohr C, Hay RJ, Langan SM, Nsoesie EO, Ferrari AJ, Erskine HE, Silverberg JI, Vos T, Naghavi M (2017) Global skin disease morbidity and mortality: an update from the global burden of disease study 2013. JAMA Dermatol 153:406–412. https://doi.org/10.1001/jamadermatol.2016.5538
Kashif M, Akhtar N, Mustafa R (2017) An overview of dermatological and cosmeceutical benefits of Diospyros kaki and its phytoconstituents. Rev Bras 27:650–662. https://doi.org/10.1016/j.bjp.2017.06.004
Kaur G, Jabbar Z, Athar M, Alam MS (2006) Punica granatum (pomegranate) flower extract possesses potent antioxidant activity and abrogates Fe-NTA induced hepatotoxicity in mice. Food Chem Toxicol 44:984–993. https://doi.org/10.1016/j.fct.2005.12.001
Kim J-E, Kang Y-G, Park JS, Lim T-G, Lee KW (2017) Review of soybean phytochemicals and their bioactive properties relevant for skin health. J Food Nutr Res 5:852–858. https://doi.org/10.12691/jfnr-5-11-9
Kour K, Sharma N, Chandan BK, Koul S, Sangwan PL, Bani S (2010) Protective effect of Labisia pumila on stress-induced behavioral, biochemical, and immunological alterations. Planta Med 76:1497–1505. https://doi.org/10.1055/s-0029-1240953
Kozlowska J, Prus W, Stachowiak N (2019) Microparticles based on natural and synthetic polymers for cosmetic applications. Int J Biol Macromol 129:952–956. https://doi.org/10.1016/j.ijbiomac.2019.02.091
Kren V, Walterová D (2005) Silybin and silymarin--new effects and applications. Biomed Pap Med Fac Univ Palacky Olomouc Czech Repub 149:29–41. https://doi.org/10.5507/bp.2005.002
Lee DH, Lim S, Kwak SS, Kim J (2024) Advancements in skin-mediated drug delivery: mechanisms, techniques, and applications. Adv Healthc Mater 13:e2302375. https://doi.org/10.1002/adhm.202302375
Limoncu ME, Balcioğlu IC, Yereli K, Ozbel Y, Ozbilgin A (1997) A new experimental in vitro culture medium for cultivation of Leishmania species. J Clin Microbiol 35:2430–2431. https://doi.org/10.1128/jcm.35.9.2430-2431.1997
Lin Y-K, Chen H-W, Leu Y-L, Yang Y-L, Fang Y, Su Pang J-H, Hwang T-L (2013) Indigo naturalis upregulates claudin-1 expression in human keratinocytes and psoriatic lesions. J Ethnopharmacol 145:614–620. https://doi.org/10.1016/j.jep.2012.11.044

Loizou S, Lekakis I, Chrousos GP, Moutsatsou P (2010) β-Sitosterol exhibits anti-inflammatory activity in human aortic endothelial cells. Mol Nutr Food Res 54:551–558. https://doi.org/10.1002/mnfr.200900012

Loney T, Paulo MS, Modenese A, Gobba F, Tenkate T, Whiteman DC, Green AC, John SM (2021) Global evidence on occupational sun exposure and keratinocyte cancers: a systematic review. Br J Dermatol 184:208–218. https://doi.org/10.1111/bjd.19152

Luongo FP, Passaponti S, Haxhiu A, Raeispour M, Belmonte G, Governini L, Casarini L, Piomboni P, Luddi A (2022) Bitter taste receptors and endocrine disruptors: cellular and molecular insights from an in vitro model of human granulosa cells. Int J Mol Sci 23:15540

Mahdi I, Fahsi N, Annaz H, Drissi B, Barakate M, Mahmoud MF, Sobeh M (2023) Thymus satureioides Coss.: mineral composition, nutritional value, phytochemical profiling, and dermatological properties. Molecules 28. https://doi.org/10.3390/molecules28124636

Matić P, Sabljić M, Jakobek L (2017) Validation of spectrophotometric methods for the determination of total polyphenol and total flavonoid content. J AOAC Int 100:1795–1803. https://doi.org/10.5740/jaoacint.17-0066

Meindl C, Öhlinger K, Zrim V, Ober J, Jeitler R, Roblegg E, Fröhlich E (2024) Skin sensitization potential of sensitizers in the presence of metal oxide nanoparticles in vitro. Nano 14:1811

Melnyk N, Vlasova I, Skowrońska W, Bazylko A, Piwowarski JP, Granica S (2022) Current knowledge on interactions of plant materials traditionally used in skin diseases in Poland and Ukraine with human skin microbiota. Int J Mol Sci 23:9644

Mendez M, Rodríguez R, Ruiz J, Morales-Adame D, Castillo F, Hernández-Castillo FD, Aguilar CN (2012) Antibacterial activity of plant extracts obtained with alternative organics solvents against food-borne pathogen bacteria. Ind Crop Prod 37:445–450. https://doi.org/10.1016/j.indcrop.2011.07.017

Mistry K, Levell NJ, Hollestein L, Wakkee M, Nijsten T, Knott CS, Steven NM, Craig PJ, Venables ZC (2023) Trends in incidence, treatment and survival of Merkel cell carcinoma in England 2004-2018: a cohort study. Br J Dermatol 188:228–236. https://doi.org/10.1093/bjd/ljac044

Młynarczyk K, Walkowiak-Tomczak D, Łysiak GP (2018) Bioactive properties of Sambucus nigra L. as a functional ingredient for food and pharmaceutical industry. J Funct Foods 40:377–390. https://doi.org/10.1016/j.jff.2017.11.025

Mocan A, Vodnar DC, Vlase L, Crişan O, Gheldiu A-M, Crişan G (2015) Phytochemical characterization of Veronica officinalis L., V. teucrium L. and V. orchidea Crantz from Romania and their antioxidant and antimicrobial properties. Int J Mol Sci 16:21109–21127

Mohd Zain FA, Shahidan N, Huda N, Zakaria Z, Septama AW (2021) Antioxidant activity of bioactive peptide derived from Pekin duck feet gelatin hydrolysate. Malays Appl Biol 49:19–24. https://doi.org/10.55230/mabjournal.v49i4.1563

Montes de Oca MK, Pearlman RL, McClees SF, Strickland R, Afaq F (2017) Phytochemicals for the prevention of photocarcinogenesis. Photochem Photobiol 93:956–974. https://doi.org/10.1111/php.12711

Murdoch ME (2021) Mapping the burden of onchocercal skin disease. Br J Dermatol 184:199–207. https://doi.org/10.1111/bjd.19143

Mwinga JL, Asong JA, Amoo SO, Nkadimeng SM, McGaw LJ, Aremu AO, Otang-Mbeng W (2019) In vitro antimicrobial effects of Hypoxis hemerocallidea against six pathogens with dermatological relevance and its phytochemical characterization and cytotoxicity evaluation. J Ethnopharmacol 242:112048. https://doi.org/10.1016/j.jep.2019.112048

Nawrot J, Budzianowski J, Nowak G, Micek I, Budzianowska A, Gornowicz-Porowska J (2021) Biologically active compounds in Stizolophus balsamita inflorescences: isolation, phytochemical characterization and effects on the skin biophysical parameters. Int J Mol Sci 22. https://doi.org/10.3390/ijms22094428

Nutho B, Tungmunnithum D (2023) Exploring major flavonoid phytochemicals from Nelumbo nucifera Gaertn. As potential skin anti-aging agents: in silico and in vitro evaluations. Int J Mol Sci 24:16571

Patel P, Hussain K (2021) Merkel cell carcinoma. Clin Exp Dermatol 46:814–819. https://doi.org/10.1111/ced.14530

Prausnitz MR (2004) Microneedles for transdermal drug delivery. Adv Drug Deliv Rev 56:581–587. https://doi.org/10.1016/j.addr.2003.10.023

Radhakrishnan J, Kennedy BE, Noftall EB, Giacomantonio CA, Rupasinghe HPV (2024) Recent advances in phytochemical-based topical applications for the management of eczema: a review. Int J Mol Sci 25:5375

Raza K, Singh B, Singal P, Wadhwa S, Katare OP (2013) Systematically optimized biocompatible isotretinoin-loaded solid lipid nanoparticles (SLNs) for topical treatment of acne. Colloids Surf B Biointerfaces 105:67–74. https://doi.org/10.1016/j.colsurfb.2012.12.043

Rosenbaum T, Gordon-Shaag A, Munari M, Gordon SE (2004) Ca2+/calmodulin modulates TRPV1 activation by capsaicin. J Gen Physiol 123:53–62. https://doi.org/10.1085/jgp.200308906

Sarikurkcu C, Locatelli M, Mocan A, Zengin G, Kirkan B (2019) Phenolic profile and bioactivities of Sideritis perfoliata L.: the plant, its most active extract, and its broad biological properties. Front Pharmacol 10:1642. https://doi.org/10.3389/fphar.2019.01642

Scalia S, Trotta V, Iannuccelli V, Bianchi A (2015) Enhancement of in vivo human skin penetration of resveratrol by chitosan-coated lipid microparticles. Colloids Surf B Biointerfaces 135:42–49. https://doi.org/10.1016/j.colsurfb.2015.07.043

Selvi B (2025) Comparative study of Pentanema verbascifolium extracts: phytochemical composition, antioxidant potential, and enzyme inhibition across plant parts. Food Biosci 68:106607. https://doi.org/10.1016/j.fbio.2025.106607

Sezen Karaoğlan E, Hancı H, Koca M, Kazaz C (2023) Some bioactivities of isolated Apigenin-7-O-glucoside and Luteolin-7-O-glucoside. Appl Sci 13:1503

Song X, Tan L, Wang M, Ren C, Guo C, Yang B, Ren Y, Cao Z, Li Y, Pei J (2021) Myricetin: a review of the most recent research. Biomed Pharmacother 134:111017. https://doi.org/10.1016/j.biopha.2020.111017

Spiker A, Mowad C (2016) Patch test negative generalized dermatitis. Dermatitis 27:259–262. https://doi.org/10.1097/DER.0000000000000217

Sroczyk EA, Tarasiuk A, Talar M, Rutledge GC, Makaro A, Misztal Z, Wołyniak M, Berniak K, Sałaga M, Fichna J, Stachewicz U (2024) Cholesterol nanofiber patches with sustainable oil delivery eliminate inflammation in atopic skin. ACS Appl Mater Interfaces 16:37783–37794. https://doi.org/10.1021/acsami.4c09400

Strzępek-Gomółka M, Gaweł-Bęben K, Kukula-Koch W (2021) Achillea species as sources of active phytochemicals for dermatological and cosmetic applications. Oxidative Med Cell Longev 2021:6643827. https://doi.org/10.1155/2021/6643827

Suedee A, Tewtrakul S, Panichayupakaranant P (2017) A validated quantitative HPLC method for proanthocyanidin A2 in Pometia pinnata leaves. Glob J Bot Sci 5:9–15. https://doi.org/10.12974/2311-858X.2017.05.01.2

Tawfeek N, Fikry E, Mahdi I, Ochieng MA, Bakrim WB, Taarji N, Mahmoud MF, Sobeh M (2023) Cupressus arizonica Greene: phytochemical profile and cosmeceutical and dermatological properties of its leaf extracts. Molecules 28. https://doi.org/10.3390/molecules28031036

Thein ZM, Seneviratne CJ, Samaranayake YH, Samaranayake LP (2009) Community lifestyle of Candida in mixed biofilms: a mini review. Mycoses 52:467–475. https://doi.org/10.1111/j.1439-0507.2009.01719.x

Toker G, Küpeli E, Memisoğlu M, Yesilada E (2004) Flavonoids with antinociceptive and anti-inflammatory activities from the leaves of Tilia argentea (silver linden). J Ethnopharmacol 95:393–397. https://doi.org/10.1016/j.jep.2004.08.008

Tomczyk M, Latté KP (2009) Potentilla--a review of its phytochemical and pharmacological profile. J Ethnopharmacol 122:184–204. https://doi.org/10.1016/j.jep.2008.12.022

Wagle A, Seong SH, Joung E-J, Kim H-R, Jung HA, Choi JS (2018) Discovery of a highly potent tyrosinase inhibitor, luteolin 5-O-β-d-glucopyranoside, isolated from Cirsium japonicum var. maackii (Maxim.) Matsum., Korean thistle: kinetics and computational molecular docking simulation. ACS Omega 3:17236–17245. https://doi.org/10.1021/acsomega.8b02694

Walendziak W, Villegas NR, Douglas TEL, Kozlowska J (2025) Phytochemical studies of plant extracts enclosed in chitosan microparticles and the effect of phytoformulations on skin condition. Eur Polym J 233:113968. https://doi.org/10.1016/j.eurpolymj.2025.113968

Wintola OA, Afolayan AJ (2011) Phytochemical constituents and antioxidant activities of the whole leaf extract of Aloe ferox Mill. Pharmacogn Mag 7:325–333. https://doi.org/10.4103/0973-1296.90414

Wölfle U, Seelinger G, Bauer G, Meinke MC, Lademann J, Schempp CM (2014) Reactive molecule species and antioxidative mechanisms in normal skin and skin aging. Skin Pharmacol Physiol 27:316–332. https://doi.org/10.1159/000360092

Wu Q, Bai P, Guo H, Guo MSS, Xia Y, Xia Y, Gao X, Wang X, Wu J, Dong TTX, Tsim KWK (2022) Capsaicin, a phytochemical from chili pepper, alleviates the ultraviolet irradiation-induced decline of collagen in dermal fibroblast via blocking the generation of reactive oxygen species. Front Pharmacol 13:872912. https://doi.org/10.3389/fphar.2022.872912

Wu X, Wanyan M-F, Shi B-B, Huang R, Yang H-X, Wang X, Liu J-K (2025) Cuphea hookeriana: phytochemical profile and the cosmeceutical and dermatological properties of its active fraction from the whole plant. Molecules 30. https://doi.org/10.3390/molecules30020311

Yamamoto T, Suzuki T, Kobayashi A, Wakabayashi J, Maher J, Motohashi H, Yamamoto M (2008) Physiological significance of reactive cysteine residues of Keap1 in determining Nrf2 activity. Mol Cell Biol 28:2758–2770. https://doi.org/10.1128/MCB.01704-07

Zengin G, Sarikurkcu C, Aktumsek A, Ceylan R, Ceylan O (2014) A comprehensive study on phytochemical characterization of Haplophyllum myrtifolium Boiss. endemic to Turkey and its inhibitory potential against key enzymes involved in Alzheimer, skin diseases and type II diabetes. Ind Crop Prod 53:244–251. https://doi.org/10.1016/j.indcrop.2013.12.043

Zillich OV, Schweiggert-Weisz U, Eisner P, Kerscher M (2015) Polyphenols as active ingredients for cosmetic products. Int J Cosmet Sci 37:455–464. https://doi.org/10.1111/ics.12218

Zou Y, Lu Y, Wei D (2004) Antioxidant activity of a flavonoid-rich extract of Hypericum perforatum L. in vitro. J Agric Food Chem 52:5032–5039. https://doi.org/10.1021/jf049571r

Phytochemicals Potentially Applied for Infectious Diseases

Aachal Lonhare, Vijayalakshmi Ghosh, and R. S. Suresh Kumar

Abstract Worldwide, infectious diseases consistently remained as one of the prime causes of mortality, endangering both economic stability and public health. An increased quest for alternative treatment agents has been motivated by the emergence of multidrug-resistant (MDR) bacteria and the sluggish pace of new antibiotic discoveries. Because of their antibacterial, antiviral, antifungal, and antiparasitic qualities, phytochemicals—a broad class of bioactive substances made by plants—have become attractive options for treating a variety of illnesses. This chapter provides a thorough overview of phytochemicals that may be used to treat infectious diseases. It examines their classifications, mechanisms of action, therapeutic options, biotechnology advancements, and challenges in clinical translation. Phenolics, flavonoids, terpenoids, alkaloids, and essential oils are given particular attention, along with how nanotechnology can enhance their pharmacokinetics and bioavailability.

Keywords Drug discovery · Natural products · Nano-phytomedicine · Infectious illnesses · Secondary metabolites · Phytochemicals

A. Lonhare · V. Ghosh (✉)
GD Rungta College of Science & Technology, Bhilai, Chhattisgarh, India

Department of Biotechnology, Rungta International Skills University, Bhilai, Chhattisgarh, India

R. S. Suresh Kumar
College of Natural and Computational Sciences, Arba Minch University, Southern Ethiopia, Ethiopia

S. Kumar Tripathi et al. (eds.), *Phytoceuticals for Sustainable Medication*, Interdisciplinary Biotechnological Advances,
https://doi.org/10.1007/978-981-95-7588-6_10

1 Introduction

The health of humans is still severely threatened by infectious diseases, which are brought on by fungi, viruses, bacteria, and parasites. The emergence of new infections like SARS-CoV-2, the recurrence of diseases like tuberculosis, and the evolution of antibiotic-resistant strains all demonstrate the immediate need for other therapeutic options (World Health Organization 2023). Plants create wide varieties of secondary metabolites called phytochemicals, which have strong antibacterial and immunomodulatory properties, as part of their defensive systems (Pandey and Rizvi 2020).

The foundation of modern medicine has long been phytochemicals. Quinine, artemisinin, and morphine are a few examples of plant-derived compounds that have revolutionised the way that illness is treated (Table 1). Interest in

Table 1 Phytochemical activities of some plant on various diseases

Diseases	Plant species	Secondary metabolites	Phytochemicals	References
Skin disease	*Azadirachta indica*	Terpenes (Sterol)	β –sitosterol,nimbin	Chanda and Ramachandra (2019)
	Acalypha indica	Alkaloid	Acalyphine	Andrade-Cetto (2003)
		Terpenes (Sterol)	Sitosterol	Andrade-Cetto (2003)
Diarrhoea	*Argyreria nervosa*	Terpenes (Sterol)	β-sitosterol, epifriedinol	Ashutosh Meher et al. (2011)
	Centella asiatica	Terpenes	β-sitosterol	Andrade-Cetto (2003)
Urinary trouble	*Costus speciosus*	Saponin	Diosgenin, trigogenin	Chanda and Ramachandra (2019)
	Cyperus rotundus	Terpenes (Sterol)	Oleanolic acid, β –Sitosterol,and others.	Andrade-Cetto (2003)
Gastrointestinal trouble	*Tinospora cordifolia*	Alkaloid	Berberne, timberine, and palmatine.	Chanda and Ramachandra (2019)
Kidney problem	*Gloriosa superba*	Terpene	Terpenoids	Ashokkumar (2015)
Jaundice	*Achyranthes aspera*	Alkaloid	Betaine, achyranthine	Andrade-Cetto (2003)
		Saponin	Saonin A&B	Andrade-Cetto (2003)
	Berberis aristata	Alkaloids	Berine, Berberine, Jatrorrhizine taxilamine, and others berbamine	Andrade-Cetto (2003)
Nervous disorder	*Syzygium cumini*	Flavonoids	Quercetin	Andrade-Cetto (2003)

ethnopharmacology and natural product chemistry is rising globally as researchers search for novel bioactive chemicals with reduced toxicity, broad-spectrum efficacy, and a lower likelihood of resistance development (Newman and Cragg 2020). Phytochemicals work through wide varieties of mechanisms, including disrupting cell membranes, blocking the production of proteins, and pathogen metabolism interference, which lower the risk of resistance developing. This contrasts the conventional antibiotics, which frequently target specific bacterial functions (Dahiru et al. 2024).

In general, identifying the compounds found in plants and their potential benefits for human health requires screening for plant phytochemicals. Infectious diseases, which affect people from all walks of life, are among the most urgent global health issues. They can spread by pathogenic microbes such as bacteria, viruses, fungi, and parasites. Urbanisation, globalisation, environmental change, and population mobility all increase the risk of infectious diseases by facilitating the spread of pathogens (Adam et al. 2023).

Infectious diseases are frequently the primary causes of death and morbidity in low- and middle-income nations, which have an effect on both social stability and economic expansion. Malaria, HIV/AIDS, tuberculosis, and a number of neglected tropical diseases (NTDs) are among the diseases that are disproportionately common in these areas (Mathew et al. 2024). In these areas, susceptibility is increased by a lack of access to healthcare, sanitation, and preventive measures.

2 Infectious Diseases and Antimicrobial Resistance

The rise of antimicrobial resistance (AMR) is one of the most significant medical issues of the twenty-first century. The World Health Organisation (WHO) estimates that by 2050, drug-resistant illnesses might cause approximately ten million annual deaths if proper precautions are not implemented (WHO 2023). Among the processes behind resistance are drug enzymatic degradation, drug target change, efflux pump activation, and biofilm formation (Ventola 2015).

Phytochemicals have shown promise in addressing AMR by simultaneously targeting many mechanisms, including microbial cell membrane rupture, quorum sensing suppression, and interference with biofilm formation (Rios and Recio 2005). They are useful scaffolds for creating novel antibacterial drugs because of these characteristics.

Over the years, microorganisms have developed resistance to given antimicrobial chemicals, giving them an innate ability to live. Antimicrobial resistance (AMR), also referred to as drug resistance, is the result of microbes such as fungi, viruses, bacteria, and parasites changing their ways so that the microbes are becoming resistant to current standard drugs, such as antivirals (H1N1 resistance to oseltamivir), antifungals (candida resistance to fluconazole), antibacterials (MRSA), and antiparasitics (chloroquine resistance to malarial parasite) (Asokan and Kasimanickam 2013). Drug-resistant diseases have become more prevalent in recent years, making them, worldwide, exceedingly deadly and impeding the achievement of the Millennium Development Goals (MDG). Furthermore, the current therapeutic arsenal is being reduced, primarily as a result of antibiotic resistance, making emerging infectious diseases incurable and unmanageable, recognising the threat to public health, and classifying AMR as the third leading risk of global health (WHO 2013).

2.1 Antimicrobial Resistance in Humans

Antimicrobials are frequently used to treat and control infectious diseases in humans, which address three of the eight MDGs: lowering child mortality rates, enhancing maternal health, and fighting HIV/AIDS, malaria, and other infections. Antimicrobials are also used to treat and prevent complicated surgeries, organ transplants, critical care, the treatment of premature infants and the elderly, and the survival of immunocompromised individuals. Multidrug-resistant tuberculosis and extensively drug-resistant tuberculosis are linked to severe AMR issues. Antimicrobials are rarely used to treat cattle mycobacterial infections, which could increase the risk of tuberculosis. Artemisinin-resistant falciparum malaria parasites are becoming more common. Several gram-negative bacteria have developed new resistance mechanisms, such as the beta-lactamase. Indian Escherichia coli strains that are resistant to beta-lactamases have spread to other nations (Thoen et al. 2008).

Such entirely antibiotic-resistant bacteria were exclusively discovered in hospitals until recently. In just 3 years, the prevalence of NDM-1 in hospitals in India increased from 3% to 20–50%, and patients were discovered to be resistant to colistin, a medication used to treat multiresistant gram-negative bacteria (Castanheira et al. 2013).

2.2 Antimicrobial Resistance in Animals and Environment

Antimicrobial resistance in animals is complicated due to the variety of animal species, the range of environmental settings in animal raising, the variations in the pathogenicity mechanisms and bacteria involved, and the intricate epidemiology. More than half of all antimicrobials produced worldwide are routinely used in animal husbandry to stimulate growth and prevent disease in animals that produce food, such as cattle, poultry, pigs, fish, and bees. Eighty percent of all antibiotics in US alone are given to food-producing animals for prophylaxis and growth promotion. Antibiotic use in fish and animals is thought to be up to 1000 times higher than that of humans. Additionally, the evolution of resistant diseases with resistance genes has been facilitated by the use of antimicrobial drugs in animals raised for food (Asokan and Kasimanickam 2013).

3 Diversity and Classification of Phytochemicals

Phytochemicals are secondary plant metabolites that can be categorised according to their solubility in different solvents. Plant secondary metabolites may be classified into chemically separate groups. These compounds may be the source of some strong medications (Chanda and Ramachandra 2019). The chemical structures and biosynthetic sources of phytochemicals are used to classify them into key groups (Fig. 1).

3.1 Phenolics

They include lignans, phenolic acids, flavonoids, and tannins. By rupturing microbial membranes and preventing the synthesis of nucleic acids, these substances exhibit antibacterial and antioxidant qualities (Balasundram et al. 2006).

3.2 Flavonoids

Their molecular structure is characterised by a variety of phenolic structures. Because of the location of the benzenoid substituent, flavonoids are divided into two classes: isoflavone (3-position) and flavone (2-position).

Flavonoids are typically produced spontaneously and can be classified as monoglycosidic, diglycosidic, or any other type of conjugated sugar. The carbohydrate unit can be galactose, L-rhamnose, Dglucose, glucorhamnose, or arabinose, and the glycosidic linkage is at 3 or 7 position. Many herbal remedies contain flavonoids as active agents (Wink 2015; Saxena et al. 2013).

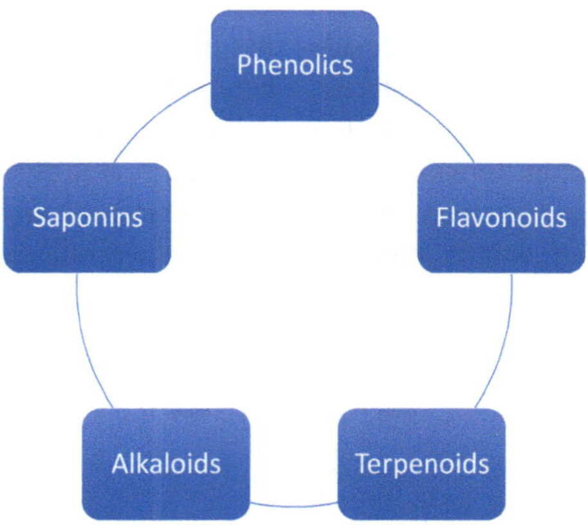

Fig. 1 Overview of phytochemicals produced by plants

3.3 Terpenoids

These substances, which include diterpenes, monoterpenes, and sesquiterpenes, interfere with microbial membranes and suppress respiratory enzymes. The largest class of secondary metabolites, terpenes, is made up of hydrocarbons. The majority of terpenoids is lipophilic, and terpenes interact with membrane proteins and biomembranes. Terpenes have been used extensively in herbal medicine to treat infections because they generally have cytotoxic actions against a variety of species. Terpenoids are modified terpenes that have had oxygen atoms added or methyl groups changed or eliminated (Wink 2015).

3.4 Alkaloids

Substances that include nitrogen, including morphine, quinine, and berberine. According to, many have potent antibacterial and antiparasitic properties. Alkaloids are generated from amino acids, which typically include nitrogen in one or more carbon rings. The location of the nitrogen atom in the carbon ring determines the kind of alkaloids and plant families. Alkaloids are crucial for plants because they prevent herbivores from grazing, shield them from pathogens, and suppress competitors. Alkaloids are important pharmacologically in a number of ways, including antihypertensive and antimalarial activity, antiarrhythmic effects, and anticancer effects. Caffeine, nicotine, morphine, and other alkaloids with stimulant properties are used as analgesics, while quinine is utilised as an anti-malarial medication (Egamberdieva et al. 2017).

3.5 Saponins

These are glycosides that increase permeability in microbial membranes by complexing with sterols. Chemically, saponins are categorised as steroid alkaloids, triterpenoids, and glycosylated steroids. The molecule that remains after a hydrogen atom replaces a glycosyl group on a glycoside is called an agylone.Furostan and spirostan are two derivatives of steroid aglycones (Saxena et al. 2013). Essential oils are volatile blends with broad-spectrum antibacterial properties that contain phenolics and terpenoids (Bakkali et al. 2008).

4 Mechanisms of Antimicrobial Action of Phytochemicals

Many of the methods that phytochemicals use to combat infections are different from those of conventional antibiotics. According to Devi et al. (2025), enzymatic degradation, efflux pump activation, drug target change, and biofilm development are some of the mechanisms that frequently lead to antibiotic resistance in bacteria (Table 2). By targeting several cellular structures and metabolic pathways at once, phytochemicals, on the other hand, demonstrate diverse antimicrobial actions that hinder the development of resistance in microorganisms (Cowan 1999; Cushnie and Lamb 2011).

Table 2 Mechanisms of antimicrobial action of phytochemicals

Mechanism of action	Representative phytochemicals	Target pathogens	Mode of action	References
Membrane disruption	Thymol, carvacrol, eugenol	*Candida albicans*, *Escherichia coli*, *Staphylococcus aureus*	Integration into lipid bilayer leading to ion and protein leakage, membrane depolarisation, and cell lysis	Burt (2004); Khan et al. (2014)
Enzyme inhibition/ Degradation	Berberine, gallic acid, phenolic acids	*Pseudomonas aeruginosa*, *Staphylococcus aureus*	Inhibits β-lactamases and bacterial oxidoreductases; disrupts antibiotic-degrading enzyme systems	Devi et al. (2025); Khameneh et al. (2019)
Quorum sensing and virulence inhibition	Flavonoids, coumarins, naringenin	*Pseudomonas aeruginosa*, *Vibrio harveyi*	Interferes with acyl-homoserine lactone (AHL) signalling and reduces virulence gene expression	Adonizio et al. (2008); Cushnie and Lamb (2011)
Induction of oxidative stress	Phenolics, tannins, curcumin	*Candida albicans*, *E. coli*, *Bacillus subtilis*	Generates (ROS) causing oxidative damage	Savoia (2012); Daglia (2012)
Biofilm disruption	Catechins, curcumin, quercetin	*Staphylococcus aureus*, *Pseudomonas aeruginosa*, *Candida* spp.	Inhibits bacterial adhesion and EPS synthesis; destabilises existing biofilms	Daglia (2012); Jafri et al. (2022)
Efflux pump inhibition	Reserpine, piperine, capsaicin	*Mycobacterium smegmatis*, *E. oli*	Blocks multidrug efflux pumps, enhancing antibiotic intracellular accumulation	Cowan (1999); Khameneh et al. (2019)
DNA and protein synthesis inhibition	Quercetin, baicalein, alkaloids	*Staphylococcus aureus*, *Bacillus cereus*	Interferes with DNA gyrase and ribosomal function, inhibiting replication and translation	Cushnie and Lamb (2011); Savoia (2012)

Membrane disruption: A lot of terpenoids and essential oils work by weakening the integrity of microbial membranes, which allows ions, proteins, and nucleotides to escape. Compounds like carvacrol and thymol, which are found in thyme and oregano oils, interact with the lipid bilayer to increase permeability and induce cytoplasmic leakage (Burt 2004). This non-specific attack on the cell membrane might result in cell lysis and death by eschewing the conventional resistance routes associated with target modification or enzyme inactivation.

Degradation and inhibition of enzymes: One of the main mechanisms of pathogen resistance is the release of enzymes such as β-lactamases, which hydrolyse the β-lactam ring in antibiotics and render them inert. Certain phytochemicals, particularly phenolic acids and alkaloids, can inhibit these enzymes or decrease their expression, restoring the efficiency of antibiotics (Devi et al. 2025). For example, it has been shown that berberine and gallic acid derivatives interfere with the bacterial enzymatic systems that produce resistance (Khameneh et al. 2019).

Quorum sensing and virulence inhibition: A microbial communication mechanism called quorum sensing (QS) is interfered with by several phytochemicals, including flavonoids and coumarins. By interfering with QS signalling molecules, such as acyl-homoserine lactones, which stop the manufacture of virulence factors and the creation of biofilms without actually killing the bacteria, these compounds reduce the likelihood of resistance emergence (Adonizio et al. 2008).

Reactive oxygen species (ROS) production: ROS are produced intracellularly by flavonoids, tannins, and other polyphenolic compounds, and they damage proteins, lipids, and DNA in cells (Savoia 2012). These chemicals lead to oxidative stress, which weakens the antioxidant defences of microorganisms and causes cell death.

Biofilm disruption: The formation of biofilms is a crucial survival strategy for bacteria under stress. Curcumin from turmeric and catechins from green tea are two examples of phytochemicals that can interfere with the extracellular polymeric substances (EPS) production and inhibit early bacterial adhesion, both of which destabilise established biofilms (Daglia 2012). This trait increases the susceptibility of bacteria to both traditional antibiotics and phytochemicals.

Together, these mechanisms give phytochemicals the antibacterial qualities. Because of their multi-targeted action, phytochemicals are less likely to cause microbial resistance than single-target antibiotics. Their unique characteristics make them promising supplements or alternatives in the fight against multidrug-resistant (MDR) diseases, as well as effective models for developing next-generation antimicrobial drugs.

5 Phytochemicals Active against Bacterial Infections

Phytochemicals derived from aromatic and medicinal plants have demonstrated strong antibacterial effects against both Gram-positive bacterial and Gram-negative bacterial diseases (Table 3). They operate by concentrating on essential bacterial structures and processes, including cell wall formation, nucleic acid replication,

Table 3 Phytochemicals active against bacterial infections

Compound	Source plant	Target organism	Mechanism of action	References
Quercetin	*Allium cepa*, *Camellia sinensis*	*Staphylococcus aureus*, *Streptococcus pneumoniae*	Inhibits nucleic acid synthesis; disrupts membrane potential; suppresses virulence gene expression	Cushnie and Lamb (2011)
Catechin	*Camellia sinensis*	*S. aureus*, *Listeria monocytogenes*	Disrupts bacterial adhesion; interferes with cell wall integrity	Cushnie and Lamb (2011)
Berberine	*Berberis vulgaris*, *Coptis chinensis*	*S. aureus*, *E. coli*	Intercalates DNA; inhibits topoisomerase; disrupts biofilm formation	Zhou et al. (2024)
Resveratrol	*Vitis vinifera*	*S. aureus*, *Listeria* spp.	Suppresses quorum sensing; inhibits toxin production	Savoia (2012)
Curcumin	*Curcuma longa*	*S. aureus*, *Enterococcus faecalis*	Disrupts cell membrane; inhibits bacterial replication enzymes	Savoia (2012)
Eugenol	*Syzygium aromaticum*	*E. coli*, *Pseudomonas aeruginosa*	Disrupts membrane permeability; inhibits ATPase activity	Gill and Holley (2006)
Thymol	*Thymus vulgaris*	*E. coli*, *Salmonella enterica*	Disintegrates outer membrane; increases ion leakage	Marchese et al. (2016)
Carvacrol	*Origanum vulgare*	*E. coli*, *P. aeruginosa*	Causes depolarisation and leakage of intracellular material	Bakkali et al. (2008)
Gallic acid	*Punica granatum*, *Camellia sinensis*	*Klebsiella pneumoniae*, *E. coli*	Chelates metal ions; disrupts oxidative stress enzymes	Daglia (2012)
Ferulic acid	*Oryza sativa*, *Triticum aestivum*	*E. coli*, *Salmonella* spp.	Inhibits cell wall synthesis and enzyme activity	Daglia (2012)
Tannins	*Acacia nilotica*, *Terminalia chebula*	*Pseudomonas aeruginosa*	Inhibits quorum sensing; reduces biofilm formation	Adonizio et al. (2008)
Linalool	*Coriandrum sativum*, *Lavandula angustifolia*	*E. coli*, *S. aureus*	Alters membrane lipid composition and permeability	Burt (2004)
Sanguinarine	*Sanguinaria canadensis*	*S. aureus*, *Streptococcus* spp.	Inhibits DNA synthesis; damages bacterial membranes	Khameneh et al. (2019)

membrane integrity, and quorum sensing (Cowan 1999; Cushnie and Lamb 2011). Unlike conventional antibiotics, phytochemicals often act across multiple pathways, reducing the likelihood of resistance. Furthermore, they complement antibiotics to enhance drug absorption and efficacy against multiple drug-resistant (MDR) bacterial strains (Khameneh et al. 2019).

5.1 Pathogens that Are Gram-Positive

Gram-positive bacteria, like *Staphylococcus aureus*, *Streptococcus pneumoniae*, and *Enterococcus faecalis*, are mostly responsible for infections contracted in hospitals and the general public. By inhibiting DNA gyrase activity and peptidoglycan cross-linking, flavonoids, e.g. catechin, quercetin, and apigenin, interfere with the nucleic acids and cell walls synthesis (Cushnie and Lamb 2011). For instance, it has been shown that quercetin reduces the expression of virulence genes and alters the potential of the S. aureus cell membrane, whereas catechin interferes with the adherence and aggregation of bacteria.

Alkaloids such as sanguinarine and berberine have bactericidal properties that stop nucleic acid replication by intercalating with DNA and inhibiting topoisomerase enzymes (Khameneh et al. 2019). Furthermore, S. aureus biofilms can be broken by berberine, increasing the bacteria's susceptibility to β-lactam antibiotics (Zhou et al. 2024). Additionally, phenolic compounds like curcumin and resveratrol have been shown to decrease quorum sensing, inhibit the formation of toxins, and block surface protein-mediated adhesion in Staphylococcus and Listeria species (Savoia 2012). Phytochemicals are interesting candidates for antibiotic adjuvant therapy because of their multitargeted actions, which make them efficient (Devi et al. 2025).

5.2 Pathogens that Are Gram-Negative

Gram-negative bacteria pose a greater treatment difficulty due to presence of outer membrane, which acts as a permeability barrier to many antimicrobial medicines (Gill and Holley 2006). Phytochemicals having lipophilic and amphipathic structures, including terpenoids, phenolic acids, and constituents of essential oils, might interact with membrane lipids to enhance permeability and facilitate the absorption of antibiotics (Burt 2004).

Clove and thyme oils contain eugenol and thymol, which have strong anti-E. coli and anti-Pseudomonas effects by dissolving the outer membrane and inhibiting ATPase enzymes essential for energy metabolism (Gill and Holley 2006; Marchese et al. 2016). Similarly, citral and carvacrol rapidly depolarise the cell membrane, causing intracellular substance to be lost, potassium ions to leak out, and ultimately the death of the bacteria (Bakkali et al. 2008).

Furthermore, a number of phenolic acids, such as gallic acid and ferulic acid, function by chelating crucial metal ions like Fe2+ and Mg2+, which prevents Klebsiella and E. coli's oxidative stress response pathways and enzymatic activity (Daglia 2012). According to Adonizio et al. (2008), other phytochemicals like flavonoids and tannins stop Pseudomonas aeruginosa from detecting quorum, which reduces the formation of biofilms and the release of virulence factors.

These findings demonstrate the value of phytochemicals as potent, multi-targeted medications that can overcome the innate and acquired resistance mechanisms of Gram-negative bacteria, offering a workable alternative in the ongoing battle against antibiotic resistance.

6 Phytochemicals Active Against Viral Infections

By obstructing viral entrance, replication, or assembly, metabolites produced from plants demonstrate antiviral activity (Fig. 2). For example, by inhibiting viral proteases, green tea's epigallocatechin gallate (EGCG) prevents the reproduction of SARS-CoV-2 and influenza (Henss et al. 2021). Viral RNA polymerases are inhibited by alkaloids like lycorine from the Amaryllidaceae.

By altering viral envelope proteins, terpenoids such as betulinic acid and glycyrrhizin suppress the hepatitis and HIV viruses, respectively (Pompei et al. 1980). These results demonstrate the potential of phytochemicals as all-purpose antivirals.

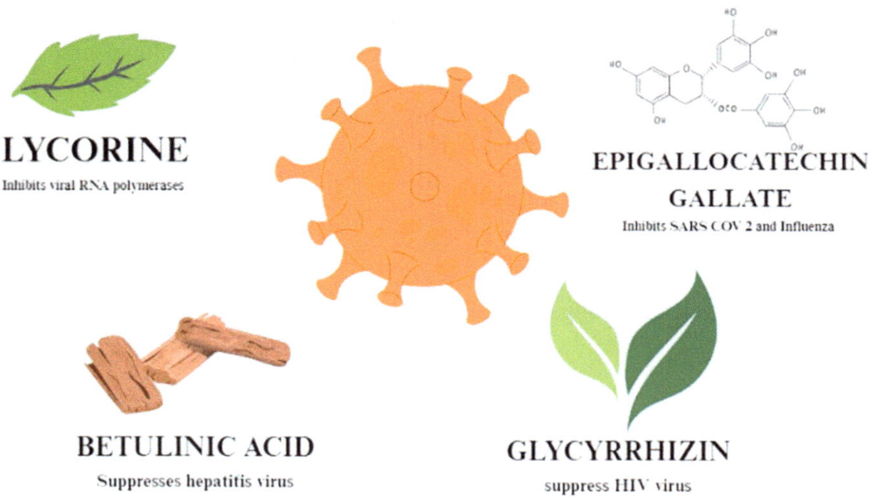

Fig. 2 Phytochemicals active against viral infections

7 Phytochemicals Active Against Fungal Infections

Phytochemicals harm the fungal cell walls and membranes, induce oxidative stress, or obstruct the synthesis of ergosterol (Table 4). Gallic acid and other phenolic acids damage Candida albicans biofilms (Khan et al. 2017). Terpenes such as citronellal and menthol affect the permeability of fungal cells. While alkaloids like sanguinarine stop fungal respiration, saponins act as organic antifungal detergents.

Naturally occurring bioactive substances derived from plants, known as phytochemicals, have shown promise as antifungal treatments, especially when used to treat drug-resistant fungal infections. Among these, phenolic substances with strong antifungal properties, such as eugenol, a key component of clove oil, have been thoroughly researched. Fungal growth and biofilm formation are eventually hampered by eugenol, which damages the integrity of fungal cell membranes, suppresses ergosterol biosynthesis, and raises membrane permeability and oxidative stress (Khan et al. 2014; Marchese et al. 2016). Similar to this, the monoterpenoid phenols thymol and carvacrol, which are present in thyme and oregano oils, have shown broad-spectrum antifungal activity by inducing hyphal deformation, inhibiting the production of ergosterol, and disrupting the fungal membrane potential (Bakkali et al. 2008; de Oliveira Pereira et al. 2017). These naturally occurring compounds have the potential to be used as supplements or substitutes for traditional antifungal treatments since they both inhibit fungal growth and lessen pathogenicity characteristics.

Alkaloids, in particular berberine, an isoquinoline derivative present in a number of medicinal plants, constitute another intriguing class of antifungal phytochemicals. According to Zhou et al. (2024), berberine has a broad spectrum of antifungal properties, with minimum inhibitory doses against filamentous fungi and yeast ranging from 64 to 128 μg/mL. In a manner akin to that of azole antifungal medications, it inhibits ergosterol manufacture by binding to the CYP51 enzyme. It also causes morphological and ultrastructural changes, including cell wall distortion and membrane rupture (Gao et al. 2023). In order to combat multidrug resistance, recent research has also shown that phytochemicals like berberine may work in concert with traditional antifungal medications (Jafri et al. 2022). All of these results show that phytochemicals derived from plants have a great deal of promise for creating safer, multi-targeted antifungal medications.

8 Phytochemicals Active Against Parasitic Infections

Traditional medicine has historically employed plant extracts to treat malaria, leishmaniasis, and trypanosomiasis. Artemisinin, which is isolated from Artemisia annua, is still a vital part of the therapy of malaria (Table 4). Quinine, which comes from the bark of the Cinchona plant, is another well-known example. Furthermore, terpenoids and alkaloids are efficient against Leishmania and Trypanosoma species

Table 4 Phytochemicals for treatment of infectious illnesses

Compound	Source plant	Target organism	Mechanism of action	References
Betulinic acid	*Betula alba*	HIV	Blocks viral protease	Pompei et al. (1980)
Artemisinin	*Artemisia annua*	*Plasmodium falciparum*	ROS generation	Kayser et al. (2003)
Eugenol	Syzygium aromaticum (Clove)	Candida albicans, Aspergillus niger	Disrupts cell membrane integrity, inhibits ergosterol biosynthesis, and suppresses biofilm formation	Khan et al. (2014); Marchese et al. (2016)
Thymol	Thymus vulgaris (Thyme)	Candida albicans, Trichophyton mentagrophytes	Alters membrane permeability and ergosterol synthesis, leading to leakage of cellular contents	Marchese et al. (2016); de Oliveira Pereira et al. (2017)
Carvacrol	Origanum vulgare (Oregano)	Candida tropicalis, Aspergillus flavus	Induces oxidative stress and morphological changes in hyphal structure	Bakkali et al. (2008)
Berberine	Berberis aristata (Indian Barberry)	Candida spp., Cryptococcus neoformans	Inhibits CYP51 enzyme, disrupts ergosterol pathway, causes membrane rupture	Zhou et al. (2024); Gao et al. (2023)
Curcumin	Curcuma longa (Turmeric)	Candida albicans, Staphylococcus aureus	Induces reactive oxygen species (ROS) generation, inhibits fungal adhesion and morphogenesis	Jafri et al. (2022)
Resveratrol	Vitis vinifera (Grapevine)	Candida albicans	Inhibits hyphal growth, impairs quorum sensing and biofilm development	Marchese et al. (2016)
Allicin	Allium sativum (Garlic)	Candida albicans, Escherichia coli	Reacts with thiol-containing enzymes, disrupting microbial metabolism	Bakkali et al. (2008)
Catechin	Camellia sinensis (Green Tea)	Candida glabrata, Pseudomonas aeruginosa	Damages membrane lipids and inhibits protein synthesis	de Oliveira Pereira et al. (2017)
Quercetin	Ocimum sanctum (Holy Basil)	Candida albicans, Staphylococcus aureus	Inhibits nucleic acid synthesis and cell wall integrity	Jafri et al. (2022)
Limonene	Citrus limon (Lemon)	Aspergillus flavus, Candida spp.	Alters cell membrane permeability and mitochondrial activity	Bakkali et al. (2008)

(Kayser et al. 2003). These chemical compounds often function by causing oxidative stress or inhibiting parasite-specific enzymes like cysteine proteases.

9 Advances in Biotechnology and Phytochemical Production

The sustainable production and improvement of phytochemicals with medicinal potential has been completely transformed by recent biotechnology breakthroughs. Low yields, protracted cultivation periods, and environmental unpredictability are common problems with traditional extraction techniques (Ramachandra Rao and Ravishankar 2002). Precursor feeding, elicitation with biotic or abiotic stresses, and growth regulator modulation to promote metabolite production are ways to optimise these cultures (Giri and Narasu 2000). For instance, cell suspensions of Catharanthus roseus have shown enhanced yields of vinblastine and vincristine, while hairy root cultures of Withania somnifera have been used to boost withanolide production.

Another revolutionary strategy that alters biosynthetic pathways to increase or reroute metabolite production is metabolic engineering. Researchers have been able to fine-tune phytochemical outputs in plants and microbial systems by overexpressing or silencing important enzymes involved in biosynthesis pathways (Sharma et al. 2020). Plant genomes may now be precisely modified to upregulate biosynthetic genes or knock off negative regulators because of advancements in genome editing technologies, especially CRISPR-Cas9 (Niu et al. 2021). For example, paclitaxel and artemisinin precursor accumulation in plant cells has been successfully enhanced by CRISPR-mediated disruption of competing pathways (Niu et al. 2021; Paddon et al. 2013).

Furthermore, microbial hosts like Saccharomyces cerevisiae and Escherichia coli may now produce plant-derived compounds heterologously, thanks to synthetic biology. A notable example of a scalable and economical model for the production of phytochemicals is the semi-synthetic production of artemisinin, a strong antimalarial compound that was first derived from Artemisia annua, through metabolic reconstitution in engineered yeast (Paddon et al. 2013). In a similar vein, systems based on yeast and algae are being investigated for the production of terpenoids, flavonoids, and alkaloids with higher yields and consistency than conventional farming (Khan et al. 2023).

Endophytic microorganisms produce phytochemicals that are either the same or very similar to those of their host plants (Singh and Dubey 2021a, b). By providing a different and sustainable source of important compounds like azadirachtin, podophyllotoxin, and camptothecin, these microbial systems lessen reliance on slow-growing or endangered plant species. Predictive models of phytochemical biosynthesis are being made possible by the combination of bioprocess optimisation and omics technologies (genomics, transcriptomics, and metabolomics), which will further improve yield, quality, and repeatability (Rai et al. 2022).

Together, these developments show a paradigm shift away from conventional plant extraction and towards sustainable and bioengineered production systems that combine synthetic biology, metabolic engineering, and molecular biology to produce phytochemicals on a large scale. In addition to guaranteeing a steady supply for pharmaceutical and nutraceutical uses, this shift is in line with sustainable and green biotechnology principles.

10 Formulation Strategies and Nano-Delivery of Phytochemicals

Despite the amazing therapeutic potential of phytochemicals, their fast metabolism, volatility, low bioavailability, and poor water solubility frequently impede their clinical translation (Yallapu et al. 2012). Traditional formulations often result in uneven pharmacokinetics and inadequate efficacy because they are unable to reach therapeutic concentrations at target locations. Delivery methods based on nanotechnology have become a game-changing method for improving the therapeutic efficacy of natural chemicals in order to get over these obstacles (Nasrollahzadeh et al. 2020a, b, c). Improved solubility, sustained release, increased stability, and increased cellular uptake are some benefits of nanocarrier formulations (Mishra et al. 2022). Through surface modification with ligands or antibodies, these nanoformulations not only shield phytochemicals from enzymatic degradation but also enable regulated release and site-specific targeting to infection or inflammatory zones (Ganesan et al. 2022).

Because liposome-based formulations are biocompatible and can encapsulate both hydrophilic and lipophilic substances, they are among the most popular phytochemical carriers. Because they may pass through microbial cell membranes more easily and have a longer systemic circulation, curcumin-loaded liposomes and nanoparticles, for example, have shown stronger antibacterial and antifungal activity than free curcumin (Nasrollahzadeh et al. 2020a, b, c). The limits of limited aqueous solubility are also overcome by quercetin- and resveratrol-loaded polymeric nanoparticles, which show improved antioxidant and anti-inflammatory effectiveness (Yadav et al. 2021). Because chitosan-based nanoparticles are cationic, they have a great affinity for negatively charged bacterial membranes, which enhances intracellular transport and drug adherence (Bilia et al. 2017).

SLNs and NLCs, which offer better encapsulation efficiency and regulated drug release patterns, are another intriguing formulation class. Bioactives such as thymol, eugenol, and berberine have benefited from the successful application of these systems, which have increased their antibacterial potency and stability in physiological settings (Rajput et al. 2021). Improved mucosal absorption and antimicrobial activity are made possible by the development of nanoemulsions, which are oil–water dispersions stabilised by surfactants and used to transport volatile phytochemicals like essential oils (Sharma et al. 2022).

Additionally, selective accumulation in sick tissues or microbial biofilms is made possible by targeted nanocarrier systems, such as ligand-functionalised nanoparticles and stimuli-responsive delivery vehicles. In acidic or enzyme-rich microenvironments, pH-sensitive and enzyme-responsive nanoparticles release their phytochemical payload, maximising medication concentration at the infection site and reducing off-target effects (Kumar et al. 2023). Furthermore, green nanotechnology techniques that use plant extracts to synthesise nanoparticles are becoming more popular since they provide biocompatible and environmentally acceptable substitutes for traditional chemical procedures (Nasrollahzadeh et al. 2020a, b, c).

All nano-delivery methods have greatly enhanced phytochemicals' pharmacokinetic, pharmacodynamic, and therapeutic results. In addition to improving solubility and stability, they offer novel approaches to combination therapy, which aims to prevent antimicrobial resistance by co-delivering several phytochemicals or phytochemical–antibiotic conjugates. The entire therapeutic potential of plant-derived bioactives in the treatment of chronic and infectious diseases is anticipated with further integration of pharmacology, material science, and nanotechnology.

11 Clinical Studies, Safety, and Pharmacological Validation

Some phytochemicals that have progressed to clinical trials and shown safety and efficacy in the treatment of infectious disorders include berberine, curcumin, and resveratrol (Kumar et al. 2022). In human studies of respiratory and gastrointestinal infections, resveratrol, a polyphenolic molecule present in grapes and berries, has demonstrated encouraging outcomes in lowering viral replication and inflammation (De Ligt et al. 2021). Likewise, several phase II and III clinical trials have shown that curcumin, which is extracted from Curcuma longa, has antibacterial and immunomodulatory activity against viral infections, Helicobacter pylori, and Candida albicans (Chainani-Wu et al. 2012; Gupta et al. 2013). Clinical research on bacterial diarrhoea and methicillin-resistant Staphylococcus aureus (MRSA) infections has shown that berberine, which is derived from Berberis species, reduces microbial load and symptom duration (Tillhon et al. 2012).

But even with these developments, it's still difficult to convert preclinical effectiveness into reliable clinical results. Pharmacological results are frequently variable because of differences in plant sources, extraction methods, and the absence of standardisation of bioactive content (Ekor 2014). Moreover, the clinical usefulness of phytochemicals is limited by their frequent low bioavailability, fast metabolism, and poor systemic absorption. To determine therapeutic windows and guarantee long-term safety, thorough toxicological, pharmacokinetic, and pharmacodynamic assessments are necessary (Yue et al. 2019). Phytochemicals may eventually be able to function as dependable substitutes or adjuvants in the treatment of infectious diseases if standardisation procedures, clinical dose optimisation, and nanotechnology-based delivery systems are combined (Nasrollahzadeh et al. 2020a, b, c).

12 Conclusion

Despite the great medicinal potential of phytochemicals, a number of obstacles prevent their broad use, including compositional heterogeneity, poor stability, and a dearth of clinical evidence. In order to maximise phytochemical-based treatments, future studies should concentrate on integrative strategies that combine computational screening, synthetic biology, and nanotechnology. Success will depend on cooperation between chemists, pharmacologists, and ethnobotanists.

A sustained and adaptable toolkit against viral illnesses is provided by phytochemicals. They are attractive options for contemporary drug discovery because of their structural diversity, multitarget activities, and low susceptibility to resistance. By combining cutting-edge formulation methods with bioengineering techniques, present constraints can be addressed and next-generation phytotherapeutics for global health issues can be developed.

References

Adam AB, Kaugama AA, Boro G, Joseph AM, Muhammad JA, Suleiman S, Mohammed H (2023) Phytochemical and antibacterial analysis of leaves extract of Pistia stratiotes. In: 9th International Mardin Artuklu Scientific Researches Conference

Adonizio A, Downum K, Bennett BC, Mathee K (2008) Anti-quorum sensing activity of medicinal plants in southern Florida. J Ethnopharmacol 105(3):427–435

Andrade-Cetto A (2003) Major herbs of Ayurveda: Elizabeth M. Williamson, Elsevier science, Churchill Livingstone, China, 2002, 70 plant monographs and color plates, 361 pp., Price£ 39.99 (hard cover), ISBN: 0-443-07203-5

Ashokkumar K (2015) Gloriosa superba (L.): a brief review of its phytochemical properties and pharmacology. Int J Pharmacogn Phytochem Res 7(6):1190–1193

Ashutosh Meher AM, Agrahari AK, Padhan AR (2011) A literature review on Argyreia nervosa (Burm. F.) Bojer

Asokan GV, Kasimanickam RK (2013) Emerging infectious diseases, antimicrobial resistance and millennium development goals: resolving the challenges through one health. Cent Asian J Glob Health 2(2):76

Bakkali F, Averbeck S, Averbeck D, Idaomar M (2008) Biological effects of essential oils. Food Chem Toxicol 46(2):446–475

Balasundram N, Sundram K, Samman S (2006) Phenolic compounds in plants and agri-industrial by-products. Food Chem 99(1):191–203

Bilia AR, Piazzini V, Guccione C, Risaliti L, Asprea M, Capecchi G, Bergonzi MC, Luceri C (2017) Improving on nature: the role of nanomedicine in the development of clinical natural drugs. Planta Med 83(5):366–381

Burt S (2004) Essential oils: their antibacterial properties and potential applications in foods—a review. Int J Food Microbiol 94(3):223–253

Castanheira M, Deshpande LM, Farrell SE, Shetye S, Shah N, Jones RN (2013) Update on the prevalence and genetic characterization of NDM-1–producing Enterobacteriaceae in Indian hospitals during 2010. Diagn Microbiol Infect Dis 75(2):210–213

Chainani-Wu N, Madden E, Lozada-Nur F, Silverman S (2012) High-dose curcumin treatment is effective in patients with oral lichen planus. J Am Acad Dermatol 66(5):752–760

Chanda S, Ramachandra TV (2019) A review on some therapeutic aspects of phytochemicals present in medicinal plants. Int J Pharm Life Sci 10(1)

Cowan MM (1999) Plant products as antimicrobial agents. Clin Microbiol Rev 12(4):564–582

Cushnie TPT, Lamb AJ (2011) Recent advances in understanding the antibacterial properties of flavonoids. Int J Antimicrob Agents 38(2):99–107

Daglia M (2012) Polyphenols as antimicrobial agents. Curr Opin Biotechnol 23(2):174–181

Dahiru S, Salele Y, Mathew TS, Adam AB (2024) Phytochemical analysis of carrot, red pepper, spinach and lettuce cultivated at Ajiwa, Batagarawa, Lambun Sarki and Dankama Vegetable Farms, Katsina State, Nigeria. Afr J Sci Tradit Med 1(1):423–427

De Ligt M, Timmers S, Schrauwen P, Eijsvogels TMH (2021) Resveratrol supplementation in humans: impact on inflammation, metabolism, and infections. Nutrients 13(9):3222

de Oliveira Pereira F, Mendes JM, de Sousa DP (2017) Bioactive compounds of essential oils: antifungal mechanisms of action and prospects for their use in the control of fungal diseases. J Essent Oil Res 29(2):1–8

Devi P, Sharma K, Kaur R (2025) Phytochemical-based strategies to combat antimicrobial resistance: mechanistic insights and therapeutic potential. Front Microbiol 16:1204567

Egamberdieva D, Mamedov N, Ovidi E, Tiezzi A, Craker L (2017) Phytochemical and pharmacological properties of medicinal plants from Uzbekistan: a review. J Med Act Plants 5(1–4)

Ekor M (2014) The growing use of herbal medicines: issues relating to adverse reactions and challenges in monitoring safety. Front Pharmacol 4:177

Ganesan P, Narayanasamy S, Rajendran S (2022) Nanotechnology-based delivery of bioactive phytocompounds against microbial infections. Front Nanotechnol 4:1007568

Gao W, Wang X, Xu Y, Zhang J, Li X (2023) Mechanistic insights into berberine-induced morphological and membrane changes in Candida species. Front Microbiol 14:1265492

Gill AO, Holley RA (2006) Disruption of Escherichia coli, Listeria monocytogenes and Lactobacillus sakei cellular membranes by plant oil aromatics. Int J Food Microbiol 108(1):1–9

Giri A, Narasu ML (2000) Production of plant secondary metabolites through cell and tissue culture. Plant Cell Tissue Organ Cult 62(1):1–17

Gupta SC, Patchva S, Aggarwal BB (2013) Therapeutic roles of curcumin: lessons learned from clinical trials. AAPS J 15(1):195–218

Henss L et al (2021) The green tea catechin epigallocatechin gallate inhibits SARS-CoV-2 infection. Antivir Res 186:104984

Jafri H, Banerjee P, Singh S (2022) Role of phytochemicals as antifungal agents and their synergistic effects with conventional drugs. Front Pharmacol 13:981374

Kayser O, Kiderlen AF, Croft SL (2003) Natural products as antiparasitic drugs. Parasitol Res 90(S2):S55–S62

Khameneh B, Iranshahy M, Soheili V, Bazzaz BSF (2019) Review on plant antimicrobials: a mechanistic viewpoint. Antimicrob Resist Infect Control 8(1):118

Khan A, Ahmad A, Manzoor N (2017) Antifungal activities of some essential oils against *Candida albicans*. Phytother Res 31(1):89–96

Khan MA, Aslam M, Ahmad A (2023) Synthetic biology approaches for the sustainable production of high-value plant secondary metabolites. Biotechnol Adv 66:108219

Khan MSA, Ahmad I, Cameotra SS, Al-Thubiani AS (2014) Formulation and characterization of eugenol-loaded solid lipid nanoparticles against Candida albicans. J Appl Microbiol 117(3):695–707

Kumar A, Singh R, Pandey A (2022) Phytochemicals in infectious disease management: clinical validation and translational challenges. Phytomedicine 98:153970

Kumar A, Singh S, Kaur R (2023) Stimuli-responsive nanocarriers for site-specific delivery of plant bioactives: recent trends and prospects. J Control Release 356:1–18

Marchese A, Orhan IE, Daglia M, Barbieri R, Di Lorenzo A, Nabavi SF, Gortzi O, Izadi M, Nabavi SM (2016) Antibacterial and antifungal activities of thymol: a brief review of the literature. Food Chem 210:402–414

Mathew TS, Chinedu EK, Haladu M, Abubakar MY, Adam AB, Shamsuddeen R (2024) Natural products as leads for neglected trophical diseases (NTDs) treatment; a chemical and biological-review. AMJSAI 1(1):552–570
Mishra V, Nayak P, Singh M, Tambuwala MM (2022) Emerging nanocarrier strategies for efficient delivery of phytochemicals in healthcare. Colloids Surf B Biointerfaces 213:112388
Nasrollahzadeh M, Sajadi SM, Sajjadi M, Issaabadi Z (2020a) An introduction to nanotechnology. In: Interface science and technology, vol 28. Elsevier, pp 1–27
Nasrollahzadeh M, Sajadi SM, Sajjadi M, Issaabadi Z (2020b) Applications of nanotechnology in food, agricultural, and pharmaceutical sciences. In: Nasrollahzadeh M et al (eds) An introduction to green nanotechnology. Elsevier, pp 1–36
Nasrollahzadeh M, Sajjadi M, Iravani S, Varma RS (2020c) Green nanotechnology for drug delivery: a review of recent advances in phytochemical-based nanocarriers. Green Chem 22(1):2162–2189
Newman DJ, Cragg GM (2020) Natural products as sources of new drugs over the nearly four decades from 1981 to 2019. J Nat Prod 83(3):770–803
Niu X, Liu Z, Tang Y, Zhang Y (2021) CRISPR/Cas-mediated metabolic engineering for plant secondary metabolite biosynthesis. Plant Biotechnol J 19(12):2421–2438
Paddon CJ, Westfall PJ, Pitera DJ, Benjamin K, Fisher K, McPhee D, Leavell MD, Tai A, Main A, Eng D, Polichuk DR, Teoh KH, Reed DW, Treynor T, Lenihan J, Fleck M, Bajad S, Dang G, Dengrove D et al (2013) High-level semi-synthetic production of the potent antimalarial artemisinin. Nature 496(7446):528–532
Pandey KB, Rizvi SI (2020) Plant polyphenols as dietary antioxidants in human health and disease. Oxidative Med Cell Longev 2020:1–15
Pompei R, Flore O, Marccialis MA, Pani A, Loddo B (1980) Glycyrrhizic acid inhibits virus growth and inactivates virus particles. Nature 281(5733):689–690
Rai A, Saito K, Yamazaki M (2022) Integrated omics for metabolic pathway engineering of plant secondary metabolites. Plant Biotechnol Rep 16(4):373–386
Rajput VD, Minkina T, Sushkova S, Mandzhieva S, Fedorenko A, Lysenko V, Rajput S (2021) Solid lipid nanoparticles: a sustainable platform for the delivery of natural bioactive compounds. Pharmaceuticals 14(12):1250
Ramachandra Rao S, Ravishankar GA (2002) Plant cell cultures: chemical factories of secondary metabolites. Biotechnol Adv 20(2):101–153
Rios JL, Recio MC (2005) Medicinal plants and antimicrobial activity. J Ethnopharmacol 100(1–2):80–84
Savoia D (2012) Plant-derived antimicrobial compounds: alternatives to antibiotics. Future Microbiol 7(8):979–990
Saxena M, Saxena J, Nema R, Singh D, Gupta A (2013) Phytochemistry of medicinal plants. J Pharmacogn Phytochem 1(6)
Sharma A, Gautam T, Pandey A (2020) Metabolic engineering strategies for enhancing secondary metabolite production in plants. Phytochem Rev 19(6):1323–1341
Sharma R, Kumar D, Mehta P (2022) Nanoemulsion-based phytochemical delivery systems for antimicrobial and therapeutic applications. Adv Colloid Interface Sci 304:102652
Singh M, Dubey S (2021a) Endophytic fungi: novel sources of bioactive secondary metabolites. Front Microbiol 12:678249
Singh S, Dubey AK (2021b) Endophytic microbes as potential source for bioactive compounds and their applications in drug discovery. Biotechnol Adv 47:107695
Thoen CO, Steele JH, Gilsdorf MJ (2008) Mycobacterium bovis infection in animals and humans. Wiley
Tillhon M, Guaman Ortiz LM, Lombardi P, Scovassi AI (2012) Berberine: new perspectives for old remedies. Biochem Pharmacol 84(10):1260–1267
Ventola CL (2015) The antibiotic resistance crisis. Pharm Therap 40(4):277–283
Wink M (2015) Modes of action of herbal medicines and plant secondary metabolites. Medicine 2(3):251–286

World Health Organization (2013) WHO expert consultation on rabies: second report, vol 982. World Health Organization

World Health Organization (2023) Global antimicrobial resistance and use surveillance system (GLASS) report. WHO, Geneva

Yadav D, Sandeep K, Pandey D, Dahiya S (2021) Nanoparticle-based drug delivery systems for improved therapeutic efficacy of natural compounds. Drug Deliv Transl Res 11(2):748–762

Yallapu MM, Jaggi M, Chauhan SC (2012) Curcumin nanoformulations: a future nanomedicine for cancer. Drug Discov Today 17(1–2):71–80

Yue GGL, Chan BCL, Hon PM, Lee MYH, Fung KP, Leung PC, Lau CBS (2019) Review on the safety and efficacy of phytochemicals in clinical practice: from experimental pharmacology to clinical pharmacokinetics. Front Pharmacol 10:1578

Zhou J, Xu Y, Liang J, Liu M (2024) Berberine as a potent antifungal agent targeting fungal CYP51 enzyme: mechanistic and structural insights. Molecules 29(21):5079

Phytochemicals Potentially Applied for Emerging Diseases

Wiwit Suttithumsatid

Abstract Phytochemicals, bioactive compounds derived from plants, present a promising therapeutic approach for emerging infectious diseases, including rapidly spreading infections like COVID-19, highly pathogenic avian influenza (H5N1), dengue fever, multidrug-resistant tuberculosis (MDR-TB), and Zika virus infection. These compounds exhibit various pharmacological activities, including antiviral, antibacterial, antifungal, anti-inflammatory, and immunomodulatory effects. Their unique chemical structures offer novel mechanisms of action, potentially overcoming limitations of conventional drugs. For example, flavonoids, terpenoids, alkaloids, and saponins have demonstrated antiviral properties by inhibiting viral entry, replication, and host cell interactions. Despite their potential, challenges remain, including the need for standardized extraction, clinical validation, and optimization of bioavailability. Nevertheless, integrating phytochemicals with modern drug discovery technologies has the potential to accelerate the development of innovative therapies for emerging diseases. This chapter aims to explore the potential clinical applications of phytochemicals, with a focus on their mechanisms, recent advances in scientific evidence, and future prospects in alternative treatments for emerging infectious diseases.

Keywords Phytochemicals · Natural products · Emerging diseases · Antiviral activity · Immunomodulation

W. Suttithumsatid (✉)
Prince of Songkla University, Faculty of Pharmaceutical Sciences, Department of Pharmacognosy and Pharmaceutical Botany, Hat-Yai, Thailand

Prince of Songkla University, Phytomedicine and Pharmaceutical Biotechnology Excellence Center, Hat-Yai, Thailand
e-mail: wiwit.su@psu.ac.th

S. Kumar Tripathi et al. (eds.), *Phytoceuticals for Sustainable Medication*, Interdisciplinary Biotechnological Advances,
https://doi.org/10.1007/978-981-95-7588-6_11

1 Introduction

The concept of 'emerging diseases' refers to illnesses that are newly recognized in a given population, or previously existed but are now spreading more rapidly or expanding their geographic distribution, e.g., severe acute respiratory syndrome (SARS), coronavirus disease 2019 (COVID-19), Zika virus, Ebola virus, and middle east respiratory syndrome (MERS). They may arise due to the discovery of previously unrecognized pathogens, known diseases spreading to new areas, or old diseases reemerging due to factors like antimicrobial resistance or gene mutation (Anderson and Gray 2019; Gharbi et al. 2025). In recent decades, several novel unknown and unidentified diseases have emerged rapidly around the world. Infectious diseases rank among the primary causes of mortality worldwide. There is an urgent need to develop effective strategy to deal with this issue.

Treatment of emerging diseases requires multidisciplinary approaches, including the development and effective use of novel therapeutics, identifying new indications for existing drugs, and supportive healthcare system strategies. However, there are significant limitations, one of which is the rapid emergence of multidrug-resistant strains and the appearance of novel microbial strains, which complicate treatment. Moreover, developing novel medications involves high research, production, and investment costs. This limits accessibility, especially in low- to middle-income countries, and delays widespread use (McCune and Reynolds 2015; Kunz Coyne et al. 2022).

Phytochemical compounds, with their unique chemical structures and resulting diverse mechanisms of action, have been playing a part in drug discovery. These bioactive compounds, derived from medicinal plants, are being investigated as potential therapeutic agents against emerging diseases, especially those of infectious origin. Their diverse biological activities, including antiviral, antibacterial, antifungal, and immunomodulatory effects, make them promising candidates. The unique structural features of phytochemicals position them as promising sources for drug discovery and alternative treatments for emerging diseases. The potential integration of phytochemicals with modern therapeutic platforms could accelerate the discovery of new alternative therapies for emerging diseases (Chihomvu et al. 2024).

Therefore, this chapter aims to provide insight into the potential applications of phytochemical compounds in treating emerging diseases. It seeks to establish a scientific foundation for those interested in phytochemicals as innovative and sustainable solutions to evolving health challenges. The potential of phytochemicals in this context is not just promising but inspiring, as it opens up new avenues for research and development.

2 Phytochemical Mechanisms and Strategic Approaches in Emerging Disease Management

Phytochemical compounds, especially plant secondary metabolites, represent a diverse group that can be categorized according to their biosynthetic pathways or chemical structures. Their distinct chemical structures allow them to interact with biological targets in different ways, resulting in multiple pharmacological activities. As phytochemicals exhibit a wide spectrum of pharmacological activities, this chapter highlights their promise in the prevention and management of emerging diseases, underscoring their significant role in modern health challenges.

2.1 Antioxidant and Anti-inflammatory Properties

Oxidative stress coupled with inflammatory processes is widely recognized as an important hallmark of many emerging diseases, especially infectious diseases. For example, in recent years, oxidative stress and dysregulated inflammation have been identified as critical factors in COVID-19. The binding of SARS-CoV-2 to its ACE2 receptor represents a starting point in the infection process, leading to oxidative stress (Beltrán-García et al. 2020). Subsequently, an excessive immune response characterized by a cytokine storm and immune-cell dysregulation contributes significantly to tissue damage and organ failure (Nazerian et al. 2022). The inflammatory and oxidative profiles of COVID-19 highlight the need for targeted interventions. It has been hypothesized that antioxidant agents can restore oxidative balance and modulate inflammatory responses, presenting a promising strategy to mitigate disease progression and improve patient outcomes (Zamparelli et al. 2025).

Phytochemical compounds, especially phenolic compounds including flavonoids and carotenoids, have been reported to possess strong antioxidant activity through various pathways, including modulating protein expression, boosting cellular defenses, and influencing epigenetic changes (Sun and Shahrajabian 2023). The anti-inflammatory effects of phytochemicals are particularly evident in flavonoids, terpenoids, alkaloids, saponins, tannins, and anthraquinones. They exert significant anti-inflammatory activity through diverse mechanisms, including inhibiting pro-inflammatory cytokines, suppressing key inflammatory signaling pathways, and enhancing anti-inflammatory cytokines. These properties make phytochemicals valuable candidates for managing emerging diseases (Sun and Shahrajabian 2023; Breda et al. 2025).

2.2 Antiviral Activities

In modern times, most emerging diseases involve microbial infection, especially viral infections. Emerging and reemerging viral epidemics lead to high morbidity and mortality and pose major global health threats. Generally, our body employs an immune system to neutralize viral invasion and prevent its spread by producing antibodies. However, some viruses have developed mechanisms to evade immune detection, enabling them to spread undetected until they cause widespread outbreaks (Nicholson 2016). Viral infections can range from mild illnesses such as the common cold to extremely debilitating diseases like HIV/AIDS and COVID-19.

Phytochemicals, naturally occurring plant substances, possess protective roles against microbial invasion. Medicinal plants have been utilized as important sources of therapeutic agents to combat infections for centuries, and scientific research has increasingly confirmed their antiviral effects. Phytochemicals exert various mechanisms of antiviral activity, including inhibition of viral entry, blocking viral replication, and immunomodulatory effects. Integrating phytochemical research with modern pharmaceutical technology could enable the discovery of powerful tools to fight current and future viral threats (Ghildiyal et al. 2020; Mehta and Pradhan 2024).

2.3 Antibacterial Activities

Emerging diseases include bacterial and antimicrobial infections, especially antibiotic-resistant infections. For example, carbapenem-resistant Gram-negative bacterial infections, particularly those caused by *Acinetobacter baumannii*, *Klebsiella pneumoniae*, and *Escherichia coli*, have been identified. These bacteria acquire resistance to carbapenems, a class of last-resort antibiotics used to treat severe infections (Mancuso et al. 2021). The World Health Organization (WHO) classifies them as critical priority pathogens due to their capacity to cause healthcare-associated outbreaks and their escalating resistance to multiple antibiotic classes (Asokan and Vanitha 2018). The current treatment for acute bacterial infections relies heavily on antibiotics. However, bacterial pathogens have developed several resistance mechanisms due to gene acquisition, mutation, antibiotic overuse, and inadequate infection control. Moreover, the development of new antibiotics has significantly slowed due to economic and regulatory challenges (Khameneh et al. 2021).

Phytochemical compounds, considered promising alternative options, may play an essential role in this crisis. Based on hypothesis, phytochemicals may provide mechanisms different from conventional antibiotics due to their unique chemical structures (Khameneh et al. 2021). Furthermore, traditional plant-based therapies offer potential pathways toward safe, low-cost, and innovative treatments, accelerating progress in identifying novel antibacterial agents.

2.4 Epigenetic Modulation

Epigenetics is the study of heritable modifications in gene expression that occur without changing the underlying DNA sequence. These changes involve mechanisms such as histone modification, DNA methylation, and regulation by noncoding RNAs. They play pivotal roles in host-pathogen interactions, immune responses, inflammation, and cellular adaptation to stress (Handel et al. 2010; Al Aboud et al. 2018). Modulating these epigenetic pathways represents a promising therapeutic strategy, particularly through the application of bioactive natural compounds.

In recent years, targeting aberrant epigenetic modifications has gained considerable attention in many diseases and conditions. Many plant-secondary metabolites, including apigenin, berberine, curcumin, genistein, lycopene, and quercetin, have shown promising abilities to modulate abnormal epigenetic modifications. These bioactive compounds can influence key mechanisms such as histone acetylation, DNA methylation, and noncoding RNA expression (Shankar et al. 2013; Khan et al. 2024). Correspondingly, they offer significant potential in addressing epigenetic vulnerabilities associated with emerging diseases, providing a foundation for novel preventive and therapeutic strategies.

2.5 Combination Therapy

The combination of phytoconstituents with conventional medications represents a promising strategy for combating emerging diseases, particularly those characterized by drug resistance, poor response to monotherapy, or rapid evolution observed in novel pandemics. The potential benefits of such combination therapy can be categorized into key mechanisms: synergistic pharmacological effects, reduction in drug resistance, decreased drug toxicity, and modulation of the immune system (Chihomvu et al. 2024).

Natural compounds such as flavonoids, terpenoids, alkaloids, and polyphenols have been thoroughly explored for their ability to enhance the therapeutic effects of existing medications. For instance, quercetin in combination with antiviral drugs demonstrates improved inhibition of viral entry and replication. Similarly, berberine combined with β-lactam antibacterial agents can potentiate antibacterial effects against resistant strains, notably Methicillin-resistant *Staphylococcus aureus* (MRSA) (Zhou et al. 2023).

Natural compounds often act through distinct mechanisms from conventional drugs, thereby reducing the likelihood of resistance development. A notable example is artemisinin, which, when used in combination with other antimalarial agents, has been shown to delay the development of resistance in *Plasmodium* species, the causative parasite of malaria (Tilley et al. 2016).

Moreover, certain phytochemicals may alleviate drug-induced toxicity through their antioxidant and anti-inflammatory properties. For example, silymarin is used as an adjuvant in antiviral therapies for its hepatoprotective effects. In addition, compounds such as andrographolide influence both innate and adaptive immunity by modulating macrophage polarization and antigen-specific antibody synthesis, thereby supporting host immunity during infections and enhancing vaccine efficacy (Xu et al. 2007; Wang et al. 2010).

Therefore, the rational integration of phytoconstituents with conventional pharmacotherapy offers substantial potential for the management of emerging diseases, particularly when multi-target approaches are required. This strategy recognizes that emerging diseases such as novel viral infections, drug-resistant bacterial outbreaks, and zoonotic pandemics often involve complex pathophysiological processes that cannot be effectively addressed by a single therapeutic agent. Conventional medications are typically designed to act on specific molecular targets, but pathogens can evolve rapidly, rendering these agents less effective over time due to the development of resistance mechanisms.

3 Scientific Evidence Supporting the Potential of Phytochemicals in Some Recent Emerging Diseases

In recent times, there has been a notable rise in newly emerging and reemerging infectious diseases, some of which pose significant public health threats due to declining vaccination rates, climate change, and increased global travel. This section provides some notable examples of emerging diseases and the potential applications of phytochemicals as therapeutic agents (Table 1).

Table 1 Summary of phytochemical classes, mechanisms of action, and therapeutic potential in emerging diseases

Phytochemical class	Mechanisms of action	Examples	Therapeutic potential for some emerging diseases
Flavonoids	Inhibition of viral entry, replication, and protein translation; immunomodulatory effects	Quercetin, Epigallocatechin gallate (EGCG), Amentoflavone, Myricetin	COVID-19, H5N1, Dengue, MDR-TB, Zika virus
Alkaloids	DNA intercalation, inhibition of viral replication, immune modulation	Berberine, Sanguinarine, Quinine, Emetine	COVID-19, MDR-TB, Malaria, Zika virus
Terpenoids	Membrane interactions, replication inhibition, cytokine modulation	Oleanolic acid, Ursolic acid, Gingerone A	H5N1, MDR-TB, Zika virus
Phenolic compounds	Antioxidant, anti-inflammatory, epigenetic modulation	Tannic acid, Chlorogenic acid, Resveratrol	COVID-19, MDR-TB, Zika virus
Saponins	Membrane disruption, inhibition of viral enzymes, immune modulation	Glycyrrhizin, Saikosaponins, Vernoniosides	COVID-19, H5N1, MDR-TB
Organosulfur compounds	Membrane disruption, enzyme inhibition, immune modulation	Allicin, Diallyl sulfide, Diallyl trisulfide	MDR-TB

3.1 Coronavirus Disease 2019 (COVID-19)

COVID-19 has been one of the most impactful pandemics in recent history, caused by SARS-CoV-2. COVID-19 can lead to a wide range of symptoms, from mild cold-like manifestations to severe, life-threatening disease. SARS-CoV-2 is characterized as a large, enveloped, single-stranded positive-sense RNA virus, approximately 125 nm in diameter, with a genome size of approximately 30 kb (Agarwal et al. 2022). Generally, understanding viral structure is essential for developing therapeutic targets. Effective antiviral strategies either directly inhibit the virus or support the host immune system in clearing infection.

During the COVID-19 pandemic in Thailand, *Andrographis paniculata* gained attention as a herbal remedy for patients with mild symptoms. It was promoted as an adjunct treatment based on its primary active compound, andrographolide, recognized for its anti-inflammatory and antiviral properties. Nevertheless, scientific evidence regarding its efficacy and safety remains limited and requires further validation (Kaewdech et al. 2022).

Many studies have reported the potential use of phytochemicals in treating COVID-19. Each type of phytoconstituent exhibits different mechanisms of antiviral activity against SARS-CoV-2, as follows:

Alkaloids are a group of plant secondary metabolites containing nitrogen-based structures with diverse physiological effects, including antiviral activity. Resoquine, a synthetic derivative of quinine traditionally used as an antimalarial drug, is suggested as a potential therapeutic agent against COVID-19 (Wink 2020). Alkaloids capable of attaching to the spike and nucleocapsid proteins of related coronaviruses, such as isoquinoline derivatives, may also be effective against SARS-CoV-2 (Jahan and Ahmet 2020). Several alkaloids including sanguinarine, quinine, cinchonine, harmine, emetine, chelidonine, coptisine, berberine, palmatine, and tetrandrine exhibit DNA-intercalating properties and may serve as promising candidates for antiviral drug development (Das et al. 2021).

Flavonoids represent one of the largest groups of polyphenolic plant compounds and have long been known to exhibit antiviral effects. They inhibit viral entry by blocking host-cell receptors and interfering with viral replication and protein synthesis. The SARS-CoV-2 main protease (Mpro), also known as 3CLpro, plays an important role in viral replication and transcription (Hu et al. 2022). Many flavonoids including amentoflavone, quercetin, isoquercetin, diosmin, epigallocatechin gallate, mangiferin, azithromycin-inspired flavonoids, and procyanidin derivatives demonstrate high binding affinities to Mpro, thereby blocking viral replication (Chauhan and Kalra 2020; Ngwa et al. 2020). Additionally, flavonoids such as hesperetin, myricetin, and caflanone have been hypothesized to target ACE2 receptors, further highlighting their potential antiviral roles (Das et al. 2021).

Several antiviral anthraquinones have been subjected to their anti-SARS-CoV-2 effect. According to in silico docking studies, several antiviral anthraquinones and related compounds including emodin, aloe-emodin, chrysophanic acid, tetrahydroaltersolanol C, aloin A and B, rhein, rubiadin, alterporriol Q, and damnacanthal as well as hypericin, pseudohypericin, and isopseudohypericin showed potential binding affinity toward the SARS-CoV-2 main protease (Mpro), a key target involved in viral replication. Collectively, these findings suggest that anthraquinones and related compounds may exert their antiviral activity through inhibition of the Mpro enzyme, highlighting Mpro as a promising molecular target for further drug discovery. Another study presents that emodin, obtained from *Rheum officinale* and *Polygonum multiflorum*, has been shown to inhibit the interaction between the spike (S) protein of SARS coronavirus and the ACE2 receptor (Das et al. 2021).

Tannins are a class of polyphenolic compounds naturally found in many plants, which commonly contain astringent taste and play important roles in plant defense mechanisms. Tannic acid and some hydrolyzable tannins such as castalin and tercatain have been identified as a potent dual inhibitor that targets both the host cell surface serine protease TMPRSS2 and the SARS-CoV-2 main protease (Mpro or 3CLpro), thereby effectively blocking viral entry and replication (Wang et al. 2020a). By inhibiting TMPRSS2, tannic acid interferes with priming the viral spike (S) protein, essential for fusion with the host cell membrane. Concurrently, the inhibition of Mpro disrupts the proteolytic processing of viral polyproteins, which is crucial for viral replication and maturation. These dual mechanisms highlight tannic acid as a promising antiviral candidate against COVID-19 (Wang et al. 2020a; Das et al. 2021). In vivo study showed that tannins derived from persimmons significantly reduced SARS-CoV-2 viral titers, alleviated the severity of COVID-19-associated pneumonia, and downregulated the expression of inflammation-related genes, including interferon-gamma (IFN-γ) (Furukawa et al. 2021). Similarly, green tea-derived tannins have demonstrated the ability to inhibit SARS-CoV-2 replication in vitro and in silico (Zhang et al. 2006; Park et al. 2021).

Saponins are a group of amphiphilic glycosides derived from steroids and triterpenes and are generally considered toxic plant secondary metabolites. Saponins have been investigated and proven for antiviral activity against various virus strains, including SARS-CoV-2. Their mechanisms of action depend on their structure, including disrupting viral envelopes, inhibiting virus-host cell binding, and blocking viral entry or replication (Mieres-Castro and Mora-Poblete 2023). Some saponins have been described for their antiviral ability, such as saikosaponins from *Bupleurum* species, glycyrrhizin from *Glycyrrhiza* spp., and vernoniosides from *Vernonia amygdalina*, which have shown potent anti-SARS-CoV-2 effects in both in vitro and in silico studies. These compounds target viral proteins like the spike (S) protein, Mpro enzyme, and nonstructural proteins (Nsps), either by binding to viral enzymes or host receptors (e.g., ACE2), thereby preventing viral replication and cell entry. Structure-activity relationship studies reveal that variations in aglycone and sugar moieties significantly influence antiviral efficacy and pharmacological potential (Cheng PeiWin et al. 2006; Mieres-Castro and Mora-Poblete 2023).

Phytoconstituents hold great promise in the fight against COVID-19 because of their various antiviral, anti-inflammatory, and immunomodulatory activities. Molecules such as flavonoids, alkaloids, terpenoids, and polyphenols blocked the main targets of the study: the main protease (Mpro), as well as the spike protein (S), which is important for SARS-CoV-2 entry and replication. Moreover, they can also regulate immune responses, mitigate oxidative stress, avoid developing into cytokine storms, and alleviate severe symptoms observed in COVID-19 patients. However, additional clinical trials and comprehensive pharmacokinetic investigations are still required to confirm their efficacy, safety, optimal dosing, and therapeutic applicability in COVID-19 management.

3.2 Highly Pathogenic Avian Influenza (H5N1)

Highly Pathogenic Avian Influenza (H5N1), commonly known as "bird flu," is caused by Influenza A virus subtypes. As of 2024, H5N1 has become globally endemic in wild bird populations and has recently caused outbreaks in poultry and dairy cattle in the United States (Ibiapina et al. 2005). Human infection cases have also been documented. Vaccination and antiviral agents form the first-line management strategy, with neuraminidase (NA) and M2 ion channels serving as major therapeutic targets. Drugs such as amantadine, rimantadine, oseltamivir, and zanamivir are widely used (Moorthy et al. 2014).

However, the emergence of drug resistance and adverse effects raises concerns, prompting interest in **natural product-based therapeutics**. Preclinical studies have identified phytochemicals with anti-H5N1 activity:

Flavonoids are the one biggest group of phytochemical compounds that have been investigated in both in vivo and in vitro studies, presenting antiviral effects by inhibiting viral entry, replication, and inflammatory responses. For example, *Capparis sinaica* (quercetin, isorhamnetin, rutin), *Camellia sinensis* (epigallocatechin gallate), and *Kaempferia parviflora* (Luteolin, Apigenin, Kaempferol) have proposed the mechanism by blocking viral entry (HA receptor interference), inhibiting replication and synthesis of viral RNA/proteins, modulating cytokines, as well as suppressing inflammatory pathways (e.g., NF-κB, MAPK) (Ibrahim et al. 2013a; Sornpet et al. 2017; Dutta et al. 2023).

Terpenoids and their derivatives exhibit strong antiviral activity, often through membrane interactions or replication inhibition. *Zingiber officinale* (Gingerone A), *Thalassodendron ciliatum* (Tetradecanamide, Diterpenoids), and *Andrographis paniculata* (1,4-deoxy-11,12-didehydroandrographolide (DAP)) have demonstrated the possible mechanism of anti-H5N1 activity through inhibition of viral replication (Janus Kinase 2, NP/NS1 protein), reduction of cytokine production, and interference with viral transcription (Ibrahim et al. 2013b; Cai et al. 2015; Wang et al. 2020b).

Only a few studies investigate the potential of alkaloids against the H5N1 virus. They found that Hemanthamine from *Lycoris radiata* exhibited favorable affinity and specificity in binding to viral neuraminidase through in silico analysis, which may have some benefit in treating H5N1 infection (Dutta et al. 2023).

Saponins are amphiphilic glycosides known for disrupting lipid membranes and modulating immunity. The *Nigella sativa* and *Kaempferia parviflora* plants have been studied and found to provide some effect against the H5N1 virus through direct virucidal activity via membrane lysis and inhibition of the neuraminidase enzyme (Dutta et al. 2023).

Phytoconstituents have the potential to be used as therapeutics for the treatment of H5N1, as they possess a variety of antiviral effects. Phytochemicals, including flavonoids, terpenoids, alkaloids, and saponins, have been found to block the viral entry, replication, and protein synthesis through binding with the essential viral proteins. The natural products also modulate the host immune response, lowering the likelihood of an excessive inflammatory response and cytokine storm, which are key causes of H5N1 mortality. Although such observations revealed the strong antiviral potential of phytoconstituents against H5N1, further in vivo studies, clinical trials, and pharmacokinetic studies are required to validate the effect and ensure safe and standardized dosing regimens for future use.

3.3 Dengue Fever

Dengue fever, classified as an infectious disease, arises from infection with an arbovirus, belonging to the family Flaviviridae and the genus *Flavivirus* (Choumet and Desprès 2015). The virus is chiefly spread via bites from diurnal mosquito species of the genus *Aedes* (Liu et al. 2023), which are mainly classified into four subtypes: dengue-1, -2, -3, and -4, depending on the species of mosquitoes (Choumet and Desprès 2015). In 2024, an estimated 13 million dengue cases were registered throughout the Americas and the Caribbean. Transmission rates in these regions remain high in this day. However, there is no treatment for dengue, but using some medications like acetaminophen may relieve fever and pain symptoms, and fluid replacement may be considered to compensate for the lost fluids (Leung et al. 2023).

Phytochemical compounds, including plant extracts, have been studied for various diseases, including dengue fever. Some herbal extracts, including *Ocimum sanctum, Andrographis paniculata, Cymbopogan citratus*, *Momordica charantia*, *Citrus limon,* and *Pelargonium citrosum*, have the ability to inhibit DENV type-1 (DENV1) growth in Vero E6 cells. The highest level of activity is observed in *A. paniculata*, with *M. charantia* coming second (Saleh and Kamisah 2021).

The dengue virus 2 (DENV2) has also been investigated for novel treatment by phytoconstituents. The essential enzyme, DENV2-NS2B-NS3 protease, an important enzyme for viral replication, is one of the main targets for discovering a novel anti-DENV2 medication. In silico study found that four novel compounds, 3′,4′-methylenedioxy-7,8-(2″,2″-dimethylpyrano)-flavone, limonianin, gnetin-B, and 5,4′-dihydroxy-3′,5′-dimethoxy-6,7-(2″,2″-dimethylpyran)flavonen presented a great binding affinities against NS2B-NS3 protease and also potential to have a good safety profile with favorable pharmacokinetic and toxicity profiles. These highlight their potential as promising leads for developing novel antiviral therapies against dengue fever (Ali et al. 2021; Bari et al. 2024).

An in vitro study demonstrated that the root extract of Eurycoma longifolia exhibited significant inhibitory activity against all four dengue virus serotypes

(DENV-1–4), suggesting its potential as a natural antiviral agent against dengue infection (He et al. 2023). Galactan isolated from *Cryptomenia crenulata* demonstrates selective activity and shows strong inhibitory action against DENV2 and DENV3. This may indicate that sulfated polysaccharides have a great potential to develop as therapeutic agents against DENV-2 and DENV-3 (Saleh and Kamisah 2021).

Over 100 plant secondary metabolites, including terpenoids, flavonoids, and alkaloids isolated from *Tanacetum parthenium* and *Silybum marianum* medical herbs from Pakistan, have been subjected to a molecular docking study. The in silico analysis is used to identify potential inhibitors of the nonstructural protein 1 (NS1) of Dengue Virus 4 (DENV4-NS1) (Qaddir et al. 2020). The phytoconstituents, including Jaceidin, Centaureidin, Artecanin, Secotanaparthenolide, Artematin, Schizolaenone B, Isopomiferin, 6,8-Diprenyleriodictyol, and Anthraxin, emerged as promising inhibitors due to the high binding affinities against NS1, which indicates strong interactions with DENV4-NS1 (Qaddir et al. 2020; Saravanan et al. 2021).

Phytoconstituents have demonstrated potential in treating prophylaxis dengue fever, owing to their broad-spectrum antiviral, immunomodulatory, and anti-inflammatory activities. Various natural products, such as flavonoids, alkaloids, terpenoids, and phenolic compounds, have exhibited antiviral activity against the dengue virus. Although the results above are promising, more animal studies, clinical trials, and pharmacokinetic studies are critical for further validating their efficacy, dose determination, and safety for their potential therapeutic use against dengue.

3.4 Multidrug Resistant Tuberculosis

Multidrug-resistant tuberculosis (MDR-TB) is an infectious condition resulting from *Mycobacterium tuberculosis* and has emerged as a world health problem, especially in the last decade. Several mechanisms contribute to mycobacterial resistance to antitubercular agents, including posttranslational modifications, the activation of efflux pumps, and the accumulation of gene mutations (Goossens et al. 2020). Several antituberculosis agents have been developed from phytochemical compounds, making plant-based agents promising anti-MDR-TB due to their different and unique chemical structures, which may provide a novel mechanism of action against MDR-TB.

Phytochemicals have demonstrated promising anti-TB activity against MDR-TB in various studies. These second metabolites can be broadly categorized into polyphenols, alkaloids, terpenes, and organosulfur compounds, each presenting unique mechanisms of action against MDR-TB.

Polyphenols are a large group of phytochemical compounds that normally contain a high antioxidant activity and show significant antimycobacterial activity. Epigallocatechin gallate (EGCG) from *Camellia sinensis* is a well-studied example, known for its ability to disrupt mycobacterial cell wall integrity and inhibit essential bacterial enzymes, thereby reducing bacterial viability. A molecular signaling study found that EGCG downregulates the NF-κB signaling pathway and upregulates cellular antioxidant defenses such as glutathione, which collectively reduce inflammation and oxidative stress in infected cells. Moreover, a combination between EGCG and rifampicin has been shown to synergist drug efficacy, making it a promising adjuvant in MDR-TB treatment (Mali and Pandey 2021; Ansari et al. 2023).

Some alkaloids have been studied and show potent antimycobacterial effects. Remarkable examples include cryptolepine from *Cryptolepis sanguinolenta*, voacangine from *Tabernaemontana* species, and biscryptolepine, which have shown potential in disrupting mycobacterial cell membranes, inhibiting essential enzymatic pathways, and reducing antibiotic resistance. These compounds have synergistic effects when combined with standard TB drugs like isoniazid and rifampicin, significantly lowering the minimum inhibitory concentrations required to suppress mycobacterial growth in preclinical study (Kishore et al. 2009; Ansari et al. 2023).

Terpenoids are known for their strong antibacterial activity against various strains of bacteria. Oleanolic acid and ursolic acid, two triterpenes commonly found in medicinal plants, have exhibited potent anti-TB activity by inhibiting bacterial growth, reducing biofilm formation, and enhancing immune responses (Jesus et al. 2015). These compounds also provide hepatoprotective benefits, potentially mitigating the liver toxicity commonly associated with prolonged anti-TB drug use (Gutiérrez-Rebolledo et al. 2016). Additionally, they can modulate the immune response by upregulating pro-inflammatory cytokines such as interferon-gamma (IFN-γ), enhancing the host's ability to clear mycobacterial infections (Jiménez-Arellanes et al. 2013).

Organosulfur compounds, predominantly found in Allium species like garlic (*Allium sativum*), have attracted attention for their potent antimicrobial and immunomodulatory properties. Allicin, diallyl sulfide, and diallyl trisulfide are key compounds in this group exhibiting strong anti-MDRTB activity. These compounds disrupt bacterial cell membranes, inhibit critical bacterial enzymes, and enhance the immune response to reduce the mycobacterial burden. Additionally, they have demonstrated synergistic effects when combined with conventional antibiotics, further highlighting their potential as adjunctive therapies for MDR-TB (Dini et al. 2011).

In conclusion, together, these phytoconstituents represent a promising antibacterial against MDR-TB, offering diverse mechanisms of action, including direct antibacterial effects, immune modulation, and synergy with conventional antibiotics. As investigations further reveal the therapeutic potential of these natural molecules, they are expected to contribute significantly to novel strategies against drug-resistant tuberculosis.

3.5 Zika Virus

Zika virus is one of mosquito (family Flavivirus)-borne diseases which causes birth defects and neurological disorders. Zika virus was first found in 1947; however, before 2007, there were no reports of large outbreaks of Zika infections, globally.

The large epidemics outbreak was identified in 2013 in French Polynesia, follow by 2015–2016 in Brazil. This prompted the World Health Organization to declare the Zika virus a Public Health Emergency of International Concern in February 2016 (Noorbakhsh et al. 2019).

The unique neurotropic characteristics of Zika virus infection and teratogenicity have upgraded it as a priority reemerging infectious disease, deserving urgent attention in vaccine development, antiviral research, and vector control. Natural products, particularly flavonoids and alkaloids, are researched for their viral replication-inhibiting ability and modulating inflammatory mechanisms, and these hold promise as therapeutic agents against Zika virus infection.

Several groups of phytochemical compounds including alkaloids, steroids, terpenoids, and polyphenols have been confirmed for their benefits against Zika virus infection. According to numerous reports, phytochemical compounds, especially the most promising compounds, including flavonoids (e.g., baicalein, isoquercitrin, myricetin, epigallocatechin gallate), alkaloids (e.g., berberine, lycorine), terpenoids (e.g., glycyrrhetinic acid derivatives, abietanes), and phenolics (e.g., ellagic acid, cinnamic acid), demonstrate significant antiviral activity against the Zika virus through various mechanisms, including inhibition of viral entry, replication, and direct virucidal effects (Pereira et al. 2023). Among a large number of phytoconstituents that have been investigated for their anti-Zika virus effect, dolastane, diterpene compounds isolated from the marine seaweed *Canistrocarpus cervicorni* (Cirne-Santos et al. 2020), and the flavonol myricetin (Lim et al. 2016) present the highest potential among other natural products with the highest selectivity index value, the ratio between cytotoxicity and antiviral activity. Epigallocatechin gallate and actephilols show affinity to target key enzymes of the Zika virus, including ZIKV NS2B-NS3 protease and NS5 RNA-dependent RNA polymerase. Furthermore, several compounds acted at multiple stages of the viral life cycle, such as entry and replication, suggesting bifunctional potential. Nonetheless, the broad-spectrum activity and structural diversity of natural products, including phytoconstituents, underscore their potential as candidates for anti-Zika virus drug development (Pereira et al. 2023).

4 Prospects of Phytoconstituents for Emerging Diseases

As global health continues to evolve, the emergence of new infectious diseases presents significant challenges for modern medicine. Novel therapeutic approaches are urgently required due to the increase in drug-resistant infections, pandemics caused by novel viral strains, and immune-evasive microorganisms. Phytoconstituents, defined as bioactive compounds found naturally in medicinal plants, represent a promising direction for the development of next-generation therapeutics due to their structural diversity, multi-target mechanisms, and generally favorable safety profiles.

Phytoconstituents demonstrate significant advantages against various emerging diseases through diverse mechanisms of action. Their potential in combating viral infection and antimicrobial-resistant pathogens positions them as valuable assets in future healthcare strategies. Phytoconstituents can provide direct antimicrobial and antiviral actions against target pathogens, as well as offer synergistic effects when combined with conventional medications.

However, the full clinical utility of phytoconstituents remains constrained by significant issues such as poor bioavailability, variability in phytochemical composition, and the requirement for comprehensive clinical validation. Future research priorities include standardizing extraction methods, conducting thorough pharmacokinetic studies, and developing delivery systems tailored to phytochemical structures in order to enhance stability, specific action, and targeted activity. Developments in high-throughput screening, bioinformatics, and molecular biology further accelerate phytochemical-based drug discovery.

In conclusion, the future of infectious disease management is likely to benefit from integrating phytoconstituents into conventional medicine as we continue to encounter novel and unpredictable pathogens. These natural substances hold substantial potential to enhance healthcare outcomes globally, particularly with continued advancements in robust preclinical and clinical research.

References

Agarwal D, Zafar I, Ahmad SU, Kumar S, Ain Q, Sundaray JK, Rather MA (2022) Structural, genomic information and computational analysis of emerging coronavirus (SARS-CoV-2). Bull Natl Res Cent 46(1):170

Al Aboud NM, Tupper C, Jialal I (2018) Genetics, epigenetic mechanism

Ali F, Chorsiya A, Anjum V, Khasimbi S, Ali A (2021) A systematic review on phytochemicals for the treatment of dengue. Phytother Res 35(4):1782–1816

Anderson B, Gray G (2019) Emerging and reemerging infectious diseases. In: Encyclopedia of microbiology, p 112

Ansari MA, Shoaib S, Alomary MN, Ather H, Ansari SMA, Hani U, Jamous YF, Alyahya SA, Alharbi JN, Imran MA (2023) Deciphering the emerging role of phytocompounds: implications in the management of drug-resistant tuberculosis and ATDs-induced hepatic damage. J Infect Public Health 16(9):1443–1459

Asokan GV, Vanitha A (2018) WHO global priority pathogens list on antibiotic resistance: an urgent need for action to integrate One Health data. Perspect Public Health 138(2):87–88

Bari MA, Ahmed S, Perveen FF, Akter M, Ahmed N, Hossain J, Nasrulla M, Akter K, Islam MN (2024) Novel antiviral phytochemicals against dengue virus 2 NS2B-NS3 protease: an in silico drug development approach. ChemistrySelect 9(47):e202404053

Beltrán-García J, Osca-Verdegal R, Pallardó FV, Ferreres J, Rodríguez M, Mulet S, Sanchis-Gomar F, Carbonell N, García-Giménez JL (2020) Oxidative stress and inflammation in COVID-19-associated sepsis: the potential role of anti-oxidant therapy in avoiding disease progression. Antioxidants 9(10):936

Breda C, Nascimento A, Meghwar P, Lisboa H, Aires A, Rosa E, Ferreira L, Barros AN (2025) Phenolic composition and antioxidant activity of edible flowers: insights from synergistic effects and multivariate analysis. Antioxidants 14(3):282

Cai W, Li Y, Chen S, Wang M, Zhang A, Zhou H, Chen H, Jin M (2015) 14-Deoxy-11, 12-dehydroandrographolide exerts anti-influenza A virus activity and inhibits replication of H5N1 virus by restraining nuclear export of viral ribonucleoprotein complexes. Antivir Res 118:82–92

Chauhan A, Kalra S (2020) Identification of potent COVID-19 main protease (MPRO) inhibitors from flavonoids

Cheng PeiWin CP, Ng LeanTeik NL, Chiang LienChai CL, Lin ChunChing LC (2006) Antiviral effects of saikosaponins on human coronavirus 229E in vitro

Chihomvu P, Ganesan A, Gibbons S, Woollard K, Hayes MA (2024) Phytochemicals in drug discovery—a confluence of tradition and innovation. Int J Mol Sci 25(16):8792

Choumet V, Desprès P (2015) Dengue and other flavivirus infections. Rev Sci Tech 34(2):473–478

Cirne-Santos CC, de Souza BC, de Oliveira MC, Rabelo VW-H, Azevedo RC, Teixeira VL, Ferreira DF, de Palmer Paixão ICN (2020) In vitro studies on the inhibition of replication of Zika and chikungunya viruses by dolastane isolated from seaweed Canistrocarpus cervicornis. Sci Rep 10(1):8263

Das A, Pandita D, Jain GK, Agarwal P, Grewal AS, Khar RK, Lather V (2021) Role of phytoconstituents in the management of COVID-19. Chem Biol Interact 341:109449

Dini C, Fabbri A, Geraci A (2011) The potential role of garlic (Allium sativum) against the multidrug resistant tuberculosis pandemic: a review. Ann Ist Super Sanita 47:465–473

Dutta AK, Gazi MS, Uddin SJ (2023) A systemic review on medicinal plants and their bioactive constituents against avian influenza and further confirmation through in-silico analysis. Heliyon 9(3):e14386

Furukawa R, Kitabatake M, Ouji-Sageshima N, Suzuki Y, Nakano A, Matsumura Y, Nakano R, Kasahara K, Kubo K, Kayano S-i (2021) Persimmon-derived tannin has antiviral effects and reduces the severity of infection and transmission of SARS-CoV-2 in a Syrian hamster model. Sci Rep 11(1):23695

Gharbi J, Rezza G, Ben M'hadheb M (2025) Emerging and re-emerging viral infections: epidemiology, pathogenesis and new methods for control and prevention. Frontiers Media SA 12:1528163

Ghildiyal R, Prakash V, Chaudhary V, Gupta V, Gabrani R (2020) Phytochemicals as antiviral agents: recent updates. In: Plant-derived bioactives: production, properties and therapeutic applications, pp 279–295

Goossens SN, Sampson SL, Van Rie A (2020) Mechanisms of drug-induced tolerance in Mycobacterium tuberculosis. Clin Microbiol Rev 34(1):10.1128/cmr. 00141-00120

Gutiérrez-Rebolledo GA, Siordia-Reyes AG, Meckes-Fischer M, Jiménez-Arellanes A (2016) Hepatoprotective properties of oleanolic and ursolic acids in antitubercular drug-induced liver damage. Asian Pac J Trop Med 9(7):644–651

Handel AE, Ebers GC, Ramagopalan SV (2010) Epigenetics: molecular mechanisms and implications for disease. Trends Mol Med 16(1):7–16

He X, Zheng Y, Tian C, Wen T, Yang T, Yu J, Fang X, Fan C, Liu J, Yu L (2023) Quassinoids from Eurycoma longifolia with antiviral activities by inhibiting dengue virus replication. Phytomedicine 110:154650

Hu Q, Xiong Y, Zhu GH, Zhang YN, Zhang YW, Huang P, Ge GB (2022) The SARS-CoV-2 main protease (Mpro): structure, function, and emerging therapies for COVID-19. MedComm 3(3):e151

Ibiapina CC, Costa GA, Faria AC (2005) Avian influenza A (H5N1): the bird flu. J Bras Pneumol 31:436–444

Ibrahim AK, Youssef AI, Arafa AS, Ahmed SA (2013a) Anti-H5N1 virus flavonoids from Capparis sinaica Veill. Nat Prod Res 27(22):2149–2153

Ibrahim AK, Youssef AI, Arafa AS, Foad R, Radwan MM, Ross S, Hassanean HA, Ahmed SA (2013b) Anti-H5N1 virus new diglyceride ester from the Red Sea grass Thallasodendron ciliatum. Nat Prod Res 27(18):1625–1632

Jahan I, Ahmet O (2020) Potentials of plant-based substance to inhabit and probable cure for the COVID-19. Turk J Biol 44(3):228

Jesus JA, Lago JHG, Laurenti MD, Yamamoto ES, Passero LFD (2015) Antimicrobial activity of oleanolic and ursolic acids: an update. Evid Based Complement Alternat Med 2015(1):620472

Jiménez-Arellanes A, Luna-Herrera J, Cornejo-Garrido J, López-García S, Castro-Mussot ME, Meckes-Fischer M, Mata-Espinosa D, Marquina B, Torres J, Hernández-Pando R (2013) Ursolic and oleanolic acids as antimicrobial and immunomodulatory compounds for tuberculosis treatment. BMC Complement Altern Med 13:1–11

Kaewdech A, Nawalerspanya S, Assawasuwannakit S, Chamroonkul N, Jandee S, Sripongpun P (2022) The use of Andrographis paniculata and its effects on liver biochemistry of patients with gastrointestinal problems in Thailand during the COVID-19 pandemic: a cross sectional study. Sci Rep 12(1):18213

Khameneh B, Eskin NM, Iranshahy M, Fazly Bazzaz BS (2021) Phytochemicals: a promising weapon in the arsenal against antibiotic-resistant bacteria. Antibiotics 10(9):1044

Khan A, Khan A, Khan MA, Malik Z, Massey S, Parveen R, Mustafa S, Shamsi A, Husain SA (2024) Phytocompounds targeting epigenetic modulations: an assessment in cancer. Front Pharmacol 14:1273993

Kishore N, Mishra BB, Tripathi V, Tiwari VK (2009) Alkaloids as potential anti-tubercular agents. Fitoterapia 80(3):149–163

Kunz Coyne AJ, El Ghali A, Holger D, Rebold N, Rybak MJ (2022) Therapeutic strategies for emerging multidrug-resistant Pseudomonas aeruginosa. Infect Dis Ther 11(2):661–682

Leung XY, Islam RM, Adhami M, Ilic D, McDonald L, Palawaththa S, Diug B, Munshi SU, Karim MN (2023) A systematic review of dengue outbreak prediction models: current scenario and future directions. PLoS Negl Trop Dis 17(2):e0010631

Lim L, Roy A, Song J (2016) Identification of a Zika NS2B-NS3pro pocket susceptible to allosteric inhibition by small molecules including qucertin rich in edible plants. bioRxiv:078543

Liu Z, Zhang Q, Li L, He J, Guo J, Wang Z, Huang Y, Xi Z, Yuan F, Li Y (2023) The effect of temperature on dengue virus transmission by Aedes mosquitoes. Front Cell Infect Microbiol 13:1242173

Mali SN, Pandey A (2021) Unveiling naturally occurring green tea polyphenol epigallocatechin-3-gallate (EGCG) targeting Mycobacterium DPRE1 for anti-Tb Drug discovery. Eng Proc 11(1):31

Mancuso G, Midiri A, Gerace E, Biondo C (2021) Bacterial antibiotic resistance: the most critical pathogens. Pathogens 10(10):1310

McCune JS, Reynolds KS (2015) Developing and using therapeutics for emerging infections., Wiley Online Library. Clin Pharmacol Ther 98:346–351

Mehta SK, Pradhan RB (2024) Phytochemicals in antiviral drug development against human respiratory viruses. Drug Discov Today:104107

Mieres-Castro D, Mora-Poblete F (2023) Saponins: research progress and their potential role in the post-COVID-19 pandemic era. Pharmaceutics 15(2):348

Moorthy N, Poongavanam V, Pratheepa V (2014) Viral M2 ion channel protein: a promising target for anti-influenza drug discovery. Mini Rev Med Chem 14(10):819–830

Nazerian Y, Ghasemi M, Yassaghi Y, Nazerian A, Hashemi SM (2022) Role of SARS-CoV-2-induced cytokine storm in multi-organ failure: molecular pathways and potential therapeutic options. Int Immunopharmacol 113:109428

Ngwa W, Kumar R, Thompson D, Lyerly W, Moore R, Reid T-E, Lowe H, Toyang N (2020) Potential of flavonoid-inspired phytomedicines against COVID-19. Molecules 25(11):2707

Nicholson LB (2016) The immune system. Essays Biochem 60(3):275–301

Noorbakhsh F, Abdolmohammadi K, Fatahi Y, Dalili H, Rasoolinejad M, Rezaei F, Salehi-Vaziri M, Shafiei-Jandaghi NZ, Gooshki ES, Zaim M (2019) Zika virus infection, basic and clinical aspects: a review article. Iran J Public Health 48(1):20

Park J, Park R, Jang M, Park Y-I (2021) Therapeutic potential of EGCG, a green tea polyphenol, for treatment of coronavirus diseases. Life 11(3):197

Pereira RS, Santos FCP, Campana PRV, Costa VV, de Pádua RM, Souza DG, Teixeira MM, Braga FC (2023) Natural products and derivatives as potential zika virus inhibitors: a comprehensive review. Viruses 15(5):1211

Qaddir I, Majeed A, Hussain W, Mahmood S, Rasool N (2020) An in silico investigation of phytochemicals as potential inhibitors against non-structural protein 1 from dengue virus 4. Braz J Pharm Sci 56:e17420

Saleh MS, Kamisah Y (2021) Potential medicinal plants for the treatment of dengue fever and severe acute respiratory syndrome-coronavirus. Biomolecules 11(1):42

Saravanan KS, Arjunan S, Kunjiappan S, Pavadai P, Sundar LM (2021) Phytoconstituents as lead compounds for anti-dengue drug discovery. In: Antiviral drug discovery and development, pp 159–193

Shankar S, Kumar D, Srivastava RK (2013) Epigenetic modifications by dietary phytochemicals: implications for personalized nutrition. Pharmacol Ther 138(1):1–17

Sornpet B, Potha T, Tragoolpua Y, Pringproa K (2017) Antiviral activity of five Asian medicinal pant crude extracts against highly pathogenic H5N1 avian influenza virus. Asian Pac J Trop Med 10(9):871–876

Sun W, Shahrajabian MH (2023) Therapeutic potential of phenolic compounds in medicinal plants—natural health products for human health. Molecules 28(4):1845

Tilley L, Straimer J, Gnädig NF, Ralph SA, Fidock DA (2016) Artemisinin action and resistance in Plasmodium falciparum. Trends Parasitol 32(9):682–696

Wang J, Prinz RA, Liu X, Xu X (2020b) In vitro and in vivo antiviral activity of gingerenone a on influenza a virus is mediated by targeting janus kinase 2. Viruses 12(10):1141

Wang S-C, Chen Y, Wang Y-C, Wang W-J, Yang C-S, Tsai C-L, Hou M-H, Chen H-F, Shen Y-C, Hung M-C (2020a) Tannic acid suppresses SARS-CoV-2 as a dual inhibitor of the viral main protease and the cellular TMPRSS2 protease. Am J Cancer Res 10(12):4538

Wang W, Wang J, Dong S-f, Liu C-h, Italiani P, Sun S-h, Xu J, Boraschi D, Ma S-p, Qu D (2010) Immunomodulatory activity of andrographolide on macrophage activation and specific antibody response. Acta Pharmacol Sin 31(2):191–201

Wink M (2020) Potential of DNA intercalating alkaloids and other plant secondary metabolites against SARS-CoV-2 causing COVID-19. Diversity 12(5):175

Xu Y, Chen A, Fry S, Barrow RA, Marshall RL, Mukkur T (2007) Modulation of immune response in mice immunised with an inactivated Salmonella vaccine and gavaged with Andrographis paniculata extract or andrographolide. Int Immunopharmacol 7(4):515–523

Zamparelli SS, Zamparelli AS, Bocchino M (2025) Immune-boosting and antiviral effects of antioxidants in COVID-19 pneumonia: a therapeutic perspective. Life 15(1):113

Zhang R, Wei D-Q, Du Q-S, Chou K-C (2006) Molecular modeling studies of peptide drug candidates against SARS. Med Chem 2(3):309–314

Zhou H, Wang W, Cai L, Yang T (2023) Potentiation and mechanism of berberine as an antibiotic adjuvant against multidrug-resistant bacteria. Infect Drug Resist 16:7313–7326

Specific Compound Classes and Mechanisms

Terpenoids in Healthcare Management

Prem Narayan Paudel, Ajaya Acharya, Vijay Kumar, Gaurav, Sheetal S. Samant, Prabodh Satyal, and Rajendra Gyawali

Abstract Terpenoids, a structurally diverse class of natural compounds derived from isoprene units, exhibit profound pharmacological potential in healthcare management. This chapter explores their classification, mechanisms of action, and therapeutic applications, emphasizing their role in modern and traditional medicine. Terpenoids demonstrate antimicrobial, anti-inflammatory, anticancer, neuroprotective, and metabolic regulatory properties, as evidenced by their ability to modulate cellular pathways (e.g., receptor interactions, enzyme inhibition, and antioxidant activity). Despite challenges like low bioavailability and standardization and advancements in drug delivery systems (e.g., nanoencapsulation), growing research on clinical validation highlights their potential. By bridging traditional knowledge and contemporary research, terpenoids offer promising avenues for developing safer, multitarget therapies for chronic and infectious diseases.

P. N. Paudel
Department of Chemical Science and Engineering, School of Engineering, Kathmandu University, Dhulikhel, Nepal

A. Acharya · R. Gyawali (✉)
Department of Pharmacy, Herbal Research Laboratory, School of Science, Kathmandu University, Dhulikhel, Nepal

V. Kumar
Department of Pharmaceutics, SPER, Jamia Hamdard, New Delhi, India

Gaurav
Department of Research and Development, Hamdard Laboratories (India), Ghaziabad, Uttar Pradesh, India

S. S. Samant
Department of Pharmacognosy, Yashwantrao Bhonsale College of Pharmacy, University of Mumbai, Mumbai, Maharashtra, India

P. Satyal
Aromatic Plant Research Center, Lehi, UT, USA
e-mail: psatyal@doterra.com

S. Kumar Tripathi et al. (eds.), *Phytoceuticals for Sustainable Medication*, Interdisciplinary Biotechnological Advances,
https://doi.org/10.1007/978-981-95-7588-6_12

Graphical Abstract

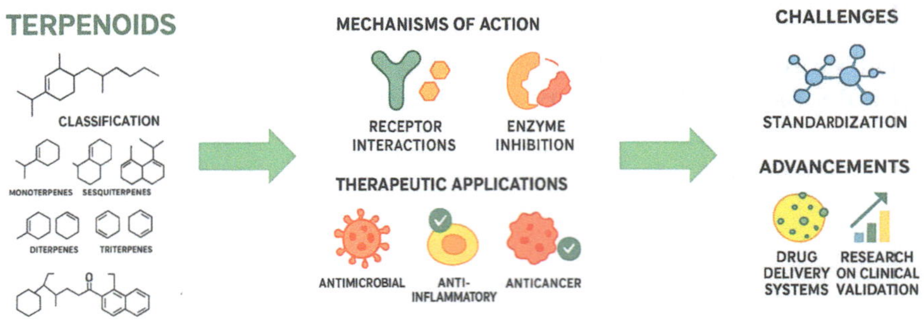

Keywords Terpenoids · Antimicrobial · Anti-inflammatory · Anticancer · Neuroprotection · Drug delivery · Traditional medicine

1 Introduction

Terpenoids, also known as isoprenoids, are a diverse class of naturally occurring organic compounds derived from five-carbon isoprene units. These compounds are widely distributed in nature, especially in plants, and are responsible for many of the characteristic odors, colors, and flavors found in fruits, flowers, and spices (Breitmaier 2006). Terpenoids are not only essential for plants in their roles as secondary metabolites involved in plant defense and attraction of pollinators but also have significant pharmacological and therapeutic potential in human health (Gershenzon and Dudareva 2007; Paduch et al. 2007). It is important to explore the role of terpenoids in healthcare management, focusing on their pharmacological properties, therapeutic applications, and how they contribute to the treatment and prevention of various diseases. Highlights on the growing body of evidence supporting their use in modern medicine and traditional healing practices are equally important.

2 Terpenoids: Classification and Structure

Terpenoids are classified based on the number of isoprene units they contain (Yang et al. 2020):

- *Monoterpenoids (C10)*: Comprising two isoprene units, they are commonly found in essential oils of plants like lavender, peppermint, and citrus fruits.
- *Sesquiterpenoids (C15)*: Made up of three isoprene units, which are abundant in plant oils and have distinct biological activities.
- *Diterpenoids (C20)*: Consisting of four isoprene units, diterpenoids are found in medicinal plants and have a wide range of biological effects.

- *Triterpenoids (C30)*: Containing six isoprene units, these compounds include saponins and sterols, which are important for human health.
- *Tetraterpenoids (C40)*: Found in pigments such as carotenoids, these are important antioxidants.
- *Polyterpenoids*: These are composed of many more than six isoprene units and are usually found in more complex compounds.

Each of these subclasses of terpenoids has unique structural features that contribute to their biological activities, making them valuable candidates for healthcare applications.

3 Mechanisms of Action in Healthcare

The therapeutic effects of terpenoids arise from their interaction with biological systems, affecting a wide range of cellular and molecular pathways (Paduch et al. 2007; Yang et al. 2020). Some of the major mechanisms by which terpenoids exert their beneficial effects are shown in Fig. 1:

- *Cell Membrane Disruption*: Many terpenoids are capable of interacting with the cell membranes of pathogens, fungi, and even human cells, altering their permeability and leading to cell death or the inhibition of replication.

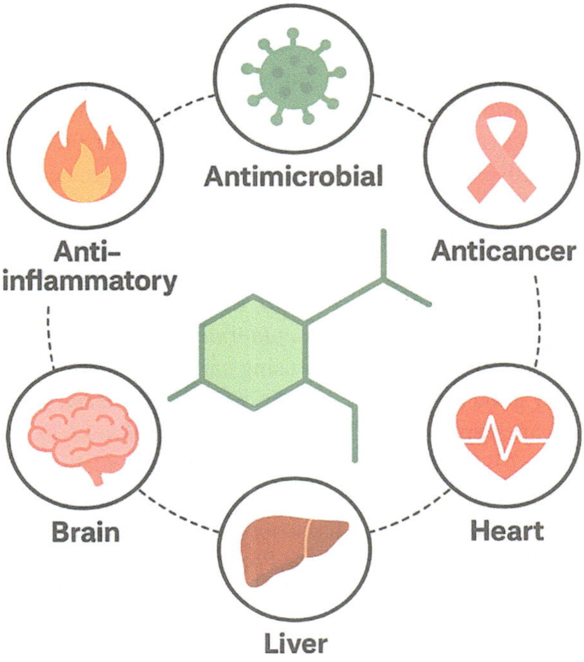

Fig. 1 Major therapeutic effects of terpenoids, including anti-inflammatory, antimicrobial, anticancer, brain, heart, and liver

- *Receptor Modulation*: Terpenoids can interact with neurotransmitter receptors and immune system receptors, modulating pain, inflammation, and mood.
- *Enzyme Inhibition or Activation*: Terpenoids can inhibit or activate enzymes involved in metabolic pathways, including those linked to oxidative stress, cancer cell proliferation, and inflammatory processes.
- *Antioxidant Activity*: By neutralizing free radicals, terpenoids reduce oxidative stress, protecting tissues from damage linked to aging and various diseases.

4 Therapeutic Applications of Terpenoids

4.1 Antimicrobial and Antifungal Properties

Terpenoids are well known for their antimicrobial properties, which include the ability to combat a range of bacterial, viral, and fungal infections. They disrupt the integrity of pathogen membranes (Nazzaro et al. 2013) or inhibit essential enzymes, leading to reduced microbial viability. Many terpenoids, mainly essential oils, are well known for their antimicrobial properties. It has been used in several industries, such as food, cosmetics, health care products, hair products, soaps, and creams. Limonene from citrus peels has synergistic effects with gentamicin drugs to inhibit *Staphylococcus aureus* and *Escherichia coli*. Thymol, eugenol, geraniol, and carvacrol have strong antimicrobial effects, making them valuable for treating respiratory infections, skin conditions, and gastrointestinal disturbances. Terpinen-4-ol, found in tea tree oil, is widely used for its antibacterial and antifungal properties, particularly in the treatment of acne (Carson et al. 2006), athletes' feet, and dandruff. Cineole, found in eucalyptus oil, works by disrupting bacterial membrane integrity, increasing oxidative stress, and altering the morphology of bacteria, leading to death. Anethole and myristicin are known for their anticancer activity and antiproliferative activity. Lower terpenoids are recognized for their ability to combat both antibiotic-susceptible and antibiotic-resistant bacteria. Disruption of the cell membrane and inhibition of protein synthesis interfere with their DNA replication. Carvacrol is one of the best antibacterial agents. Microorganisms like Serratia spp., *Enterobacter* spp., *pneumonia, Escherichia coli, Streptococcus pneumonia, Proteus mirabilis, Staphylococcus epidermis, Staphylococcus aureus,* and *Klebsiella pneumonia* can be inhibited by using carvacrol (Alagawany et al. 2015). Carvacrol has a very good antifungal effect. It can inhibit *Alternaria alternata, Trichoderma viride, Candida* spp., *Penicillium rubrum, Aspergillus niger,* and dermatophytes (Alagawany et al. 2015). Bakuchiol also has a very significant role in oral healthcare. It has good antibacterial properties and hence can be used in different products (Nizam et al. 2023). Bakuchiol also has a very strong antimicrobial effect on microbes. *Bakuchiol can be used to promote good oral health* (Katsura et al. 2001). Geraniol has a very good antifungal and antibacterial property. Geraniol inhibits microbes like *Streptococcus agalactia, Neisseria gonorrhoeae, Streptococcus pneumoniae,* and

Haemophilus influenzae. Fungi like *Candida albicans* and *C. glabrata* are inhibited by geraniol, thus exhibiting a very strong antifungal effect (Fajdek-Bieda et al. 2025a).

4.2 Anti-inflammatory Effects

Chronic inflammation is implicated in many diseases, including arthritis, cardiovascular disease, and metabolic disorders. Terpenoids can help manage inflammation through the modulation of key inflammatory mediators. Caryophyllene, found in black pepper and cloves, acts on cannabinoid receptors, providing anti-inflammatory and analgesic effects (Gertsch et al. 2008). Limonene, a citrus-derived compound, reduces pro-inflammatory cytokines and enhances the activity of antioxidant enzymes, contributing to reduced inflammation (d'Alessio et al. 2013). *Artemisia annua* L contains compounds like Deoxyartemisinin and Artemisinin. These compounds can be used to treat inflammation. Artemisinin shows a very good anti-inflammatory effect. Deoxyartemisinin also shows good anti-inflammatory effects, but it has good antinociceptive properties (de Faveri Favero et al. 2024). Anti-inflammatory effects are exerted by pentacyclic terpenoids like oleanolic acid and ursolic acid. The anti-inflammatory property is achieved by downregulating various molecular targets, including NF-κB and STAT3/6 pathways (Kashyap et al. 2016). Cannabidiol is also a very good anti-inflammatory compound. It reduces the levels of pro-inflammatory cytokines. Cannabidiol induces T cells and inhibits T-cell proliferation (Atalay et al. 2019). Ginkgolide B shows a very strong antioxidant property. It can also be used to treat inflammation (Zhu et al. 2019). *G. biloba contains a bioactive compound, bilobalide. This bilobalide is a* sesquiterpenoid lactone. It can be used to treat colitis. It also has a good anti-inflammatory effect (Xiang et al. 2021). Menthol can treat wounds. It also has good anti-inflammatory and antioxidant properties. It reduces the mRNA expression of inflammatory cytokines during the inflammatory phase (Rozza et al. 2021). Linalool has a good anti-inflammatory property, so it can be used to treat arthritis. When linalool is taken orally, it reduces inflammation and symptoms related to arthritis. Linalool reduces lipid peroxidation. It also reduces pro-inflammatory (Riaz et al. 2025). Thymol shows good anticancer. It also has antioxidant and anti-inflammatory properties (Li et al. 2015). Eugenol has anti-inflammatory properties. It exhibits anti-inflammatory properties by inhibiting the synthesis of pro-inflammatory cytokines (IL-6 and TNF) and NF-B signaling (Abdou et al. 2024). Eugenol can be used to treat diseases that are associated with inflammatory response and oxidative stress (Barboza et al. 2018). Carvacrol can also be used to inhibit bacteria. Carvacrol can be used to treat inflammation. It also has good antioxidant properties (Cicalău et al. 2021). Carvacrol reduces symptoms of PCOS. It affects oxidative stressors and the NLRP3/NF-ĸB dependent pathway, thus reducing symptoms of PCOS. It also has antioxidant properties. It is a very good candidate that can be included in PCOS therapy (Siddiqua et al. 2025). Strong hepatoprotective is shown by carvacrol (Barzan et al. 2023). Ursolic acid is found in peppermint, rosemary, apples, basil, cranberries, oregano, and prunes. It has anticancer properties. It also has good anti-inflammatory properties. It suppresses NF-κB (Checker et al. 2012). Ursolic acid shows good antioxidant properties along with anti-inflammatory properties (Zhao et al. 2023a). Betulinic acid shows anti-inflammatory properties. It inhibits the NF-kB and MAPK pathways. The production of IL-10 is promoted by betulinic acid, which helps to modulate several immune cell types (Oliveira-Costa et al. 2022). Ginsenosides are obtained from ginseng plants. It is a type of steroidal glycoside. Its anti-inflammatory property is exhibited by targeting reactive oxygen species. It reduces oxidative stress (Paik et al. 2023). Asiatic acid is a pentacyclic triterpene. It possesses good anti-inflammatory and antioxidant properties. It also exhibits hepato-protective properties by inhibiting oxidative stress and inflammatory responses. It can be used to prevent and treat liver injury (Lv et al. 2017a). Geraniol induces the degradation of NF-κB p65, thus showing a good anti-inflammatory effect (Su et al. 2010). Pro- and anti-inflammatory mediators and pathways are targeted by squalene. This modulates macrophages, neutrophils, and monocytes by preventing their overactivation (Cárdeno et al. 2015). Farnesol modulates inflammation. It can be used to treat asthma and chronic inflammation (Jung et al. 2018). Inflammatory conditions can be treated by using bakuchiol. Bakuchiol is also used to treat diabetes, psoriasis, asthma, nephritis, and Alzheimer's disease (Nizam et al. 2023). Myrcene shows good analgesic and anti-inflammatory effects. It is also used to treat inflammatory joint disease. It activates articular cannabinoid receptors and exhibits anti-inflammatory effects. It is also used to treat arthritis (McDougall and Reid 2022). Zerumbone suppresses eicosanoid signaling and thus exhibits anti-inflammatory properties (Uppin et al. 2024).

4.3 *Anticancer Effects*

The anticancer potential of terpenoids is an area of intense research. Many terpenoids have demonstrated the ability to inhibit the proliferation of cancer cells, induce apoptosis (programmed cell death), and limit metastasis. Taxol (paclitaxel), derived from the Pacific yew tree, is a highly effective chemotherapeutic agent used to treat various cancers, including breast, ovarian, and lung cancer (Cragg and Newman 2005). Curcumin, a yellow pigment in turmeric, exhibits anticancer properties by modulating numerous pathways involved in cell survival, apoptosis, and inflammation (Aggarwal et al. 2007). Carvacrol decreases the expression of matrix metalloproteases 2 and 9 and exhibits good anticancer properties (Subramaniyan et al. 2014). Farnesol is used to treat lung cancer, pancreatic cancer, breast cancer and prostate cancer. It acts by inhibiting cell proliferation and suppressing the growth of tumors (Jung et al. 2018). Bakuchiol is used to treat cancer. Bakuchiol acts by inhibiting cell proliferation (Nizam et al. 2023). Artemisinin also acts as a potent anticancer agent. It arrests the cell cycle by inhibiting cancer proliferation and metastasis. This causes changes in signaling pathways. Artemisinin acts by following different mechanisms like inhibiting cell proliferation, promoting cell cycle arrest, suppressing angiogenesis, inhibiting glycolysis, and regulating immunity (Wen et al. 2024). The *Ginkgo biloba* contains *Ginkgolide B. Ginkgolide B* has potent anticancer properties. It can be used to treat lung cancer. It avoids inflammation by inhibiting NLRP3 (Wang et al. 2020). *Ginkgolide B is also used to treat liver cancer, breast cancer, and ovarian cancer* (Papadopoulos et al. 2000; Zhi et al. 2016). Bilobalide is a sesquiterpenoid. It is used to treat gastric carcinoma. It inhibits the PI3K signaling pathway and thereby arrests the cell cycle. Gastric carcinoma can be cured by bilobalide (Liu et al. 2021a). Menthol is used to treat cancer. It shows anticancer properties by following different mechanisms. It promotes the death of cancer cells. The invasion, metastasis, and proliferation of cancer cells are inhibited by menthol. Menthol has fewer side effects, which is why it is very safe (Zhao et al. 2023b). Skin cancer, liver cancer, kidney cancer, and breast cancer can be treated by using D-limonene. D-limonene shows good cytotoxic effects on malignant cancer cells. It induces apoptosis. The growth of lung cancer is also suppressed by D-limonene (Yu et al. 2018). Lung cancer, skin cancer, hepatic cancer, and gastric cancer can be treated by using Linalool (Cherng et al. 2007; Usta et al. 2009). Linalool is also used to treat colon cancer. Linalool is also cost-effective, so it can be used in cancer therapy (Iwasaki et al. 2016). Carvacrol shows good anticancer properties. It targets the cancer cells and hinders their growth. It also reduces oxidative stress. It follows mitochondrial-mediated apoptosis in cancer cells. Carvacrol prevents the progression of tumors by regulating the cell cycle. Angiogenesis, cell migration, and invasion in cancer cells are inhibited by carvacrol. Carvacrol targets the major signaling pathways (Singh et al. 2023). Geraniol is a monoterpene that is used to treat anticancer properties by inhibiting the NF-κB, MAPK, and JAK-STAT-3 signaling pathways (E Silva et al. 2022; Yang et al. 2022). Citral is a monoterpene that is used to manage cancer in many studies. Geranial, Nerol, and Neral also have good anticancer properties (E Silva et al. 2022). Myrcene also exhibits anticancer activity by enhancing Bax expression and repressing Bcl-2 expression. It can be used to treat oral cancer (Wu et al. 2022).

4.4 Neuroprotective Effects

Terpenoids, especially those found in traditional herbs, have shown promise in managing neurological disorders such as Alzheimer's disease, Parkinson's disease, and general cognitive decline. *Ginkgo biloba*, rich in ginkgolides, has been used for centuries to improve memory and cognitive function, and recent studies suggest that it may help protect against age-related neurodegeneration (Smith and Luo 2004). Turmerones, found in turmeric, possess neuroprotective effects and have been studied for their potential in treating conditions like Alzheimer's disease by inhibiting amyloid plaque formation and promoting neurogenesis (Hucklenbroich et al. 2014). Neurological diseases can be treated by using ginkgolide B, which shows good neuroprotective and anti-inflammatory properties (Sun et al. 2021). Bilobalide can be used to prevent Alzheimer's disease. It inhibits inflammation. The expression of Aβ-degrading enzymes in astrocytes is promoted by bilobalide. Amyloid and inflammation are reduced by bilobalide (Xiang et al. 2021). Menthol protects the dopaminergic neurons in Parkinson's disease (Du et al. 2020). Linalool is found in essential oils. Therefore, it can be seen as a potential drug to treat neurological disorders (Li et al. 2015). Carvacrol also has a good neuroprotective effect. Cell death was reduced by carvacrol (Guan et al. 2019). Memory capacities, cognitive functions, and spatial learning were improved by carvacrol (Shahrokhi Raeini et al. 2020). Bakuchiol can be used to treat neuroinflammatory diseases. Microglial inflammatory responses are suppressed by bakuchiol. Bakuchiol may be used as a potential drug for inflammatory-mediated neurodegenerative diseases (Lim et al. 2019). Thymol is a monoterpene that exhibits neuroprotective effects. It attenuates dopaminergic neuronal loss. It prevents oxidative stress and inflammation. It can be used as a potential candidate in therapy for Parkinson's disease (Javed et al. 2019). Carvacrol is obtained from essential oils. It can be used as a neuroprotective agent. It can be included in the treatment of Parkinson's disease, Alzheimer's disease, behavioral disorders, and multiple sclerosis (Tareen et al. 2024). Ursolic acid shows neuroprotective effects by suppressing oxidative stress and inflammation. It can be used in the management of seizures and epilepsy. Ursolic acid improves cognitive improvement (Liu et al. 2022). Oleanolic acid shows a good neuroprotective effect by reducing oxidative stress and the level of pro-inflammatory cytokines (Sharma et al. 2024). Betulinic acid can be used in the management of Parkinson's disease. Betulinic acid reduces oxidative stress, ferroptosis, apoptosis, and glial activation. Betulinic acid improves motor function and cognition. It reduces oxidative stress and neuroinflammation (Pandey et al. 2025). Oleanolic acid is used in the management of anxiety and depression. It is used to treat traumatic brain injury. It acts by reducing oxidative stress, pro-inflammatory cytokines, and brain edema (Sharma et al. 2024). Inflammatory CNS diseases can be managed by using oleanolic acid. It can be used to treat ischemic stroke (Sapkota and Choi 2022). Neurological conditions can be managed by using ginsenosides. It follows anti-inflammatory, antioxidant, and antiapoptotic mechanisms to show neuroprotective effects (Zhou et al. 2024). Geraniol can be used in the management of depression, epilepsy, and Parkinson's disease. It binds to GABA and glycine receptors and exhibits neuroprotective effects (Bagheri et al. 2022). Neuropathic pain can be mitigated by using Ginkgolide B. Neuralgia can be treated by ginkgolide B (Liu et al. 2013).

4.5 Pain and Anxiety Management

Several terpenoids have been identified as having analgesic and anxiolytic (anxiety-reducing) effects, making them useful in the management of both acute and chronic pain conditions. Menthol, derived from peppermint, has been used for centuries in topical formulations for pain relief, particularly in musculoskeletal pain, headaches, and gastrointestinal discomfort (Patel et al. 2007). Linalool, found in lavender, is widely used in aromatherapy to reduce stress and anxiety and even improve sleep quality (Koulivand et al. 2013). Injured neurons can be repaired by ursolic acid. It also regulates the immune system. It shows good antioxidant and anti-inflammatory activity (Liang et al. 2024). Geraniol is a monoterpene that shows good anti-inflammatory and antioxidant properties. It has a calming effect on the brain (Nisar et al. 2024). Neuropathic pain can be reduced with geraniol (Lv et al. 2017b). The symptoms of PTSD can be reduced by using artemisinin (Liu et al. 2024). Cloves contain Eugenol. Myalgia can be managed using Eugenol. It reduces pain and inflammation. It inhibits production of inhibit prostaglandin E2. It also reduces cyclooxygenase-2. It shows analgesic action by interacting with TRPV1, HVACC, and α2-adrenergic receptors (Mochtar et al. 2025). Nerolidol is an acyclic sesquiterpene. It is found in essential oils. It can be used to treat pain due to its analgesic property. It shows good anti-inflammatory properties. Nerolidol suppressed TNF-α and IL-1β pro-inflammatory cytokines (Fonsêca et al. 2016). Anxiety disorders can be treated using farnesol. It can also be used as a sedative (Shahnouri et al. 2016). β-elemene has good analgesic property. It can be used to treat chronic pain. It reduces neuropathic pain by reversing the process of spinal neuroinflammation. It also has good antioxidant properties (Ma et al. 2022). Zerumbone can be used to treat neuropathic pain. It has a very good analgesic activity. Production of nitric oxide is inhibited, which reduces NOS activation (Zulazmi et al. 2017).

4.6 Cardiovascular Health

Terpenoids can also play a role in cardiovascular health by reducing cholesterol levels, enhancing blood flow, and reducing the risk of atherosclerosis. Hesperidin, found in citrus fruits, has been shown to improve blood circulation and reduce blood pressure, thus benefiting heart health (Roohbakhsh et al. 2015). Betulinic acid, found in birch bark, may help lower cholesterol and reduce the formation of plaques in blood vessels. Carvacrol shows a cardioprotective effect. It can be used to treat myocardial ischemia. It protects heart function. It enhances SOD and CAT levels. It reduces the MDA level. The apoptosis of cardiomyocytes can be reduced by using carvacrol (Chen et al. 2017). Carvacrol can be used to treat myocardial ischemia. Carvacrol acts by different mechanisms to exhibit its cardioprotective action. It reduces the size of cardiac infarct (Yu et al. 2013). α-Bisabolol can be used to ameliorate damage caused by myocardial infarction. It reduces serum lactate dehydrogenase. It also shows good antioxidant effects (Eddin et al. 2022). D-limonene shows good cardioprotective effects. Myocardial infarction can be managed by using D-limonene. It has antioxidant properties. D-limonene stabilizes myocardial membranes. It improves the scavenging of free radicals. It also inhibits membrane lipid peroxidation (Saifullah et al. 2025).

Menthol has cardioprotective properties and can be used to manage various cardiovascular diseases (Nagarajan and Doss 2023). Linalool has cardioprotective properties. It has good anti-inflammatory and antioxidant properties. The cardiac antioxidant activity is enhanced by Linolool (Mohamed et al. 2021). Thymol also exhibits good cardioprotective effects. It shows good cardioprotective action (El-Marasy et al. 2020). Increased arterial blood pressure, hyperglycemia, thrombosis, arrhythmia, heart failure, and hyperlipidemia can be treated by using Eugenol. Eugenol has good cardioprotective effects. It improves cardiac function and modulates the cardiac rate and rhythm (Liu et al. 2025). Ursolic acid is a pentacyclic triterpenoid that shows very good cardioprotective effects. It exhibits its cardioprotective property by following different mechanisms. It has antioxidant, anti-inflammatory, and antiapoptotic properties. It improves lipid peroxidation. It also reduces oxidative stress. Inflammatory pathways are inhibited by downregulating pro-inflammatory cytokines. These actions help to protect cardiac tissues. Energy metabolism and mitochondrial function can be promoted by Ursolic acid (Roudi et al. 2025). Ginsenosides are present in Ginseng. It can be used to manage CHD. It exhibits good cardioprotective effects. It shows antiatherosclerotic, antithrombotic, and antihyperlipidemic effects (Parmar et al. 2024). Hypertrophic cardiomyopathy can be treated using forskolin (Wang et al. 2024b). Nerolidol also shows good cardioprotective activity, and it can be used in the management of hypertension. It acts by targeting the TLR4/NF-κB signaling pathway (Lin et al. 2021). β-Myrcene has a good cardioprotective effect and can be used to treat ischemic stroke (Burcu et al. 2016). Geraniol also shows good cardioprotective effects and is used to manage different heart-reacted diseases (Crespo et al. 2017).

4.7 Metabolic Regulation

Some terpenoids can influence metabolic processes in the body, helping to regulate blood sugar, cholesterol levels, and other markers associated with metabolic diseases like diabetes and obesity. Cinnamon oil, rich in cinnamaldehyde, has been shown to help lower blood sugar levels in individuals with type 2 diabetes. Berberine, found in several plants, including goldenseal, has a range of metabolic benefits, including lowering cholesterol and improving insulin sensitivity. Oleanolic acid is a triterpenoid compound. It can be used to treat inflammation. It is used to manage obesity and diabetes. The insulin resistance can be reduced by using oleanolic acid. It also reduces the adipose tissue hypertrophy. Suppression of MAPK signaling is carried out by oleanolic acid. It activates the NLRP3 inflammasome (Li et al. 2021). Metabolic disorders can be treated by using bilobalide. It can also help improve liver injury. Diabetes can be maintained by using bilobalide. It regulates the HMGB1/TLR4/NF-κB signaling pathway to improve liver injury (Zhao et al. 2021). Citrus peels contain Limonene. Lipid metabolism is enhanced by limonene. It metabolizes fatty acids (Wang et al. 2024a). The essential oils contain carvacrol. It has potent antidiabetic activity. It exhibits its antidiabetic activity by following different mechanisms. It affects the glucose uptake. It also affects insulin sensitivity and insulin resistance. The antioxidant and anti-inflammatory mechanisms also enhance the antidiabetic activity of carvacrol (Hoca et al. 2024). Bilobalide reduces oxidative stress and inflammation, thereby promoting its antidiabetic activity (Su et al. 2022). Linalool also has good antidiabetic and antioxidant effects (Bar and Kara 2024). Thymol has very good antidiabetic properties. Plasma triglycerides can be reduced by using Linalool. It can be used in the management of diabetes. It enhances glycogen synthesis (Sun et al. 2017).

4.8 Cosmetic and Dermatological Applications

Terpenoids are commonly used in skincare products due to their anti-inflammatory, antimicrobial, and antioxidant properties. They help with conditions like acne, eczema, and skin irritation. Tea tree oil, containing terpinen-4-ol, is commonly used for acne treatment because of its antibacterial properties (Carson et al. 2006). Lavender oil is used in skin care for its calming effects and ability to promote wound healing (Koulivand et al. 2013). Eugenol has antibacterial and anti-inflammatory properties. It is present in essential oils. It has very soothing property. This is why it is used in different skincare products like tonics, creams, gels, and soap. It is used to treat toothache. Upper respiratory infections can be treated by using Eugenol (Fajdek-Bieda et al. 2025b). Menthol is present in Mint. It is a type of monoterpene alcohol. It is used in a variety of cosmetic products. It has cooling properties. It also has aromatic and analgesic properties. It is used in shampoos and conditioners. It is also used in cleaners, shaving cream, and ointments. It gives fresh and energized feelings to the skin. It is mostly used in balms and lotions. Menthol is also used in solid formulations to enhance palatability (El Boukhari and Fatimi 2024). Cosmetic products use ginsenosides. It is obtained from Ginseng. Ginsenosides have skin-whitening and antiwrinkle effects. It also has moisturizing and skin-whitening effects. It helps to reduce wrinkles on the skin. It also increases the content of collagen. It can also be used in sun-screen products to protect skin against sun damage (Kim et al. 2024a). Bakuchiol is used in cosmetic products due to its various beneficial properties. It can prevent and treat hyperpigmentation. It has antiaging and antimelanogenesis properties. It can also be used as an antiaging agent. It has inti-inflammatory and antioxidant properties. Acne can be treated by using Bakuchiol. Bakuchiol is formulated into cleansers. Serums, creams, and nanoemulsions (Putriana et al. 2024). Squalene is a triterpenoid that has many cosmeceutical applications. Rice bran oil, olive oil, wheat germ oil, and amaranth oil contain squalene. It has antioxidant properties. Squalene acts as an emollient. It also promotes skin hydration. It can also be used to treat cancer (Huang et al. 2009). It has a moisturizing property. Various skin disorders like dermatitis, acne, psoriasis, atopic dermatitis, and seborrheic dermatitis can be treated by using Squalene (Wołosik et al. 2013). Detergents and cleansers contain geraniol. The perfume industry uses geraniol. It is nonirritant and nontoxic. It also enhances the permeation of other ingredients. Toilet soap, shampoos, perfumes, and cosmetics contain geraniol (Lapczynski et al. 2008). Antitanning formulations contain forskolin, as it can protect the skin from skin damage. Skin cancer can be managed by using forskolin, as it protects the skin from harmful UV rays of the sun (Passeron et al. 2009).

4.9 Dietary Supplements

Due to their wide array of health benefits, many terpenoids are incorporated into dietary supplements and functional foods. These include extracts from plants like turmeric, ginger, ginseng, and citrus fruits, all of which contain terpenoids with various health-promoting properties (Gershenzon and Dudareva 2007). Essential oils contain carvacrol. It is a type of phenolic monoterpene that has many health benefits. It has good anti-inflammatory and antioxidant properties (Beninca et al. 2024). Limonene has a calming effect on the body. It is used in a variety of cosmetic products. Various diseases can be treated by using Limonene. It can be taken as a supplement to promote good health. The signaling pathways linked to several diseases can be modulated by using limonene (Vieira et al. 2018). Different skin disorders can be treated by using *G. biloba*. It can be used as a supplement to treat fever and skin issues. It can be used to treat a toothache. The neurodegenerative diseases can be prevented by taking *G. biloba* supplements (Das et al. 2022). Linalool shows the antioxidant properties of shoes. It can be used as a functional food to prevent different diseases. It promotes immunity. It can be used as a sedative. It can be used as an anticonvulsant, and it also has good anticancer properties (Kasper et al. 2010). *Thymus vulgaris* contains thymol. It has antioxidant and anti-inflammatory effects. It can be used as a dietary supplement to promote immunity. It has antimicrobial properties (Hafsan et al. 2022). *Eugenol helps in lipid metabolism. The lipid profile of blood is regulated by Eugenol* (Nie et al. 2025). Ursolic acid can be used to treat different health issues. It can be taken as a dietary supplement and functional food. It can be used to prevent skin aging and neurodegenerative diseases. Metabolic diseases and inflammation can be treated by using ursolic acid (Arulnangai et al. 2025). Weight loss can be promoted by using betulinic acid. Obesity can be treated using betulinic acid. The accumulation of abdominal fat is inhibited by betulinic acid (Azevedo et al. 2025). Oleonolic acid can also be used to promote weight loss. It has antiobesity and antidiabetic properties. Insulin sensitivity is improved by Oleonolic acid. It improves lipid homeostasis. It promotes body weight regulation. The absorption of glucose is reduced by Oleonolic acid. It also increases insulin sensitivity (Silva et al. 2016). Immunity can be enhanced by using ginsenosides. It is used to treat skin issues (Tang et al. 2024). Squalene can be taken as a supplement to prevent different diseases. It can promote cardiovascular health. It also has lipid-lowering effects (Ibrahim et al. 2020). *Psoralea corylifolia* contains Bakuchiol. It has good antioxidant and anti-inflammatory properties. It is used to treat cancer (Nizam et al. 2023). Geraniol has cardioprotective and hepatoprotective effects. It can be used to enhance the skin penetration of different ingredients. It has antioxidant and anti-inflammatory properties (Chen and Viljoen 2022).

5 Terpenoids in Traditional Medicine

For centuries, terpenoids have played a vital role in traditional medicine systems across the world. In Ayurveda, terpenoid-rich plants such as Tulsi (*Ocimum sanctum*) and Neem (*Azadirachta indica*) have been used for their antimicrobial, anti-inflammatory, and healing properties. Similarly, in traditional Chinese medicine (TCM), terpenoid-containing herbs like ginseng (*Panax ginseng*) and camphor are valued for promoting vitality, improving circulation, and relieving pain. Indigenous and folk medicine systems in Africa, South America, and Europe have also relied on aromatic and resinous plants rich in terpenoids for treating infections, wounds, and respiratory ailments. The widespread historical use of these compounds highlights their pharmacological importance and provides a foundation for modern scientific validation. By bridging ancient wisdom and contemporary research, terpenoids continue to inspire the development of safe, effective, and nature-derived therapeutic agents (Efferth and Koch 2011):

- **Lavender** (*Lavandula angustifolia*): Known for its calming effects, lavender oil, rich in linalool, has been used for its anxiolytic and sedative properties (Koulivand et al. 2013).
- **Turmeric** (*Curcuma longa*): Curcumin, a compound belonging to the curcuminoid class of terpenoids, is revered for its anti-inflammatory and antioxidant activities (Hucklenbroich et al. 2014).
- **Ginseng** (*Panax ginseng*): Ginsenosides, the active terpenoid compounds in ginseng, are used for their adaptogenic properties, helping the body resist stress and improve overall vitality (Smith and Luo 2004).

6 Modern Pharmaceutical Applications of Terpenoids

The pharmaceutical importance of terpenoids has received much attention in recent years because of their diversity and the great number of bioactivities. In recent years, significant advances in biotechnology as well as synthetic biology have provided a means to produce and chemically modify terpenoids on a large scale, leading to the improvement of their stability, bioavailability, and therapeutic effectiveness. Several terpenoid-derived compounds like artemisinin (antimalarial), Taxol/paclitaxel (anticancer), and menthol (analgesics cooling agent) are already in clinical use or currently at the stage of clinical trials. In addition, the current trend of utilization is also directed toward the development of nanoformulation and controlled release systems for improved pharmacological activity (Table 1). The incorporation of terpenoids into modern drug discovery and formulation technology is evidence of the promise of these naturally occurring molecules present for the management of infectious, inflammatory, and chronic ailments in Table 2 (Efferth and Koch 2011).

Table 1 Summary of prominent terpenoids, their natural sources, and significant activities in health care management

S. No.	Terpenoid (common name)	Class (mono/di/tri/other)	Natural source	Therapeutic use	References
1	Artemisinin	Sesquiterpene lactone	*Artemisia annua* (sweet wormwood)	Artemisinin-based combination therapy (rapid parasite clearance) is based on a powerful antimalarial	Henry (2014)
2	Paclitaxel (Taxol)	Diterpenoid (taxane)	*Taxus* spp. (Pacific yew)	Chemotherapy for malignancies of the breast, ovaries, and lungs that uses microtubule stabilizers	Weaver (2014)
3	Cannabidiol (CBD)	Terpenophenol/ meroterpenoid-like	*Cannabis sativa*	FDA-approved (Epidiolex) for many epilepsies (LGS, TSC, Dravet); has anxiolytic and anticonvulsant properties	de Araújo-Filho et al. (2021) and Kumar (2025)
4	Ginkgolide B	Diterpene trilactone	*Ginkgo biloba* leaves	Neuroprotective benefits of a platelet-activating factor (PAF) antagonist; utilized in vascular and cognitive supplements	Li et al. (2022)
5	Bilobalide	Sesquiterpene (terpene trilactone)	*Ginkgo biloba*	Neuroprotective, protective of mitochondria; investigated for support of cognition	Kim et al. (2024b)

(continued)

6	Menthol	Monoterpenoid alcohol	Peppermint oil (*Mentha piperita*)	Inhalants and topical pain/itch compositions employ a topical analgesic/cooling (TRPM8 agonist)	Masyita et al. (2022)
7	Limonene	Monoterpene	Citrus peels	Anti-inflammatory, with potential for chemoprevention and anticancer effects; utilized as an excipient and in aromatherapy	Masyita et al. (2022)
8	Linalool	Monoterpenoid alcohol	Lavender, many essential oils	Preclinical and aromatherapy investigations have shown anxiolytic/sedative effects, along with anti-inflammatory qualities	Del Prado-Audelo et al. (2021)
9	Thymol	Monoterpenoid phenol	Thyme (*Thymus vulgaris*)	Antimicrobial, antiseptic (oral rinses, topical antiseptics); anti-inflammatory	Del Prado-Audelo et al. (2021)
10	Carvacrol	Monoterpenoid phenol	Oregano (*Origanum vulgare*)	Antimicrobial and anti-inflammatory; researched for gastrointestinal and respiratory applications	Del Prado-Audelo et al. (2021)
11	Eugenol	Phenylpropanoid/terpenoid (in essential oils)	Clove oil (*Syzygium aromaticum*)	Antimicrobial, anti-inflammatory, and dental analgesic/antiseptic qualities	Masyita et al. (2022)

Table 1 (continued)

S. No.	Terpenoid (common name)	Class (mono/di/tri/other)	Natural source	Therapeutic use	References
12	Ursolic acid	Triterpenoid	Apple peel, rosemary, many plants	Anti-inflammatory, antioxidant, and anticancer potential; investigated for effects on wound healing and metabolism	Câmara et al. (2024)
13	Oleanolic acid	Triterpenoid	Olive, many plants	Hepatoprotective, anti-inflammatory, and metabolic advantages; investigated as a therapeutic framework	Câmara et al. (2024)
14	Betulinic acid/betulin	Triterpenoid	Birch bark and woody plants	Anticancer (selective cytotoxicity), antiviral, and anti-inflammatory properties (preclinical/early investigations)	Lou et al. (2021)
15	Celastrol	Triterpenoid (quinone methide triterpene)	*Tripterygium wilfordii*	Investigational because of toxicity; strong anti-inflammatory and anticancer efficacy in preclinical animals	Lou et al. (2021)
16	Ginsenosides (e.g., Rb1, Rg1)	Triterpenoid saponins	*Panax ginseng*	Claims of cardioprotection, neuroprotection, and adaptogenicity; many mechanisms (antioxidant, signaling regulation)	Lou et al. (2021)

17	Asiatic acid/asiaticoside	Triterpenoid/saponin derivatives	*Centella asiatica*	Increases wound healing, collagen production; has anti-inflammatory and neuroprotective properties	Diniz et al. (2023)
18	Perillyl alcohol	Monoterpenoid (alcohol)	Lavender, mint, citrus	Investigated in preclinical and early clinical studies as a chemopreventive and anticancer drug	Yang et al. (2020)
19	Geraniol	Monoterpenoid alcohol	Rose, geranium, citronella	Antimicrobial and anti-inflammatory properties; preliminary evidence of chemopreventive and anticancer action	Yang et al. (2020)
20	Phytol	Acyclic diterpene alcohol	–	Antioxidant, anti-inflammatory, and immunomodulatory properties; preclinical research and formulation application	Devi et al. (2024)
21	Zingiberene	Sesquiterpene hydrocarbon	Ginger (*Zingiber officinale*)	Antioxidant and anti-inflammatory qualities are included in the bioactivity profile of ginger	Devi et al. (2024)
22	Forskolin (coleonol)	Labdane diterpenoid	*Coleus forskohlii* root	Activates adenylate cyclase → cAMP; shown to have little clinical evidence for glaucoma (IOP), cardioprotective, and metabolic benefits	Pateraki et al. (2017)

(continued)

Table 1 (continued)

S. No.	Terpenoid (common name)	Class (mono/di/tri/other)	Natural source	Therapeutic use	References
23	Andrographolide	Diterpene lactone	Andrographis paniculata (king of bitters)	Traditional medicine uses anti-inflammatory, antiviral, and immunomodulatory drugs, and pharmacological research is ongoing	Pateraki et al. (2017)
24	Perseitol/(taxane derivatives)	Diterpenoids (taxane family)	*Taxus* spp. and semisynthetic derivatives	Oncological use of certain semisynthetic taxanes (mechanism: Microtubule stabilization)	Subramaniam et al. (2021)
25	Celery/apigenin-adjacent terpenoids (e.g., limonene-related)	Monoterpenes/diterpenes (various)	–	Broad-spectrum properties: antibacterial, anti-inflammatory, and antioxidant; often utilized as excipients and nutraceuticals	Masyita et al. (2022)

Table 2 An extensive summary of medicine-related terpenoids including their sources, chemical classifications, bioactivities, and mechanisms

S. No.	Terpenoid	Source	Class	Pharmacological activity	Mechanism	References
1	Menthol	Peppermint (*Mentha* spp.)	Monoterpene alcohol	Analgesic, antitussive, anti-inflammatory, permeation enhancer	Activation of TRPM8 causes cooling and pain relief; it also affects inflammation and ion channels	Li et al. (2022)
2	D-limonene	Citrus peel oils	Monoterpene hydrocarbon	Anti-inflammatory, antioxidant, anticancer, gastroprotective	Regulates cytokines, promotes apoptosis in neoplastic mice; has antioxidant properties	Anandakumar et al. (2021)
3	Linalool	Lavender, many essential oils	Monoterpene alcohol	Anxiolytic, analgesic, anti-inflammatory, antimicrobial	Neuroactive: reduces inflammation; alters GABAergic/serotonergic transmission	dos Santos et al. (2021)
4	α-Pinene	Pine oils, conifers	Monoterpene hydrocarbon	Anti-inflammatory, antimicrobial, bronchodilator, neuroprotective	Inhibits NF-κB/COX, an inflammatory signaling pathway, and alters transmission	dos Santos et al. (2021)
5	1,8-Cineole (Eucalyptol)	Eucalyptus, rosemary	Monoterpene ether	Bronchodilator, mucolytic, anti-inflammatory, antimicrobial	Regulates NF-κB/Nrf2; facilitates bronchodilation and mucus clearance	Cai et al. (2021)
6	Thymol	Thyme (*Thymus vulgaris*)	Monoterpene phenol	Antimicrobial, anti-inflammatory, antioxidant	Reduces inflammatory mediators and is membrane-active against microorganisms	Nagoor Meeran et al. (2017)

(continued)

Table 2 (continued)

S. No.	Terpenoid	Source	Class	Pharmacological activity	Mechanism	References
7	Carvacrol	Oregano, thyme	Monoterpene phenol	Antimicrobial, anti-inflammatory, antioxidant, anticancer	Interferes with microbial membranes and controls inflammation and oxidative stress	Nagoor Meeran et al. (2017)
8	β-Caryophyllene (BCP)	Clove, black pepper, cannabis	Sesquiterpene	Anti-inflammatory, analgesic, CB2 agonist (nonpsychoactive)	Immunomodulation and analgesia using selective CB2 receptor agonists	Francomano et al. (2019)
9	Nerolidol	Many floral essential oils	Sesquiterpene alcohol	Anti-inflammatory, antioxidant, antimicrobial, skin-penetration enhancer	Suppresses inflammatory cytokines; improves transdermal medication administration	Francomano et al. (2019)
10	Farnesol	Essential oils (e.g., citronella)	Sesquiterpene alcohol	Antimicrobial, antifungal (Candida quorum sensing), anticancer	Disrupts fungal development; regulates apoptosis and oxidative stress	Delmondes et al. (2020)
11	Squalene	Olive oil, amaranth, shark liver (traditional)	Triterpene hydrocarbon	Antioxidant, emollient (dermatology), immunostimulant adjuvant	Lipoperoxides are scavenged; it is employed as a skin protector and vaccination adjuvant	Huang et al. (2009)
12	Ursolic acid	Apples, rosemary, many plants	Pentacyclic triterpenoid	Anti-inflammatory, anticancer, cardioprotective, neuroprotective	Modulates NF-κB, induces apoptosis in tumors, antioxidant effects	Huang et al. (2009)
13	Oleanolic acid	Olive, many herbs	Pentacyclic triterpenoid	Hepatoprotective, antioxidant, anti-inflammatory, antitumor	Anti-inflammatory signaling and detox mechanisms are altered	Wasim and Bergonzi (2024)

14	Betulinic acid	Birch bark (*Betula* spp.)	Pentacyclic triterpenoid	Anticancer, anti-inflammatory, antiviral	Anti-inflammatory signaling and detoxification pathways are modified	Lou et al. (2021)
15	Glycyrrhizin/ lycyrrhetinic acid	Licorice (*Glycyrrhiza glabra*)	Triterpenoid saponin	Anti-inflammatory, antiviral (e.g., hepatitis C), hepatoprotective	Inhibits NF-κB, modifies the metabolism of cortisol, and has antiviral properties	Graebin (2018)
16	Asiatic acid	*Centella asiatica*	Pentacyclic triterpenoid	Wound healing, neuroprotective, anti-inflammatory, anticancer	Regulates apoptosis, antioxidant enzymes, and collagen formation, so facilitating wound healing	Dong et al. (2025)
17	Ginsenosides (e.g., Rb1, Rg1, Re)	Panax ginseng (*ginseng root*)	Triterpenoid saponins	Neuroprotective, cardioprotective, antidiabetic, adaptogenic	Antioxidant, anti-inflammatory, and it also affects insulin signaling and neurotransmitters	Liu et al. (2021b)
18	Artemisinin (and derivatives)	*Artemisia annua*	Sesquiterpene lactone	Potent antimalarial; investigated anticancer, antiviral	The endoperoxide moiety combines with iron to produce free radicals, which kill parasites and have extra anticancer effects	Ho et al. (2014)
19	Paclitaxel (Taxol)	Pacific yew (*Taxus* spp.)	Diterpenoid (taxane)	Cytotoxic anticancer drug (breast, ovarian, lung)	Microtubule stabilization leads to mitotic arrest and apoptosis	Cidon and Ballesteros (2016)
20	Ginkgolides/ Bilobalide	*Ginkgo biloba* leaves	Diterpenoid trilactones	Neuroprotective, anti-ischemic, platelet-activating factor (PAF) antagonists	Ginkgolides inhibit PAF, whereas bilobalide has mitochondrial and neuroprotective properties	Kim et al. (2024b)

(continued)

Table 2 (continued)

S. No.	Terpenoid	Source	Class	Pharmacological activity	Mechanism	References
21	Steviol glycosides (stevioside, rebaudioside A)	Stevia rebaudiana	Diterpenoid glycosides	Noncaloric sweetener with antihyperglycemic/ antihypertensive potential	Regulates insulin signaling, glucose metabolism, and safe sweetening	Momtazi-Borojeni et al. (2016)
22	Tocopherols (Vitamin E—α/γ-tocopherol)	Vegetable oils, nuts	Tocols (terpenoid family)	Antioxidant, neuroprotective, cardioprotective (mixed clinical evidence)	Antioxidant lipid that regulates inflammation and signaling	Peh et al. (2016)
23	α-Bisabolol	Chamomile, candeia oil	Sesquiterpene alcohol	Anti-inflammatory, wound healing, antitumor, skin-soothing	Inhibition of NF-κB/ MAPK signaling and reduction of pro-inflammatory cytokines	Eddin et al. (2022)
24	α-Humulene	Hops, basil, coriander	Sesquiterpene hydrocarbon	Anti-inflammatory, analgesic, antimicrobial	Inhibits pro-inflammatory cytokines; possible interactions with CB1 and CB2 receptors identified	Dalavaye et al. (2023)
25	Zerumbone	*Zingiber zerumbet* (ginger)	Sesquiterpene	Anticancer, anti-inflammatory, antioxidant	Apoptosis and inflammatory mediators (ROS pathways, NF-κB) are altered	Kalantari et al. (2017)
26	Bakuchiol	Psoralea (*P. corylifolia) seeds*	Meroterpenoid (phenolic terpenoid)	Retinol-like antiaging effects, antioxidant, anti-inflammatory	Regulates gene expression akin to retinol; has favorable topical tolerability	Nizam et al. (2023)

27	Sclareol	Clary sage (*Salvia sclarea*)	Diterpene alcohol	Antitumor, anti-inflammatory, antimicrobial	Regulates inflammatory pathways; investigated for anticancer efficacy	Zhou et al. (2022)
28	Geraniol	Rose, palmarosa, citronella	Monoterpene alcohol	Antitumor, antimicrobial, anti-inflammatory	Apoptosis in neoplastic cells, modulates antioxidants and enzymes	Lei et al. (2019)
29	β-Myrcene	Hops, lemongrass, cannabis	Monoterpene hydrocarbon	Analgesic, sedative, anti-inflammatory, antioxidant	Regulates nociceptive pathways and inflammation; induces sedation via central nervous system actions	Surendran et al. (2021)
30	β-Elemene	Curcuma species (e.g., *Curcuma wenyujin*)	Sesquiterpene	Anticancer (investigational), chemosensitizer	Induces cell cycle arrest and apoptosis; investigated in nanoparticle delivery methods	Feng et al. (2024)
31	Sabinene	Several essential oils (e.g., Norway spruce)	Monoterpene	Antimicrobial, antioxidant, may protect muscle	Antioxidant effects; in atrophy models, it affects ROS/MAPK	Judžentienė et al. (2024)
32	Terpinen-4-ol	Tea tree oil (*Melaleuca alternifolia*)	Monoterpene alcohol	Antimicrobial (broad), anti-inflammatory	Disrupts microbial membranes and diminishes inflammatory mediators	Prerna et al. (2024)

(continued)

Table 2 (continued)

S. No.	Terpenoid	Source	Class	Pharmacological activity	Mechanism	References
33	Tocotrienols (Vitamin E family)	Palm oil, rice bran	Tocols (terpenoid family)	Neuroprotective, cholesterol-lowering, antioxidant	Antioxidant and signaling regulation; exclusive advantages of tocopherols	Ahsan et al. (2014)
34	β-Pinene (β- and α-isomers)	Conifer oils, many plants	Monoterpene hydrocarbon	Antimicrobial, anti-inflammatory, bronchodilator	Analogous to α-pinene; has antioxidant and anti-inflammatory properties	Park et al. (2021)
35	Sclareolide/related diterpenes (sclareol derivatives)	Clary sage and derivatives	Diterpenoid/lactone derivatives	Studied for anti-inflammatory, anticancer actions; perfumery and cosmetics ingredient	Several processes, include the stimulation of apoptosis and regulation of inflammation	Zanotti et al. (2023)

- *Menthol*: Found in peppermint oil, menthol has cooling and analgesic effects, often used in topical treatments for pain and muscle discomfort (Patel et al. 2007).
- *Artemisinin*: Derived from *Artemisia annua*, artemisinin is a potent antimalarial agent and has been one of the most effective treatments for malaria (Tu 2011).
- *Taxol (Paclitaxel)*: A diterpenoid derived from the Pacific yew tree, Taxol, is widely used in the treatment of cancers, particularly ovarian and breast cancer (Cragg and Newman 2005).

Furthermore, with growing interest in plant-based medicine, terpenoids are increasingly being explored as natural alternatives to synthetic drugs, offering a lower risk of side effects and better compatibility with the human body.

7 The Future of Terpenoids in Healthcare Management

The role of terpenoids in medical and health care is looking encouraging, mainly due to breakthrough advancements in molecular biology, pharmacology, and biotechnology. As the various molecular activities that underlie the therapeutic effects of terpenoids are clarified, consideration for this class in personalized medicine approaches becomes more feasible. This type of compound represents a sort of lead-like molecule that is potentially useful in the prevention and/or treatment of different human diseases, from infectious and inflammatory pathologies to neoplastic and neurodegenerative ones (Efferth and Koch 2011). New approaches for terpenoid delivery are represented by innovative nanotechnology-based drug delivery systems, such as nanoencapsulation, liposomes, and polymeric nanoparticles. These systems improve the bioavailability, stability, and target delivery of the formulation to facilitate greater therapeutic effectiveness with fewer side effects. Moreover, the reports emphasize that there may be a higher synergistic effect of terpenoids used together with other bioactive compounds and classic drugs, which suggests that the combinations of these could be more effective to treat applications such as cancer metabolic syndromes or autoimmune diseases. Prospect In the future, the combination of computational simulation, omics technologies, and network pharmacology methods would further advance our understanding of molecular interactions for terpenoids. Application of these integrative strategies should further a rational development of multicomponent, plant-based medicine with multiple targets, thereby facilitating the leap into the future of evidence-based natural medicine.

8 Challenges and Limitations

Pharmacological prospects Despite terpenoids having significant pharmacological potential, several drawbacks and limitations exist that restrict their extensive usage in modern healthcare. The low retention of many terpenoids by the tissue is also an impediment to delivering them at a desired location and through consumption as part of eating mentholiums or dietary supplements with limited systemic availability. These properties restrict their absorption and distribution to the systemic circulation, having an effect on therapeutic responses. In this light, new drug delivery systems like nanoencapsulation, liposomal formulations, and polymer-based carriers are under study to enhance the water solubility, stability, and targeted release of terpenoid compounds (Yang et al. 2020). A second essential subject is that of standardization and quality control. Plant-derived materials were varied in bioactive terpenoid content and composition originating from plant species, geographical area, harvest season, and so forth. Intrinsic heterogeneity among stem cells also poses challenges for dosing, reproducibility, and therapeutic efficacy. To this end, the current trends are using established extraction protocols and chromatographic profile bioprofiling methods to be equipped with a reliable quality assurance system for the consistency and reproducibility of terpenoid-based product strategies. There are also some hard regulatory challenges. Drugs: The difficulty in providing drugs derived from terpenoids is more pronounced, mainly because of the lack of published clinical studies combined with source-to-source variation (including genetic markers), and countries show very different criteria for the approval of herbal or natural products. However, the tremendous acceptance of herbal products globally and their experimental affirmation is gradually modifying perceptions about integrating herbal medicines with formal healthcare. To overcome these challenges and to fully exploit the theoretical potential of terpenoids, an interdisciplinary, state-of-the-art in formulation technology and harmonized concepts for their regulatory as well as post-registration development application in modern medicine will be required (Efferth and Koch 2011).

9 Conclusion

Terpenoids are among the world's most commercially important natural products having a wide range of medicinal values. Their pharmacological activities, such as antimicrobial, anti-inflammatory, cardiovascular, anticancer, neuroprotective, and analgesic activity, prove their important role in current drug discovery and health care technologies. Advances in basic science have provided increasing insight into the molecular mechanisms of these effects—terpenoids are shown to target cellular pathways, enzymes, and receptors, which may be critical for disease progression. Terpenoids are likely to become increasingly important in both orthodox and complementary medicine as the evidence of their effectiveness and safety grows. The use of such compounds (especially of plant origin) in medication holds promise for improved therapeutic outcomes by decreasing the dependence on synthetic pharmaceuticals and their side effects. In addition, progress in biotechnology, nanomedicine, and pharmacognosy has led to the development of better formulations able to bypass the drawbacks of existing poorly bioavailable and unstable ones. In conclusion, the inclusion of terpenoid drugs in modern medicine could revolutionize disease prevention and treatment by creating natural multitargeted alternatives that are consistent with the current worldwide transition toward holistic personalized medicine.

References

Abdou A, Ennaji H, Maaghloud FE, El Azhary K, Badou A, Elmakssoudi A, Aboulmouhajir A, Ibenmoussa S, JamalEddine J, Dakir M (2024) In silico and in vivo anti-inflammatory effect of eugenol and acetyleugenol. Sci Afr 24:e02205

Aggarwal BB, Sundaram C, Malani N, Ichikawa H (2007) Curcumin: the Indian solid gold. Adv Exp Med Biol 595:1–75. https://doi.org/10.1007/978-0-387-46401-5_1

Ahsan H, Ahad A, Iqbal J, Siddiqui WA (2014) Pharmacological potential of tocotrienols: a review. Nutr Metab. https://doi.org/10.1186/1743-7075-11-52

Alagawany M, El-Hack M, Farag MR, Tiwari R, Dhama K (2015) Biological effects and modes of action of carvacrol in animal and poultry production and health-a review. Adv Anim Vet Sci 3(2s):73–84

Anandakumar P, Kamaraj S, Vanitha MK (2021) D-limonene: a multifunctional compound with potent therapeutic effects. J Food Biochem. https://doi.org/10.1111/jfbc.13566

Arulnangai R, Thabassoom HA, Banu HV, Thirugnanasambandham K, Ganesamoorthy R (2025) Recent developments on ursolic acid and its potential biological applications. Toxicol Rep 14:101900

Atalay S, Jarocka-Karpowicz I, Skrzydlewska E (2019) Antioxidative and anti-inflammatory properties of cannabidiol. Antioxidants (Basel) 9(1):21. https://doi.org/10.3390/antiox9010021. PMID: 31881765; PMCID: PMC7023045

Azevedo L, Ferraz R, Vieira M, Prudêncio C, Fernandes S (2025) Betulinic acid and obesity-related disorders. Front Pharmacol 16:1674713

Bagheri S, Salehi I, Ramezani-Aliakbari F, Kourosh-Arami M, Komaki A (2022) Neuroprotective effect of geraniol on neurological disorders: a review article. Mol Biol Rep 49(11):10865–10874. https://doi.org/10.1007/s11033-022-07755-w. Epub 2022 Jul 28 PMID: 35900613

Bar S, Kara M (2024) Linalool exerts antioxidant activity in a rat model of diabetes by increasing catalase activity without antihyperglycemic effect. Exp Ther Med 28(3):359. https://doi.org/10.3892/etm.2024.12648. PMID: 39071903; PMCID: PMC11273359

Barboza JN, da Silva Maia Bezerra Filho C, Silva RO, Medeiros JVR, de Sousa DP (2018) An overview on the anti-inflammatory potential and antioxidant profile of eugenol. Oxid Med Cell Longev 2018:3957262. https://doi.org/10.1155/2018/3957262. PMID: 30425782; PMCID: PMC6217746

Barzan M, Heydari M, Mirshekari-Jahangiri H, Firouzi H, Dastan M, Najafi M, Khaledi M, Nouri A, Shah-Abadi ME (2023) Carvacrol exerts anti-inflammatory, anti-oxidative stress and hepatoprotective effects against diclofenac-induced liver injury in male rats. Int J Prev Med 14(1):61

Beninca T, Schmidt L, Cardoso LT, Augusti PR, da Silva Malheiros P (2024) Carvacrol as a food additive: toxicological aspects and the role of nanotechnology in enhancing its antimicrobial and antioxidant properties. Food Res Int 197:115256

Breitmaier E (2006) Terpenes: flavors, fragrances, pharmaca, pheromones. Wiley-VCH

Burcu GB, Osman C, Aslı C, Namik OM, Neşe BT (2016) The protective cardiac effects of B-myrcene after global cerebral ıschemia/reperfusion in C57BL/J6 mouse. Acta Cir Bras 31(7):456–462. https://doi.org/10.1590/S0102-865020160070000005. PMID: 27487280

Cai ZM, Peng JQ, Chen Y, Tao L, Zhang YY, Fu LY, De Long Q, Shen XC (2021) 1,8-cineole: a review of source, biological activities, and application. J Asian Nat Prod Res. https://doi.org/10.1080/10286020.2020.1839432

Câmara JS, Perestrelo R, Ferreira R, Berenguer CV, Pereira JAM, Castilho PC (2024) Plant-derived terpenoids: a plethora of bioactive compounds with several health functions and industrial applications—a comprehensive overview. Molecules 29. https://doi.org/10.3390/molecules29163861

Cárdeno A, Aparicio-Soto M, Montserrat-de la Paz S, Bermúdez B, Muriana FJ, Alarcón-de-la-Lastra C (2015) Squalene targets pro-and anti-inflammatory mediators and pathways to modulate over-activation of neutrophils, monocytes and macrophages. J Funct Foods 14:779–790

Carson CF, Hammer KA, Riley TV (2006) Melaleuca alternifolia (tea tree) oil: a review of antimicrobial and other medicinal properties. Clin Microbiol Rev 19(1):50–62. https://doi.org/10.1128/CMR.19.1.50-62.2006

Checker R, Patwardhan RS, Sharma D, Menon J, Thoh M, Bhilwade HN, Konishi T, Sandur SK (2012) Schisandrin B exhibits anti-inflammatory activity through modulation of the redoxsensitive transcription factors Nrf2 and NF-κB. Free Radic Biol Med 53(7):1421–1430

Chen W, Viljoen AM (2022) Geraniol – a review update. S Afr J Bot 150:1205–1219

Chen Y, Ba L, Huang W, Liu Y, Pan H, Mingyao E, Shi P, Wang Y, Li S, Qi H, Sun H (2017) Role of carvacrol in cardioprotection against myocardial ischemia/reperfusion injury in rats through activation of MAPK/ERK and Akt/eNOS signaling pathways. Eur J Pharmacol 796:90–100

Cherng JM, Shieh DE, Chiang W, Chang MY, Chiang LC (2007) Chemopreventive effects of minor dietary constituents in common foods on human cancer cells. Biosci Biotechnol Biochem 71(6):1500–1504

Cicalău GIP, Babes PA, Calniceanu H, Popa A, Ciavoi G, Iova GM, Ganea M, Scrobotă I (2021) Anti-inflammatory and antioxidant properties of carvacrol and magnolol, in periodontal disease and diabetes mellitus. Molecules 26(22):6899. https://doi.org/10.3390/molecules26226899. PMID: 34833990; PMCID: PMC8623889

Cidon EU, Ballesteros A (2016) Paclitaxel: taxol. In: The easy book of cancer pharmacology. https://doi.org/10.1056/nejm199504133321507

Cragg GM, Newman DJ (2005) Plants as a source of anti-cancer agents. J Ethnopharmacol 100(1–2):72–79. https://doi.org/10.1016/j.jep.2005.05.011

Crespo R, Wei K, Rodenak-Kladniew B, Mercola M, Ruiz-Lozano P, Hurtado C (2017) Effect of geraniol on rat cardiomyocytes and its potential use as a cardioprotective natural compound. Life Sci 172:8–12. https://doi.org/10.1016/j.lfs.2017.01.008. Epub 2017 Jan 25 PMID: 28131760

d'Alessio PA, Ostan R, Bisson J-F, Schulzke JD, Ursini MV, Béné MC (2013) Oral administration of d-limonene controls inflammation in rat colitis and displays anti-inflammatory properties as diet supplementation in humans. Life Sci 92(24–26):1151–1156. https://doi.org/10.1016/j.lfs.2013.04.013

Dalavaye N, Nicholas M, Pillai M, Erridge S, Sodergen MH (2023) The clinical translation of α-humulene – a scoping review. Planta Med:664–674. https://doi.org/10.1055/a-2307-8183

Das R, Lami MS, Chakraborty AJ, Mitra S, Tallei TE, Idroes R, Mohamed AA, Hossain MJ, Dhama K, Mostafa-Hedeab G, Emran TB (2022) Ginkgo biloba: a treasure of functional phytochemicals with multimedicinal applications. Evid Based Complement Alternat Med 2022(1):8288818

de Araújo-Filho HG, dos Santos JF, Carvalho MTB, Picot L, Fruitier-Arnaudin I, Groult H, Quintans-Júnior LJ, Quintans JSS (2021) Anticancer activity of limonene: a systematic review of target signaling pathways. Phytother Res. https://doi.org/10.1002/ptr.7125

de Faveri Favero F, Basting RT, de Freitas AS, Rabelo LD, Nonato FR, Zafred RR, de Oliveira Sousa IM, Queiroz ND, Napimoga JT, de Carvalho JE, Foglio MA (2024) Artemisinin and deoxyartemisinin isolated from Artemisia annua L. promote distinct antinociceptive and anti-inflammatory effects in an animal model. Biomed Pharmacother 178:117299

Del Prado-Audelo ML, Cortés H, Caballero-Florán IH, González-Torres M, Escutia-Guadarrama L, Bernal-Chávez SA, Giraldo-Gomez DM, Magaña JJ, Leyva-Gómez G (2021) Therapeutic applications of terpenes on inflammatory diseases. Front Pharmacol. https://doi.org/10.3389/fphar.2021.704197

Delmondes GDA, Santiago Lemos IC, Dias DDQ, Da Cunha GL, Araújo IM, Barbosa R, Coutinho HDM, Felipe CFB, Barbosa-Filho JM, De Lima NTR, De Menezes IRA, Kerntopf MR (2020) Pharmacological applications of farnesol (C15H26O): a patent review. Expert Opin Ther Pat. https://doi.org/10.1080/13543776.2020.1718653

Devi M, Bamrah PK, Goyal R, Choudhary M, Chopra H (2024) Insights on the emerging therapeutic potential of terpenoids as anti-inflammatory agents: a scoping review. J Bio-X Res 7. https://doi.org/10.34133/jbioxresearch.0006

Diniz LRL, Calado LL, Duarte ABS, de Sousa DP (2023) Centella asiatica and its metabolite Asiatic acid: wound healing effects and therapeutic potential. Metabolites. 13(2):276. https://doi.org/10.3390/metabo13020276

Dong X, Wang T, Gao C, Cui Y, Li L (2025) Multi-target pharmacological effects of Asiatic acid: advances in structural modification and novel drug delivery systems. Molecules (Basel, Switzerland) 30:1–37. https://doi.org/10.3390/molecules30183688

dos Santos ÉRQ, Maia JGS, Fontes-Júnior EA, do Socorro Ferraz Maia C (2021) Linalool as a therapeutic and medicinal tool in depression treatment: a review. Curr Neuropharmacol. https://doi.org/10.2174/1570159x19666210920094504

Du J, Liu D, Zhang X, Zhou A, Su Y, He D, Fu S, Gao F (2020) Menthol protects dopaminergic neurons against inflammation-mediated damage in lipopolysaccharide (LPS)-evoked model of Parkinson's disease. Int Immunopharmacol 85:106679

E Silva GD, de Jesus Marques JN, Linhares EP, Bonora CM, Costa ET, Saraiva MF (2022) Review of anticancer activity of monoterpenoids: geraniol, nerol, geranial and neral. Chem Biol Interact 362:109994

Eddin LB, Jha NK, Goyal SN, Agrawal YO, Subramanya SB, Bastaki SMA, Ojha S (2022) Health benefits, pharmacological effects, molecular mechanisms, and therapeutic potential of α-bisabolol. Nutrients 14(7):1370. https://doi.org/10.3390/nu14071370. PMID: 35405982; PMCID: PMC9002489

Efferth T, Koch E (2011) Complex interactions between phytochemicals: the multi-target therapeutic concept of phytotherapy. Curr Drug Targets 12(1):122–132. https://doi.org/10.2174/138945011793591626

El Boukhari R, Fatimi A (2024) Patent landscape and applications of organic menthol crystals: An in-depth analysis of emerging trends and industrial applications. Chem Proc 15(1):2. https://doi.org/10.3390/chemproc2024015002

El-Marasy SA, El Awdan SA, Hassan A, Abdallah HMI (2020) Cardioprotective effect of thymol against adrenaline-induced myocardial injury in rats. Heliyon 6(7):e04431. https://doi.org/10.1016/j.heliyon.2020.e04431. PMID: 32715125; PMCID: PMC7378581

Fajdek-Bieda A, Pawlińska J, Wróblewska A, Żwierełło W, Łuś A, Michalska A (2025a) Antibacterial and anticancer properties of geraniol in the context of clinical applications. Appl Sci 15(17):9669. https://doi.org/10.3390/app15179669

Fajdek-Bieda A, Pawlińska J, Wróblewska A, Żwierełło W, Łuś A, Klimowicz A (2025b) Antibacterial and preservative potential of eugenol and isoeugenol in cosmetics: a natural solution for product stability. Appl Sci 15(4):2129. https://doi.org/10.3390/app15042129

Feng Y, An Q, Zhao Z, Wu M, Yang C, Liang WY, Xu X, Jiang T, Zhang G (2024) Beta-elemene: a phytochemical with promise as a drug candidate for tumor therapy and adjuvant tumor therapy. Biomed Pharmacother. https://doi.org/10.1016/j.biopha.2024.116266

Fonsêca DV, Salgado PR, de Carvalho FL, Salvadori MG, Penha AR, Leite FC, Borges CJ, Piuvezam MR, Pordeus LC, Sousa DP, Almeida RN (2016 Feb) Nerolidol exhibits antinociceptive and anti-inflammatory activity: involvement of the GABA ergic system and proinflammatory cytokines. Fundam Clin Pharmacol 30(1):14–22

Francomano F, Caruso A, Barbarossa A, Fazio A, La Torre C, Ceramella J, Mallamaci R, Saturnino C, Iacopetta D, Sinicropi MS (2019) β-caryophyllene: a sesquiterpene with countless biological properties. Appl Sci (Switz). https://doi.org/10.3390/app9245420

Gershenzon J, Dudareva N (2007) The function of terpene natural products in the natural world. Nat Chem Biol 3(7):408–414. https://doi.org/10.1038/nchembio.2007.5

Gertsch J, Leonti M, Raduner S, Racz I, Chen J-Z, Xie X-Q, Altmann K-H, Karsak M (2008) Beta-caryophyllene is a dietary cannabinoid. Proc Natl Acad Sci 105(26):9099–9104. https://doi.org/10.1073/pnas.0803601105

Graebin CS (2018) The pharmacological activities of glycyrrhizinic acid ("glycyrrhizin") and glycyrrhetinic acid. In: Reference series in phytochemistry. Springer, Cham. https://doi.org/10.1007/978-3-319-27027-2_15

Guan X, Li X, Yang X, Yan J, Shi P, Ba L, Cao Y, Wang P (2019) The neuroprotective effects of carvacrol on ischemia/reperfusion-induced hippocampal neuronal impairment by ferroptosis mitigation. Life Sci 235:116795

Hafsan H, Saleh MM, Zabibah RS, Obaid RF, Jabbar HS, Mustafa YF, Sultan MQ, Gabr GA, Ramírez-Coronel AA, Khodadadi M, Dadras M (2022) Dietary thymol improved growth, body composition, digestive enzyme activities, hematology, immunity, antioxidant defense, and resistance to Streptococcus iniae in the rainbow trout (Oncorhynchus mykiss). Aquac Nutr 2022:3288139. https://doi.org/10.1155/2022/3288139. PMID: 36860433; PMCID: PMC9973134

Henry R (2014) Etymologia. Emerg Infect Dis. https://doi.org/10.3201/eid2007.ET2007

Ho WE, Peh HY, Chan TK, Wong WSF (2014) Artemisinins: pharmacological actions beyond anti-malarial. Pharmacol Ther. https://doi.org/10.1016/j.pharmthera.2013.12.001

Hoca M, Becer E, Vatansever HS (2024) Carvacrol is potential molecule for diabetes treatment. Arch Physiol Biochem 130(6):823–830. https://doi.org/10.1080/13813455.2023.2288537. Epub 2023 Nov 29 PMID: 38019023

Huang ZR, Lin YK, Fang JY (2009) Biological and pharmacological activities of squalene and related compounds: potential uses in cosmetic dermatology. Molecules 14(1):540–554. https://doi.org/10.3390/molecules14010540. PMID: 19169201; PMCID: PMC6253993

Hucklenbroich J, Klein R, Neumaier B, Graf R, Fink GR, Schroeter M, Rueger MA (2014) Aromatic-turmerone induces neural stem cell proliferation in vitro and in vivo. Stem Cell Res Ther 5(4):100. https://doi.org/10.1186/scrt500

Ibrahim N'I, Fairus S, Zulfarina MS, Naina Mohamed I (2020) The efficacy of squalene in cardiovascular disease risk-a systematic review. Nutrients 12(2):414. https://doi.org/10.3390/nu12020414

Iwasaki K, Zheng YW, Murata S, Ito H, Nakayama K, Kurokawa T, Sano N, Nowatari T, Villareal MO, Nagano YN, Isoda H, Matsui H, Ohkohchi N (2016) Anticancer effect of linalool via cancer-specific hydroxyl radical generation in human colon cancer. World J Gastroenterol 22(44):9765–9774. https://doi.org/10.3748/wjg.v22.i44.9765. PMID: 27956800; PMCID: PMC5124981

Javed H, Azimullah S, Meeran MFN, Ansari SA, Ojha S (2019) Neuroprotective effects of thymol, a dietary monoterpene against dopaminergic neurodegeneration in rotenone-induced rat model of Parkinson's disease. Int J Mol Sci 20(7):1538. https://doi.org/10.3390/ijms20071538. PMID: 30934738; PMCID: PMC6480243

Judžentienė A, Pečiulytė D, Nedveckytė I (2024) In situ antimicrobial properties of sabinene hydrate, a secondary plant metabolite. Molecules 29. https://doi.org/10.3390/molecules29174252

Jung YY, Hwang ST, Sethi G, Fan L, Arfuso F, Ahn KS (2018) Potential anti-inflammatory and anti-cancer properties of farnesol. Molecules 23(11):2827. https://doi.org/10.3390/molecules23112827. PMID: 30384444; PMCID: PMC6278318

Kalantari K, Moniri M, Moghaddam AB, Rahim RA, Ariff AB, Izadiyan Z, Mohamad R (2017) A review of the biomedical applications of zerumbone and the techniques for its extraction from ginger rhizomes. Molecules. https://doi.org/10.3390/molecules22101645

Kashyap D, Sharma A, Tuli HS, Punia S, Sharma AK (2016) Ursolic acid and oleanolic acid: pentacyclic terpenoids with promising anti-inflammatory activities. Recent Patents Inflamm Allergy Drug Discov 10(1):21–33. https://doi.org/10.2174/1872213X10666160711143904

Kasper S, Gastpar M, Müller WE, Volz HP, Möller HJ, Dienel A, Schläfke S (2010) Efficacy and safety of silexan, a new, orally administered lavender oil preparation, in subthreshold anxiety disorder–evidence from clinical trials. Wien Med Wochenschr 160(21):547–556

Katsura H, Tsukiyama RI, Suzuki A, Kobayashi M (2001) In vitro antimicrobial activities of bakuchiol against oral microorganisms. Antimicrob Agents Chemother 45(11):3009–3013

Kim JH, Lee R, Hwang SH, Choi SH, Kim JH, Cho IH, Lee JI, Nah SY (2024a) Ginseng and ginseng byproducts for skincare and skin health. J Ginseng Res 48(6):525–534

Kim H, Kang S, Go GW (2024b) Exploring the multifaceted role of ginkgolides and bilobalide from Ginkgo biloba in mitigating metabolic disorders. Food Sci Biotechnol 33:2903–2917. https://doi.org/10.1007/s10068-024-01656-3

Koulivand PH, KhaleghiGhadiri M, Gorji A (2013) Lavender and the nervous system. Evid Based Complement Alternat Med 2013:681304. https://doi.org/10.1155/2013/681304

Kumar V (2025) A comprehensive review of risk factors, diagnosis, and treatment options for oral squamous cell carcinoma. Curr Cancer Ther Rev 21:1–8. https://doi.org/10.2174/0115733947379301250703053245

Lapczynski A, Bhatia SP, Foxenberg RJ, Letizia CS, Api AM (2008) Fragrance material review on geraniol. Food Chem Toxicol 46(11):S160–S170

Lei Y, Fu P, Jun X, Cheng P (2019) Pharmacological properties of geraniol-a review. Planta Med. https://doi.org/10.1055/a-0750-6907

Li Y, Lv O, Zhou F, Li Q, Wu Z, Zheng Y (2015) Linalool inhibits LPS-induced inflammation in BV2 microglia cells by activating Nrf2. Neurochem Res 40(7):1520–1525

Li W, Zeng H, Xu M, Huang C, Tao L, Li J, Zhang T, Chen H, Xia J, Li C, Li X (2021) Oleanolic acid improves obesity-related inflammation and insulin resistance by regulating macrophages activation. Front Pharmacol 12:697483

Li Z, Zhang H, Wang Y, Li Y, Li Q, Zhang L (2022) The distinctive role of menthol in pain and analgesia: mechanisms, practices, and advances. Front Mol Neurosci. https://doi.org/10.3389/fnmol.2022.1006908

Liang JH, Yu H, Xia CP, Zheng YH, Zhang Z, Chen Y, Raza MA, Wu L, Yan H (2024) Ginkgolide B effectively mitigates neuropathic pain by suppressing the activation of the NLRP3 inflammasome through the induction of mitophagy in rats. Biomed Pharmacother 177:117006

Lim HS, Kim YJ, Kim BY, Jeong SJ (2019) Bakuchiol suppresses inflammatory responses via the downregulation of the p38 MAPK/ERK signaling pathway. Int J Mol Sci 20(14):3574. https://doi.org/10.3390/ijms20143574. PMID: 31336605; PMCID: PMC6678636

Lin YM, Badrealam KF, Kuo WW, Lai PF, Shao-Tsu Chen W, Hsuan Day C, Ho TJ, Viswanadha VP, Shibu MA, Huang CY (2021) Nerolidol improves cardiac function in spontaneously hypertensive rats by inhibiting cardiac inflammation and remodelling associated TLR4/ NF-κB signalling cascade. Food Chem Toxicol 147:111837. https://doi.org/10.1016/j.fct.2020.111837. Epub 2020 Nov 17 PMID: 33212213

Liu B, Liu Y, Yang G, Xu Z, Chen J (2013) Ursolic acid induces neural regeneration after sciatic nerve injury. Neural Regen Res 8(27):2510–2519. https://doi.org/10.3969/j.issn.1673-5374.2013.27.002. PMID: 25206561; PMCID: PMC4145935

Liu J, Geng Z, Zhang Y, Alharbi SA, Shi Y (2021a) Sesquiterpenoid bilobalide inhibits gastric carcinoma cell growth and induces apoptosis both in vitro and in vivo models. J Biochem Mol Toxicol 35(5):e22723. https://doi.org/10.1002/jbt.22723. Epub 2021 Jan 28 PMID: 33511709

Liu M-Y, Liu F, Gao Y-L, Yin J-N, Yan W-Q, Liu J-G, Li H-J (2021b) Pharmacological activities of ginsenoside Rg5 (review). Exp Ther Med. https://doi.org/10.3892/etm.2021.10272

Liu KM, Huang Y, Wan PP, Lu YH, Zhou N, Li JJ, Yu CY, Chou JJ, Zhang L, Zhang C, Qiang YY (2022) Ursolic acid protects neurons in temporal lobe epilepsy and cognitive impairment by repressing inflammation and oxidation. Front Pharmacol 13:877898

Liu Q, Ding X, Wang Y, Chu H, Guan Y, Li M, Sun K (2024) Artemisinin reduces PTSD-like symptoms, improves synaptic plasticity, and inhibits apoptosis in rats subjected to single prolonged stress. Front Pharmacol. 15:1303123. https://doi.org/10.3389/fphar.2024.1303123.

Erratum in: Front Pharmacol 2024 Jun 18;15:1427681. doi:10.3389/fphar.2024.1427681. PMID: 38379899; PMCID: PMC10876839
Liu XY, Nie YK, Liu Y, Chen M (2025) Cardiovascular protective properties of the natural product eugenol. Eur J Pharmacol:177929
Lou H, Li H, Zhang S, Lu H, Chen Q (2021) A review on preparation of betulinic acid and its biological activities. Molecules. https://doi.org/10.3390/molecules26185583
Lv H, Qi Z, Wang S, Feng H, Deng X, Ci X (2017a) Asiatic acid exhibits anti-inflammatory and antioxidant activities against lipopolysaccharide and d-Galactosamine-induced fulminant hepatic failure. Front Immunol 8:785. https://doi.org/10.3389/fimmu.2017.00785. PMID: 28736552; PMCID: PMC5500632
Lv Y, Zhang L, Li N, Mai N, Zhang Y, Pan S (2017b) Geraniol promotes functional recovery and attenuates neuropathic pain in rats with spinal cord injury. Can J Physiol Pharmacol 95(12):1389–1395. https://doi.org/10.1139/cjpp-2016-0528. Epub 2017 Mar 23 PMID: 28334550
Ma LT, Bai Y, Cao P, Ren KX, Chen J, Zhang T, Fan BY, Qiao Y, Yan HY, Wang JJ, Li YQ, Zheng J (2022) The analgesic effects of β-elemene in rats with neuropathic pain by inhibition of spinal astrocytic ERK activation. Mol Pain 18:17448069221121562. https://doi.org/10.1177/17448069221121562. PMID: 35976914; PMCID: PMC9393702
Masyita A, Mustika Sari R, Dwi Astuti A, Yasir B, Rahma Rumata N, Emran TB, Nainu F, Simal-Gandara J (2022) Terpenes and terpenoids as main bioactive compounds of essential oils, their roles in human health and potential application as natural food preservatives. Food Chemistry: X. https://doi.org/10.1016/j.fochx.2022.100217
McDougall JJ, Reid AR (2022) Joint damage and neuropathic pain in rats treated with lysophosphatidic acid. Front Immunol 13:811402
Mochtar CF (2025) Therapeutic potential of eugenol for muscle pain management in athletes: a scoping review. J Basic Med Vet 14(1):89–103
Mohamed ME, Abduldaium MS, Younis NS (2021) Cardioprotective effect of linalool against isoproterenol-induced myocardial infarction. Life (Basel) 11(2):120. https://doi.org/10.3390/life11020120. PMID: 33562483; PMCID: PMC7915311
Momtazi-Borojeni AA, Esmaeili S-A, Abdollahi E, Sahebkar A (2016) A review on the pharmacology and toxicology of Steviol glycosides extracted from Stevia rebaudiana. Curr Pharm Des. https://doi.org/10.2174/1381612822666161021142835
Nagarajan A, Doss VA (2023) Antihypertrophic effect of menthol from Mentha x Piperita concerning cardiac hypertrophy: a review. Nat Prod J 13(2):40–54
Nagoor Meeran MF, Javed H, Al Taee H, Azimullah S, Ojha SK (2017) Pharmacological properties and molecular mechanisms of thymol: prospects for its therapeutic potential and pharmaceutical development. Front Pharmacol. https://doi.org/10.3389/fphar.2017.00380
Nazzaro F, Fratianni F, De Martino L, Coppola R, De Feo V (2013) Effect of essential oils on pathogenic bacteria. Pharmaceuticals 6(12):1451–1474. https://doi.org/10.3390/ph6121451
Nie L, Qiu Y, Chen X, Zheng P, Luo Y, Yu B, Chen D, Huang Z (2025) Dietary supplementation with eugenol modulates lipid metabolism in finishing pigs through the TRPV1/AMPK signaling pathway. J Nutr Biochem:110027
Nisar R, Inamullah A, Ghalib AUF, Nisar H, Sarkaki A, Afzal A, Tariq M, Batool Z, Haider S (2024) Geraniol mitigates anxiety-like behaviors in rats by reducing oxidative stress, repairing impaired hippocampal neurotransmission, and normalizing brain cortical-EEG wave patterns after a single electric foot-shock exposure. Biomed Pharmacother 176:116771. https://doi.org/10.1016/j.biopha.2024.116771. Epub 2024 May 24 PMID: 38795639
Nizam NN, Mahmud S, Ark SMA, Kamruzzaman M, Hasan MK (2023) Bakuchiol, a natural constituent and its pharmacological benefits. F1000Res 12:29. https://doi.org/10.12688/f1000research.129072.2. PMID: 38021404; PMCID: PMC10683784
Oliveira-Costa JF, Meira CS, Neves MV, Dos Reis BP, Soares MB (2022) Anti-inflammatory activities of betulinic acid: a review. Front Pharmacol 13:883857

Paduch R, Kandefer-Szerszeń M, Trytek M, Fiedurek J (2007) Terpenes: substances useful in human healthcare. Arch Immunol Ther Exp 55(5):315–327. https://doi.org/10.1007/s00005-007-0039-1

Paik S, Song GY, Jo EK (2023) Ginsenosides for therapeutically targeting inflammation through modulation of oxidative stress. Int Immunopharmacol 121:110461

Pandey SK, Nanda A, Gautam AS, Singh RK (2025) Betulinic acid protects against lipopolysaccharide and ferrous sulfate-induced oxidative stress, ferroptosis, apoptosis, and neuroinflammation signaling relevant to Parkinson's disease. Free Radic Biol Med (233):340–354

Papadopoulos V, Kapsis A, Li H, Amri H, Hardwick M, Culty M, Kasprzyk PG, Carlson M, Moreau JP, Drieu K (2000) Drug-induced inhibition of the peripheral-type benzodiazepine receptor expression and cell proliferation in human breast cancer cells. Anticancer Res 20(5A):2835–2847

Park BB, An JY, Park SU (2021) Recent studies on pinene and its biological and pharmacological activities. EXCLI J. https://doi.org/10.17179/EXCLI2021-3714

Parmar SA, Mayasa V, Nelson VK, Divecha J (2024) A systemic review of ginseng and its activity on coronary heart disease. Pharmacol Res-Mod Chin Med 12:100480

Passeron T, Namiki T, Passeron HJ, Le Pape E, Hearing VJ (2009) Forskolin protects keratinocytes from UVB-induced apoptosis and increases DNA repair independent of its effects on melanogenesis. J Invest Dermatol 129(1):162–166. https://doi.org/10.1038/jid.2008.182. Epub 2008 Jun 26. PMID: 18580960; PMCID: PMC2654621

Patel T, Ishiuji Y, Yosipovitch G (2007) Menthol: a refreshing look at this ancient compound. J Am Acad Dermatol 57(5):873–878. https://doi.org/10.1016/j.jaad.2007.04.008

Pateraki I, Andersen-Ranberg J, Jensen NB, Wubshet SG, Heskes AM, Forman V, Hallström B, Hamberger B, Motawia MS, Olsen CE, Staerk D, Hansen J, Møller BL, Hamberger B (2017) Total biosynthesis of the cyclic AMP booster forskolin from Coleus forskohlii. Elife. https://doi.org/10.7554/eLife.23001

Peh HY, Tan WSD, Liao W, Wong WSF (2016) Vitamin E therapy beyond cancer: tocopherol versus tocotrienol. Pharmacol Ther. https://doi.org/10.1016/j.pharmthera.2015.12.003

Prerna, Chadha J, Khullar L, Mudgil U, Harjai K (2024) A comprehensive review on the pharmacological prospects of Terpinen-4-ol: from nature to medicine and beyond. Fitoterapia 176:4–11. https://doi.org/10.1016/j.fitote.2024.106051

Putriana NA, Husni P, Mita SR (2024) Recent advance Bakuchiol application as a potential alternative to retinol in skincare and cosmetics

Riaz R, Younis W, Uttra AM, Malik MN, Manzoor W, Qasim S, Hasan UH, Mushtaq MN, Kluck AJ, dos Reis Lívero FA, Junior AG (2025) Anti-arthritic and anti-inflammatory activity of linalool against formaldehyde and complete Freund's adjuvant induced arthritis in rats. Biochem Biophys Res Commun 752:151462

Roohbakhsh A, Parhiz H, Soltani F, Rezaee R, Iranshahi M (2015) Molecular mechanisms behind the biological effects of hesperidin and hesperetin for the prevention of cardiovascular diseases. Life Sci 124:64–74. https://doi.org/10.1016/j.lfs.2014.12.030

Roudi HS, Safaei R, Dabbaghi MM, Fadaei MS, Saberifar M, Sakhaee K, Rahimi VB, Askari VR (2025) Mechanistic insights on cardioprotective properties of ursolic acid: regulation of mitochondrial and non-mitochondrial pathways. Curr Pharm Des 31(13):1037–1056. https://doi.org/10.2174/0113816128344497241120025757. PMID: 39710917

Rozza AL, Beserra FP, Vieira AJ, Oliveira de Souza E, Hussni CA, Martinez ERM, Nóbrega RH, Pellizzon CH (2021) The use of menthol in skin wound healing-anti-inflammatory potential, antioxidant defense system stimulation and increased epithelialization. Pharmaceutics 13(11):1902. https://doi.org/10.3390/pharmaceutics13111902. PMID: 34834317; PMCID: PMC8620938

Saifullah M, Mahmood T, Ahsan F, Bano S, Zaidi SMH, Khan MMU (2025) Cardioprotective potential of d-limonene against isoproterenol induced myocardial infarction in rats. Cell Biochem Biophys 83(2):2389–2403. https://doi.org/10.1007/s12013-024-01649-3. Epub 2024 Dec 31 PMID: 39738843

Sapkota A, Choi JW (2022) Oleanolic acid provides neuroprotection against ischemic stroke through the inhibition of microglial activation and NLRP3 inflammasome activation. Biomol Ther Seoul 30(1):55–63. https://doi.org/10.4062/biomolther.2021.154. PMID: 34873072; PMCID: PMC8724842

Shahnouri M, Abouhosseini Tabari M, Araghi A (2016) Neuropharmacological properties of farnesol in Murine model. Iran J Vet Res. 17(4):259–264. PMID: 28224010; PMCID: PMC5309458

Shahrokhi Raeini A, Hafizibarjin Z, Rezvani ME, Safari F, Afkhami Aghda F, Zare MF (2020) Carvacrol suppresses learning and memory dysfunction and hippocampal damages caused by chronic cerebral hypoperfusion. Naunyn Schmiedeberg's Arch Pharmacol 393(4):581–589

Sharma S, Vasudeva N, Hooda T (2024) Neuroprotective effects of oleanolic acid against secondary cascades of traumatic brain injury in mice. Brain Disorders 16:100173

Siddiqua A, Malik A, Iqbal U, Sial NT, Mehmood MH, Rehman MFU (2025) Antioxidative and anti-inflammatory effects of Carvacrol against polycystic ovary syndrome associated complications using high fat diet and Letrozole challenged rat model: a multidisciplinary study cascading in vivo, in vitro, in silico and network pharmacology approaches. Inflammopharmacology 33:1–22

Silva FS, Oliveira PJ, Duarte MF (2016) Oleanolic, ursolic, and betulinic acids as food supplements or pharmaceutical agents for type 2 diabetes: promise or illusion? J Agric Food Chem 64(15):2991–3008

Singh J, Luqman S, Meena A (2023) Carvacrol as a prospective regulator of cancer targets/signalling pathways. Curr Mol Pharmacol 16(5):542–558. https://doi.org/10.2174/1874467215666220705142954. PMID: 35792130

Smith JV, Luo Y (2004) Studies on molecular mechanisms of Ginkgo biloba extract. Appl Microbiol Biotechnol 64(4):465–472. https://doi.org/10.1007/s00253-003-1527-9

Su YW, Chao SH, Lee MH, Ou TY, Tsai YC (2010) Inhibitory effects of citronellol and geraniol on nitric oxide and prostaglandin E_2production in macrophages. Planta Med 76(15):1666–1671. https://doi.org/10.1055/s-0030-1249947. Epub 2010 May 26 PMID: 20506077

Su Q, Dong J, Zhang D, Yang L, Roy R (2022) Protective effects of the bilobalide on retinal oxidative stress and inflammation in streptozotocin-induced diabetic rats. Appl Biochem Biotechnol 194(12):6407–6422. https://doi.org/10.1007/s12010-022-04012-5. Epub 2022 Aug 6 PMID: 35932369

Subramaniyan J, Krishnan G, Balan R, Mgj D, Ramasamy E, Ramalingam S, Veerabathiran R, Thandavamoorthy P, Mani GK, Thiruvengadam D (2014) Carvacrol modulates instability of xenobiotic metabolizing enzymes and downregulates the expressions of PCNA, MMP-2, and MMP-9 during diethylnitrosamine-induced hepatocarcinogenesis in rats. Mol Cell Biochem 395(1):65–76

Subramaniam N, Poptani H, Schache A, Bhat V, Iyer S, Sunil HV, Chandrasekhar NH, Pillai V, Chaturvedi P, Krishna SH, Krishnamurthy A, Kekatpure V, Kuriakose MA, Iyer NG, Thakkar A, Kantharia R, Sonkar A, Shetty V, Rangappa VB, Kolur T, Vidhyadharan S, Murthy SP, Kudpaje A, Srinivasalu VK, Mahajan A (2021) Imaging advances in oral cavity cancer and perspectives from a population in need: consensus from the UK-India Oral Cancer Imaging Group. J Head Neck Physicians Surg 9:10.4103/jhnps.jhnps_10_21

Sun W, Xu G, Guo X, Luo G, Wu L, Hou Y, Guo X, Zhou J, Xu T, Qin L, Fan Y, Han L, Matsabisa M, Ma X, Liu T (2017) Protective effects of asiatic acid in a spontaneous type 2 diabetic mouse model. Mol Med Rep 16(2):1333–1339. https://doi.org/10.3892/mmr.2017.6684. Epub 2017 Jun 2. PMID: 28586016; PMCID: PMC5562101

Sun M, Sheng Y, Zhu Y (2021) Ginkgolide B alleviates the inflammatory response and attenuates the activation of LPS-induced BV2 cells in vitro and in vivo. Exp Ther Med 21(6):586. https://doi.org/10.3892/etm.2021.10018. Epub 2021 Apr 2. PMID: 33850558; PMCID: PMC8027720

Surendran S, Qassadi F, Surendran G, Lilley D, Heinrich M (2021) Myrcene—what are the potential health benefits of this flavouring and aroma agent? Front Nutr. https://doi.org/10.3389/fnut.2021.699666

Tang P, Liu S, Zhang J et al (2024) Ginsenosides as dietary supplements with immunomodulatory effects: a review. Appl Biol Chem 67:27. https://doi.org/10.1186/s13765-024-00881-y

Tareen FK, Catenacci L, Perteghella S, Sorrenti M, Bonferoni MC (2024) Carvacrol essential oil as a neuroprotective agent: a review of the study designs and recent advances. Molecules 30(1):104. https://doi.org/10.3390/molecules30010104. PMID: 39795159; PMCID: PMC11721141

Tu Y (2011) The discovery of artemisinin (qinghaosu) and gifts from Chinese medicine. Nat Med 17(10):1217–1220. https://doi.org/10.1038/nm.2471

Uppin V, Zarei M, Acharya P, Nair D, Kempaiah B, Talahalli R (2024) Zerumbone exhibits anti-inflammatory effects by suppressing eicosanoid signaling: evidence from LPS-induced peripheral blood leukocytes. Prostaglandins & Other Lipid Mediators 173:106852

Usta J, Kreydiyyeh S, Knio K, Barnabe P, Bou-Moughlabay Y, Dagher S (2009) Linalool decreases HepG2 viability by inhibiting mitochondrial complexes I and II, increasing reactive oxygen species and decreasing ATP and GSH levels. Chem Biol Interact 180(1):39–46

Vieira AJ, Beserra FP, Souza MC, Totti BM, Rozza AL (2018) Limonene: aroma of innovation in health and disease. Chem Biol Interact 283:97–106

Wang X, Shao QH, Zhou H, Wu JL, Quan WQ, Ji P, Yao YW, Li D, Sun ZJ (2020) Ginkgolide B inhibits lung cancer cells promotion via beclin-1-dependent autophagy. BMC Complement Med Ther 20(1):194. https://doi.org/10.1186/s12906-020-02980-x. Retraction in: BMC Complement Med Ther 2023 Jul 20;23(1):251. doi:10.1186/s12906-023-04095-5. PMID: 32576183; PMCID: PMC7310550

Wang QS, Li M, Gao Y, Feng Y, Xu Y, Liu W, Zhang ZF, Ren JN, Yang J, Fan G, Pan S (2024a) Limonene alleviates hepatic lipid accumulation by regulating fatty acids metabolism: insights from the transcriptome. Food Biosci 62:105391

Wang W, Xue Y, Li D, Shao C, Wu K, Sun N, Chen Q (2024b) Forskolin is an effective therapeutic small molecule for the treatment of hypertrophic cardiomyopathy through ADCY6/cAMP/PKA pathway. Eur J Pharmacol 978:176770

Wasim M, Bergonzi MC (2024) Unlocking the potential of oleanolic acid: integrating pharmacological insights and advancements in delivery systems. Pharmaceutics 16. https://doi.org/10.3390/pharmaceutics16060692

Weaver BA (2014) How taxol/paclitaxel kills cancer cells. Mol Biol Cell. https://doi.org/10.1091/mbc.E14-04-0916

Wen L, Chan BC-L, Qiu M-H, Leung P-C, Wong C-K (2024) Artemisinin and its derivatives as potential anticancer agents. Molecules 29(16):3886. https://doi.org/10.3390/molecules29163886

Wołosik KA, Knaś M, Zalewska A, Niczyporuk M, Przystupa AW (2013) The importance and perspective of plant-based squalene in cosmetology. J Cosmet Sci 64(1):59–66

Wu Z, Li Z, Liang Y (2022) Myrcene exerts anti-tumor effects on oral cancer cells in vitro via induction of apoptosis. Trop J Pharm Res 21(5):933–938

Xiang J, Yang F, Zhu W, Cai M, Li XT, Zhang JS, Yu ZH, Zhang W, Cai DF (2021) Bilobalide inhibits inflammation and promotes the expression of Aβ degrading enzymes in astrocytes to rescue neuronal deficiency in AD models. Transl Psychiatry 11(1):542

Yang W, Chen X, Li Y, Guo S, Wang Z, Yu X (2020) Advances in pharmacological activities of terpenoids. Nat Prod Commun 15(3):1–14. https://doi.org/10.1177/1934578X20903555

Yang H, Zhang Y, Cui J, Hao Z (2022) Apoptosis-mediated anticancer activity of geraniol inhibits NF-κB, MAPK, and JAK-STAT-3 signaling pathways in human thyroid cancer cells. Pharmacogn Mag 18(80)

Yu W, Liu Q, Zhu S (2013) Carvacrol protects against acute myocardial infarction of rats via anti-oxidative and anti-apoptotic pathways. Biol Pharm Bull 36(4):579–584

Yu X, Lin H, Wang Y, Lv W, Zhang S, Qian Y, Deng X, Feng N, Yu H, Qian B (2018) D-limonene exhibits antitumor activity by inducing autophagy and apoptosis in lung cancer. Onco Targets Ther 11:1833–1847. https://doi.org/10.2147/OTT.S155716. PMID: 29670359; PMCID: PMC5894671

Zanotti A, Baldino L, Scognamiglio M, Reverchon E (2023) Supercritical fluid extraction of essential oil and sclareol from a clary sage concrete. Molecules. https://doi.org/10.3390/molecules28093903

Zhao M, Qin J, Shen W, Wu A (2021) Bilobalide enhances AMPK activity to improve liver injury and metabolic disorders in STZ-induced diabetes in immature rats via regulating HMGB1/TLR4/NF-κB signaling pathway. BioMed Res Int 2021:8835408. https://doi.org/10.1155/2021/8835408. PMID: 33959665; PMCID: PMC8075671

Zhao M, Wu F, Tang Z, Yang X, Liu Y, Wang F, Chen B (2023a) Anti-inflammatory and antioxidant activity of ursolic acid: a systematic review and meta-analysis. Front Pharmacol 14:1256946. https://doi.org/10.3389/fphar.2023.1256946. PMID: 37841938; PMCID: PMC10568483

Zhao Y, Pan H, Liu W, Liu E, Pang Y, Gao H, He Q, Liao W, Yao Y, Zeng J, Guo J (2023b) Menthol: an underestimated anticancer agent. Front Pharmacol 14:1148790. https://doi.org/10.3389/fphar.2023.1148790. PMID: 37007039; PMCID: PMC10063798

Zhi Y, Pan J, Shen W, He P, Zheng J, Zhou X, Lu G, Chen Z, Zhou Z (2016) Ginkgolide B inhibits human bladder cancer cell migration and invasion through microRNA-223-3p. Cell Physiol Biochem 39(5):1787–1794

Zhou J, Xie X, Tang H, Peng C, Peng F (2022) The bioactivities of sclareol: a mini review. Front Pharmacol. https://doi.org/10.3389/fphar.2022.1014105

Zhou L, Tan F, Zhang X, Li Y, Yin W (2024) Neuroprotection and mechanisms of ginsenosides in nervous system diseases: progress and perspectives. IUBMB Life 76(11):862–882

Zhu PC, Tong Q, Zhuang Z, Wang ZH, Deng LH, Zheng GQ, Wang Y (2019) Ginkgolide B for myocardial ischemia/reperfusion injury: a preclinical systematic review and meta-analysis. Front Physiol 10:1292

Zulazmi NA, Gopalsamy B, Min JC, Farouk AA, Sulaiman MR, Bharatham BH, Perimal EK (2017) Zerumbone alleviates neuropathic pain through the involvement of l-arginine-nitric oxide-cGMP-K^+ ATP channel pathways in chronic constriction injury in mice model. Molecules 22(4):555. https://doi.org/10.3390/molecules22040555

Medicinal Plants for Sustainable Healthcare

Priti Jana, Suvechchha Jana, Melford Egbujor, Sankhadip Bose, and Subas Chandra Dinda

Abstract India has a vast and broad collection of medicinal plants that have long been used in its healthcare system, especially by rural and indigenous people. The application of medicinal plants that have their roots in traditional knowledge systems has made a significant contribution to sustainable healthcare by providing natural, affordable, and culturally appropriate treatment solutions. The ethnobotanical importance of medicinal plants in India is discussed in this review, which also highlights the plants' pharmacological potential and impact on sustainable healthcare practices. Because it is easily available and has lower side effects than synthetic alternatives, plant-based medicine is still used. However, the conservation and incorporation of traditional medical knowledge are endangered by issues including habitat degradation, overharvesting, and the requirement for scientific proof. Additionally, policy frameworks that ensure the standardization, control, and ethical use of medicinal plant resources are becoming more and more important to close the gap between traditional and modern healthcare systems. Solving these problems will increase the sustainable use of medicinal plants for future medical needs and at the same time help preserve indigenous knowledge. This article discusses the importance of maintaining ethnobotanical traditions, along with promoting the use of medicinal plants in a sustainable and science-supported modern healthcare system.

Keywords Medicinal plant · Sustainable healthcare · Conservation · Ethnobotany · Pharmacological activity · Biotechnological technique

P. Jana (✉) · S. Jana · S. Bose · S. C. Dinda
School of Pharmacy, The Neotia University, Sarisa, West Bengal, India
e-mail: subaschandra.dinda@tnu.in

M. Egbujor
Department of Chemistry, Federal University Otuoke, Otuoke, Bayelsa State, Nigeria

S. Kumar Tripathi et al. (eds.), *Phytoceuticals for Sustainable Medication*, Interdisciplinary Biotechnological Advances,
https://doi.org/10.1007/978-981-95-7588-6_13

1 Introduction

Thousands of years have been spent on medicinal plants to treat human diseases. Increasing numbers of people are recognizing traditional health systems and medicinal plants as having benefits in solving health issues across the world. The result of this new interest is that the world is being exposed to a surge in the research of medicinal plants. Medicinal herbs have been used by people as a form of treatment over thousands of years. The reality is that thousands of years ago, the ancient man used all his medicinal needs, prevention, healing, and other forms of drugs wholly supported by plants. As human society has evolved, the role of medicinal plant use in human society has played a mysterious and profound role, and many opinions exist about the concept of infection and health within each culture (Oyewole et al. 2018).

Plant-based medicines are heavily utilized in Ayurveda, Siddha, and Unani medicine, and India as a country with a very rich biodiversity has traditionally been a depository of traditional medicine. The native people in the country have amassed sophisticated ethnobotanical information, and this is what can be used to make sure that therapeutic plants are utilized in a sustainable manner (Jain 1983).

In India, approximately 80% of rural population use herbal medicines as their main healthcare needs, which shows that the country has high dependency of using plant-based formulations in the traditional healthcare systems. Ayurveda is considered to be one of the oldest medical systems that significantly emphasize the holistic use of medicinal herbs to assist the body in restoring its balance. Equally, a significant number of plant-based preparations utilized in Siddha medicine, primarily practiced in Tamil Nadu, are made of local plants. The unani medicine that began in Greek traditions but is more successful in India uses medicinal plants in concoctions that are supposed to enhance body balance (Sharma 2019).

The ethnobotanical practice by the native societies has contributed significantly to the sustainable use and conservation of medicinal plants. In India, there are numerous tribes, including the Bhil, Gond, and Santhal tribes, who have large traditional bodies of knowledge on the medicinal properties of diverse plant species (Jain 1983). The information is often transferred orally across the generations and ensures the preservation of the plant-based treatments. Also, other ethnobotanical studies indicate that such approaches would be useful in identifying new bioactive chemicals, which could be used in pharmaceutical applications (Singh and Singh 2025).

Over the last few years, there has been increased concern in integrating traditional knowledge of medicinal plants and modern healthcare systems. The world healthcare has been emphasized by the world health organization (WHO) to uphold the role of traditional medicine in augmenting modern healthcare services, and particularly in underdeveloped countries where the availability of allopathic medicines might be limited. Government programs in India such as the National Medicinal Plants Board (NMPB) are making efforts to promote the sustainability and conservation of medicinal plant species. Also, the presence of pharmacological studies confirming the traditional herbal remedies has enhanced their acceptability in healthcare today (Sharma 2019).

Although there is much potential in the use of medicinal plants as sustainable healthcare approaches, challenges such as overharvesting, destruction of habitats, and lack of proper regulatory measures pose a risk to the future existence of the medicinal plants (Chen et al. 2016). To ensure the sustainable utilization of these priceless resources, addressing these issues calls for a multidisciplinary approach combining ethnobotanists, conservationists, and legislators (Sharma 2019). As such, preservation of traditional knowledge and promotion of sustainable practices are needed to keep medicinal plants valuable in the health care.

2 Role of Medicinal Plants in Human Health

Due to their numerous pharmacological properties, medicinal plants have played a major role in traditional and modern medicine. The traditional use of these plants has been proved by current modern scientific research which has revealed that there is much potential in terms of medicinal values of many bioactive chemicals which have been extracted out of the plants.

Medicinal plants are being used more all over the world due to the massive expansion of the traditional medicine and the rising popularity of herbal preparations. Plants are also used to cure some diseases and conditions as well as to sustain and promote moral, emotional, and physical wellbeing in medicine. The medicinal plants do this in an integrated or probiotic manner with minimal or no side effects to the human body as compared to the chemically prepared drugs whose side effects are long-lasting and detrimental to the human body (Sandberg and Corrigan 2013).

This part discusses the pharmacology properties of some selected medicinal herbs including Curcuma longa (turmeric), Azadirachta indica (neem), and Withania somnifera (ashwagandha) focusing on their adaptogenic, anti-inflammatory, and antibacterial properties (Table 1).

3 Sustainable Utilization of Medicinal Plants

The availability of these valuable resources is in danger due to the significant loss of biodiversity caused by the uncontrolled use of medical herbs (Hamilton 2004). A sustainable use of medicinal plants requires the adoption of environmentally sound harvesting practices and conservation that are in tandem with the national and international policies (Schippmann et al. 2002). To maintain the biodiversity of medicinal plants in India, this section discusses significant sustainable ways of harvesting and conservation programs, along with regulatory methods.

Table 1 Pharmacology properties of some medicinal herbs

Plants name	Parts used	Active constituents	Pharmacological activity	References
Curcuma longa (Turmeric)	Rhizome	Curcumin	Anti-inflammatory, antioxidant	Aggarwal and Sung (2009)
Aloe barbadensis miller (Aloe vera)	Leaf	Aloin, aloesin, barbaloin	Anti-inflammatory, wound healing	Sandeep Kumar Verma (2011)
Ocimum sanctum (Tulsi)	Leaves, seed, and root	Eugenol, ursolic acid	Antimicrobial, adaptogenic	Pandey and Madhuri Sharma (2010)
Azadirachta indica (Neem)	Leaves, bark, seed, flower, and root	Azadirachtin, nimbin	Antibacterial, antifungal	Atawodi and Atawodi (2025)
Withania somnifera (Ashwagandha)	Root	Withanolides	Adaptogenic, antistress	Mishra et al. (2000)
Zingiber officinale (Ginger)	Rhizome	Gingerols, shogaols	Antiemetic, anti-inflammatory	Dissanayake (2020)
Emblica officinalis (Amla)	Fruit	Ascorbic acid, tannins	Antioxidant, immunomodulator	Dasaroju S and Gottumukkala K Mohan (2025)
Catharanthus roseus (Vinca)	Leaves and stems	Vincristine, vinblastine	Anticancer	Gautam Kumar et al. (2025)
Allium sativum (Garlic)	Bulb	Allicin	Hypolipidemic, antimicrobial	Harris et al. (2001)
Rauwolfia serpentina (Rauwolfia)	Roots and rhizomes	Reserpine	Antihypertensive, sedative	Vakil (1955)
Mentha piperita (Peppermint)	Leaves	Menthol	Carminative, analgesic	Herro and Jacob (2010)
Glycyrrhiza glabra (Liquorice)	Roots and rhizomes	Glycyrrhizin	Antiulcer, expectorant	Kalsi et al. (2016)
Tinospora cordifolia (Guduchi)	Stem	Tinosporin, berberine	Immunomodulatory, antipyretic	Kirti Sinha et al. (2025)
Adhatoda vasica (Vasaka)	Leaves	Vasicine	Expectorant, bronchodilator	Kumar et al. (2010)
Plantago ovata (Isabgol)	Husk	Mucilage, psyllium	Laxative	Sohani (2021)

(continued)

Table 1 (continued)

Plants name	Parts used	Active constituents	Pharmacological activity	References
Vitex negundo (Nirgundi)	Leaves	Casticin, Negundoside, Agnuside	Anti-inflammatory, antioxidant, analgesic, antipyretic, antibacterial, and anticancer effects	Sohani (2021)
Urginea indica (Jangli pyaj)	Bulb	Proscillaridin A, Scillaren A	Anticancer, antioxidant, anti-inflammatory, anthelmintic	Sohani (2021)
Tylophora indica (Antamool)	Leaves	Tylophorine, Quercetin, Kaempferol	Anticancer, anti-inflammatory, antimicrobial, anti-asthmatic, immunomodulatory.	Sohani (2021)
Syzygium cumini (Jamun)	Seed	Jamboline, Ellagic acid, Jambosine	Antioxidant, antidiabetic, antimicrobial, and anti-inflammatory properties	Sohani (2021)
Solanum nigrum (Makoy)	Leaves	Solamargine, Solasonine, and Solanine	Antioxidant, anti-inflammatory, antitumor and antimicrobial activities.	Sohani (2021)
Phyllanthus amarus (Bhuiamla)	Plant	Phyllanthin, Hypophyllanthin, Quercetin	Antioxidant, anti-inflammatory, antidiabetic, antimicrobial, diuretic	Sohani (2021)
Gymnema sylvestre (Gurmar)	Leaves	Gymnemic acids, Gymnemasaponins Gymnemagenin, Quercetin	Antioxidant, antimicrobial, anti-inflammatory, hypolipidemic, antidiabetic	Sohani (2021)
Datura metal (Dhatura)	Seeds	Atropine, Scopolamine (Hyoscine), Hyoscyamine	Anticholinergic, antispasmodic, antioxidant, and anti-inflammatory activity	Sohani (2021)
Cyperus scariosus (Nagarmotha)	Tubers	Cyperene, Cyperotundone, Cyperone, Quercetin	Anti-inflammatory, antioxidant, antidiarrheal, astringent, antipyretic	Sohani (2021)
Curcuma caesia (Kali Haldi)	Rhizomes	Curcumin, Ar-turmerone, Camphor	Anti-inflammatory, antimicrobial, antioxidant, anticancer activities	Sohani (2021)

(continued)

Table 1 (continued)

Plants name	Parts used	Active constituents	Pharmacological activity	References
Curculigo orchoides (Kali Musli)	Root	Curculigoside A, Curculigoside B, Curculigosaponin	Antioxidant, adaptogenic, aphrodisiac	Sohani (2021)
Chlorophytum spp. (Safed Musli)	Roots	Saponin A, Saponin B, Saponin C, Protodioscin, Diosgenin, Chlorophytoside A–F	Aphrodisiac, adaptogenic, immunomodulatory effects, antioxidant and anti-inflammatory actions	Sohani (2021)
Catharanthus roseus (Sadabahar)	Leaves and white flowers	Vincristine and Vinblastine	Anticancer, antihypertensive, antidiabetic, and sedative properties	Sohani (2021)
Boerhaavia diffusa (Punarnava)	Plant	Punarnavine, Boeravinone B and E, Quercetin	Diuretic, antispasmodic, antioxidant, antihypertensive, and antimicrobial activity	Sohani (2021)
Argemone mexicana (Pili Katari)	Extract of leaves	Sanguinarine, Berberine	Antimicrobial, analgesic, anti-inflammatory	Sohani (2021)
Anogeissus latifolia (Dhawra)	Leaves	Ellagic acid, Gallic acid, Anogeissumin	Antioxidant, and antimicrobial activity	Sohani (2021)
Anisomelos indica (Bhandari)	Leaves	Anisomelic acid, Ovatodiolide	Antiviral, anticancer, anti-inflammatory, and antimalarial activities	Sohani (2021)
Andrographis paniculata (Kalmegh)	Plant	Andrographolide, Neoandrographolide	Hepatoprotective, anti-inflammatory, immunomodulatory, and antipyretic effects	Sohani (2021)
Acacia catechu (Khair)	Bark	Catechin, Epicatechin, Catechutannic acid	Antioxidant and antimicrobial effects	Sohani (2021)
Acacia nilotica (Babul)	Twig	Gallic acid, Catechin, Ellagic acid	Antioxidant and antimicrobial activities	Sohani (2021)
Abutilon indicum (Kanghi)	Seeds	Abutiline (alkaloid), β-sitosterol (sterol), Quercetin (flavonoid)	Bronchodilator, expectorant, and antimicrobial properties	Sohani (2021)

3.1 Sustainable Harvesting Techniques

Maintaining plant populations and assuring their availability for future generations depends heavily on sustainable harvesting practices (Ticktin 2004). Selective harvesting minimizes ecological harm by only collecting mature plants or specific plant parts (Kala 2005). Furthermore, rotational harvesting reduces the pressure on a single species by harvesting various plant species or populations in cycles (Schippmann et al. 2002). Another successful conservation strategy that reduces reliance on wild populations is the regulated cultivation of highly sought-after medicinal plants. The World Health Organization (WHO) and other ethical harvesting guidelines put a strong emphasis on causing the least amount of harm to the plant' s natural habitat. Plant sustainability can be maintained by increasing regeneration rates through harvesting during nonreproductive seasons. In addition, community-based strategies that utilize indigenous and local knowledge greatly support ethical harvesting while maintaining customs (Ross 2005).

3.2 *Strategies of Conservation*

Increasing amounts of medicinal plant resources, mainly from wild populations, are being gathered. In fact, during the past few decades, the demand for wild resources has risen by 8–15% annually in Europe, North America, and Asia (Ross 2005). Numerous sets of guidelines for the conservation of medicinal plants have been developed, including ones that address both in situ and ex situ conservation. Botanic gardens and seed banks are significant models for ex situ conservation, while natural reserves and wild nurseries are common examples to conserve the medicinal effectiveness of plants in their native environments (Figueiredo and Grelle 2009) (Fig. 1). The geographic distribution and biological characteristics of medicinal plants must be known to guide conservation activities, e.g., to assess whether species conservation should take place in nature or in a nursery.

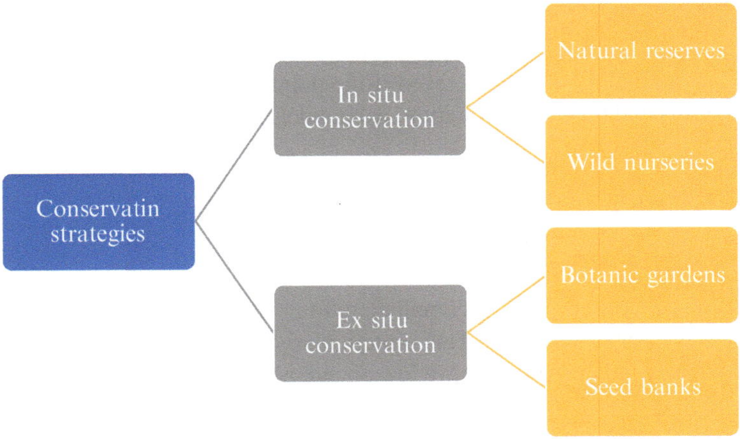

Fig. 1 Diagram of different methods involved in the conservation of medicinal plants

3.2.1 In Situ Conservation

Most of the medicinal plants are indigenous species, and the primary source of their medicinal qualities is the presence of secondary metabolites that react to stimuli in their natural habitats but might not manifest in cultivation (Figueiredo and Grelle 2009). We can conserve native flora and natural ecosystems, as well as their complex web of interrelationships, by practicing in situ conservation of entire communities. Furthermore, in situ conservation reinforces the connection between resource conservation and sustainable use and expands the amount of diversity that can be conserved (Long et al. 2003) worldwide; in situ conservation initiatives have concentrated on creating protected areas and adopting an ecosystem-oriented technique as opposed to a species-oriented one. The rules, regulations, and possible compliance of medicinal plants within growth habitats are important for successful in situ conservation (Volis and Blecher 2025).

Natural Reserves

One of the primary reasons for a shortage of resources for medicinal plants is habitat degradation and destruction (Camm et al. 2002). Protected areas containing significant wild resources are known as natural reserves, and they were created to maintain biodiversity. Over 12,700 protected areas have been established worldwide, covering 13.2 million km^2, or 8.81% of the planet's land. Evaluating the contributions and ecosystem functions of individual habitats is required to conserve medicinal plants by conserving important natural habitats (Liu et al. 2001).

Wild Nurseries

Wild nurseries can be a useful method for in situ conservation of rare, endangered, and in-demand medicinal plants, even if the populations of many wild species are severely impacted by overexploitation, habitat degradation, and invasive species (Li and Chen 2007).

3.2.2 Ex Situ Conservation

Ex situ conservation is a useful complement to in situ conservation, even if it is not always clearly separate from it. This is particularly true for medicinal plants that are overfished and endangered and have low abundance, lack of growth, and a high risk of replanting diseases (Havens et al. 2006). Ex situ conservation, often a direct action to preserve medicinal plant resources, tries to propagate and naturalize threatened plants to guarantee their steady existence and sometimes generate large amounts of planting material needed in the production of drugs (Swarts and Dixon 2009). Besides retaining their high levels of efficiency when planted in gardens outside their natural habitats, certain species of medicinal plants that had been wild can have their reproductive resources selected and placed in seed banks that can be replanted in the future (Hamilton 2004).

Botanic Gardens

Besides maintaining ecosystems to enhance the survival of endangered and rare plant species, botanic gardens also play an important role in ex situ conservation (Havens et al. 2006). Both botanical gardens have several unique features, although in general, living collections may contain a limited number of individuals of a particular species, making them useless for genetic conservation. They include an extensive variety of plant species that are cultivated in similar environments and frequently include plants that are both ecologically and taxonomically varied (Primack and Miller-Rushing 2009). By developing cultivation and propagation guidelines and implementing domestication and variety breeding programs, botanic gardens may contribute even more to the conservation of medicinal plants (Maunder et al. 2001).

Seed Banks

To help preserve the biological and genetic diversity of wild plant species, seed banks are recommended as a better choice to the botanic gardens to store the genetic diversity of a large number of therapeutic plants ex situ. The most striking seed bank is the Millennium Seed Bank Project in the Royal Botanic Gardens in Britain. The samples of plants can be acquired in seed banks quite fast to evaluate their properties, which provides helpful data to save the rest of the existing natural population. The hard tasks relating to seed banking are the reintroduction of the plant species into the wild and the active participation in the restoration of the wild populations (Schoen and Brown 2001).

4 Biotechnological Approaches

While many medicinal plant species are protected in situ due to the value and practicality of natural plant resources, ex-situ conservation is used instead. In vitro techniques or biotechnological approaches are becoming more and more important in the conservation of endangered or threatened plants.

This is particularly true for plants that have reproductive issues and/or a very low population. For the important genotype of medicinal plants to be conserved and multiplied quickly, biotechnological methods are important. There are some techniques shown in Fig. 2.

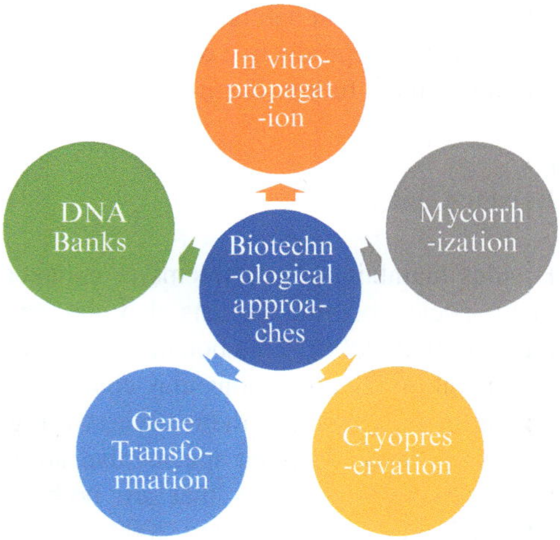

Fig. 2 Different biotechnological approaches

4.1 *In Vitro Propagation*

In vitro propagation involves the regeneration or micropropagation of several plants from their parts, leaves, seeds, nodes, and tubers, and other materials. Novel plant regeneration and multiplication are accomplished using in vitro propagation. Micropropagation has been shown to be an important method for large-scale plant multiplication.

It is commonly achieved by either the production of callus by an auxillary explant after which the rooting process is done or by production of an explant after which shoots and roots are produced. In vitro propagation under controlled conditions yields a complete plantlet using a single explant which can be transported to the field after acclimatizing (Rai 2010).

4.2 *Mycorrhization*

Mycorrhization is the process by which mycorrhizal fungus is introduced into plant roots. Arbuscular Mycorrhizal fungus (AMF) and ectomycorrhizal fungi are the two types of mycorrhial fungus. Ninety percent of plants have this symbiotic fungus (Williams et al. 1994). By improving the intake of nutrients in general and phosphorus in particular, the AMF helps the plant partner. AMF' s varied roles in plant growth have been the subject of much research (Chandra et al. 2010).

4.3 Cryopreservation

Transferring biological material at a very low temperature is called freeze-preservation, cryogenic storage, or cryopreservation (Here liquid nitrogen is used for cryopreservation). Time-related biochemical phenenoma are eliminated since all forms of cellular metabolism are halted at this low temperature zone. Getting to and from the storage temperature is still a challenge in cryopreservation.

The process of cryopreservation increases the amount of bound water in the material being kept while reducing the amount of free water. *Atropa belladonna*, *Digitalis lanata*, *Hyoscyamus* sp., and *Rauwolfia serpentina* have all shown great benefit from the approach.

4.4 Gene Transformation

One effective technique for increasing the productivity of novel secondary metabolites with limited yield is genetic transformation. Because of their stable and high output under hormone-free growing conditions, hairy roots transformed with Agrobacterium rhizogenes have been found to be appropriate for the production of secondary metabolites. The production of therapeutic plants with several long-lasting resistances to pests and illnesses is facilitated by genetic transformation. Additionally, transgenes or marker-assisted selection could help develop insect, pest, drought, and salinity-resistant plants—all of which are important to fulfill global demand and conserve land for the preservation of plant biodiversity in their natural environments.

4.5 DNA Banks

DNA banks maintain a library of the "DNA sample" in a way much similar to the "Gene Library". These provide important information to the conservation scientists. DNA samples may be of three kinds such as total genomic DNA, DNA libraries, and individual cloned DNA fragments. DNA banks were established as a substitute to conventional techniques for genetic resource conservation. This is important because the preservation of whole genotypes for future use as living beings is very different from the preservation of genome fragments or individual genes (Jain et al. 2025).

5 Challenges in Medicinal Plant Research

Medicinal plants have an impressive array of benefits, but their applications in healthcare systems are filled with restrictions like environmental harm, unsustainable harvesting practices, lack of standardization, and the lack of sufficient scientific results. Besides posing a threat to biodiversity, the issues complicate the successful adoption of herbal medicine into traditional healthcare systems. To solve these problems, a complex approach of conservation strategies, law reforms, and better scientific studies is required.

Habitat degradation and deforestation is a major setback to sustainable use of medicinal herbs. Due to the rapid urbanization, agricultural development as well as industrialization, the number of medicinal plant species to be used has reduced drastically through the degradation of the natural habitats (Kala 2005). Most plant species are also highly vulnerable to environmental destruction since most of them are also only found in specific biological zones. The conservation activity, including the establishment of protected zones and botanical gardens, is the only way to keep these invaluable resources alive.

The other problem that is pressing is overharvesting of the medicinal plants which jeopardizes the survival of a large number of species. Another urgent issue is the overharvesting of medicinal plants which threatens the existence of many species. Overexploitation is usually caused by uncontrolled trade and poor harvesting practices like cutting down entire plants instead of picking the necessary ones like leaves or bark. This problem can be reduced through funding community conservation projects and promoting sustainable harvesting practices (Hamilton 2004).

Another serious issue of medicinal plant products is that there are no quality control and standardization. This is because the effects of the variations in climate, geography, and harvesting methods affect the safety and efficacy of herbal remedies due to the variations in their plant composition (Wichtl 2004). Medical vegetation products are also very often inconsistent in their active constituents, unlike synthetic drugs, which undergo a rigorous quality control process. The standardized cultivation, processing, and formulation processes should be developed so as to ensure reliability and consistency of herbal medication.

Another major issue that still remains is scientific validation of medicinal herbs. A large number of therapeutic plants have been in use over a long period of time, yet they have not all been subjected to rigorous pharmacological and clinical studies (Fabricant and Farnsworth 2001). The lack of empirical information on their effectiveness, safety, and potential side effects limits their use in modern healthcare. To seal this gap, intensive research studies on the virtues of medicinal plants should be done by interdisciplinary scientists consisting of pharmacologists, ethnobotanists as well as medical experts (Basisht 2014).

To overcome such hindrances, the ancient knowledge should be integrated with modern scientific techniques. To gain greater credibility in the medical field, government policies ought to promote conservation and sustainable harvesting techniques and research investment on medicinal plants. Conservation and proper use could also be achieved through education projects and education campaigns. Modern scientific methods must be combined with ancient knowledge in order to overcome these obstacles. For medicinal plants to be more credible in the medical field, government policies should encourage conservation efforts, sustainable harvesting methods, and research funding. Education initiatives and public awareness campaigns can also significantly contribute to conservation and appropriate use. The use of medicinal plants as a resource for viable medical care can be protected by managing these issues.

6 Future Prospects

Remarkable developments in the study of medicinal plants are expected in India in the future, particularly given the combination of phytochemistry, biotechnology, and nanotechnology. Since environmentally friendly healthcare systems are growing more and more crucial globally, botanical expertise has become even more crucial for developing medicines and clinical inventions (Pullaiah 2023). Three main areas are anticipated to be the focus of future research in this context: multidisciplinary medical models, plant-derived therapies, and nanotechnology. Natural health care is experiencing an innovation due to nanotechnology, which improves drug delivery, bioavailability, and potency. Chronic conditions like cancer, diabetes, and neurological disorders have showed promising responses to biological nanotechnology made from therapeutic plants. Traditional herbal treatments become more effective and forceful because of these compounds' higher solubility, stability, and controlled release. For results to ensure the safety and effectiveness of nanotechnology systems, future research should concentrate in enhancing them and carrying out complete research studies.

Manufacturing pharmaceuticals originating from plants comprise another fascinating field. It is now possible to identify new bioactive chemicals from medicinal plants because of developments in metabolomics and molecular biology (Sharma 1998). The herbal industry continues to face major difficulties with standardization and quality control, which calls for the invention of exacting standards for formulation, extraction, and cultivation. Applying scientific methods like tissue culture and synthetic biology can also improve the synthesis of vital phytochemicals, maintaining a steady supply of resources for beneficial plants.

Also, integrative healthcare treatments that blend traditional beliefs with technological healthcare techniques are becoming more and more popular. Indian healthcare historically utilized the Ayurvedic, Siddha, and Unani systems; when mixed with evidence-based medicine, these systems can offer broad treatment options. Therapeutic approval, safety examinations, and rules and regulations should be the primary topics of future study on the affinities between herbal and traditional treatments in order to promote the adoption of integrative therapies into mainstream healthcare.

Extended traditional herbal systems' longevity also depends on the wide variety of medicinal plants being conserved successfully. Many plant species are in risk due to excessive collection and environment damage, which calls for methods of protection including agroforestry and community-based farming. Digital sources for traditional knowledge and pharmacological information can also help preserve indigenous medicinal methods and promote multidisciplinary collaboration.

The future of India's studying medicinal plants depends on complementary partnerships that combine traditional knowledge with modern technologies. Scientists can fully realize the promise of plant medicine in sustainable resource management by tackling issues with clinical validation, standardization, and effective resource management medical care (Basisht 2014).

A medicinal chemistry perspective is also essential. The phytoconstituents of medicinal plants have been linked to the therapeutic effects of these plants due to their structural diversities (Kumar et al. 2023). These phytoconstituents, which include terpenoids, alkaloids, phenolic acids, glycosides, terpenoids, flavonoids, and many more, possess a wide range of pharmacological activities as a result of unique functional groups and redox properties. The structure-activity relationship analysis of some phytoconstituents such as flavonoids and phenolic acids has shown that the phenolic hydroxyl groups in these phytoconstituents contribute to their antioxidant activities by improving their radical scavenging and NRF2-inducing activities (Sun and Shahrajabian 2023; Tiranakwit et al. 2023). Alkaloids, which are nitrogen-containing phytoconstituents, have been linked to receptor binding or enzyme inhibition mechanisms of medicinal plants (Zandavar and Afshari Babazad 2023). Thus, to increase potency and pharmacokinetic stability, phytoconstituents originating from medicinal plants can be subjected to SAR and semisynthetic modification. Furthermore, computational chemistry analysis, including molecular docking, QSAR modeling, and LC-MS/MS, can be employed to elucidate active principles and optimize lead compounds. These medicinal chemistry techniques can be applied to improve rational extraction, design green synthetic analogues, and support molecular optimization and drug development.

7 Conclusion

In India's sustainable healthcare system, medicinal plants are important because they offer a wealth of therapeutic resources with a strong ethnobotanical foundation. Developing innovative and comprehensive healthcare solutions is made possible by fusing traditional knowledge with current scientific research. The safety and effectiveness of medicinal plants can be further confirmed through promoting a synergistic strategy that blends conventional wisdom with evidence-based validation, increasing their acceptance in mainstream healthcare. However, ethical use, effective legal frameworks, and efficient conservation techniques are necessary for the sustainability of medicinal plant-based healthcare. The availability of these important botanical resources is endangered by overharvesting, habitat degradation, and climate change. Therefore, to conserve the ecological balance and maintain the long-term existence of medicinal plant species, coordinated efforts toward sustainable harvesting, cultivation, and biodiversity conservation are important. To preserve and advance ethnobotanical techniques, collaboration between traditional healers, scientists, and legislators is important. Enhancing this partnership can help regulate and standardize herbal medicines, encourage clinical research, and facilitate the sharing of knowledge. Furthermore, maintaining traditional medicine systems and encouraging their integration into modern healthcare frameworks depend heavily on institutional support, community involvement, and public knowledge. Medicinal plants have a lot of potential to solve contemporary healthcare issues and promote sustainability. To ensure that medicinal plant-based healthcare continues to be a useful concept in India, the multidisciplinary approach involving integration of scientific findings with ethnobotanical knowledge, proactive conservation, and policy programs is needed.

References

Aggarwal BB, Sung B (2009) Pharmacological basis for the role of curcumin in chronic diseases: an age-old spice with modern targets. Trends Pharmacol Sci 30(2):85–94. https://doi.org/10.1016/j.tips.2008.11.002

Atawodi SE, Atawodi JC (2025) Azadirachta indica (neem): A plant of multiple biological and pharmacological activities | request PDF. ResearchGate https://doi.org/10.1007/s11101-009-9144-6

Basisht G (2014) Exploring insights towards definition and laws of health in Ayurveda: global health perspective. Ayu 35(4):351–355. https://doi.org/10.4103/0974-8520.158975

Camm JD, Norman SK, Polasky S, Solow AR (2002) Nature reserve site selection to maximize expected species covered. Oper Res 50(6):946–955+1076. https://doi.org/10.1287/opre.50.6.946.351

Chandra S, Bandopadhyay R, Kumar V, Chandra R (2010) Acclimatization of tissue cultured plantlets: from laboratory to land. Biotechnol Lett 32(9):1199–1205. https://doi.org/10.1007/s10529-010-0290-0

Chen S-L, Yu H, Luo H-M, Wu Q, Li C-F, Steinmetz A (2016) Conservation and sustainable use of medicinal plants: problems, progress, and prospects. Chin Med 11:37. https://doi.org/10.1186/s13020-016-0108-7

Dasaroju S, Gottumukkala KM (2025) Current trends in the research of Emblica officinalis (Amla): a pharmacological perspective. ResearchGate

Dissanayake KGC (2020) A review on medicinal uses of Zingiber officinale (Ginger)

Fabricant DS, Farnsworth NR (2001) The value of plants used in traditional medicine for drug discovery. Environ Health Perspect 109(Suppl 1):69–75. https://doi.org/10.1289/ehp.01109s169

Figueiredo MSL, Grelle CEV (2009) Predicting global abundance of a threatened species from its occurrence: implications for conservation planning. Divers Distrib 15:117–121. https://doi.org/10.1111/j.1472-4642.2008.00525.x

Hamilton AC (2004) Medicinal plants, conservation and livelihoods. Biodivers Conserv 13(8):1477–1517. https://doi.org/10.1023/B:BIOC.0000021333.23413.42

Harris JC, Cottrell SL, Plummer S, Lloyd D (2001) Antimicrobial properties of Allium sativum (garlic). Appl Microbiol Biotechnol 57(3):282–286. https://doi.org/10.1007/s002530100722

Havens K, Vitt P, Maunder M, Guerrant EO, Dixon K (2006) Ex situ plant conservation and beyond. Bioscience 56(6):525–531. https://doi.org/10.1641/0006-3568(2006)56[525:ESPCAB]2.0.CO;2

Herro E, Jacob SE (2010) Mentha piperita (peppermint). Dermatitis 21(6):327–329
Jain SK (1983) Ethnobotany in India: an overview. Botanical Survey in India, Department of Environment, Government of India
Jain M, Johnson TS, Prakash (2025) (PDF) Biotechnological approaches to conserve the wealth of nature: endangered and rare medicinal plant species, a review. ResearchGate. https://doi.org/10.18311/jnr/2012/261
Kala CP (2005) Indigenous uses, population density, and conservation of threatened medicinal plants in protected areas of the Indian Himalayas. Conserv Biol 19(2):368–378. https://doi.org/10.1111/j.1523-1739.2005.00602.x
Kalsi S, Verma DSK, Neha, Kaur A, Singh N (2016) A review on Glycyrrhiza glabra (Liquorice) and its pharmacological activities. Int J Pharma Drug Anal:234–239
Kumar KPS, Bhowmik D, Tiwari P, Kharel R (2010) Indian traditional herbs Adhatoda vasica and its medicinal application
Kumar A, P N, Kumar M, Jose A, Tomer V, Oz E, Proestos C, Zeng M, Elobeid T, K S, Oz F (2023) Major phytochemicals: recent advances in health benefits and extraction method. Molecules 28(2):887. https://doi.org/10.3390/molecules28020887
Gautam Kumar, Ravi Kumar, Girendra Kumar Gautam, Harshit Rana (2025) (PDF) Phytochemical and pharmacological properties of Catharanthus roseus (Vinca). ResearchGate. https://doi.org/10.52152/spr/2021.164
Li X-W, Chen S-L (2007) Conspectus of ecophysiological study on medicinal plant in wild nursery. Zhongguo Zhong Yao Za Zhi 32(14):1388–1392
Liu J, Linderman M, Ouyang Z, An L, Yang J, Zhang H (2001) Ecological degradation in protected areas: the case of Wolong Nature Reserve for giant pandas. Science 292(5514):98–101. https://doi.org/10.1126/science.1058104
Long C-L, Li H, Ouyang Z, Yang X, Li Q, Trangmar B (2003) Strategies for agrobiodiversity conservation and promotion: a case from Yunnan, China. Biodivers Conserv 12:1145–1156. https://doi.org/10.1023/A:1023085922265
Maunder M, Higgins S, Culham A (2001) The effectiveness of botanic garden collections in supporting plant conservation: a European case study. Biodivers Conserv 10(3):383–401
Mishra LC, Singh BB, Dagenais S (2000) Scientific basis for the therapeutic use of Withania somnifera (ashwagandha): a review. Altern Med Rev 5(4):334–346
Oyewole SO, Akinyemi O, Jimoh KA (2018) Medicinal plants and sustainable human health: a review. HIJ 2(4). https://doi.org/10.15406/hij.2018.02.00051
Pandey G, Madhuri Sharma (2010) (PDF) Pharmacological activities of Ocimum sanctum (Tulsi): a review. https://www.researchgate.net/publication/270220228_Pharmacological_activities_of_Ocimum_sanctum_Tulsi_A_review. Accessed 17 Oct 2025
Primack RB, Miller-Rushing AJ (2009) The role of botanical gardens in climate change research. New Phytol 182(2):303–313. https://doi.org/10.1111/j.1469-8137.2009.02800.x
Pullaiah T (2023) Phytochemistry and pharmacology of medicinal plants
Rai MK (2010) Review: biotechnological strategies for conservation of rare and endangered medicinal plants. Biodiversitas 11(3):157–166
Ross IA (2005) Medicinal plants of the world, volume 3: chemical constituents, traditional and modern medicinal uses. ResearchGate https://www.researchgate.net/publication/321878372_Medicinal_Plants_of_the_World_Volume_3_Chemical_Constituents_Traditional_and_Modern_Medicinal_Uses. Accessed 17 Oct 2025
Sandberg F, Corrigan D (2013) Natural remedies: their origins and uses
Schippmann U, Leaman DJ, Cunningham AB (2002) (PDF) Impact of cultivation and gathering of medicinal plants on biodiversity: global trends and issues. ResearchGate
Schoen DJ, Brown AHD (2001) The conservation of wild plant species in seed banks: attention to both taxonomic coverage and population biology will improve the role of seed banks as conservation tools. Bioscience 51(11):960–966. https://doi.org/10.1641/0006-3568(2001)051[0960:TCOWPS]2.0.CO;2
Sharma P.V (1998) Charaka Samhita text with English translation

Sharma DA (2019) Role of medicinal plants in sustainable healthcare: a review of ethnobotanical practices in India. 5(3)

Singh A, Singh PK (2025) An ethnobotanical study of medicinal plants in Chandauli District of Uttar Pradesh, India | request PDF. ResearchGate. https://doi.org/10.1016/j.jep.2008.10.018

Kirti Sinha, N. P. Mishra, Suman P S Khanuja (2025) (PDF) Tinospora cordifolia (Guduchi): a reservoir plant for therapeutic applications: a review. ResearchGate

Sohani S (2021) Role of medicinal plant in human health perspective. Acta Sci Agric 5(6):65–68. https://doi.org/10.31080/ASAG.2021.05.1006

Sun W, Shahrajabian MH (2023) Therapeutic potential of phenolic compounds in medicinal plants-natural health products for human health. Molecules 28(4):1845. https://doi.org/10.3390/molecules28041845

Swarts ND, Dixon KW (2009) Terrestrial orchid conservation in the age of extinction. Ann Bot 104(3):543–556. https://doi.org/10.1093/aob/mcp025

Ticktin T (2004) The ecological implications of harvesting non-timber forest products. J Appl Ecol 41:11–21. https://doi.org/10.1111/j.1365-2664.2004.00859.x

Tiranakwit T, Puangpun W, Tamprasit K, Wichai N, Siriamornpun S, Srisongkram T, Weerapreeyakul N (2023) Phytochemical screening on phenolic, flavonoid contents, and antioxidant activities of six indigenous plants used in traditional Thai medicine. Int J Mol Sci 24(17):13425. https://doi.org/10.3390/ijms241713425

Vakil RJ (1955) Rauwolfia serpentina in the treatment of high blood pressure; a review of the literature. Circulation 12(2):220–229. https://doi.org/10.1161/01.cir.12.2.220

Sandeep Kumar Verma (2011) (PDF) Aloe vera their chemicals composition and applications: a review. In: ResearchGate. https://www.researchgate.net/publication/48347118_Aloe_vera_their_chemicals_composition_and_applications_A_review. Accessed 17 Oct 2025

Volis S, Blecher M (2025) (PDF) Quasi in situ: a bridge between ex situ and in situ conservation of plants. ResearchGate. https://doi.org/10.1007/s10531-010-9849-2

Wichtl M (2004) Herbal drugs and phytopharmaceuticals: a handbook for practice on a scientific basis. CRC Press

Williams PG, Roser DJ, Seppelt RD (1994) Mycorrhizas of hepatics in continental Antarctica. Mycol Res 98(1):34–36. https://doi.org/10.1016/S0953-7562(09)80332-8

Zandavar H, Afshari Babazad M (2023) Secondary metabolites: alkaloids and flavonoids in medicinal plants. IntechOpen. https://doi.org/10.5772/intechopen.108030

MIX
Papier aus verantwortungsvollen Quellen
Paper from responsible sources
FSC® C105338

If you have any concerns about our products,
you can contact us on
ProductSafety@springernature.com

In case Publisher is established outside the EU,
the EU authorized representative is:
Springer Nature Customer Service Center GmbH
Europaplatz 3, 69115 Heidelberg, Germany

Printed by Libri Plureos GmbH
in Hamburg, Germany